O₂ER	Oxygen extraction ratio
O₂ sat	Oxygen saturation
PA	Pulmonary artery
PAD	Pulmonary artery diastolic
Pao₂	Arterial oxygen tension or partial pressure
PAo₂	Alveolar oxygen tension or partial pressure
P(A-a)o₂	Alveolar-arterial O₂ tension difference
P(a/A)o₂	Arterial-alveolar tension ratio or oxygen exchange index
PAP	Pulmonary artery pressure
PAS	Pulmonary artery systolic
PAWP	Pulmonary artery wedge pressure
Petco₂	End tidal carbon dioxide
PP	Pulse pressure
PT	Prothrombin
PTT	Partial thromboplastin time
PVR	Pulmonary vascular resistance
PVRI	Pulmonary vascular resistance index
Qs/Qt	Physiological shunt
RPP	Rate pressure product
RR	Respiratory rate
RVSWI	Right ventricular stroke work index
Sao₂	Oxygen saturation of the hemoglobin of arterial blood
SBP	Systolic blood pressure
SI	Stroke index
SOB	Shortness of breath
Spo₂	Oxygen saturation measured by pulse oximetry
SV	Stroke volume
Svo₂	Mixed venous oxygen saturation
SVR	Systemic vascular resistance
SVRI	Systemic vascular resistance index
u/o	Urine output
VC	Vital capacity
VO₂	Oxygen consumption
VS	Vital signs
Vт	Tidal volume
WNL	Within normal limits

Mosby's Critical Care Nursing Reference

Mosby's Critical Care Nursing Reference

Susan B. Stillwell, RN, MSN, CCRN

Consultant,
Emtek Health Care Systems, Inc.,
Lecturer, School of Nursing,
Arizona State University,
Tempe, Arizona

with 84 illustrations

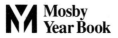

**Mosby
Year Book**

St. Louis   Baltimore   Boston   Chicago   London   Philadelphia   Sydney   Toronto

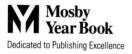

**Mosby
Year Book**
Dedicated to Publishing Excellence

Editors: Don Ladig, Terry Van Schaik
Developmental Editor: Jeanne Rowland
Production Manager: Carol Sullivan Wiseman
Production Editor: Linda McKinley
Manuscript Editor: Suzanne Seeley Wakefield
Designer: Susan Lane

Printed in the United States of America

Mosby–Year Book, Inc.
11830 Westline Industrial Drive
St. Louis, Missouri 63146

The authors and publisher have made a conscientious effort to ensure that the drug information and recommended dosages in this book are accurate and in accord with accepted standards at the time of publication. However, pharmacology is a rapidly changing science, so readers are advised to check the package insert before administering any drug.

International Standard Book Number 0-8016-6118-8

93 94 95 96 CL/VH 9 8 7 6 5 4 3 2

Contributors

Bonnie M. Cegles, MS, RN, CCRN
Faculty Associate,
Arizona State University,
Tempe, Arizona
Chapters 2, 5, and 6

Kerry H. Cheever, MSN, RN, CCRN, CEN
Partner, Consultation and Research Educational Systems, Inc., :.,
Winter Park, Florida
Chapters 2, 5, and 6

Kathie Clarke, BSN, RN, CVNS, CCRN
Critical Care Nurse Clinician,
Maryvale Samaritan Medical Center,
Phoenix, Arizona
Chapters 2, 5, and 6

Colleen Counsell, MSN, RN, CCRN
Nursing Supervisor, Neuroscience,
Shands Hospital at the University of Florida,
Gainesville, Florida
Chapter 7

Mary Ann Cammy House, MSN, RN, CCRN, CS
Assistant Professor, Graduate Program,
College of Nursing,
University of Florida,
Gainesville, Florida
Chapters 2, 5, and 6

Adele A. Large, MSN, RN, CEN, CCRN
Clinical Instructor—Staff Development,
Presbyterian University Hospital,
Pittsburgh, Pennsylvania
Chapters 2, 5, and 6

Dianne Lepley-Frey, MS, RN, CCRN
Critical Care Clinical Nurse Specialist,
Mesa Lutheran Hospital,
Mesa, Arizona
Chapter 3

Ronald J. Lynch, MSN, RN, CCRN
Education Specialist,
Orlando Regional Medical Center,
Sand Lake Hospital,
Orlando, Florida
Chapters 2, 5, and 6

Patricia A. Moloney-Harmon, MS, RN, CCRN
Pediatric Clinical Nurse Specialist,
University of Maryland Medical Center,
Baltimore, Maryland
Chapter 8

Virginia Prendergast, MSN, RN, CNRN
Neuroscience Clinical Specialist,
Barrow Neurological Institute,
St. Joseph's Hospital,
Phoenix, Arizona
Chapters 2, 5, and 6

Marla J. Prizant-Weston, MS, RN, CCRN
Critical Care Clinical Nurse Specialist,
Desert Samaritan Medical Center,
Mesa, Arizona
Chapters 2, 5, and 6

Sharon L. Roberts, PhD, RN, FAAN
Professor, Department of Nursing,
California State University—Long Beach,
Long Beach, California
Chapter 4

Cathy H. Rosenthal, MN, RN, CCRN
Clinical Nurse Specialist Pediatric Critical Care,
Critical Care Nursing Service,
National Institutes of Health,
Bethesda, Maryland
Chapter 8

Susan B. Stillwell, RN, MSN, CCRN
Consultant, Emtek Health Care Systems, Inc.,
Lecturer, School of Nursing,
Arizona State University,
Tempe, Arizona
Chapters 1, 2, 5, and 6

Laura A. Talbot, PhD, RNC
Assistant Professor,
Texas Christian University,
Fort Worth, Texas
Chapters 5 and 6

Consultants

Lynn M. Feeman, MSN, RN, CS, CCRN
Clinical Nurse Specialist,
Trauma/Critical Care,
Detroit Receiving Hospital,
University Health Center,
Detroit, Michigan

Dorrie Fontaine, DNSc, RN, CCRN
Assistant Professor—Trauma/Critical Care Nursing,
School of Nursing,
University of Maryland,
Baltimore, Maryland

Doris M. Gates, MS, RN, CCRN
Critical Care Clinical Educator,
Sharp Memorial Hospital,
San Diego, California

Lori Geisman, MSN(R), RN, CCRN
Head Nurse—Medical Intensive Care Unit South,
Barnes Hospital,
St. Louis, Missouri

Teresa Heise Halloran, MSN, RN, CCRN
Critical Care Clinical Specialist,
St. John's Mercy Medical Center,
St. Louis, Missouri

Virginia Byrn Huddleston, MSN, RN, CCRN
Adjunct Faculty,
Vanderbilt University,
Nashville, Tennessee;
Associate, Barbara Mims Clark Associates,
Dallas, Texas

Elizabeth L. Hughes, MSN, RN, CDE
Diabetes Clinical Nurse Specialist,
Barnes Hospital,
St. Louis, Missouri

Ainslie T. Nibert, MSN, RN, CCRN
Assistant Professor,
College of Nursing,
Houston Baptist University,
Houston, Texas

Sally A. Palmer, MS, RNC
Nurse Practitioner—Adult Medicine,
Health Services Association,
Syracuse, New York

Donna Prentice, MSN, RN, CCRN
Critical Care Clinical Nurse Specialist,
Barnes Hospital,
St. Louis, Missouri

Edith McCarter Randall, MS, RN, CCRN
Clinical Nurse Specialist,
St. Luke's Medical Center,
Phoenix, Arizona

Deborah Shpritz, MS, RN, CCRN
Faculty,
School of Nursing,
University of Maryland,
Baltimore, Maryland

Marilyn Sawyer Sommers, PhD, RN, CCRN
Assistant Professor,
College of Nursing and Health,
University of Cincinnati,
Cincinnati, Ohio

Robert E. St. John, BA, BSN, RN, RRT
Cardiopulmonary Nurse Clinician,
Jewish Hospital at Washington University Medical Center,
St. Louis, Missouri

Preface

Mosby's Critical Care Nursing Reference was developed to provide the nurse with a resource for accessing information about the multiple aspects involved in the acute care management of a patient hospitalized in the adult ICU. The reference is not intended to be a critical care textbook or a procedure manual and assumes that the nurse is familiar with critical care technology and the pathophysiology associated with life-threatening illnesses.

Clinical briefs are used throughout the reference to describe diagnostic tests, clinical disorders, invasive monitoring, and therapeutic modalities. *Mosby's Critical Care Nursing Reference* also includes nursing diagnoses and patient outcomes for clinical disorders and for the complications associated with diagnostic tests, invasive monitoring, and therapeutic modalities. In addition, aspects of critical care nursing common to all ICU patients are presented in nursing diagnosis format.

Although the majority of this reference contains physiological nursing diagnoses, a separate chapter has been devoted to the management of behavioral manifestations that can occur in the critically ill patient, regardless of the medical diagnosis.

Mosby's Critical Care Nursing Reference includes a variety of clinical disorders organized by body systems. Although the major focus is acute care patient management, the Goals of Treatment sections provide the reader with an overview of the potential medical plan of care. Clinical sequelae are listed in tables for quick access to complications and signs and/or symptoms the nurse should assess. All priority nursing diagnoses are listed to provide the reader with an overview of the life-threatening or most immediate patient problems. The care required for a critically ill patient can be complex; thus the nursing care has been organized into patient monitoring, which includes specialized equipment and physiological parameters requiring calculations; physical assessment; diagnostics assessment, which includes the test results the nurse should monitor frequently; and patient management, which includes independent and collaborative nursing functions.

The drugs most commonly found on any adult emergency code cart are discussed according to classification, effects, indications, contraindications, administration, and patient management. Vasoactive drug dosage charts are also included.

A unique aspect of this reference is the pediatric component. A PEDS framework is used to discuss a variety of pertinent topics for modifying the adult ICU environment, as well as practical hints in approaching the child in an adult ICU.

Other additions that make this reference a useful tool include ACLS algorithms, a BSA nomogram, brain-death criteria and organ donation guidelines, cardiopulmonary formulas, and conversion factors.

Novice ICU nurses, students in a critical care course, and seasoned ICU nurses who "float" will find *Mosby's Critical Care Nursing Reference* a valuable resource in unfamiliar patient situations.

Susan B. Stillwell

Contents

6 *Therapeutic Modalities,* 437

7 *Pharmacology: Emergency Drugs,* 547

8 *Nursing Care Modifications for the Child in the Adult ICU,* 588

CHAPTER 1

Critical Care Patient Assessment Guides

PATIENT ASSESSMENT GUIDES

Analyzing a Symptom

A positive finding can be analyzed using the following guide. It is equally important to obtain pertinent negative information about the patient's health status.

Location: Site, including any radiation of the symptom
Timing: Onset, progression and duration of the symptom
Setting: Place the symptom began
Quality: Characteristics or properties of the symptom
Quantity: Degree of symptom—amount, extent, size
Alleviating factors: Factors that improve/relieve the symptom
Aggravating factors: Factors that make the symptom worse
Associated factors: Concomitant symptoms

Self-Report Scales

A visual analogue scale or a modified Borg Scale[1] are self-report instruments that can be used to assess subjective sensations such as pain and dyspnea (Figure 1-1 and the box on p. 2).

Head-to-Toe Survey

When a critically ill patient is admitted to the unit, a routine assessment should be performed and repeated at least every 4 hours thereafter. A more frequent and more selective or detailed assessment may be necessary, depending on the patient's clinical disorder and/or a change in his condition.

Neurological Assessment

Level of consciousness (LOC)

Note the patient's state of wakefulness and awareness. First, observe the patient for spontaneous activity; if none is noted, verbally stimulate the patient. If the patient is unresponsive to verbal stimuli, use noxious stimuli such as applying pressure to the nail bed, pinching the trapezius muscle, or pinching the inner aspect of the arm or thigh. Avoid rub-

```
No                                              Extreme
difficulty  ——————————————  difficulty
breathing                                       breathing


No        ————————————————        Intolerable
pain                                            pain
```

Figure 1-1   Sample visual analogue scales. Patient places an X on the line that indicates the severity of the symptom.

Modified Borg Scale

0	None/nothing at all
0.5	Very, very _____ * (just noticeable)
1	Very _____
2	_____
3	Moderate
4	Somewhat severe
5	Severe
6	
7	Very severe
8	
9	Very, very severe (almost maximal)
10	Maximal

Modified from Borg GAV: Psychological bases of perceived exertion, Med Sci Sports Exercise 14(5): 377-381, 1982.
*Descriptors such as mild, weak, or slight can be inserted to assess symptoms such as pain, exertion, or breathlessness. Patients rate the symptom on a scale of 1 to 10 according to the descriptor that best indicates the severity of the symptom.

---

bing the sternum with knuckles, applying pressure to the supraorbital area, and pinching the nipples or testicles.

The Glasgow coma scale (GCS)[16] is a tool for assessing consciousness (Table 1-1). The best or highest response is recorded for the purpose of assessing the degree of altered consciousness. If a patient's abilities cannot be evaluated, a notation of the condition should be documented, and the subscore should be labeled untestable.

Pupillary reaction and reflexes

Check position, size, shape, and response of the pupils. Photophobia may be associated with increased intracranial pressure or meningeal irritation. No direct pupillary response

TABLE 1-1 Glasgow Coma Scale

Ability	Response	Score*
Best eye response	Spontaneously (as nurse approaches)	4
	To verbal stimulus (nurse speaks/shouts)	3
	To painful stimulus (pressure on nail bed)	2
	No response to painful stimulus	1
Best motor response	Obeys simple command	6
	Localizes pain (locates and attempts to remove pain source)	5
	Withdrawal (attempts to withdraw from pain source)	4
	Flexion (Figure 1-2)	3
	Extension (Figure 1-2)	2
	No response to painful stimulus	1
Best verbal response	Oriented to time, person, place	5
	Confused, but able to converse	4
	Inappropriate words—makes little or no sense; words are recognizable	3
	Incomprehensible sounds—groans or moans; words are not recognizable	2
	No verbal response	1

*Possible score ranges between 3 and 15. 15 = Alert and oriented; less than 8 = coma.

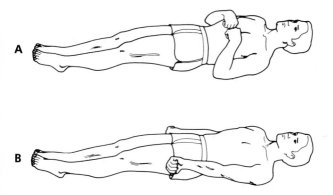

Figure 1-2 Flexion and extension. **A,** Flexion or decorticate rigidity. **B,** Extension or decerebrate rigidity. (From Budassi SA: Mosby's manual of emergency care, ed 3, St Louis, 1990, The CV Mosby Co.)

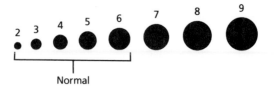

Figure 1-3   Pupil gauge in millimeters.

will occur in a blind eye; however, a consensual response can occur in the blind eye when the light is shined in the normal eye. Pinpoint pupils can result from miotic drugs, opiate drugs, or a pontine hemorrhage. Dilated pupils may result from use of cycloplegic drugs (atropine) or pressure on cranial nerve III (e.g., from a tumor or clot). Fixed pupils may be the result of barbiturate coma or hypothermia. Irregularly shaped pupils may occur as a result of cataract surgery.

Position: Pupils should be midposition.

Size: Note size in millimeters (Figure 1-3).

Shape: Pupils are normally round.

Direct light reflex: The tested pupil should constrict briskly.

Consensual light reflex: Nontested pupil constricts as light is shined in other eye.

Accommodation: Pupils constrict and eyes converge as the patient focuses on an object moved toward the nose.

Corneal reflex: An absent reflex (lack of blinking or eyelid closure) indicates trigeminal or facial nerve damage, necessitating eye protection with artificial tears and eye shields.

Cranial nerve assessment
Table 1-2 lists the cranial nerves and components to test.

Motor function
Observe the patient's resting posture and note any spontaneous or involuntary movement; also note any rigidity, spasticity, and flaccidity. Test gross muscle strength by assessing hand grasp and testing dorsiflexion and plantar flexion of the lower extremities. Compare both sides of the body and note any lateralizing signs (unilateral deterioration). A quick screening for weakness would include lifting the patient's arms off the bed and releasing them simultaneously. Observe for arm drifting, which indicates a weakness on one side of the body. A hemiparetic side falls more quickly and limply than the normal side. The GCS can evaluate motor function.

TABLE 1-2 Cranial Nerves

Nerve	Evaluate
Olfactory (I)	Sense of smell
Optic (II)	Vision: visual fields and acuity
Oculomotor (III), trochlear (IV), and abducens (VI)	Pupil reactions, EOMs: III—evaluate eye movement up and outward, down and outward, and up and inward; IV—evaluate eye movement down and inward; VI—evaluate eye movement outward
Trigeminal (V)	Sensation on both sides of face, opening and closing of jaw, corneal reflex
Facial (VII)	Facial muscle movement: eye brows, smile, frown, eyelid closing; taste sensation
Acoustic (VIII)	Hearing
Glossopharyngeal (IX) Vagus (X)	Gag reflex, swallowing, soft palate elevation
Spinal accessory (XI)	Shoulder shrug and head movement
Hypoglossal (XII)	Tongue position, movement, and strength

Sensory function

A gross evaluation of sensory function would include light touch to the forehead, cheeks, hands, lower arms, abdomen, lower legs, and feet. Other types of sensations can be used, e.g., pain, heat/cold, vibration, position changes, and deep pressure pain. Compare both sides of the body.

Spinal cord assessment

The motor strength of each muscle group should be evaluated in patients with spinal cord dysfunction (Table 1-3). A 5-point system can be used to assess overall muscle strength of the extremities (Table 1-4). A less complex system, such as 0 = absent, 1 = weak, and 2 = strong, may be used.

Specific dermatomal areas (Figure 1-4) should be evaluated in the patient with a spinal cord dysfunction. Terms used to describe sensory dysfunction can be found below.

Analgesia: Loss of pain
Anesthesia: Complete loss of sensation
Dysesthesia: Impaired sensation
Hyperesthesia: Increased sensation

TABLE 1-3 Spinal Cord Assessment

Level of innervation	Function	Reflex
C4	Neck movement, diaphragmatic breathing	
C5	Abduction of the shoulder	Biceps (C5)
C5-6	Elbow flexion	Brachioradialis (C6)
C7-8	Elbow extension	Triceps (C7)
C6,7,8	Wrist dorsiflexion	
C8	Hand grip	
C6-8,T1	Finger extension and flexion	
L2-4	Hip flexion	
L4,5,S1	Hip extension	
L2-4	Knee extension	
L4,5-S1	Knee flexion	Patellar (L4)
L5	Dorsiflexion of the foot	
S1	Plantar flexion of the foot	

TABLE 1-4 Muscle Strength Scale

Description	Score
Normal power or muscle strength in extremities	5
Weak extremities, but patient can overcome resistance applied by examiner	4
Patient can overcome gravity (can lift extremities) but cannot overcome resistance applied by examiner	3
Weak muscle contraction, but not enough to overcome gravity (movement, but cannot lift extremities)	2
Palpable or visible muscle flicker or twitch, but no movement	1
No response to stimulus, complete paralysis	0

Hypesthesia: Decreased sensation
Paresthesia: Burning, tingling sensation
Peripheral neurovascular assessment
Peripheral nerve and circulation should be evaluated in patients with injury (e.g., fractures, burns) to upper or lower

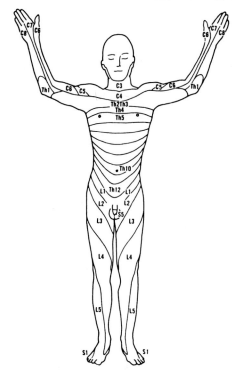

The dermatomes from the anterior view.

Figure 1-4 Dermatomes. Landmarks are: Clavicle—C4; deltoid—C5; nipples—T4; navel—T10; knee—L3-L4; great toe—L5; little toe—S1; sole of foot—S1. (From Thelan L et al: Textbook of critical care nursing, St Louis, 1990, Mosby–Year Book, Inc, p. 528.)

Continued.

extremities. Both sensory and motor function of the ulnar, radial, median, and peroneal nerves should be assessed.

5 P's: Pain, paresthesia, paralysis, pulse, and pallor.

Circulation: Check presence and amplitude of pulses, capillary refill, and skin temperature.

Movement: Upper extremities—have patient hyperextend the thumb or wrist (radial), oppose the thumb and little finger (median), and abduct all fingers (ulnar).

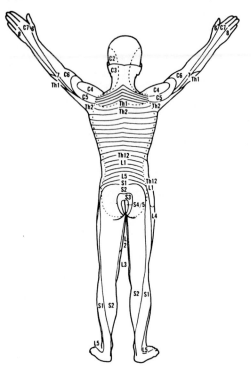

The dermatomes from the posterior view.

Figure 1-4 cont'd. Dermatomes. Landmarks are: Clavicle—C4; deltoid—C5; nipples—T4; navel—T10; knee—L3-L4; great toe—L5; little toe—S1; sole of foot—S1. (From Thelan L et al: Textbook of critical care nursing, St Louis, 1990, Mosby–Year Book, Inc, p. 528.)

Lower extremities: have patient dorsiflex the foot (peroneal) and plantarflex the foot (tibial).

Sensation: Upper extremities—use a pin to prick the webbed space between the thumb and index finger (radial), distal fat pad of small finger (ulnar), and distal fat pad of index/middle finger (median).

Lower extremities: use a pin to prick the dorsal surface of the foot near the webbed space between the great and second toes.

TABLE 1-5 Scale for Deep Tendon Reflexes

Score	Description
0	Absent
1+	Diminished
2+	Normal
3+	Increased, more brisk than average
4+	Hyperactive, clonus

Reflexes

Abnormal reflexes may be early signs of upper motor neuron disease, lower motor neuron disease, or disease of the afferent sensory component of muscles.

Deep tendon reflexes: Jaw, biceps, brachioradialis, triceps, patellar, and achilles reflexes can be assessed on a scale from 0 to 4+ (Table 1-5).

Pathological reflexes: Positive Babinski sign—great toe pointing upward (extension) and fanning of the other toes. Grasp reflex—patient does not release an object that has been placed in the patient's hand. Snout reflex—pursing of lips when the mouth is tapped above or below the midline.

Brainstem function

An alteration in brainstem function can affect the state of consciousness; respiratory, circulatory, and vasomotor activities; and a number of reflexes.

DERM mnemonic: The mnemonic device *DERM* can be used to assess brainstem functioning; *D* = Depth of coma; *E* = Eye assessment; *R* = Respiration assessment; *M* = Movement assessment (Table 1-6).

Oculocephalic reflex—doll's eye maneuver: Tested in the comatose patient to assess brainstem function. Positive doll's eyes sign (both eyes move in the direction opposite to the head rotation) is normal and indicates an intact brainstem. If this response is absent, the patient's airway may not be protected by gag and cough reflexes.

Oculovestibular reflex—caloric testing: Usually tested in the comatose patient to assess brainstem function. With an intact brainstem, eyes deviate with nystagmus toward the ear that is irrigated with cold water. An absent reflex

TABLE 1-6 Assessing Brainstem Function Using the DERM Mnemonic

The brainstem levels	Herniation levels	D = Depth of coma	E = Eyes	R = Respirations	M = Motor function	Posturing
	Thalamus	Painful stimulus causes nonpurposeful response	Small; reaction to light	Eupnea / Cheyne-Stokes respirations	Hyperactive deep tendon reflexes	Decorticate
	Midbrain	Painful stimulus causes no response	Midpoint to dilated; fixed; no reaction to light	Central neurogenic breathing	Decreased deep tendon reflexes	Decerebrate
	Pons	Painful stimulus causes no response	Pinpoint; no reaction to light	Biot's respirations	Flaccid	No tone
	Medulla	Painful stimulus causes no response	Midpoint to dilated; fixed; no reaction to light	Ataxic/apneustic	Flaccid	No tone

From Budassi SA, Marvin JA, and Jimmerson CL: Manual of clinical trauma care, ed 1, St. Louis 1989, The CV Mosby Co.

(both eyes remain fixed in midline position) may indicate impending brain death. Neuromuscular blocking agents, barbiturates, and antibiotic agents can inhibit this reflex.

Determining brain death: Reversible conditions such as sedation, neuromuscular blockade, shock, hypothermia, and metabolic imbalances must be excluded. The clinical examination is most important; however, laboratory tests may be used in conjunction with the clinical examination to confirm brain death. The absence of recordable brain waves on the EEG is associated with brain death. However, EEGs may produce false positive and false negative results. A cerebral blood flow (CBF) study is more useful than the EEG. The absence of cerebral circulation is diagnostic of brain death regardless of cause.

CLINICAL EXAMINATION

The following findings must be present on examination of the patient:

- Patient must be comatose.
- Pupils must be nonreactive.
- Corneal reflex must be absent.
- Gag reflex must be absent.
- Cough reflex must be absent.
- Oculocephalic reflex must be absent.
- Oculovestibular reflex must be absent.
- Spontaneous respirations must be absent (see Apnea testing).

APNEA TESTING

To test for the presence of apnea, 100% oxygen is administered to the patient for 10 to 20 minutes. The ventilator is withdrawn while the patient receives passive flow of oxygen. Lack of spontaneous respirations in the presence of adequate carbon dioxide stimulus ($Paco_2 > 60$ mm Hg for 3 min) indicates that the brainstem is nonfunctioning.

Incisions, drainage, and equipment

Assess the condition of incisional sites from neurosurgical surgeries and procedures. Assess for the presence of cerebral spinal fluid drainage, e.g., rhinorrhea or otorrhea. Assess ventriculostomy site and other equipment and devices for proper functioning and complications.

Intracranial monitoring

Obtain ICP and calculate CPP. (See p. 74 for ICP monitoring and p. 31 for formula.)

Pattern		Description
Eupnea	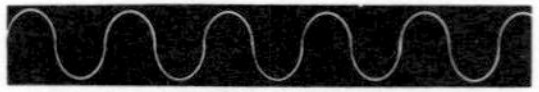	Rhythm is smooth and even with expiration longer than inspiration.
Tachypnea	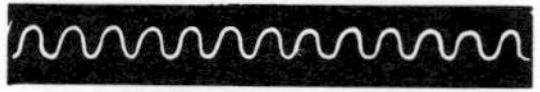	Rapid superficial breathing; regular or irregular rhythm.
Bradypnea	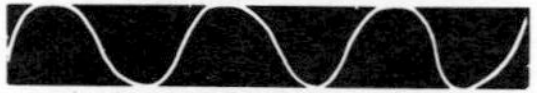	Slow respiratory rate; deeper than usual depth; regular rhythm.
Apnea		Cessation of breathing.
Hyperpnea	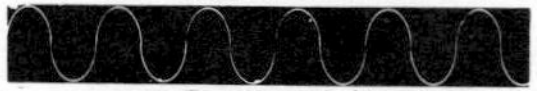	Increased depth of respiration with a normal to increased rate and regular rhythm.
Cheyne-Stokes respiration	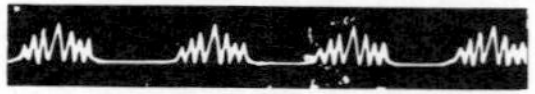	Periodic breathing associated with periods of apnea, alternating regularly with a series of respiratory cycles; the respiratory cycle gradually increases, then decreases in rate and depth.
Ataxic breathing	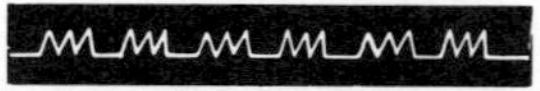	Periods of apnea alternating irregularly with a series of shallow breaths of equal depth.
Kussmaul's respiration	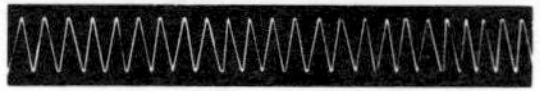	Deep regular sighing respirations with an increase in respiratory rate.
Apneusis	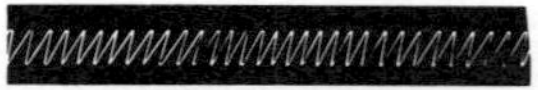	Long, gasping inspiratory phase followed by a short, inadequate expiratory phase.
Obstructed breathing	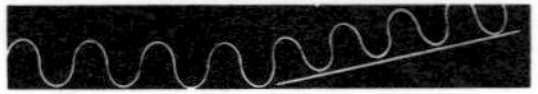	Long, ineffective expiratory phase with shallow, increased respirations.

Figure 1-5 Respiratory patterns. (Modified from Talbot L and Marquardt M: Pocket guide to critical care assessment, St Louis, 1989, The CV Mosby Co.)

Pulmonary Assessment
Respirations

Determine respiratory rate and rhythm (Figure 1-5). Assess chest for depth of respirations, paradoxical movement, and symmetry of respirations. Note use of accessory muscles, nasal flaring, tracheal deviation, and cough.

Breath sounds

Auscultate all lung fields (Figure 1-6).

Bronchial sounds: High-pitched and normally heard over the trachea. Timing includes an inspiration phase less than the expiration phase. If heard in lung fields, this usually indicates consolidation (Figure 1-7).

Vesicular sounds: Low-pitched and normally heard in the

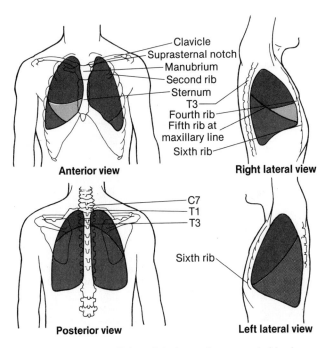

Figure 1-6 Location of lobes of the lung using anatomical landmarks. (From Talbot L and Marquardt M: Pocket guide to critical care assessment, St Louis, 1989, The CV Mosby Co.)

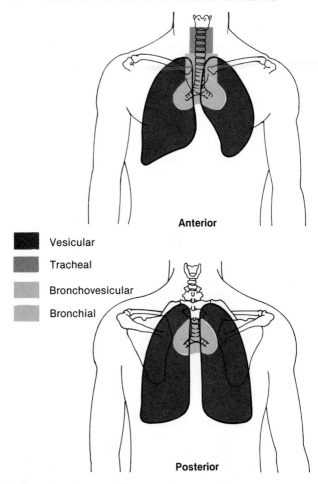

Anterior

- ■ Vesicular
- ■ Tracheal
- ■ Bronchovesicular
- ■ Bronchial

Posterior

Figure 1-7 Location of normal breath sounds. (From Talbot L and Marquardt M: Pocket guide to critical care assessment, St Louis, 1989, The CV Mosby Co.)

periphery of the lungs. Timing includes an inspiration phase greater than the expiration phase (see Figure 1-7).
Bronchovesicular sounds: Medium-pitched, with a muffled quality. Timing includes an inspiration phase equal to the expiration phase (see Figure 1-7).

Adventitious sounds

Assess breath and voice sounds.

Crackles: Discontinuous sounds heard during inspiration that can be classified as "fine" (similar to rubbing strands of hair together next to the ear) or "coarse" (bubbling quality similar to carbonated soda). Generally not cleared with coughing.

Wheezes: High-pitched sounds that may be heard during inspiration or expiration.

Rhonchi: Low, coarse sounds of a "snoring" quality. Generally clears with coughing.

Pleural friction rub: Grating, harsh sound, located in an area of intense chest wall pain.

Bronchophony: Spoken words (have patient say "99") that are heard clearly and distinctly are indicative of lung consolidation.

Whispered pectoriloquy: Extreme bronchophony, such that a voice sound (have patient whisper "99") is heard clearly and distinctly.

Egophony: Spoken word assumes a nasal quality (have patient say "E"; it is heard as "A") indicative of consolidation or pleural effusion.

Intubation and mechanical ventilation

Check endotracheal tube placement, cuff pressure, and ventilator settings and alarms (see Mechanical ventilation, p. 463).

Respiratory equipment

Check equipment, such as pulse oximeters, for proper functioning and alarms.

Chest drainage

Assess system for proper functioning and note the amount, color, and character of chest drainage.

Oxygenation calculations

Calculate relevant oxygen parameters (see Cardiopulmonary parameters, p. 25).

Cardiovascular Assessment

Heart rate and rhythm

Note monitor lead placement and obtain a rhythm strip to determine rate and rhythm (see Rhythm strip analysis, p. 113).

Integument

Note color, temperature, and moisture. Check anterior chest wall for capillary refill (>3 sec reflects poor tissue perfusion). Evaluate severity of edema (Table 1-7).

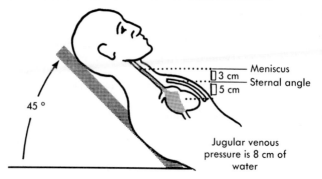

Figure 1-8 Estimation of central venous pressure. Identify the highest level of pulsations in the internal jugular vein (meniscus). Determine the vertical distance between the sternal angle and meniscus. Add that distance to the constant 5 cm (sternal angle is 5 cm above mid-RA level).

TABLE 1-7 Grading Scale for Edema

Depth of pitting edema	Score
0-¼ in	+1
¼-½ in	+2
½-1 in	+3
> 1 in	+4

Central venous pressure (CVP)
Check neck veins to estimate CVP (Figure 1-8). Note presence of Kussmaul's sign (level of pulsation in internal jugular increases on inspiration). Test hepatojugular reflex (HJR). An increase in venous level >1 cm = positive HJR.

Pulses
Check pulses bilaterally *except* for carotids. Note rate, rhythm, equality, and amplitude. Figure 1-9 shows variations in arterial pulses. The following scale can be used to describe pulses: 0 = absent, +1 = weak, +2 = normal, +3 = bounding.

Heart sounds
Systematically auscultate each area of the precordium (Figure 1-10), concentrating on one component of the cardiac

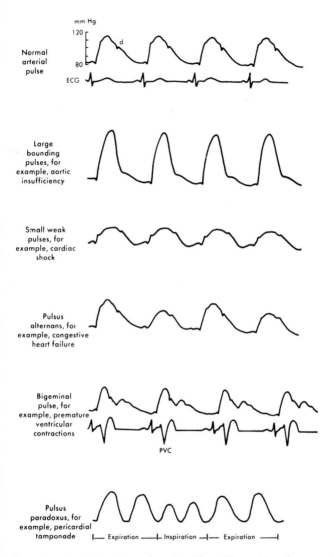

Figure 1-9 Variations in arterial pulse. (From Kinney M et al: Comprehensive cardiac care, ed 7, St Louis, 1991, Mosby-Year Book, Inc.)

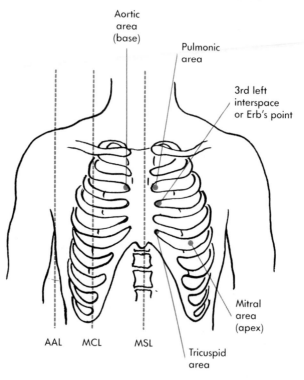

Figure 1-10 Cardiac auscultatory sites. S_1 is heard loudest at mitral and tricuspid areas. S_2 is heard loudest at aortic and pulmonic areas. S_3 and S_4 are heard best at mitral area.

cycle at a time. The bell of the stethoscope accentuates lower frequency sounds, e.g., S_3, S_4. The diaphragm of the stethoscope accentuates high-pitched sounds, e.g., S_1, S_2. Figure 1-11 illustrates heart sounds in relation to ECG. Table 1-8 lists the various heart sounds and differentiating components.

Heart murmurs
Describe murmurs according to location, e.g., distance from midsternal, midclavicular, or axillary lines; radiation—where the sound is transmitted; loudness—grades I to VI (Table 1-9); pitch—high or low; shape—crescendo, decrescendo, crescendo-decrescendo, plateau; and quality—harsh, rumbling, musical, blowing.

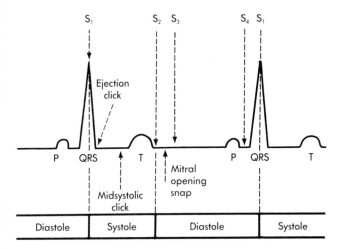

Figure 1-11   Heart sounds in relation to the ECG.

TABLE 1-8 Differentiating Heart Sounds

Heart sound	Best area to auscultate	Timing
S_1	Apex	Systole
S_2	Base	Diastole
S_3	Apex, LSB	Early diastole, after S_2
S_4	Apex, LSB	Late diastole, before S_1
Split S_1	4ICS, LSB	Systole
Split S_2	2ICS, LSB	End of systole
Aortic ejection sound	2ICS, RSB; apex	Early systole
Pulmonic ejection sound	2ICS, LSB	Early systole
Midsystolic click	Apex	Mid to late systole
Opening snap	Lower LSB, 4ICS	Early diastole
Pericardial friction rub	Loudest along LSB	Systole and diastole

ICS, intercostal space. LSB, left sternal border. RSB, right sternal border.

TABLE 1-9 Murmur Grading Scale

Grade	Description
I/VI	Faint, barely audible
II/VI	Quiet, heard immediately on auscultation
III/VI	Moderately loud, no thrill
IV/VI	Loud, thrill
V/VI	Very loud, requires a stethoscope; thrill present
VI/VI	Same as V/VI but can be heard with stethoscope off the chest

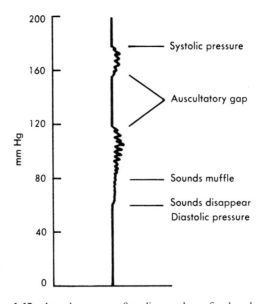

Figure 1-12 Auscultatory gap. Systolic sounds are first heard at 180 mm Hg. They disappear at 160 mm Hg and reappear at 120 mm Hg; the silent interval is known as the *auscultatory gap*. Korotkoff sounds muffle at 80 mm Hg and disappear at 60 mm Hg. Blood pressure is recorded as 180/80/60 with auscultatory gap. If the cuff was inflated to 150 mm Hg, the reading may have been interpreted as normotensive. (From Kinney M et al: Comprehensive cardiac care, ed 7, St Louis, 1991, Mosby-Year Book, Inc.)

Blood pressure

Assess blood pressure on both arms. Use a blood pressure cuff 20% wider than the diameter of the limb to avoid false high or low pressures.

Auscultatory Gap

Determine the presence of an auscultatory gap (Figure 1-12).

Pulsus Paradoxus

Determine the presence of pulsus paradoxus. Slowly deflate the BP cuff (1 mm Hg per respiratory cycle); note when the first sound is heard, which will be on expiration. Note when sounds begin again and are heard continuously (during inspiration and expiration). If the difference between the first sound and the continuous sound is > 10 mm Hg, pulsus paradoxus is present.

Hemodynamic monitoring

Obtain readings and calculate cardiopulmonary parameters. (See p. 78 for Hemodynamic monitoring and p. 25 for Cardiopulmonary formulas.)

Pacemaker

Validate settings. Assess for failure to capture and failure to sense. Assess what percentage of the patient's rhythm is paced.

Gastrointestinal Assessment

Bowel sounds

Auscultate all quadrants (Figure 1-13).

Absent sounds: May be associated with intestinal obstruction, paralytic ileus, or peritonitis. Listen for at least 5 minutes.

Intensified or gurgling sounds: May be associated with early intestinal obstruction, increased peristalsis, or diarrhea.

Abdomen

Note size, shape, and symmetry. Measure abdominal girth. Palpate for tenderness or masses.

Bowel elimination

Note characteristics of stool; guaiac stool for occult blood.

Nasogastric tube

Check placement, patency, drainage, and amount of suction. Check pH of gastric secretions, guaiac secretions. If the NG tube is used for enteral feeding, check placement and residual. Note skin condition.

Drains

Note type and location of drain. Check for proper function-

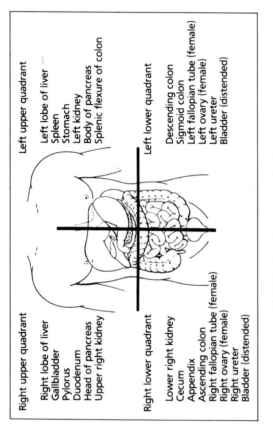

Right upper quadrant

Right lobe of liver
Gallbladder
Pylorus
Duodenum
Head of pancreas
Upper right kidney

Left upper quadrant

Left lobe of liver
Spleen
Stomach
Left kidney
Body of pancreas
Splenic flexure of colon

Right lower quadrant

Lower right kidney
Cecum
Appendix
Ascending colon
Right fallopian tube (female)
Right ovary (female)
Right ureter
Bladder (distended)

Left lower quadrant

Descending colon
Sigmoid colon
Left fallopian tube (female)
Left ovary (female)
Left ureter
Bladder (distended)

Figure 1-13 Topography of abdomen.

ing of drainage system and the characteristics and amount of drainage. Assess skin condition.

Incisions and stomas

Check condition of incisions and stomas.

Genitourinary Assessment

Genitalia

Check external genitalia for any drainage, inflammation, or lesions.

Fluid status

Check weight daily. An increase of 0.5 kg/day suggests fluid retention. Measure I & O; 1 L fluid ~ 1 kg of body weight. Table 1-10 lists findings associated with volume excess or deficit.

TABLE 1-10 Signs and Symptoms Associated with Volume Disturbances

	Hypovolemia	Hypervolemia
Weight	Acute loss	Acute gain
Pulse	Decrease pulse pressure Tachycardia	Bounding
Blood pressure	Postural hypotension	Hypertension
Mucous membranes	Dry	Moist
Turgor	Decreased skin elasticity	Pitting edema
Peripheral veins	JVP flat when supine Slow filling hand veins	JVP elevated
Hemodynamics	CVP < 2 cm H_2O Decreased PAWP	CVP > 12 cm H_2O Increased PAWP
Other	Thirst Urine output < 30 ml/hr	Cough Dyspnea Crackles S_3
Laboratory data	Increased hemoglobin Increased hematocrit Increased serum osmolality Increased specific gravity Increased BUN/ creatinine ratio	Decreased hemoglobin Decreased hematocrit Decreased serum osmolality Decreased specific gravity

JVP, Jugular venous pressure; *CVP*, central venous pressure, *PAWP*, pulmonary artery wedge pressure.

Bladder

Percuss the abdomen for bladder distention.

Urine

Measure urinary output. Note color and consistency.

Anuria: <100 ml/24 hr

Oliguria: 100-400 ml/24 hr

Catheters

Identify type of urinary drainage tube and assess proper functioning.

Shunts

Assess patency of shunt by palpation and auscultation. Inspect external shunts for color and for clots.

SCORING SYSTEMS FOR THE ICU PATIENT

Apache III

The Acute Physiology and Chronic Health Evaluation (APACHE III) is a prognostic scoring system[10] (see Appendix D). The score, which can range from 0 to 299, is determined from physiological values, age, and the presence of chronic illness. The APACHE III risk equation can be used to calculate a predicted risk of hospital mortality and takes into account the patient's APACHE III score, major disease category, and treatment location before the ICU admission.

Trauma Score

The trauma score (see Appendix D, p. 691) is a system for estimating the severity of patient injury.[3,4] The patient's LOC (using the GCS) and cardiopulmonary function are assessed. A numerical value is assigned to each of the assessment parameters. The total score reflects the severity of the injury and a survival estimate for the patient can be projected from the score.

Therapeutic Intervention Scoring System (TISS)

TISS has been used to determine severity of illness, establish nurse/patient ratios, and assess current bed utilization and need.[9] Patient classification of severity of illness is based on points: class I, under 10 points; class II, 10 to 19 points; class III, 20 to 39 points; and class IV, 40 or more points (see Appendix D).

It has been proposed that class IV patients receive a 1:1 nurse/patient ratio and that an accomplished critical care nurse should be capable of managing 40 to 50 patient TISS points.

FORMULAS

Cardiopulmonary Parameters

Coronary perfusion pressure (CPP)

CPP is the driving pressure influencing coronary blood flow. Coronary blood flow ceases when CPP reaches 40 mm Hg.

EQUATION: CPP = DBP − PAWP (LVEDP)

NORMAL: 60-80 mm Hg

Pulse pressure (PP)

PP reflects stroke volume and arterial compliance. Widened PP is associated with a decrease in peripheral resistance and/or increased stroke volume. Narrowed PP is associated with an increase in peripheral resistance and/or decreased stroke volume.

EQUATION: PP = SBP − DBP

NORMAL: 30-40 mm Hg

Rate pressure product (RPP)

RPP is also known as double product (DP); it is an indirect measurement of myocardial oxygen demand. Activities performed at lower heart rates and systolic blood pressures are better tolerated by individuals with coronary artery disease.

EQUATION: RPP = HR × SBP

NORMAL: < 12000

Mean arterial pressure (MAP)

MAP is a measure of the average arterial perfusion pressure, which determines blood flow to the tissues.

EQUATION: MAP = ⅓ PP + DBP

$$MAP = \frac{2(DBP) + SBP}{3}$$

NORMAL: 70-105 mm Hg

Cardiac output (CO)

CO is the measurement of the amount of blood ejected by the ventricles each minute. It reflects pump efficiency and is a determinant of tissue perfusion.

EQUATION: CO = HR × SV

NORMAL: 4-8 L/min

Cardiac index (CI)

CI is a measurement of the cardiac output adjusted for body size. It is a more precise measurement of pump efficiency than CO.

$$EQUATION: \quad CI = \frac{CO}{BSA}$$

NORMAL: 2.5-4.0 L/min/m²

Stroke volume (SV)

SV represents the volume of blood ejected from the ventricle with each cardiac contraction. It is influenced by preload, afterload, and contractility.

$$EQUATION: \quad SV = \frac{CO \ (ml/min)}{HR}$$

NORMAL: 60-80 ml/beat

Stroke index (SI)

SI is a measurement of SV adjusted for body size.

$$EQUATION: \quad SI = \frac{SV}{BSA} \text{ or } \frac{CI \ (ml/min)}{HR}$$

NORMAL: 40-50 ml/beat/m²

Systemic vascular resistance (SVR)

SVR is a measurement of left ventricular afterload. A diseased aortic valve and resistance in the systemic arterial circulation increase left ventricular afterload.

$$EQUATION: \quad SVR = \frac{MAP - CVP}{CO} \times 80$$

NORMAL: 900-1400 dynes/sec/cm⁻⁵

$NORMAL:$ 900-1400 dynes/sec/cm^{-5}

Systemic vascular resistance index (SVRI)

SVRI is a measurement of left ventricular afterload, adjusted for body size.

$$EQUATION: \quad SVRI = \frac{MAP - CVP}{CI} \times 80$$

NORMAL: 1700-2600 dynes/sec/cm^{-5}/m²

Pulmonary vascular resistance (PVR)

PVR is a measurement of right ventricular afterload. A diseased pulmonic valve and resistance in pulmonary arterial circulation increase right ventricular afterload.

$$EQUATION: \quad PVR = \frac{PAM - PAWP}{CO} \times 80$$

NORMAL: 100-250 dynes/sec/cm^{-5}

Pulmonary vascular resistance index (PVRI)

PVRI is a measurement of right ventricular afterload, adjusted for body size.

$$EQUATION: \quad PVRI = \frac{PAM - PAWP}{CI} \times 80$$

NORMAL: 200-450 dynes/sec/cm^{-5}/m^2

Left ventricular stroke work index (LVSWI)

LVSWI is a measurement of amount of work the left ventricle does per cardiac contraction, adjusted for body size. It is an indirect method of measuring myocardial contractility.

EQUATION: LVSWI = SVI × (MAP − PAWP) × 0.0136

NORMAL: 45-60 g-m/m^2

Right ventricular stroke work index (RVSWI)

RVSWI is a measurement of amount of work the right ventricle does per cardiac contraction, adjusted for body size. It is an indirect method of measuring myocardial contractility.

EQUATION: RVSWI = SVI × (PAM − CVP) × 0.0136

NORMAL: 8.5−12 g-m/m^2

Ejection fraction (EF)

EF is a measurement of the ratio of the amount of blood ejected from the left ventricle to the amount of blood remaining in the ventricle at end diastole. It is an indirect measurement of contractility.

$$EQUATION: \quad EF = \frac{SV}{EDV} \times 100$$

NORMAL: 60% or greater

EDV = End diastolic volume

Alveolar air equation (PAo$_2$)

PAo$_2$ is a measurement of alveolar partial pressure of oxygen.

$$EQUATION: \quad PAo_2 = Fio_2 (Pb - PH_2O) - \frac{Paco_2}{0.8}$$

Pb = Barometric pressure

$$PH_2O = \text{Water vapor pressure}$$
$$Pb - PH_2O = 713$$

NORMAL: 100 mm Hg

Expected Pao$_2$ (Pao$_2$)

Pao$_2$ is a measurement of lung function when the expected Pao$_2$ is compared with the actual Pao$_2$. For persons older than 60 years of age, subtract 1 mm Hg for each year over 60.

EQUATION: $Pao_2 = Fio_2 \times 5$

Alveolar-arterial oxygen gradient (P[A−a]o$_2$) or (A-a gradient)

P(A-a)o$_2$ is a measurement of the difference between partial pressure of oxygen in the alveoli and arterial blood and an indication of oxygen transfer in the lung. However, supplemental oxygen and age can affect the gradient in individuals who do not have an acute condition of the lung.

EQUATION: $P(A-a)o_2 = Pao_2 - Pao_2$

NORMAL: < 15 mm Hg (room air) 10-65 mm Hg (100% O_2)

Arterial-alveolar oxygen tension ratio (P[a/A]o$_2$ ratio)

P(a/A)o$_2$ ratio is a measurement of the efficiency of gas exchange in the lung. Supplemental oxygen does not affect the ratio. A value less than 0.75 can indicate ventilation/perfusion (V/Q) inequalities, shunt abnormalities, or diffusion problems.

EQUATION: $\dfrac{Pao_2}{Pao_2}$

NORMAL: 0.75-0.90

Arterial oxygen content (Cao$_2$)

Cao$_2$ is a measurement of oxygen content in arterial blood, including oxygen bound to hemoglobin and oxygen dissolved in blood. A decreased value may indicate a low Pao$_2$, Sao$_2$, and/or hemoglobin (Hgb).

EQUATION: $Cao_2 = (Sao_2 \times Hgb \times 1.34) + (Pao_2 \times 0.003)$

NORMAL: 18-20 ml/100 ml

Venous oxygen content (Cvo$_2$)

Cvo$_2$ is a measurement of oxygen content in venous blood. It takes into account Svo$_2$, Pvo$_2$, and hemoglobin; thus any change in these indices affects the Cvo$_2$.

EQUATION: $Cv_{O_2} = (Sv_{O_2} \times Hgb \times 1.34) + (Pv_{O_2} \times 0.003)$

NORMAL: 15.5 ml/100 ml

Arteriovenous oxygen content difference (C[a-v]o_2)

$C(a-v)_{O_2}$ is a measurement that reflects oxygen uptake at the tissue level. An increased value indicates inadequate cardiovascular functioning. A decrease in CO results in more O_2 extracted, thus reducing the O_2 content of venous blood. A decreased value indicates poor tissue utilization of oxygen.

EQUATION: $C(a-v)_{O_2} = Ca_{O_2} - Cv_{O_2}$

NORMAL: 4-6 ml/100 ml

Arterial oxygen delivery (DO$_2$) or oxygen transport

DO_2 is a measurement of volume of O_2 delivered to tissues every minute. A decrease in DO_2 may be due to a decrease in oxygen content or decrease in cardiac output.

EQUATION: $DO_2 = CO \times 10 \times Ca_{O_2}$

NORMAL: 900-1200 ml/min

Arterial oxygen delivery index (DO$_2$I)

DO_2I is a measurement of DO_2 adjusted for body size.

EQUATION: $DO_2I = CI \times 10 \times Ca_{O_2}$

NORMAL: 500-600 ml/min/m^2

Oxygen consumption (VO$_2$)

VO_2 is a measurement of volume of oxygen used by tissues every minute. A decreased value may indicate that metabolic needs of tissues are not being met, usually as a result of inadequate O_2 transport.

EQUATION: $VO_2 = CO \times 10 \times C(a-v)_{O_2}$

NORMAL: 200-250 ml/min

Oxygen consumption index (VO$_2$I)

VO_2I is a measurement of VO_2 adjusted for body size.

EQUATION: $VO_2I = CI \times 10 \times C(a-v)_{O_2}$

NORMAL: 115-165 ml/min/m^2

Oxygen utilization coefficient or oxygen extraction ratio (O$_2$ER)

O_2ER is a measurement that indicates the balance between oxygen supply and demand. It is the fraction of available O_2 that is utilized by the tissues. Values greater than 25% indicate that an increased O_2 supply is needed.

$$EQUATION: \quad O_2ER = \frac{C(a\text{-}v)o_2}{Cao_2}$$

NORMAL: 25%

Physiological shunt (Qs/Qt)

Qs/Qt is a measurement of the efficiency of the oxygenation system. It reflects the portion of venous blood that is not involved in gas exchange. High values are indicative of lung dysfunction, e.g., atelectasis or pulmonary edema.

$$EQUATION: \quad Qs/Qt = \frac{Cco_2 - Cao_2}{Cco_2 - Cvo_2}$$

NORMAL: 0%-8%

$Cco_2 = O_2$ content in capillary blood
$Cco_2 = (Hgb \times 1.34) + (P_{AO_2} \times 0.003)$

Qs/Qt approximation

$$EQUATION: \quad \frac{Pao_2}{Fio_2}$$

VALUES: 500 = 10%

300 = 15%

200 = 20%

Dynamic compliance

Dynamic compliance is a measure of maximum airway pressure required to deliver a given tidal volume. It reflects lung elasticity and airway resistance during the breathing cycle. A low value reflects a reduced compliance (bronchospasm, secretions in airway).

$$EQUATION: \quad \frac{V_T}{PIP - PEEP}$$

NORMAL: 35-55 ml/cm H_2O

V_T = Tidal volume; PIP = peak inspiratory pressure; PEEP = positive end-expiratory pressure

Static compliance

Static compliance is a measurement of airway pressure required to hold the lungs at end inspiration (after a tidal volume has been delivered and no air flow is present). It reflects only lung elasticity not affected by gas flow. A low value reflects lung stiffness.

$$EQUATION: \quad \frac{V_T}{\text{Plateau pressure} - \text{PEEP}}$$

NORMAL: 50-100 ml/cm H_2O

Neurological Parameters
Cerebral perfusion pressure (CPP)

CPP is a measurement of the pressure necessary to provide adequate cerebral blood flow. A value < 60 mm Hg is associated with cerebral ischemia.

EQUATION: $CPP = MAP - ICP$

NORMAL: 60-100 mm Hg

Metabolic Parameters
Anion gap (GAP) or delta

GAP is a measurement of excess unmeasurable anions used to differentiate the mechanisms of metabolic acidosis. GAP will remain normal in metabolic acidosis resulting from bicarbonate loss.

EQUATION: $GAP = Na - (HCO_3 + CL)$

NORMAL: 8-16 mEq/L

Basal energy expenditure (BEE)

BEE is a measurement of basal energy expenditure required to support vital life functions.

EQUATION: Men: $= (66.47 + 13.7W + 5H) - (6.76A)$
Women: $= (655.1 + 9.56W + 1.8H) - (4.68A)$
$W = wt(kg); H = ht(cm); A = age$

Total energy expenditure (TEE) $= BEE \times AF \times IF$
AF = Activity factor (bed rest = 1.2; ambulatory = 1.3)
IF = Injury factor (surgery = 1.2; trauma = 1.35; sepsis = 1.6; burn = 2.1)

Respiratory quotient (RQ)

RQ is a measurement of the state of nutrition. The relationship of oxygen consumption and carbon dioxide production reflects the oxidative state of the cell and energy consumption.

EQUATION: $RQ = \dfrac{CO_2 \text{ production}}{O_2 \text{ consumption}}$

VALUES: 0.8-1.0 (normal)
0.7 = Lipolysis or starvation
0.8 = Protein is primary source of energy

0.85 = Carbohydrates, protein, and fat are
energy sources
1.0 = Carbohydrate is primary source of energy
> 1.0 = Lipogenesis; state of being overfed

Renal Parameters

Glomerular filtration rate (GFR)

GFR is a measurement of amount of blood filtered by glomeruli each minute. GFR is affected by blood pressure and glomerular capillary membrane permeability. A decreased value may indicate renal disease or decreased perfusion to the kidneys.

EQUATION: Male: $\dfrac{(140 - age) \times wt\ (kg)}{75 \times serum\ Cr}$

Female: $\dfrac{(140 - age) \times wt\ (kg)}{85 \times serum\ Cr}$

NORMAL: 80-120 ml/min

Osmolality

Osmolality is a measurement of solute concentration per volume of solution. An increased value is associated with dehydration, a decreased value with overhydration. Renal concentrating ability can be assessed with simultaneous urine and serum osmolality measurements.

EQUATION: $(2Na) + K + \dfrac{BUN}{3} + \dfrac{Glucose}{18}$

NORMAL: 275-295 mOsm (serum)

BIBLIOGRAPHY

1. Borg G: Psychophysical bases of perceived exertion, Med Sci Sports Exercise 14(5):377-381, 1982.
2. Budassi SA: Mosby's manual of emergency care, ed 3, St Louis, 1990, The CV Mosby Co.
3. Champion HR et al: Trauma score, Crit Care Med 9(9):672-676, 1981.

4. Champion HR, Gainer PS and Yackee E: A progress report on the trauma score in predicting a fatal outcome, J Trauma 26(10):927-931, 1986.
5. Daily E and Schroeder J: Techniques in bedside hemodynamic monitoring, ed 4, St Louis, 1989, The CV Mosby Co.
6. Deepak V, Babcock R and Magilligan D: A simplified concept of complete physiological monitoring of the critically ill patient, Heart Lung 10(1):75-82, 1981.
7. Gould K (editor): Crit Care Nurs Clin North Am 1(3):539-628, 1989.
8. Guidelines for the determination of death: report of the Medical Consultants in the Diagnosis of Death to the President's Commission for the Study of Ethical Problems in Medicine and Biomedical and Behavioral Research, JAMA 246:2184-2186, 1981.
9. Keene R and Cullen D: Therapeutic intervention scoring system: update 1983, Crit Care Med 11(1):1-3, 1983.
10. Knaus WA et al: APACHE III prognostic system, Chest (in press).
11. Mlynczak B: Assessment and management of the trauma patient in pain, Crit Care Nurs Clin North Am 1(1):55-65, 1989.
12. Palmer P: Advanced hemodynamic assessment, Dim Crit Care Nurs 1(3):139-144, 1982.
13. Pollard D and Seliger E: An implementation of bedside physiological calculations, Waltham, Mass, Hewlett-Packard Monograph, 1985.
14. Stillwell S and Randall E: Pocket guide to cardiovascular care, St Louis, 1990, The CV Mosby Co.
15. Talbot L and Marquardt M: Pocket guide to critical care assessment, St Louis, 1989, The CV Mosby Co.
16. Teasdale G and Jennett B: Glasgow coma scale, Lancet 2:81-83, 1974.
17. Thelan L et al: Textbook of critical care nursing, St Louis, 1990, The CV Mosby Co.
18. Transplant challenge, E Hanover NJ, 1988, Sandoz Pharmaceuticals Corp.
19. Zisfein J: Brain death in perspective, Hosp Phys 22(1):11-16, 1986.

CHAPTER 2

Diagnostic Tests and Patient Management

ANGIOGRAPHY

Clinical Brief

Angiography involves the injection of a contrast medium via a percutaneously inserted catheter in the area to be studied. Radiographs are then taken of the flow of the contrast material.

Digital subtraction angiography involves a computerized technique that subtracts images that block visualization of arteries.

Cardiac catheterization

Catheterization of the left side of the heart allows evaluation of mitral and aortic valvular function, ventricular function and structure, hemodynamics, and coronary artery patency. It also provides a means for percutaneous transluminal coronary angioplasty and intracoronary thrombolytic therapy.

Catheterization of the right side of the heart allows for an evaluation of tricuspid and pulmonic valvular function, the presence and degree of shunts, and hemodynamics.

The contrast medium that is injected to visualize cardiac chambers, valves, coronary arteries, and the great vessels can cause hemodynamic loading, decreased contractility (thus increasing the risk for congestive heart failure), and renal toxicity.

Once the catheter is in place, pressures are measured and blood samples obtained.

	Values
Pressures (mm Hg)	$\overline{RA}$ −1-+8
	LA 4-12
	RV 15-28/0-8
	LV 90-140/4-12
	$\underline{PAP}$ 15-28/5-16
	$\overline{PAWP}$ 6-15

O_2 saturation (abnormally low values are indicative of shunting)	75% (R heart) 95% (L heart) 70% (SVC) 80% (IVC) 75% (PA) 20% (coronary sinus)
O_2 content	14-15 vol% (R heart) 19 vol% (L heart)
CO	4-8 L/min
O_2 consumption	250 ml/min
CI	2.5-4 L/min/M^2
SI	30-60 ml/beat/M^2
EF	65% ± 10%
Volume	LVED 70 +/− 20 ml/M^2 LVES 24 +/− 10 ml/M^2 RVED 81 +/− 12 ml/M^2 LA 63 +/− 16 ml/M^2
Mass	LV wall thickness 9 mm (females) LV wall thickness 12 mm (males) LV wall mass 76 g/M^2 (females) LV wall mass 99 g/M^2 (males)
Wall motion	Normal
Valve orifice areas (critical values)	Aortic valve = 0.7 cm^2 Mitral valve = 1.0 cm^2
Valve gradient	None

Cerebral angiography

Cerebral angiography allows for identification and evaluation of vascular abnormalities such as aneurysms, arteriovenous malformations (AVMs), spasm, atherosclerosis, and intracerebral hemorrhages. For suspected tumors, an angiogram can illustrate both the vascular supply to the tumor and the relationship of surrounding blood vessels to the mass.

Gastrointestinal angiography

Gastrointestinal angiography provides a view of the anatomical structures and locates the source of bleeding. GI hemorrhage presents as extravasation of the contrast medium into the interstitium. Once located, vasopressin or artificial embolization can then be initiated. Portal pressure can also be measured during angiography.

Pulmonary angiography

Pulmonary angiography allows visualization of pulmonary vessels and the measurement of pressures, cardiac output, and pulmonary vascular resistance. Angiography allows identification of abnormalities in pulmonary perfusion, aiding in the diagnosis of thrombi, aneurysms, or blood vessel defects. Angiography may also be performed for preoperative patient evaluation or after an inconclusive lung scan.

Renal angiography

Renal angiography allows for visualization and identification of abnormalities of the renal circulation and to assess patency of dialysis shunts and fistulas. It also provides a means for balloon dilation angioplasty, thrombolytic therapy, or embolization.

▶ Complications and related nursing diagnoses

General	
Contrast reaction	Impaired skin integrity Decreased cardiac output Ineffective breathing pattern Impaired gas exchange Fluid volume deficit
Hematoma/hemorrhage at catheter insertion site	Altered tissue perfusion: peripheral Decreased cardiac output Fluid volume deficit
Arterial occlusion	Altered tissue perfusion: peripheral, cerebral, renal, gastrointestinal, cardiopulmonary
Renal failure	Altered pattern in urinary elimination Fluid volume excess
Osmotic diuresis	Altered pattern in urinary elimination Fluid volume deficit
Organ specific	
Brain—cerebral embolism	Altered tissue perfusion: cerebral
Cardiac—myocardial ischemia	Pain Decreased cardiac output

Cardiopulmonary—dysrhythmias	Decreased cardiac output
Myocardial perforation/tamponade	Decreased cardiac output

Special Patient Management
Pretest
1. Obtain baseline vital signs (VS) and rhythm strip.
2. Assess the quality of pulses and mark pulse sites.
3. Check for allergies to iodine and seafood.
4. Check for previous history of contrast reaction.
5. Check laboratory results for BUN and creatinine (renal function); and PT, PTT, platelets (coagulation).
6. Assess hydration status and ensure that the patient is well hydrated for angiography.
7. GI angiography may require bowel preparation.

Posttest
PATIENT OUTCOMES
1. HR 60-100
2. SBP 90 to 140 mm Hg
3. Eupnea; RR 12-20
4. Hemostasis at catheterization insertion site
5. Peripheral pulses unchanged
6. Affected extremity warm
7. Urine output $\geq$ 25 to 30 ml/hr
8. Absence of systemic or pulmonary vascular engorgement
9. Alert and oriented; neurological examination unchanged
10. Absence of hives, flushing, diaphoresis

INTERVENTIONS
1. Keep patient on bed rest for 6 to 12 hours (or as ordered).
2. Prevent flexion of affected extremity.
3. Encourage fluids (if not contraindicated).
4. Monitor hemodynamic status:
   VS q15" × 2-4h
   q30" × 2h
   q1h until stable
5. Check dressing with VS checks; if bleeding occurs, apply pressure to the site.
6. Assess tissue perfusion with VS checks:
   Peripheral: For arterial puncture, assess the quality of the pulse (use Doppler if unable to palpate pulse), skin

temperature, color, and sensation of the extremity. For venous puncture, assess for swelling, redness, pain, or any increase in skin temperature.

Cerebral: Assess the level of consciousness, motor strength and sensation, and speech.

Renal: Assess urine output hourly (profound diuresis, secondary to contrast medium, and electrolyte disturbances may occur). If dialysis access was studied, assess for thrill and bruit with VS checks.

7. Apply ice to the puncture site prn for pain and hematoma.

8. Observe for delayed hypersensitivity reaction: decreased BP, increased HR, flushing, diaphoresis, hives, decreased urine output.

CONSULT WITH PHYSICIAN

- Vascular insufficiency: cold, pale, mottled extremity, absent or diminished pulse, or sudden pain
- Allergic reaction: hives, flushing, diaphoresis, increased HR, and decreased BP
- Renal insufficiency: decreased u/o, increased BUN and Cr
- Hemorrhage: uncontrolled bleeding at puncture site
- Dysrhythmias compromising CO: syncope, irregular rhythm, decreased in BP
- Cerebral ischemia: change in neurological status or worsening neurological deficits

CARDIAC CATHETERIZATION OR PULMONARY ANGIOGRAPHY

- Cardiac tamponade: hypotension, tachycardia, pallor or cyanosis, JVD, decrease in pulse pressure, decrease in heart sounds, tachypnea
- Myocardial ischemia: severe chest discomfort, ST segment changes
- Heart failure: S_3, crackles, increased HR, decreased u/o

BARIUM ENEMA

Clinical Brief

A barium enema is used to examine the colon. Radiographic barium sulfate is instilled into the rectum and x-ray films are taken. Barium and air, which produce a more clear picture of the integrity of the bowel lining, can also be used. This test should only be performed after all GI bleeding has stopped. A barium enema is routinely scheduled before an upper GI series. Other diagnostic tests such as ultrasonography or CT scans must be performed before any barium study. Abnormal findings will suggest areas of probable bleeding or tumors. A barium enema should not be performed if there is a possibility that a bowel perforation or obstruction exists.

▶ **Complications and related nursing diagnoses**

Retained barium	Constipation
Perforated bowel	Pain
	High risk for infection

Special Patient Management
Pretest
1. Ensure hydration.
2. Check to see that patient has received and responded to the bowel prep, and if ordered, has remained NPO since midnight.
3. Validate narcotic withholding, since narcotics may interfere with intestinal motility.
4. Validate routine medication administration of the patient when NPO.

Posttest
PATIENT OUTCOME
1. Barium will be evacuated.

INTERVENTIONS
1. Administer laxatives after the test and assess bowel evacuation; barium should pass in 24 to 72 hours following the test.
2. Encourage fluids if not contraindicated.

CONSULT WITH PHYSICIAN
- Bowel perforation: abdominal pain, rigid abdomen, hypoactive bowel sounds
- Constipation: absence of stools, palpable mass in abdomen, hypoactive bowel sounds

BARIUM SWALLOW
Clinical Brief
A barium swallow is used to examine the mucous membranes of the esophagus, stomach, and small intestines. Barium is ingested and serial x-ray films are taken that may reveal areas of ulcerations, hiatal hernia, varices, strictures, tumors, or motility abnormalities. This test is contraindicated if the patient has an intestinal obstruction or is actively bleeding.

▶ **Complications and related nursing diagnoses**

Retained barium	Constipation

Special Patient Management
Pretest
1. Validate withholding anticholinergic agents and narcotics, since these agents affect motility.
2. Check to see that the patient has received and responded to bowel prep, and if ordered, has remained NPO.
3. Validate routine medication administration if the patient is NPO.

Posttest
PATIENT OUTCOME
1. Barium will be evacuated.

INTERVENTIONS
1. Administer laxatives after the test and assess bowel evacuation; barium should pass in 24 to 72 hours following the test.
2. Encourage fluids if not contraindicated.

CONSULT WITH PHYSICIAN
- Bowel perforation: abdominal pain, rigid abdomen, hypoactive bowel sounds
- Constipation: absence of stools, palpable mass in abdomen, hypoactive bowel sounds

BIOPSY

Clinical Brief
A biopsy involves the percutaneous or surgical insertion of a needle, under the guide of ultrasound, fluoroscopy, or CT scan, to obtain tissue for analysis. *Bone* biopsies are used to evaluate developmental stages of blood cells and diagnose leukemias and anemias. *Liver* biopsies are used to diagnose parenchymal disorders of the liver. *Renal* biopsies are used to diagnose or stage various renal disorders and to assess transplant functioning.

▶ Complications and related nursing diagnoses

Hemorrhage   Decreased cardiac output
                                   Altered tissue perfusion

Special Patient Management
Pretest
1. Check to see that the results of the patient's clotting studies are normal and that hemoglobin and hematocrit levels are stable.
2. Obtain baseline vital signs.

Posttest

PATIENT OUTCOMES
1. Hemostasis at insertion site
2. Alert and oriented
3. SBP 90-140 mm Hg
4. HR 60-100

INTERVENTIONS
1. Apply a pressure dressing to the biopsy site.
2. If bleeding occurs, apply pressure to the puncture site.
3. Monitor hemodynamic status: VS q15″ × 2-4h; check dressing q15″ × 2-4h.
4. Keep the patient on bed rest. Renal biopsy—keep the patient lying supine for 24 hours (or as ordered); liver biopsy—keep the patient lying on the right side for 4 hours after the biopsy (or as ordered).
5. Monitor u/o after renal biopsy; urine should clear within 8 hours after biopsy.

CONSULT WITH PHYSICIAN
• Hemorrhage: uncontrolled bleeding at puncture site
• Abdominal and flank hematoma or pain
• Gross hematuria
• Decreasing BP or increasing HR

CHEST RADIOGRAPH

Clinical Brief

A chest radiograph is used to provide information about gross anatomical proportions and the location of cardiac structures, including the great vessels; to evaluate lung fields; and to confirm placement of airways, central venous catheters, pulmonary artery catheters, chest tubes, and transvenous pacemaker leads.

The least dense (air-filled) structures, e.g., lungs, absorb fewer x-rays and appear black on the radiographic film. Structures that are as dense as water, e.g., heart and blood vessels, appear gray. Bone and contrast material are most dense and appear white on the radiograph.

Figure 2-1 depicts a normal chest radiograph with underlying structures outlined; Figures 2-2, 2-3, and 2-4 identify conditions commonly evaluated in ICU patients. Normal findings are identified in Table 2-1.

Serial assessments of endotracheal tube, central lines, and chest tube placement should be done. An endotracheal tube

Text continued on p. 47.

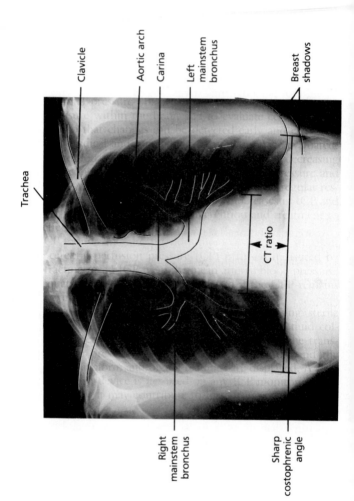

Respiratory Assessment

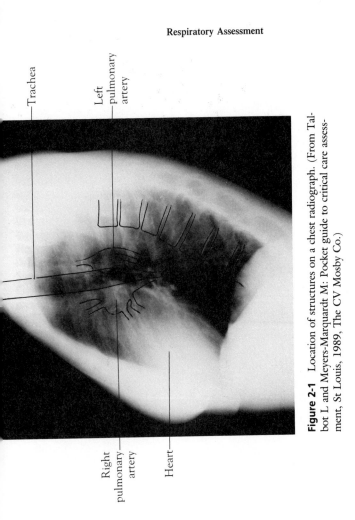

Figure 2-1 Location of structures on a chest radiograph. (From Talbot L and Meyers-Marquardt M: Pocket guide to critical care assessment, St Louis, 1989, The CV Mosby Co.)

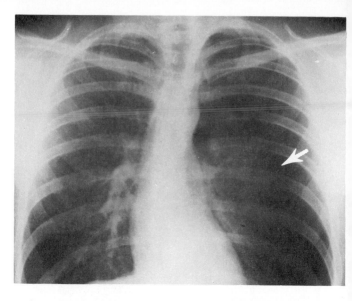

Figure 2-2 Radiograph of a spontaneous pneumothorax. (From Sahn SA: Pneumothorax and pneumomediastinum. In Mitchell RS and Petty TL (editors): Synopsis of clinical pulmonary disease, ed 4, St Louis, 1989, The CV Mosby Co.)

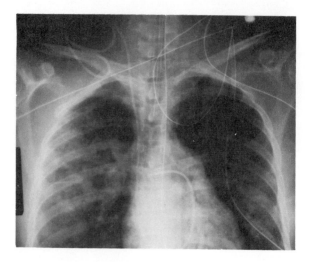

Figure 2-3 Radiograph of patient admitted with acute respiratory distress syndrome. (From Petty TL: Adult respiratory distress syndrome. In Mitchell RS and Petty TL (editors): Synopsis of clinical pulmonary disease, ed 4, St Louis, 1989, The CV Mosby Co.)

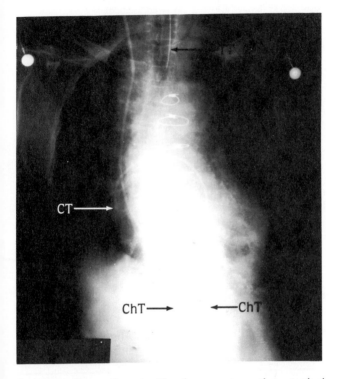

Figure 2-4 Chest radiograph with pulmonary artery catheter, tracheal tube, and chest tube. Pulmonary artery catheter (Swan-Ganz catheter) in its usual position in the right lower lung field. This view does not indicate whether catheter is anterior or posterior within the chest. Catheter tip *(CT)*; tracheal tube *(TT)*; chest tube *(ChT)*. (From Sheldon RL: Clinical application of the chest radiograph. In Wilkins RL, Sheldon RL and Krider SJ (editors): Clinical assessment in respiratory care, St Louis, 1990, The CV Mosby Co.)

TABLE 2-1 Normal Findings on Chest Radiograph

Assessed area	Usual adult findings
Trachea	Midline, translucent, tubelike structure found in the anterior mediastinal cavity
Clavicles	Equally distant from the sternum
Ribs	Thoracic cavity encasement
Mediastinum	Shadowy-appearing space between the lungs that widens at the hilum
Heart	Solid-appearing structure with clear edges visible in the left anterior mediastinal cavity; cardiothoracic ratio should be less than half the width of the chest wall on a PA film; cardiac shadow appears larger in an AP film
Carina	Lowest tracheal cartilage at the bifurcation
Mainstem bronchus	Translucent, tubelike structure visible approximately 2.5 cm from the hilum
Hilum	Small, white, bilateral densities present where the bronchi join the lungs; left should be 2 to 3 cm higher than the right
Bronchi	Not usually visible
Lung fields	Usually not completely visible except for "lung markings" at periphery
Diaphragm	Rounded structures visible at the bottom of the lung fields; right side is 1 to 2 cm higher than the left; costophrenic angles should be clear and sharp

Adapted from Talbot L and Meyers-Marquardt M: Pocket guide to critical care assessment, St Louis, 1990, The CV Mosby Co.

TABLE 2-2 Abnormal Radiographic Findings

Finding	Possible diagnosis
Nondistinct or widened aortic knob	Aortic dissection
Silhouette sign (loss of border visibility)	Infiltrates or consolidation of RML or lingula
Enlarged cardiac silhouette	CHF, pericardial effusion, pulmonary edema
Blackened area without tissue markings	Pneumothorax
Patchy infiltrates or streaky densities	Pneumonia, atelectasis
Fluffy infiltrates (Kerley B lines)	Pulmonary edema
Loss of costophrenic angle sharpness	Pleural effusion

should be 2 to 3 cm above the carina. Table 2-2 lists abnormal radiographic findings common to ICU patients.

Complications and related nursing diagnoses
None

Special Patient Management
None

COMPUTED TOMOGRAPHY (CT) OR COMPUTED AXIAL TOMOGRAPHY (CAT)

Clinical Brief

CT or CAT scans are used to obtain rapid and more definitive visualization of body structures than radiographs provide. X-ray beams are passed through substances of varying densities and a computer makes calculations to provide cross-sectional images of the specific body part being studied. A contrast medium, which enhances vascular areas, may or may not be used. White-appearing images reflect more dense substances such as bone; black-appearing images reflect less dense substances such as air or CSF. Soft tissue appears as shades of gray.

Complications and related nursing diagnoses   (contrast CT)

Reaction to contrast	Impaired skin integrity
	Ineffective breathing pattern
	Decreased cardiac output
	Altered pattern in urinary elimination

Special Patient Management

Pretest
1. Check for allergy to iodine or seafood.
2. Verify NPO status and need for bowel prep.

Posttest

PATIENT OUTCOME
1. Absence of contrast reaction: hives, rash, pruritis, wheeze, laryngospasm, hypotension, oliguria or change in level of consciousness

INTERVENTIONS
1. Obtain VS.
2. Encourage fluids if not contraindicated.
3. Monitor for reaction to contrast.

CONSULT WITH PHYSICIAN
• Delayed contrast reaction: hives, rash, pruritis, wheeze,

laryngospasm, hypotension, oliguria, and change in level of consciousness
- Renal failure: decreased u/o, increased BUN and creatinine

TWELVE-LEAD ELECTROCARDIOGRAPHY
Clinical Brief
Twelve-lead ECG is used as a diagnostic tool in determining overall electrical functioning of the heart and can aid in targeting pathological conditions. Normal and abnormal activity, as evidenced by examining individual waves, deflections, intervals, and segments can be evaluated.
Twelve leads
The 12 leads are either bipolar or unipolar. The precordial leads (V_1 to V_6) are unipolar and provide information about anterior, posterior, right and left electrical forces. The bipolar limb leads (I, II, III) consist of a + and − electrode and compose Einthoven's triangle. Leads aV_R, aV_L, and aV_F are unipolar limb leads representing augmented vector right, left, and foot. The limb leads provide information about vertical electrical forces as well as left and right forces.
Deflections
Deflections signify individual cardiac cycle events and their electrical direction in relation to a positive electrode. When the electrical current moves in the general direction of a positive electrode, an upward or positive deflection is recorded. Conversely, a downward or negative deflection signifies movement away from the positive electrode. Major deflections are referred to as the P, Q, R, S, T, and U waves.
Waves, intervals, and segments
See Table 2-3 for components of a normal ECG.
Electrical axis
An imaginary line drawn between two electrodes is called the axis of the lead. A vector signifies a quantity of electrical force that has both a given magnitude and direction. When the cardiac vector is parallel to the axis of the lead recording it, the ECG deflection is either the most upright or the most negative (Figure 2-5). When the direction of the electrical activity is perpendicular to the axis of the lead recording it, an equiphasic deflection will be recorded.
Hexaxial reference system
The mean vector, or axis of the heart, can be measured in degrees using the hexaxial reference system. A normal QRS

TABLE 2-3 Components of Normal ECG

Component	Criteria	Comment
Rhythm	Atrial and ventricular are same; R-R and P-P intervals vary less than 0.16 sec	
Rate	Atrial and ventricular rates are equal; 60-100 cycles/min	
P wave	Present; only one P for each QRS	
Direction	Upright in I, II, aV$_F$, and V$_4$ to V$_6$; inverted in aV$_R$; biphasic, flat or inverted in III, V$_1$, and V$_2$	Upright and notched in I, II, V$_4$ to V$_6$ suggests left atrial abnormality
Shape	Rounded, symmetrical, without notches, peaks	
Amplitude	<3.0 mm	
Width	1.5 to 2.5 mm (0.06-0.10 sec)	Tall and peaked in II, III, aV$_F$ suggests lung disease
Axis	0 to +90 degrees	
PR interval	0.12 to 0.20 sec	>0.20 = AVB
QRS interval	0.06 to 0.10 sec	>0.12 = BBB V$_1$, V$_2$ are best to measure QRS
QT interval	< Half the preceding R-R interval in normal rates $Q\text{-}Tc = \dfrac{Q\text{-}t \text{ (measured)}}{\sqrt{R\text{-}R \text{ interval(s)}}}$ Normal = 0.30 – 0.40 sec	Prolonged QT interval is associated with torsade de pointes

Kinney M, Packa D, and Dunbar S: AACN's clinical reference for critical-care nursing, New York, 1988, McGraw Hill Book Co.
Continued.

TABLE 2-3 Components of Normal ECG—cont'd

Component	Criteria	Comment
QRS complex Configuration	Follows each P	Upper- and lower-case letters indicate the relative sizes of the QRS components
	qRs Rs qR rSR' QS	
ST segment	Isoelectric, but may be elevated <1 mm in limb leads and <2 mm in some precordial leads Not depressed more than 0.05 mm Curves gently into proximal limb of T wave	Elevation associated with vasospasm or acute injury; depression suggests ischemia
T wave Direction	Upright in I, II, and V_3 to V_6; inverted in aV_R; and varies in III, aV_L, aV_F, V_1 and V_6	Tall T wave is associated with hyperkalemia, ischemia
Shape	Slightly rounded and asymmetrical	
Height	<5 mm in limb leads; <10 mm in precordial leads	
Axis	Left and inferior	

Q wave	Width: <0.039 sec	Significant if 0.04 sec
	Depth: 1-2 mm in I, aV_L, aV_F, V_5, and V_6; deep QS or Qr in aV_R and possibly in III, V_1, and V_2	
Amplitude	>5 mm and <25 mm in limb leads; 5 to 30 mm in V_1 and V_6; 7 to 30 mm in V_2 and V_5; 9 to 30 mm in V_3 and V_4	
R progression	Progressive rise in R wave amplitude from V_1 to V_6	
Axis	−30 to +120 degrees	
Transition	V_3 or V_4	
Intrinsicoid deflection	<0.02 sec in V_1; <0.04 sec in V_6	Delayed in BBB and chamber enlargement
U wave Direction	Upright	Increases in amplitude in hypokalemia
Amplitude	0.33 mm in precordial leads (average); 2.5 mm (maximum)	
Width	<0.24 sec	

Kinney M, Packa D, and Dunbar S: AACN's clinical reference for critical-care nursing, New York, 1988, McGraw Hill Book Co.

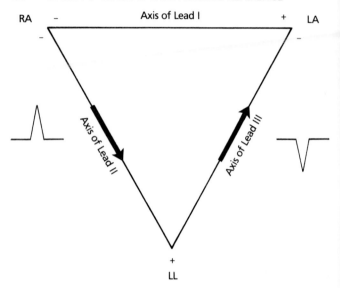

Figure 2-5 Axis. When a mean vector is parallel to the axis of a lead, the tallest (electrical current flowing toward the positive lead) or the deepest (electrical current flowing away from the positive lead) complex will result in that lead.

vector should lie between -30 and $+120$. Left axis deviation can be caused by left anterior hemiblock, left bundle branch block, left ventricular hypertrophy, obesity, or inferior myocardial infarction. Right axis deviation can be caused by left posterior hemiblock, right ventricular hypertrophy, limb lead reversal, dextrocardia, or lateral myocardial infarction.

Quick method to axis determination
See Figure 2-6.

ECG pattern associated with ischemia
Reduced blood supply is characterized by inverted T waves, transient ST depression during anginal episodes, and transient ST elevation during anginal episodes that are vasospastic (Figure 2-7).

ECG pattern associated with injury
Acuteness of an infarction is represented by ST segment elevation. ST segment elevation without Q wave may indicate

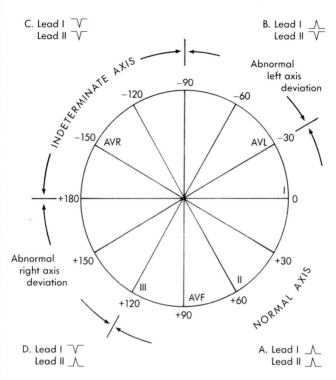

C. Lead I ⊽
Lead II ⊽

B. Lead I ⋏
Lead II ⊽

Abnormal
left axis
deviation

INDETERMINATE AXIS

−90
−120   −60
−150   AVR   AVL   −30
+180   I   0
+150   +30
AVF
III   +120   +90   +60   II
NORMAL AXIS

Abnormal
right axis
deviation

D. Lead I ⊽
Lead II ⋏

A. Lead I ⋏
Lead II ⋏

Figure 2-6 Estimating axis using leads I and II. **A,** If the QRS is upright in both I and II, the axis is normal. **B,** If the QRS is upright in I and down in II, left axis deviation is present. **C,** If the QRS is down in both I and II, indeterminate axis is present. **D,** If the QRS is down in I and upright in II, right axis deviation is present.

Ischemia
Symmetrically
inverted T waves

Injury
ST elevation
(indicates acuteness)

Infarction
Diagnosed by large
Q wave—0.04 sec wide
or 1/3 size of QRS

Figure 2-7 Patterns of infarction, injury, and ischemia.

V_2-V_3

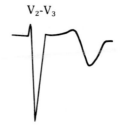

Figure 2-8 ECG changes associated with critical stenosis of the proximal LAD. (From Conover M: Pocket guide to electrocardiography, St Louis, 1990, The CV Mosby Co.)

non–Q wave infarction. Persistent ST segment depression can indicate non–Q wave infarction.

ECG pattern associated with Q wave infarction

Indicative changes, significant Q waves, ST elevation, and T wave inversion can be found in leads over infarcted myocardium:

- Anterior MI—leads V_1-V_4
- Lateral MI—leads I, aV$_L$, and V_5 and V_6
- Inferior MI—leads II, III, and aV$_F$
- Posterior MI—reciprocal changes in anterior leads(e.g., tall R wave, ST depression, and tall symmetrical T wave in V_1-V_4)

Right ventricular infarction is represented by lead V_{4R} and will exhibit ST elevation>1 mm.

Critical stenosis of proximal LAD

Signs associated with critical stenosis of the proximal LAD and impending infarction include unstable angina; little or no cardiac enzyme elevation; an ECG that demonstrates ST segment turning down into a deeply inverted and symmetrical T wave, no significant Q waves in precordial leads, and little or no ST elevation in V_2 and V_3 (Figure 2-8).

Differentiating bundle branch block

LBBB characteristics include a mainly downward QRS deflection in V_1; upright QRS deflection in V_6; and R wave and no Q or S wave in leads I, aV$_L$, and V_6. RBBB characteristics include an upright QRS in V_1; intrinsicoid deflection 0.07 sec or later in V_1; and small Q wave and broad S wave in leads I, aV$_L$, and V_6. See Figure 2-9 for quick identification of BBB.

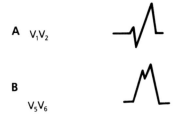

Figure 2-9   Right and left bundle branch block (BBB). **A,** Check right precordial leads (V_1, V_2) for RR′, suggesting RBBB. **B,** Check left precordial leads (V_5, V_6) for RR′, suggesting LBBB.

TABLE 2-4 Chamber Enlargement

Chamber	Changes
RA	Tall peaked P wave (>2.5 mm) in II, III, aVF; low or isoelectric P wave in I; P waves in V_1, V_2 may be upright with increased amplitude
LA	P wave duration >0.12 sec, P wave notched and upright in I, II, V_4-V_6; wide, deep, negative component to P wave in V_1
RV	Right axis deviation, R/S ratio >1 in V_1; ST segment depression and T wave inversion in V_1 or V_2
LV*	Increased voltage; R or S wave in limb leads >20 mm or S wave in V_1 or V_2 >30 mm or R wave in V_5 or V_6 >30 mm, 3 points
	ST changes; with digitalis, 1 point; without digitalis, 2 points
	LA enlargement, 3 points
	Left axis deviation, 2 points (−30 or more)
	QRS duration >0.09 sec, 1 point
	Intrinsicoid deflection in V_5 or V_6 >0.05 sec, 1 point

*4 points, LVH likely; 5 points, LVH present.

Chamber enlargement
Table 2-4 outlines changes on ECG indicative of chamber enlargement.

Ventricular ectopy versus aberrant ventricular conduction
Wide QRS complexes with bizarre morphology generally signify either a source of ventricular ectopy or an aberrancy.

Complexes are called premature ventricular complexes (PVCs) when they are a source of ventricular ectopy. If the complexes result from an aberrancy in ventricular conduction (AVC), they usually signify a block in one of the bundle branches.

Characteristics that can distinguish PVCs from AVC can be derived by examining the 12-lead ECG.

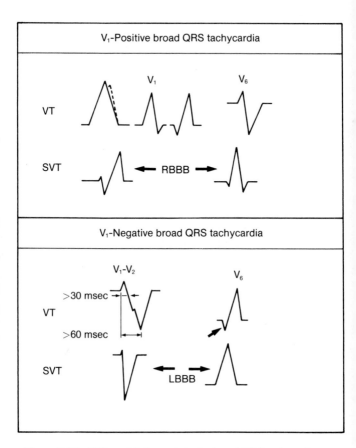

Figure 2-10 Differential diagnosis in the broad QRS tachycardia. (From Conover M: Pocket guide to electrocardiography, St Louis, 1990, The CV Mosby Co.)

In V₁-positive broad QRS tachycardia (Figure 2-10): Characteristics of QRS complex favoring aberrancy include an rsR′ configuration in V_1 and qRs in V_6. Characteristics of QRS favoring ectopy include monophasic or biphasic QRS complex in V_1; taller left rabbit ear in V_1; and R/S ratio in $V_6 < 1$ (deep S).

In V₁-negative broad QRS tachycardia: Characteristics of QRS complex favoring aberrancy include a swift, clean downstroke of the QRS complex; narrow r. Characteristics of QRS complex favoring ectopy include broad R wave (>0.03 sec); notched downslope of S wave; S nadir delay (>0.06 sec); and any Q wave in V_6. Other characteristics favoring aberrancy include QRS interval 0.12 to 0.14 sec; P waves (if identifiable) precede normal QRS complexes. Other characteristics favoring ectopy include a QRS interval >0.14 sec; P waves independent of QRS.

Systematic Approach to Twelve-Lead Electrocardiogram

Review all 12 leads to determine (1) underlying rhythm; (2) patterns of ischemia, injury, or infarction; (3) chamber enlargement; and (4) ventricular axis.

1. Determine rate.
2. Examine P-P and R-R intervals for regularity in rhythm.
3. Analyze P waves in each lead.
4. Measure PR, QRS, and QT intervals.
5. Analyze QRS complex.
6. Identify leads having significant Q waves.
7. Determine presence of R wave progression and identify lead associated with transition.
8. Measure intrinsicoid deflection.
9. Determine axis.
10. Identify leads displaying ST segment elevation or depression.
11. Analyze T wave for increased amplitude.
12. Identify presence of U wave.

ELECTROENCEPHALOGRAPHY

Clinical Brief

Electroencephalography is used to detect and/or localize abnormal electrical findings, which may be caused by hemorrhage, tumor, abcess, or infarction. EEG can also help identify seizure types and aid in the diagnosis of brain death.

Electrodes are placed over the scalp and connected to a main recording system that provides a printout of the electrical activity of the brain.

▶ Complications and related nursing diagnoses
None

Special Patient Management
Verify withholding anticonvulsants, stimulants, depressants, or tranquilizers, since these drugs can affect electrical activity of the brain.

ENDOSCOPY

Clinical Brief
Endoscopy is used to visualize an organ, structure, or system via a rigid or flexible scope. *Esophagogastroduodenoscopy,* or *panendoscopy,* refers to visualizing the esophagus, stomach, and duodenum. *Proctoscopy* and *sigmoidoscopy* refer to visualizing the rectum and sigmoid colon. *Colonoscopy* refers to visualizing the large intestine. *Endoscopic retrograde cholangiopancreatography (ERCP)* refers to a contrast procedure visualizing the pancreatic duct and hepatobiliary tree. *Bronchoscopy* refers to visualization of the trachea and bronchi.

Ulcers, sites of hemorrhage, or neoplasms can be confirmed with GI endoscopy. Pancreatic, gallbladder, and liver disorders such as stones, strictures, and tumors or growths can often be visualized with ERCP. Tumors, sites of hemorrhage and lesions can be visualized with bronchoscopy.

Endoscopy also allows a means to remove specimens or foreign bodies, cauterize or sclerose bleeding vessels, and obtain biopsies.

▶ Complications and related nursing diagnoses

General	
Perforation of the GI/ respiratory tract	Pain
	High risk for infection
	Decreased cardiac output
Postprocedural bleeding	Fluid volume deficit
Oversedation	High risk for injury
	Ineffective breathing pattern
	High risk for aspiration

Bronchoscopy, ERCP, panendoscopy	
Aspiration	High risk for infection
	Impaired gas exchange

Bronchoscopy

Laryngospasm/bronchospasm	Ineffective breathing pattern
	Impaired gas exchange

ERCP

Cholangitis	Altered body temperature
	Hyperthermia
	Pain

Special Patient Management
Pretest
1. Obtain baseline VS.
2. Check clotting studies.
3. If a proctoscopy, sigmoidoscopy, or colonoscopy is to be performed, check to see whether the patient has received and responded to bowel prep, if it was ordered.
4. Check to see that the patient has remained NPO.
Posttest
PATIENT OUTCOMES
1. Patient is pain free
2. SBP 90-140 mm Hg
3. HR 60-100
4. Absence of bleeding
5. Alert and oriented
6. Gag reflex present (following bronchoscopy, panendoscopy, ERCP)
7. Lungs clear when auscultated

INTERVENTIONS
1. Assess VS for fever, hemodynamic instability, and respiratory compromise.
2. Determine presence of gag reflex (after the appropriate test) and keep the patient NPO until the reflex returns.
3. Monitor for bleeding or perforation.

CONSULT WITH PHYSICIAN
- Perforation or bleeding: decreased BP, increased HR, pain, fever, abdominal tenderness, difficulty breathing
- Oversedation: inability to arouse, decreased respirations

GATED BLOOD POOL SCAN (MUGA)
Clinical Brief
A gated blood pool scan is similar to myocardial infarct imaging. Technetium-99m pyrophosphate is used to tag the red blood cells; however, the patient's ECG is synchronized

to the imaging equipment, and multiple images are obtained. Ventricular ejection fractions and regional wall motion abnormalities can be evaluated. The "first pass" technique analyzes the radiotracer as it first transits the right heart, lungs, and the left heart. The "gated" technique analyzes radiotracer volume within a given cardiac chamber over 200 to 300 cardiac cycles, estimating chamber performance. "Gated" scans are frequently obtained after first passes and can better estimate chamber volumes, left and right ventricular ejection fractions, and rates of ventricular filling. These scans can be performed with or without exercise "stress" testing. The normal left ventricular response to exercise is for the ejection fraction to increase by at least 5%. Failure to accomplish this and/or the development of one or more regional wall abnormalities may indicate significant coronary artery disease.

▶ **Complications and related nursing diagnoses**
See Special patient management.

Special Patient Management
If stress testing is performed, monitor VS and ECG as per protocol. MI, sustained V-tach, or cardiac arrest may occur during the stress test.

GI BLOOD LOSS SCAN
Clinical Brief
A GI blood loss scan is used to detect and localize the site of bleeding. Once the radioactive material is injected, imaging is begun. Delayed repeated imaging may be performed if the patient exhibits clinical signs of active bleeding and results of the initial scan were negative.

▶ **Complications and related nursing diagnoses**
None

Special Patient Management
Determine whether the patient has received barium in the last 24 hours, since barium may interfere with imaging and obscure the site of bleeding.

INTRACARDIAC ELECTROPHYSIOLOGICAL STUDY
Clinical Brief
An intracardiac electrophysiological study is used to diagnose and evaluate the conduction system of the heart. Percutaneous endocardial electrodes are placed via right-sided heart catheterization, and the heart is electrically stimulated

to evaluate recurrent lethal ventricular and supraventricular tachydysrhythmias. Pharmacological agents can be administered to evaluate their efficacy in controlling the dysrhythmia.

▶ Complications and related nursing diagnoses

Cardiac perforation	Decreased cardiac output
Thrombosis formation at catheter and arterial emboli	Altered tissue perfusion: peripheral, cerebral, renal, coronary
Hematoma/bleeding at catheter insertion site	Pain Altered tissue perfusion: peripheral Fluid volume deficit
Lethal dysrhythmia	Decreased cardiac output

Special Patient Management
Pretest
1. Obtain baseline VS and rhythm strip.
2. Verify withholding antidysrhythmic administration with physician.

Posttest
PATIENT OUTCOMES
1. Absence of life-threatening dysrhythmias
2. Alert and oriented
3. SBP 90-140 mm Hg
4. Hemostasis at catheter insertion site

INTERVENTIONS
1. Keep patient on bed rest for 6-12 hours as ordered.
2. Prevent flexion of affected extremity.
3. Monitor hemodynamic status:
   VS q15″ × 2-4h
   q30″ × 2h
   q1h until stable
4. Check dressing with VS checks; if bleeding occurs, apply pressure.
5. Assess tissue perfusion: level of consciousness, urinary output, peripheral pulses.
6. Check for thrombophlebitis of affected extremity: swelling, redness, pain, or any increase in skin temperature.

CONSULT WITH PHYSICIAN
- Dysrhythmias compromising CO: syncope, decreased BP
- Cardiac perforation: hypotension, tachycardia, pallor/cyanosis, JVD, decreased pulse pressure, diminished heart sounds, tachypnea

- Arterial emboli: chest pain, change in level of consciousness, dyspnea, diminished pulses
- Thrombophlebitis: swelling, redness, pain, increased skin temperature
- Bleed at site of catheter insertion: hematoma, swelling, pain, blood

INTRAVENOUS PYELOGRAM (IVP)
Clinical Brief
An intravenous pyelogram is used to assess the renal system structure and excretory function. Contrast medium is injected intravenously, followed by serial x-ray films; CT may also be done. Films can be taken after the patient voids to assess residual urine volume. A retrograde pyelogram involves cystoscopy to inject dye through catheters placed into the ureters.

▶ Complications and related nursing diagnoses

Contrast reaction	Impaired skin integrity
	Ineffective breathing pattern
	Decreased cardiac output
	Altered pattern in urinary elimination
Osmotic diuresis secondary to contrast medium	Fluid volume deficit
Infection from catheterization	High risk for infection

Special Patient Management
Pretest
1. Check for allergy to iodine or seafood.
2. Check to see that the patient has received and responded to bowel prep and, if it was ordered, has remained NPO for 4 to 6 hours before the procedure.
3. Check BUN; IVP is contraindicated if levels are >40 mg/dl.

Posttest
PATIENT OUTCOMES
1. SBP 90-140 mm Hg
2. Urine output >30 ml/hr
3. Absence of contrast reaction; hives, rash, pruritis, wheeze, hypotension, oliguria

INTERVENTIONS
1. Obtain VS and measure urine hourly.
2. Encourage fluids if not contraindicated.

3. Monitor for reaction to contrast.

CONSULT WITH PHYSICIAN

- Reaction to contrast medium: hives, rash, difficulty breathing, decreased BP
- Renal failure (new onset): decreased urine output, increasing BUN and creatinine
- Urinary tract infection: cloudy urine, pain with voiding, increased temperature

LIVER/SPLEEN SCAN

Clinical Brief

A liver/spleen scan is used to evaluate size, shape, and position of the liver, gallbladder, common bile duct, and spleen. Space-occupying lesions, metastatic disease, infarctions, and damage to organs can be determined. These studies are performed in conjunction with computed tomography to provide a three-dimensional view of the radioactive material distribution.

Complications and related nursing diagnoses

None

Special Patient Management

Determine whether the patient has received barium within the last 24 hours, since barium may interfere with imaging.

MAGNETIC RESONANCE IMAGING (MRI)

Clinical Brief

MRI is a noninvasive technique used to obtain biochemical information from body tissues and produce tomographic images without the use of ionizing radiation. The hydrogen atom is the proton studied. Hydrogen reflects water content of tissue; thus the varying densities of hydrogen atoms and their interactions with other tissues can be evaluated and distinctions between tissues can be made. Images are generated as hydrogen atoms change alignment of their nuclei when exposed to radiowaves and are generally displayed in one of three planes: axial, sagittal, or coronal. MRI is most beneficial in evaluating body structures that have little or no motion; it is superior to radiographs and ultrasonography because distortion from surrounding bone is nonexistent. A hazard does exist if some types of metal are present in the environment, necessitating careful screening of patients.

Brain

MRI visualizes cerebral lesions such as brain abscesses, brainstem tumors, and small hemorrhages not evident on

CT scans, identifies areas of infarction within a few hours of the incident, and localizes lesions in white matter.

Cardiac

In cardiac evaluation, MRI has had limited usefulness thus far.

Renal

MRI can be used to identify renal structures and differentiate such abnormalities as cyst contents, tumor stages, and the status of renal transplants.

▶ **Complications and related nursing diagnoses**

None

Special Patient Management

Screen the patient for metallic implants such as a pacemaker, an implantable defibrillator, prosthetic heart valves, neurostimulators, aneurysm clips, cochlear implants, or an insulin pump. Hip implants, dental fillings and braces, sternal wire sutures, and intrauterine devices are not dangerous for the study.

MYELOGRAPHY

Clinical Brief

Myelography is used to visualize the spinal canal and nerve roots. A contrast material is injected through a lumbar or cisternal puncture, and areas in question are visualized on radiographs or by CT scanning. Lesions that block subarachnoid space, e.g., intervertebral discs, tumors, or anomalies can be identified.

▶ **Complications and related nursing diagnoses**

Contrast reaction	Impaired skin integrity
	Ineffective breathing pattern
	Decreased cardiac output
	Altered pattern in urinary elimination
Headache	Pain
Seizures	High risk for injury

Special Patient Management

Pretest

1. Obtain baseline VS and neurological assessment.
2. Verify the type of contrast material to be used; patients who are receiving water-soluble contrast should be well hydrated.

Posttest

PATIENT OUTCOMES

1. SBP 90-100 mm Hg
2. Neurological assessment appropriate for patient
3. Absence of seizures and headache

INTERVENTIONS

1. Obtain VS every 30″ for 2 hr, every 60″ for 2 hr, then every 4 hr for 24 hr.
2. If a water-soluble contrast is used, maintain patient upright at 30 to 45-degree angle for first 12 hr, then bed rest either upright or flat for 12 hr. Increase fluids if not contraindicated. Avoid phenothiazines for nausea and vomiting, since these agents can increase symptoms of toxicity.
3. If an oil-based contrast is used, keep the patient flat for 4-6 hr.

CONSULT WITH PHYSICIAN

- Nausea/vomiting
- Severe headache, change in level of consciousness, or seizure activity

MYOCARDIAL PERFUSION IMAGING

Clinical Brief

Myocardial perfusion imaging is used to identify areas of stress-induced ischemia or old infarction. Myocardial uptake of thallium-201, which concentrates in normal tissue (not ischemic or infarcted tissue), is analyzed after intravenous injection. Normal myocardial imaging should result in a homogeneous appearance of all structures. Ischemic or scarred areas would have a lessened uptake of thallium-201, resulting in a "cold" appearance, rather than an enhanced uptake or "hot" appearance of healthy tissue. If exercise stress testing is performed with this technique, a 4-hour postinjectate image is typically obtained to ascertain whether "cold" areas begin to appear "hot," which could indicate transient ischemia rather than infarction.

Myocardial perfusion imaging with exercise "stress" testing is more sensitive and specific than exercise "stress" testing alone and can be useful in detecting ischemia in patients with exercise-induced ECGs that are difficult to interpret.

▶ Complications and related nursing diagnoses
See Special patient management.

Special Patient Management

If stress testing is performed, monitor VS and ECG as per protocol. MI, sustained V-tach, or cardiac arrest may occur during stress test.

MYOCARDIAL INFARCT IMAGING

Clinical Brief

Myocardial infarct imaging is useful when it is suspected that the patient has had an MI several days before a diagnostic workup was begun or when cardiac enzymes cannot be obtained. It is sensitive in visualizing Q wave infarcts but less sensitive in visualizing non–Q wave infarcts. Myocardial uptake of technetium-99m pyrophosphate, which binds with the calcium within damaged myocardial cells, is analyzed after intravenous injection. Necrotic areas are visualized as "hot"; healthy areas appear "cold." Cardioversion or chest wall trauma may result in false-positive uptake.

▶ **Complications and related nursing diagnoses**

See Special patient management

Special Patient Management

If stress testing is performed, monitor VS and ECG as per protocol. MI, sustained V-tach, or cardiac arrest may occur during the stress test.

PULMONARY FUNCTION TESTS

Clinical Brief

Spirometry is used to measure lung volumes, capacities, and flow rates to quantify the performance of the respiratory system. Spirometry can be performed at the bedside or in the pulmonary function laboratory. More sophisticated tests, such as body plethysmography and gas dilution techniques, require testing in the pulmonary function laboratory; these tests measure lung volumes and diffusion capacities.

Pulmonary function tests can be used to predict the need for mechanical ventilation and the likelihood of success at weaning a critically ill patient from mechanical ventilation. A commonly measured lung volume is the vital capacity (VC), which correlates with the patient's ability to deep breathe and cough. A vital capacity of >15 ml/kg is generally needed for spontaneous breathing. Another useful test to predict successful weaning is the negative inspiratory force (NIF). A negative inspiratory force of at least -20 cm H_2O is necessary to maintain spontaneous ventilation.

Other measurements that provide an assessment of lung function in the mechanically ventilated patient include maximal voluntary ventilation (MVV), which is reflective of muscle strength, lung mechanics, and patient effort; the V_D/V_T ratio, which represents wasted ventilation; and compliance, or the stiffness of the lungs and chest wall, which is often decreased in the presence of air flow obstruction, increased lung stiffness, or limited chest wall mobility. A discussion of the mechanically ventilated patient can be found in Chapter 6. Pulmonary function tests are also used to differentiate obstructive from restrictive lung disorders and to assess patient response to therapy (e.g., before and after use of a bronchodilator). Restrictive lung disorders have little or no effect on air flow; however, lung volumes and capacities are decreased. Restrictive defects are commonly caused by chest wall deformity, e.g., scoliosis, and neuromuscular weakness. Patients with obstructive lung disorders, which affect the patient's ability to exhale, have decreased flow rates with normal or decreased lung volumes and capacities. The most common obstructive diseases leading to respiratory failure are emphysema and chronic bronchitis.

Pulmonary function tests can also be used to assess high-risk patients undergoing thoracic or abdominal surgery. Patients who smoke or experience pulmonary symptoms or who will undergo thoracic or abdominal surgery are at a high risk for developing postoperative pulmonary complications, such as atelectasis, pneumonia, and prolonged ventilation. Assessing lung function in these patients is helpful to identify patients who will benefit from intense respiratory care. A patient with an FEV_1 less than 2 L has little respiratory reserve and if not supported meticulously postoperatively is at risk for developing respiratory failure. Table 2-5 lists pulmonary function assessment parameters.

Complications and related nursing diagnoses
See Special patient management.

Special Patient Management
Monitor for development of bronchospasm.

RENAL SCAN
Clinical Brief
A renal scan is used to assess perfusion to and functioning of the kidneys; it is especially helpful to differentiate acute tubular necrosis (ATN) from rejection in transplanted kidneys.

TABLE 2-5 Pulmonary Function Assessment Parameters

Parameter	Description
Tidal volume (V_T)	Volume of gas inspired or expired with each quiet breath; normally ~ 500 ml
Inspiratory reserve volume (IRV)	Additional volume of gas that can be inspired after a normal tidal volume inspiration; normally ~ 3000 ml
Inspiratory capacity (IC)	Maximum volume of gas inspired after a normal exhalation; includes V_T + IRV; normally ~ 3500 ml
Expiratory reserve volume (ERV)	Additional volume of gas that can be forcefully exhaled after a normal expiration; normally ~ 1000 ml
Vital capacity (VC)	Maximum volume of gas exhaled after a maximal inspiration; includes V_T + IRV + ERV; normally ~ 4500 ml
Residual volume (RV)	Volume of gas remaining in the lungs after a maximal expiration; normally ~ 1500 ml
Functional residual capacity (FRC)	Volume of gas remaining in the lungs after a normal expiration; includes RV + ERV; normally ~ 2500 ml
Total lung capacity (TLC)	Sum of all of the lung volumes, which includes IRV + V_T + ERV + RV; normally ~ 6000 ml

Forced vital capacity (FVC)
Maximum volume of gas forcibly and rapidly exhaled after a forceful inspiration; normally ~ 4500 ml

Forced expiratory volume (FEV)
FEV$_1$
Amount of FVC that has been exhaled at a timed measurement
Amount of gas exhaled in the first second during maximal exhalation; most commonly used test to measure obstruction; also expressed as a ratio: FEV$_1$/FVC; a ratio <75% indicates airway obstruction

FEF $_{25\%-75\%}$
The forced expiratory flow between 25% and 75% vital capacity; reflects small airways function

Maximal voluntary ventilation (MVV)
Volume of gas exhaled during a specified time (usually 1 min) while performing repetitive maximal efforts; normally ~ 50-250 L/min

Minute ventilation ($\dot{V}_E$)
Volume of gas inhaled and exhaled during quiet breathing per minute: (V_T) × respiratory rate per minute; normally ~ 6-7 L/min

Deadspace (V_D)
Volume of gas that never reaches the alveoli; normally ~ 1 ml/lb

Deadspace to tidal volume ratio (V_D/V_T)
Amount of V_T used to ventilate areas of the lung that do not participate in gas exchange; normally ~ <0.4

Compliance (Δ Volume/Δ Pressure)
Increase in volume for a given pressure change; normally ~ 50-100 ml/cm H_2O

Negative inspiratory force (NIF)
Pressure the respiratory muscles must generate to maintain spontaneous ventilation; normally ~ −20 cm H_2O or greater.

▶ Complications and related nursing diagnoses
None
Special Patient Management
Check that the patient is adequately hydrated prior to test.

SKULL AND SPINE RADIOGRAPHS
Clinical Brief
X-ray films of the skull are used to evaluate the head-injured patient for skull fractures and detect air-fluid levels in the skull or sinus, which may indicate a possible CSF leak. Spine radiographs are helpful to evaluate trauma patients for any fractures/subluxation of the cervical, thoracic, and lumbar regions.
▶ Complications and related nursing diagnoses
See Special patient management.
Special Patient Management
Patients should be maintained in a neutral position. Prevent any movement that could result in further neurological deterioration until the initial spine films have been read.

ULTRASONOGRAPHY
Clinical Brief
Ultrasonography is a noninvasive procedure in which high-frequency sound waves are reflected off tissue to produce images of internal organs. Structure and function of organs can be visualized and evaluated.
Echocardiogram
An echocardiogram is used to assess left ventricular function, cardiac motion wall abnormalities, and valvular function. Currently three methods can be used. (1) M-mode echocardiography involves a single beam to sweep across cardiac structures. Valvular mobility, chamber size, pericardial effusions, and septal size can be evaluated. (2) Two-dimensional (cross-sectional) echocardiography involves an ultrasonic beam that oscillates across viewed cardiac structures. Valvular vegetations, septal defects, wall motion, chamber size, the presence of a pericardial effusion, valve motion, and wall thickness can be evaluated. (3) Doppler echocardiography analyzes blood flow velocity and turbulence. Cross-valvular pressure gradients, blood flow patterns, and specific valve orifices can be evaluated.
Gastrointestinal ultrasonogram
A GI ultrasonogram is useful for confirming gallbladder, pancreas, or liver diseases; differentiating obstructive versus

nonobstructive jaundice; localizing tumors and hematomas; and guiding biopsies and drainage of abcesses. A gaseous filled bowel or a dehydrated state may render this test inconclusive.

Renal ultrasonogram

Renal ultrasonography is used to identify and locate renal structures and abnormalities such as ureteral leaks, abscesses, and obstructions; to differentiate cysts from solid masses (tumors); and to guide biopsies, aspiration, and drain insertion.

Transcranial Doppler flow study

Doppler flow studies are used to assess velocity of cerebral blood flow and the degree of stenosis, occlusion, collateral blood flow, and vasospasm of the internal carotid, anterior cerebral, middle cerebral, posterior cerebral, and occasionally the basilar arteries. Flow rates are increased in cases of vasospasm or vessel disease because the vessel lumen is narrowed.

Normal velocity rates are as follows:

ICA 40-60 cm/sec
ACA 20-40 cm/sec
MCA 60-80 cm/sec
PCA 20-40 cm/sec

► Complications and related nursing diagnoses
None

Special Patient Management
Patients should be adequately hydrated before GI and renal ultrasonograms are performed.

VENTILATION-PERFUSION SCAN (V/Q SCAN)

Clinical Brief
A ventilation-perfusion scan is used to diagnose pulmonary emboli. After a radioactive material is injected intravenously, pulmonary vascular supply and air flow movement in the lungs are evaluated. The V/Q scan is compared with the chest radiograph. A high probability of pulmonary emboli is present if the V/Q scan has a perfusion defect larger than the radiograph or multiple segmental or lobar mismatch defects.

► Complications and related nursing diagnoses
None

Special Patient Management
None

XENON CEREBRAL BLOOD FLOW
Clinical Brief
This study is used to estimate cerebral blood flow. Xenon-133 is inhaled and brain tissue is monitored for isotope clearance. Probes that are externally positioned around the head provide information to a computer, which calculates blood flow. Conditions of increased or decreased blood flow are evaluated, e.g., injured brain, vasospasm, or during and after neurosurgery. Normal cerebral blood flow is 50-75 ml/100 g/min.

▶ Complications and related nursing diagnoses
None
Special Patient Management
None

REFERENCES
1. Barrow DL: Cerebral AVMs, Neurosurg Consultations 4:1, 1990.
2. Beare PG, Rahr VA and Ronshausen CA: Nursing implications of diagnostic tests, ed 2, Philadelphia, 1985, JB Lippincott Co.
3. Conover MB: Pocket guide to electrocardiography, ed 2, St Louis, 1990, The CV Mosby Co.
4. Conover MB: Understanding electrocardiography, ed 5, St Louis, 1988, The CV Mosby Co.
5. Elkin M: Radiology of the urinary system, Boston, 1980, Little, Brown & Co.
6. Fischbach F: A manual of laboratory diagnostic tests, Philadelphia, 1988, JB Lippincott Co.
7. Karnes N: Differentiation of aberrant ventricular conduction from ventricular ectopic beats, Crit Care Nurse 7(4):56, 1987.
8. Makow LS: Magnetic resonance imaging: a brief review of image contrast. In Sonn PM and Shapiro MD (editors): The radiologic clinics of North America 195:(2)27, 1989.

9. McConnell EA and Zimmerman MF: Care of patients with urologic problems, Philadelphia, 1983, JB Lippincott Co.
10. Moon KL and Hricak H: NMR imaging of the urinary tract, Applied Radiology 13:21, 1984.
11. Newman F, Ogburn-Russell L and Rutledge, JN: Magnetic resonance imaging: the latest in diagnostic technology, Nursing 87(1):44, 1987.
12. Petty TL: Adult respiratory distress syndrome. In Mitchell RS, Petty TL and Schwarz MI (editors): Synopsis of clinical pulmonary disease, ed 4, St Louis, 1989, The CV Mosby Co.
13. Ramsey RG: Neuroradiology, ed 2, 1987, WB Saunders Co.
14. Rau J and Pearce D: Understanding chest radiographs, Denver, 1984, Multi-Media Publishing, Inc.
15. Ruppel G: Manual of pulmonary function testing, ed 4, St Louis, 1986, The CV Mosby Co.
16. Sahn SA: Pneumothorax and pneumomediastinum. In Mitchell RS, Petty TL and Schwarz MI (editors): Synopsis of clinical pulmonary disease, ed 4, St Louis, 1989, The CV Mosby Co.
17. Samuels BI and Blane CE: The expanding role of renal ultrasonography, Applied Radiology 16:74, 1987.
18. Sheldon Rl: Clinical application of the chest radiograph. In Wilkins RL, Sheldon RL and Krider SJ (editors): Clinical assessment in respiratory care, St. Louis, 1990, The CV Mosby Co.
19. Talbot L and Meyers-Marquardt M: Pocket guide to critical care assessment, St Louis, 1989, The CV Mosby Co.
20. Thelan L, Davie J and Urden L: Textbook of critical care nursing, diagnosis and management, St Louis, 1990, The CV Mosby Co.
21. Tilkian S, Conover M and Tilkian A: Clinical implications of laboratory tests, ed 4, St Louis, 1987, The CV Mosby Co.
22. Unkle DW et al: Interpretation of the cervical spine x-ray: a simplified approach, Crit Care Nurse 48(8):10, 1990.
23. Willis D and Harbit MD: Transcatheter arterial embolization of cerebral arteriovenous malformations, J Neuroscience Nurs 280(5):22, 1990.

Monitoring the Critically Ill Patient

INTRACRANIAL PRESSURE MONITORING

Clinical Brief

Intracranial pressure (ICP) monitoring is used to measure the pressure within the brain and to evaluate cerebral compliance so that changes can be detected early and effects of various medical and nursing interventions can be evaluated. The traditional clinical signs of increased ICP (decreasing level of consciousness, increased systolic blood pressure and widening pulse pressure, bradycardia, and slow irregular respirations) do not accurately reflect early increases in ICP and in fact may occur too late for intervention and treatment to be effective.

ICP monitoring also provides the necessary data to calculate cerebral perfusion pressure (CPP); this is measured by subtracting mean ICP from the mean arterial blood pressure. Adequate cerebral circulation is ensured if the CPP remains approximately 70 to 90 mm Hg.

A pressure transducer setup is connected, using sterile normal saline (without preservative) to provide a fluid column between the CSF within the ventricles and the transducer. The pressure is transmitted to a monitor, and the pressure waveform and digital readings are displayed. A continuous flush device is *not* used on any ICP monitoring system, because it may contribute to further increased intracranial pressure.

Indications

The Monro-Kellie hypothesis states that the volume of the intracranium is equal to the volume of the brain plus the volume of the blood within the brain plus the volume of the cerebrospinal fluid (CSF) within the brain. Therefore, any condition that results in an increase in the volume of one or more of these will increase the ICP.

Types

The *intraventricular catheter* is placed in the lateral ventricle of the nondominant hemisphere. When ICP is severely elevated, CSF can be drained using this type of system. This is the most invasive method of monitoring ICP, yet it is also the most accurate, because the catheter is placed directly into the ventricle.

The *subarachnoid screw* is a screw device that is inserted approximately 1 mm into the subarachnoid space. No appreciable amounts of CSF can be drained with the subarachnoid screw. This system is less accurate than the intraventricular catheter at high pressures.[17]

The *epidural sensor* is a transducer placed between the skull and dura. It is less invasive than the intraventricular catheter and the subarachnoid screw, so it may be less accurate. Once it is placed, recalibration is not necessary. Drainage of CSF cannot be performed with this system.

The *fiberoptic transducer–tipped catheter* can be placed in the ventricle, subarachnoid or subdural spaces, or in the parenchyma. With ventricular placement, CSF can be drained. Once it is placed, it cannot be recalibrated.

Values
Normal
0-15 mm Hg
Significance of abnormal values
Consistently elevated ICP suggests that the compensatory mechanisms of cerebral autoregulation (arterial constriction and dilation) have failed. Patients usually become symptomatic with an ICP of 20 to 25 mm Hg, and a sustained ICP greater than 60 mm Hg is usually fatal. Factors that increase ICP include hypercapnea ($Paco_2$ greater than 42 mm Hg); hypoxia (Pao_2 less than 50 mm Hg); excessive fluid intake; head, neck, and extreme hip flexion; head rotation of 90 degrees to either side; Valsalva maneuver (straining, coughing); and continuous activity without adequate rest. Additionally, arousal from sleep, REM sleep, emotional upset, and noxious stimuli are known to increase ICP.

Patient Care Management
Preinsertion
The patient is placed in a supine position with the head of the bed elevated 30 to 45 degrees for insertion. A twist drill is used to insert the device. Strict aseptic technique is essential, as is a sterile environment during the procedure.

▶ Complications and related nursing diagnoses

Infection of the central nervous system	High risk for infection

It is imperative that strict aseptic technique be followed during insertion, and manipulation of the pressure line and during dressing changes. Assess for signs of infection, drainage, swelling, or irritation. The site must be kept clean and dry and should be covered with an occlusive dressing at all times.

The entire pressure transducer setup must remain a closed system to prevent contamination. Risk factors that influence infection rate include the patient's age and diagnosis, the duration of monitoring, the consistency of maintaining a closed system, the insertion environment and technique, and the type of device used.

Postinsertion

The ICP waveform should be continuously displayed on the monitor, and alarms should be set to coincide with the patient's clinical status. The ICP should be monitored and recorded as ordered, and the mean arterial blood pressure should be monitored to determine CPP.

The patient should be positioned with the head of the bed elevated 15 to 30 degrees (unless this is contraindicated) and maintained in a neutral position with minimal hip and knee flexion to facilitate venous drainage from the brain and prevent further increases in ICP.

Additional measures to prevent sustained intracranial hypertension should be taken: avoid hypothermia and hyperthermia; hyperventilate the patient's lungs, keeping $Paco_2$ at 25 to 30 mm Hg; instruct the patient to avoid Valsalva's maneuver; and restrict fluids as ordered.

Obtaining accurate measurements

1. Zero the transducer by opening the transducer to air and adjusting the monitor to read zero; this eliminates the pressure contributions from the atmosphere, and only pressures within the chamber being monitored will be measured.
2. Balance the air reference port of the transducer to the foramen of Monro (Figure 3-1) every 4 hours and with each position change.
3. Check the pressure and transducer setup frequently for air, since this will alter readings.
4. Obtain ICP readings at end-expiration to avoid the effects of thoracic pressures on the cerebral venous system.

Waveform interpretation

The ICP waveform (Figure 3-2) is very similar in appearance to that of the central venous pressure. It has small sys-

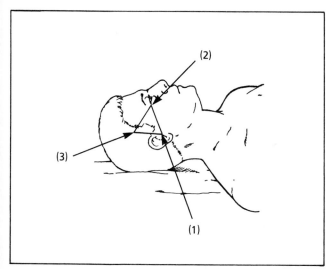

Figure 3-1 Location of foramen of Monro for transducer placement. Map an imaginary equilateral triangle from the external auditory meatus *(1)* to the outer canthus of the eye *(2)* to behind the hairline *(3)*. Point 3 is the location of the foramen of Monro.

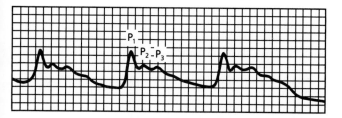

Figure 3-2 ICP waveform.

tolic and diastolic fluctuations, but the *mean* is monitored, since the ventricles of the brain are relatively low-pressure chambers. The waveform consists of at least three peaks (see Figure 3-2), although additional peaks may be present in some individuals. An increase in ICP will cause an increase in all waveform components initially; as ICP progresses, there is an elevation of P_2.

TABLE 3-1 Troubleshooting Intracranial Pressure Monitoring Lines

Problem	Cause	Solution
ICP waveform damped or absent	Air in transducer system	Eliminate air
	Loose connections	Tighten connections
	Occlusion of monitoring device	Flush device only as directed by physician
False high-pressure reading	Transducer too low	Place transducer at level of foramen of Monro and zero balance
	Air in transducer system	Eliminate air
False low-pressure reading	Transducer too high	Place transducer at level of foramen of Monro and zero balance
	Air in transducer system	Eliminate air

A P_2 equal to or higher than P_1 suggests decreased compliance, which may precede an actual increase in ICP. This signifies that compensatory mechanisms are failing and that a small increase in the volume can increase ICP significantly.

The intraventricular catheter and subarachnoid screw may develop a damped waveform as a result of tissue, blood, or debris blocking the transmission of the pressure. The line is irrigated only when ordered by a physician (Table 3-1).

Removal

The ICP monitoring device is removed by a physician. A wrench is required for the bolt. Sterile technique is used to prevent contamination of the insertion site. A sterile dressing is applied to the site for at least 24 hours; after this, the site is left open to air. If there is evidence of a CSF leak, additional sutures may be required.

ARTERIAL PRESSURE MONITORING

Clinical Brief

Arterial pressure monitoring provides a continuous display of the arterial blood pressure waveform and digital readings of the systolic, diastolic, and mean pressures. Mean arterial pressure (MAP) is the average pressure throughout the cardiac cycle; it is an important indicator of tissue perfusion. MAP is determined by cardiac output and systemic vascular resistance. MAP can be calculated using the following formula:

$$MAP = \frac{Systolic\ BP + 2\ (Diastolic\ BP)}{3}$$

When a pressure monitoring system is used, the bedside monitor displays the MAP, and it does not have to be calculated.

An indwelling arterial line provides continuous access to arterial blood for serial sampling, such as for blood gas analysis and/or serum laboratory tests.

Indications

Arterial pressure monitoring may be used in the following situations: (1) patients with unstable blood pressure, (2) administration of vasoactive drugs to measure trends and effects of therapy, (3) long-term ventilatory support or weaning, requiring frequent blood gas sampling, (4) extensive burns with limited intravascular access through intact skin for blood sampling, and (5) shock states in which vasoconstriction is so severe that Korotkoff sounds are difficult to hear with a conventional blood pressure cuff and stethoscope. In addition, arterial pressure monitoring allows ease in obtaining MAP readings, a measurement reflective of tissue perfusion.

Description

An arterial catheter, usually a Teflon catheter around a needle, is inserted into an artery through a percutaneous or cutdown method. The radial artery is preferred because of its accessibility, although the axillary, femoral, brachial, or pedal arteries can be used. The catheter is then attached to a pressure transducer setup with a continuous flush of heparinized saline. When the fluid is pressurized to 300 mm Hg, 3 ml/hr will be delivered through the line, thus ensuring patency of the line. The pressure transducer is connected to the monitor, and a continuous waveform is displayed on the oscilloscope. Digital display of the pressure is also available.

Values

Normal

Systolic blood pressure 100-140 mm Hg
Diastolic blood pressure 60-80 mm Hg
Mean arterial pressure 70-105 mm Hg

Significance of abnormal values

Systolic blood pressure values can be abnormal from changes in stroke volume (as occurs with hypervolemia, hypovolemia, or congestive heart failure), changes in wall compliance (as occurs with arteriosclerosis and hypertension), changes in the rate of ejection of blood from the left ventricle (as occurs with sympathetic nervous system stimulation and with some vasoactive drugs) or when there is aortic insufficiency (elevated systolic blood pressure) or aortic stenosis (lowered systolic blood pressure).

Diastolic blood pressure may be elevated as a result of increased stroke volume or systemic vascular resistance, and it may be lowered as a result of hypovolemia, peripheral dilation of blood vessels, or aortic insufficiency.

Changes in mean arterial pressure are caused by changes in cardiac output and/or changes in systemic vascular resistance.

Patient Care Management

Preinsertion

Before insertion of a radial arterial line, an Allen test should be performed to assess adequacy of collateral circulation to the hand (Figure 3-3).

The insertion of the arterial catheter is done under aseptic conditions. The transducer must be connected to the monitor prior to arterial cannulation, so that the waveform is immediately visible once the pressure tubing is connected to the arterial catheter.

▶ Complications and related nursing diagnoses

Hemorrhage   Fluid volume deficit

Hemorrhage can occur if the arterial catheter inadvertently becomes disconnected from the transducer. To prevent this, the alarm system must be activated at all times, and Luer-Lok connections should be used at all connections in the pressure setup. If the patient is restless or confused and is at risk for accidental dislodgement of the tubing or catheter, sedation or restraint should be considered.

Clot formation   Altered tissue perfusion: peripheral

Clot formation can occur at the insertion site or at the tip of the catheter. Patients with peripheral vascular disease or arteriosclerosis are particularly prone to clot formation and

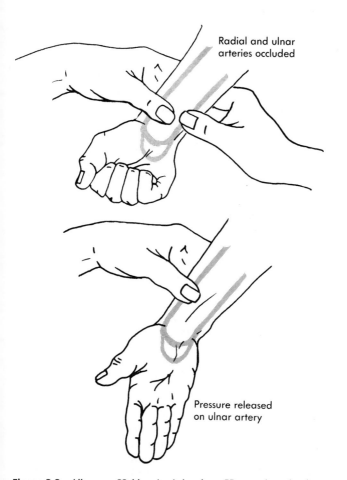

Radial and ulnar
arteries occluded

Pressure released
on ulnar artery

Figure 3-3   Allen test. Hold patient's hand up. Have patient clench
and unclench hand while occluding the radial and ulnar arteries. The
hand will become pale. Lower the hand and have the patient relax the
hand. While continuing to hold the radial artery, release pressure on
the ulnar artery. Brisk return of color (5 to 7 seconds) demonstrates
adequate ulnar blood flow. If pallor persists for more than 15 seconds,
ulnar flow is inadequate and radial artery cannulation should not be
attempted.

embolization. Use of the femoral artery is associated with a higher incidence of distal embolic complications than other sites.[23] To prevent this from occurring, a continuous infusion (3 ml/hr) of heparinized saline is connected to the arterial catheter. After each blood sample, the line must be flushed thoroughly to clear the catheter of blood. The tracing on the monitor must be observed frequently for loss of amplitude, which may be caused by clot formation. Assess capillary refill, color and temperature of the skin, as well as sensation and movement of the extremity distal to the cannulation site at least every 2 hours. Signs of decreased circulation that result from embolization of a clot include pain, pallor, and cyanosis in the distal extremity.

Infection   High risk for infection

Infection can occur with any invasive monitoring line; it can occur within the system setup, at the cannulation site, or within the catheter. Flush solution containing glucose should be avoided to decrease the risk of bacterial growth. Strict aseptic technique is used during the system setup, during insertion of the catheter, while drawing blood samples, and during site dressing changes. The site should be inspected daily for redness, swelling, or exudate. The tubing and flush solution should be changed at least every 72 hours and when contamination of the line or solution is suspected, and the dressing should be changed at least every 48 hours. Sterile deadender caps should be placed on all open ports of the stopcocks.

Vessel damage   High risk for injury

Vessel damage results from trauma to the vessel at the time of cannulation or from friction of the catheter in the vessel. The catheter should be handled gently at all times to minimize the friction on the wall of the vessel. If a clot is suspected, it should be drawn back instead of being flushed into the artery. Vessel spasm can occur if too much force is used during blood sampling procedures; only minimal pressure should be used to draw blood into the syringe. If a radial catheter is used, support the patient's wrist on an armboard or other supportive device to prevent flexion and movement of the catheter.

Air embolus   High risk for injury
                                              Altered tissue perfusion

Air that is trapped in the tubing can be inadvertently flushed into the artery and the systemic circulation. All air must be purged from the tubing during the setup of the system. Also, the tubing should be frequently inspected for air, especially before fast-flushing the line. Observe the arterial waveform for decreased amplitude, which may indicate air in the line or in the transducer.

Electric shock   High risk for injury

Electric shock is a potential risk with any fluid-filled monitoring system. It can occur if current leaks from an electrical device to the fluid-filled catheter, which provides a low resistance pathway directly to the heart. All electrical equipment used in patient rooms should be adequately grounded and have three-pronged plugs. Electrical devices used in the critical care unit should be checked by the biomedical department at regular intervals.

Postinsertion

With centrally located catheters (such as the femoral artery), the air reference port of the transducer should be balanced with the tip of the catheter, which is approximately at the level of the right atrium. This point is the *phlebostatic axis* (Figure 3-4), and the landmark for this is the intersection of the fourth intercostal space and the mid-axillary line. By balancing the air reference port of the transducer in this manner, the effects of hydrostatic pressure within the fluid-filled system are eliminated. Mark the phlebostatic axis with ink or tape on the patient's skin and use this same point for taking readings consistently; failure to do so will result in inaccurate readings.

When the arterial catheter is located peripherally (such as the radial artery), it is more accurate to place the air refer-

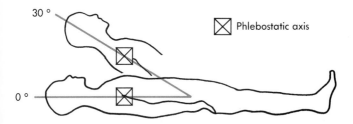

Figure 3-4   Phlebostatic axis.

ence port of the transducer at the level of the tip of the catheter (e.g., the patient's wrist); this eliminates the effects of hydrostatic pressure within the fluid-filled column and provides an accurate measurement of the static pressure within the artery itself.[10] The line must also be zeroed to eliminate the effect of atmospheric air on the pressure readings.

Alarm parameters should be set (usually 10 to 20 mm Hg above and below the patient's baseline pressure) and activated. The alarms should be maintained at all times so that sudden changes in pressure and/or disconnection of the line is immediately noted.

The cuff blood pressure should be checked and compared with the monitor readings periodically to determine the accuracy of the monitor. Usually the cuff reading is 5 to 20 mm Hg less than the intraarterial reading. The blood pressure should be auscultated in the same arm as the arterial catheter is placed to ensure accuracy.

Obtaining accurate measurements

Rezero and balance the line every 4 hours and each time the patient is repositioned. Prevent kinks in the catheter by stabilizing securely. Observe the line frequently for air, which may damp the waveform. Flush the line thoroughly each time blood is drawn. Peripheral arterial catheters are often positional, and the waveform may be damped if the extremity is flexed. Use of an armboard or splint will eliminate this.

Waveform interpretation

Systole is apparent on the waveform as a sharp rise in pressure; this is the anacrotic limb, and it signifies the rapid ejection of blood from the ventricle through the open aortic valve. If there is a delay in this rapid rise, it could suggest a decrease in myocardial contractility, aortic stenosis, or damped pressure movement secondary to catheter position or clot formation. A steep rate of rise along with a high peak systolic pressure and a poorly defined dicrotic notch may be seen with aortic insufficiency.

Diastole follows closure of the aortic valve (seen as the dicrotic notch on the waveform) and continues until the next systole. The location of the dicrotic notch should be one third or greater the height of the systolic peak; if it is not, suspect a decreased cardiac output (Figure 3-5). Table 3-2 offers methods for troubleshooting invasive hemodynamic monitoring lines.

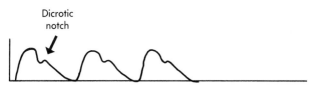

Figure 3-5 Arterial waveform. Dicrotic notch represents closure of the aortic valve.

Obtaining a blood sample

1. Attach a sterile 10 ml syringe to the arterial catheter stopcock that is closest to the patient.
2. Open the stopcock to the syringe and catheter; aspirate enough blood to clear the line (the amount depends on the length of the tubing and catheter; usually 5 ml is sufficient).
3. Close the stopcock to the halfway position; remove the syringe and discard.
4. Attach the blood sample syringe (a heparinized syringe is necessary for a blood gas sample) to the catheter stopcock; open the stopcock to the syringe and catheter and gently aspirate the blood sample.
5. Turn the stopcock to the halfway position and remove the blood sample syringe. Expel the air from the blood gas syringe to ensure accurate measurement of oxygen saturation.
6. Attach a sterile syringe; open the stopcock to the syringe and activate the fast flush until all blood is removed from the stopcock and port.
7. Open the stopcock to the catheter; activate fast flush until all blood is removed from the tubing (1 to 3 seconds).
8. Ensure return of a normal arterial waveform on the monitor.

Removal of arterial catheter

1. Close the stopcock closest to the patient off to the patient and disconnect the transducer from the monitor.
2. Remove the arterial line dressing from the site and remove any sutures.
3. Gently withdraw the catheter from the artery and apply direct, firm pressure to the site with sterile gauze while

TABLE 3-2 Troubleshooting Invasive Hemodynamic Monitoring Lines

Problem	Cause	Solution
Bleed back into tubing	Loose connections	Tighten connections
	Stopcock open to patient	Close stopcock
	Inadequate pressure in bag	Inflate pressure bag to 300 mm Hg
Damped pressure tracing	Air bubbles in system	Purge air from system
	Clot formation	Aspirate blood from catheter and briefly flush system*
	Loose connections	Tighten connections
	Compliant tubing	Use stiff (high-pressure) tubing
No waveform	Transducer not open to catheter	Check system
	Transducer not connected to monitor	Connect transducer to monitor
	Incorrect scale selection	Select appropriate scale for physiological pressure
	Kink in catheter	Reposition catheter; use armboard to prevent wrist flexion

Inaccurate readings	Change in transducer reference level:	Keep transducer at phlebostatic axis or catheter tip level when obtaining readings
	Transducer *above* reference point results in false low readings	
	Transducer *below* reference point results in false high readings	
	Air or clotting within system	Check system: flush air from system, aspirate clots from system
Noise or fling in pressure waveform ("whip")	Excessive catheter movement: occurs when catheter in large vessel	Reposition catheter; use damping device to remove fling from waveform
	Excessive tubing length	Eliminate excessive tubing

*Do *not* flush ICP, LAP.

continuously assessing the circulation of the distal extremity. Maintain pressure for a minimum of 5 minutes or until bleeding stops.

4. Apply a pressure dressing to the site.
5. Assess the dressing and distal circulation to the extremity frequently.
6. Remove the dressing 8 hours after the removal of the catheter.

CENTRAL VENOUS PRESSURE MONITORING

Clinical Brief

This type of monitoring line is used to obtain intermittent or continuous central venous pressure (CVP) to evaluate right-sided heart function. It can also be used to assess efficacy of fluid replacement therapy.

Indications

CVP monitoring may be used to assess (1) volume replacement therapy, (2) right-sided heart failure (acute left ventricular failure will eventually elevate the CVP from the backup of blood in the pulmonary vasculature but by the time the pressure is reflected in the right atrium the consequence, pulmonary edema, is already well established), and (3) response to intravenous vasoactive drugs.

Description

The CVP catheter is inserted into a large vein by percutaneous or cutdown method. The catheter may be single lumen, or it may be a multilumen catheter that allows the infusion of several different or incompatible drugs or fluids simultaneously. The most common sites for insertion are the jugular (internal or external), subclavian, basilic, or femoral veins. Once the catheter is inserted, it is placed so that the tip ends in the superior vena cava, approximately 2 cm above the right atrium. The pressure waveform is displayed on the monitor oscilloscope with a digital readout.

Values

Normal

2-6 mm Hg

The waveform has systolic (positive) and diastolic (negative) variations, but the fluctuations are small (since the right atrium is a low-pressure chamber); thus the *mean* pressure is monitored.

Significance of abnormal values

Increased CVP may be caused by fluid overload or retention, tricuspid or pulmonic valvular disease, ventricular septal defect with left-to-right shunting, constrictive pericarditis, right ventricular infarction, myocarditis, cardiac tamponade, chronic obstructive lung disease, pulmonary embolus, pulmonary hypertension, or *chronic* left ventricular failure.

Decreased CVP may be caused by hypovolemia, excessive diuresis, or systemic venodilation secondary to sepsis, drugs, or neurogenic causes.

Patient Care Management

Preinsertion

The patient is placed in the Trendelenburg position if the subclavian or jugular approach is to be used; this will facilitate filling of the vessel and will diminish the risk of air embolism. In addition, the patient should be instructed to hold a breath at peak expiration at the moment of catheter insertion. This will increase the intrathoracic pressure and diminish the risk for an air embolism.

Complications and related nursing diagnoses

Similar to the arterial catheter, CVP monitoring can result in air embolism, clot formation, hemorrhage, electrical shock, and infection (interventions to prevent these are the same as those described in Arterial pressure monitoring: patient care management, p. 80). Additionally, the following complication may occur with CVP monitoring:

Catheter tip migration   Decreased cardiac output

The tip of the catheter may move forward to the right ventricle and irritate the endocardium, causing ventricular dysrhythmias. If the tip migrates far enough that the heart wall is perforated, cardiac tamponade can result if bleeding into the pericardial sac occurs.

Postinsertion

Following the subclavian or jugular insertion of the catheter, both lung fields must be auscultated for symmetrical breath sounds since pneumothorax or hemothorax can occur. A chest radiograph is obtained to verify catheter placement and to rule out pneumothorax. A hydrothorax can occur if large amounts of fluids are infused through the catheter before a radiograph rules out the possibility of a pneumothorax.

A sterile occlusive dressing is applied to the site. The dressing should be changed every 48 hours, and the site should be inspected for signs of infection or phlebitis. The flush system and tubing are changed every 72 hours. During tubing changes, place the patient in Trendelenburg position and instruct the patient to hold a breath to prevent air from entering the catheter.

The waveform should be monitored continuously or at regular intervals to ensure that the catheter tip has not migrated into the right ventricle; this would be apparent by a much taller waveform associated with higher pressures (25 to 30 mm Hg). Additionally, the ECG waveform must be monitored for ventricular dysrhythmias.

Alarm parameters should be set and maintained at all times.

Obtaining accurate measurements

Zero and balance the transducer every 4 hours and each time the patient is repositioned. The transducer should be kept at the level of the phlebostatic axis during readings (the phlebostatic axis should be marked with ink or tape on the patient's skin to ensure consistency). The waveform may fluctuate with respirations; readings should be taken at end-expiration to minimize the influence of intrathoracic pressure (see Pulmonary artery pressure monitoring: obtaining accurate measurements, pp. 97-99).

Waveform interpretation

The CVP waveform (Figure 3-6) has positive waves and negative descents. The *a* wave indicates right atrial systole; it is followed by the *x* descent, which indicates the drop in pressure that occurs during right atrial relaxation. The *c* wave, which may not be distinguishable on the waveform, is caused by bulging of the closed tricuspid valve into the atrium during right ventricular systole; the *x'* descent follows the *c* wave. The *v* wave indicates right atrial diastole, when blood is filling the atrium; it is followed by the *y* descent, which indicates the passive right atrial emptying of blood into the right ventricle through the open tricuspid valve.

Various changes in the CVP waveform can indicate pathophysiological changes in the heart and pulmonary vasculature. An elevated *a* wave is seen with tricuspid stenosis, right ventricular hypertrophy secondary to pulmonic valve stenosis, or pulmonary hypertension, constrictive pericarditis, and cardiac tamponade, all of which impede right atrial emptying. Tricuspid insufficiency, with backflow of blood into the right atrium during ventricular systole, will cause increased pressure and an elevated *v* wave on the right atrial waveform. Tricuspid insufficiency can also cause an absence

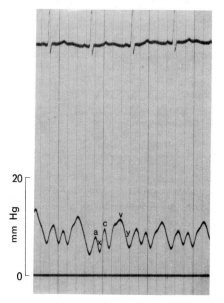

Figure 3-6 CVP waveform. (From Daily EK and Schroeder JS: Techniques in bedside hemodynamic monitoring, ed 4, St Louis, 1989, The CV Mosby Co.)

of the *c* wave on the waveform, since the valve is incompetent and will not bulge back into the right atrium during ventricular systole.

Cannon waves (combined *a* and *c* waves) occur whenever the atrium contracts against a closed valve; for example, when junctional or ventricular beats occur, the atria contract out of sequence and the valve is closed because of ventricular systole. The cannon waves are large and obscure the *v* waves.

Troubleshooting

Table 3-2 offers troubleshooting suggestions for invasive hemodynamic monitoring lines.

Removal of CVP catheter

1. Place the patient in Trendelenburg position to prevent air embolism during catheter removal from the jugular or subclavian veins.
2. Turn the stopcock off to the patient and disconnect the transducer from the monitor.

3. Remove the dressing and remove the sutures.
4. Instruct the patient to hold a breath at full expiration and remove the catheter slowly; inspect the tip to ensure the catheter is intact.
5. Apply pressure to the site until the bleeding has stopped, being careful not to compress any arteries (e.g., carotid) and impair blood flow.
6. Apply a sterile occlusive dressing to the site and leave in place for 24 hours.
7. Observe the site frequently for bleeding or hematoma.

PULMONARY ARTERY PRESSURE MONITORING

Clinical Brief

The pulmonary artery (PA) catheter is used to continuously monitor right intracardiac and pulmonary artery pressures. Since it is situated in the pulmonary artery, it can measure left-sided heart pressures reflected across the pulmonary vasculature; therefore, left ventricular end-diastolic pressure (LVEDP) can be estimated and the hemodynamic response to fluid or drug therapy can be assessed. The PA catheter also allows for the sampling of mixed venous blood from the pulmonary artery in order to measure oxygen saturation (see discussion under Svo_2 monitoring, pp. 103-105). Finally, the PA catheter enables the measurement of cardiac output via the thermodilution technique.

Indications

The PA catheter may be used in the following clinical situations: (1) left-sided heart failure, (2) valvular disease, (3) titration of vasoactive drugs or fluids, (4) severe respiratory failure, and (5) perioperative and postoperative monitoring of surgical patients with cardiovascular or pulmonary dysfunction.

Description

The PA catheter has four ports: (1) the proximal lumen ends in the right atrium and is used for infusion of fluids or monitoring of right atrial pressure, and the injection of a bolus of fluid to measure cardiac output; (2) the distal lumen ends in the pulmonary artery, allowing measurement of left-sided heart pressures reflected across the pulmonary vasculature; (3) the balloon port leads to an inflatable balloon at the tip of the catheter; when the balloon is inflated it blocks pressures behind it (the right side of the heart) and senses pressures through the pulmonary vasculature from the left side of the heart; and (4) the thermodilution port terminates 4 to 6 cm proximal to the tip of the catheter and senses temperature changes during cardiac output measurement. Some PA catheters have additional ports for the infusion of fluids or for insertion of a temporary pacing wire.

The catheter is inserted into a large vein (the same sites as those used for CVP catheters) via percutaneous or cutdown method. Upon entry into the right atrium, the balloon is inflated and the catheter is flow-directed into position in the pulmonary artery. Continuous pressure monitoring of the waveform during insertion shows the anatomical location of the tip of the catheter, based on the characteristic waveforms of the right atrium, the right ventricle, and the pulmonary artery (Figure 3-7). Once the pulmonary artery has been reached, the balloon tip "wedges" into a small branch of the pulmonary artery.

Values
Normal
RV: 15-28/0-8 mm Hg. Right ventricular pressure is measured during catheter insertion only; this value provides information about the function of the right ventricle as well as the tricuspid and pulmonic valves.

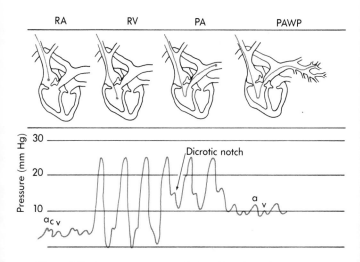

Figure 3-7 Pressure waveforms during PA catheter insertion.

PAS: 15-30 mm Hg. The pulmonary artery systolic pressure indicates the pressure in the pulmonary artery during right ventricular contraction, when the pulmonic valve is open.

PAD: 5-15 mm Hg. Pulmonary artery diastolic (PAD) pressure reflects the resistance to flow by the pulmonary vasculature. It indirectly measures the LVEDP, because the pulmonic valve is closed during diastole (thereby eliminating right heart pressure influences) and the mitral valve is open, so that the catheter "sees" the pressure in the left atrium and the left ventricle. PAD can be used in place of the pulmonary artery wedge pressure (PAWP) to estimate LVEDP when there is no pulmonary vascular obstruction, thereby decreasing the number of balloon inflations and potential patient risk. The PAD is normally 1 to 4 mm Hg higher than the PAWP because of the slight resistance to forward blood flow from the pulmonary vasculature; when the catheter is "wedged" there is no forward flow distal to the catheter tip and the effects of pulmonary vascular resistance do not affect the PAWP reading. The PAD/PAWP gradient is greater anytime there is increased pulmonary vascular resistance (pulmonary embolus, hypoxia, chronic lung disease). Neither PAD nor PAWP accurately reflects LVEDP in the presence of mitral valve disease because the pressure is increased by the altered blood flow between the atrium and the ventricle.

PAWP: 4-12 mm Hg. PAWP, also known as pulmonary artery occlusive pressure (PAOP), reflects the LVEDP most accurately because the pressures from the right side of the heart are blocked by the inflated balloon so that the tip of the catheter (distal to the balloon) senses pressures only forward of the catheter (Figure 3-8). The PAWP waveform has small fluctuations similar to the CVP waveform, thus the *mean* pressure is monitored.

Significance of abnormal values

RV: Right ventricular systolic pressures may be elevated as a result of pulmonic stenosis, pulmonary hypertension, pulmonary vascular volume overload, ventricular septal defect with left-to-right shunting, chronic lung disease, pulmonary embolism, hypoxemia, or adult respiratory distress syndrome (ARDS). Decreased right ventricular systolic pressures may be the result of right ventricular failure secondary to infarction or ischemia, as a result of myopathy, or secondary to hypovolemia.

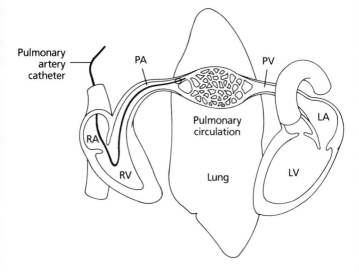

Figure 3-8 Pulmonary artery catheter in the wedged position. Balloon inflation allows for recording of pressures in left heart as it "sees" the left atrium.

Right ventricular diastolic pressure may be elevated because of pulmonic valve insufficiency, right ventricular failure, pulmonary hypertension, cardiac tamponade, constrictive pericarditis, or intravascular volume overload. Decreased right ventricular diastolic pressure occurs with hypovolemia.

PAS: Pulmonary artery systolic pressure may be elevated due to increased pulmonary blood volume or increased pulmonary vascular resistance secondary to pulmonary embolism, hypoxemia, lung disease, or ARDS. Decreased pulmonary artery systolic pressure occurs with hypovolemia.

PAD: Pulmonary artery diastolic pressure is elevated in the same circumstances as the PA systolic pressure, as well as left heart dysfunction (from any cause), mitral stenosis/insufficiency, cardiac tamponade, or increased intravascular volume. Hypovolemia causes a decrease in pulmonary diastolic pressure.

PAWP: Pulmonary artery wedge pressure is increased in any situation in which there is left ventricular dysfunction: mitral stenosis/insufficiency, left ventricular failure, decreased left ventricular compliance, increased systemic vascular resistance, cardiac tamponade, or fluid volume overload. Decreased pulmonary artery wedge pressure is seen with hypovolemia or vasodilation with resulting decreased afterload.

Patient Care Management

Preinsertion

The patient is prepared in the same manner as for CVP insertion. Prior to insertion, the inflated balloon is tested for integrity by submerging it in saline and checking for air leaks. The transducer must be zeroed prior to catheter insertion because the waveforms and pressure readings used to evaluate catheter placement as it is advanced through the heart must be accurate. (see Figure 3-6). The pressures of the right atrium, right ventricle, and pulmonary artery are documented during insertion. It is important to monitor for ventricular dysrhythmias during insertion, especially during passage through the right ventricle.

▶ Complications and related nursing diagnoses

Pulmonary artery pressure monitoring is associated with the risk of developing the same complications as those seen with arterial and central venous pressure monitoring (air embolus, clot formation, hemorrhage, electrical shock, infection, and catheter tip migration [see pp. 80-83]). In addition, the following complications may occur with pulmonary artery pressure monitoring.

Perforation of the pulmonary artery by the catheter	High risk for injury

Perforation of the pulmonary artery can occur during catheter positioning; it is for this reason that the balloon should be inflated anytime the tip is repositioned, since the balloon provides some protection to the wall of the vessel.

Pulmonary artery infarction, hemorrhage, or embolism	High risk for injury
	Impaired gas exchange

Pulmonary artery infarction or hemorrhage can occur if the balloon is inadvertently left inflated or if the catheter spontaneously wedges, blocking blood flow to that branch of the vessel. The PA waveform must be monitored continuously so that inadvertent wedging of the catheter can be recognized immediately. If the PA waveform spontaneously develops a wedge appearance, the catheter has likely migrated forward into a smaller branch of the pulmonary artery. To regain a PA waveform, the line should be aspirated then flushed; if the problem continues, have the patient cough and/or turn to the side because this may help the catheter move back into a larger branch of the pulmonary artery. The catheter may have to be pulled back slightly if these measures do not correct the problem. Pulmonary embolism can occur if a clot breaks off the tip of the catheter.

Ventricular dysrhythmias   Decreased cardiac output

Ventricular dysrhythmias, secondary to irritation of the ventricular wall by the catheter tip, can occur during insertion of the catheter or if the catheter falls back into the right ventricle after placement in the pulmonary artery. If this occurs, the catheter should be floated into the pulmonary artery by a physician or it should be removed. The chest radiograph should be used as a guide in determining correct placement.

Balloon rupture   High risk for injury

The balloon of the catheter can rupture and cause an air embolus. The balloon should never be overinflated, and deflation should be passive (pulling back the air may damage the balloon). If balloon rupture is suspected (no resistance is felt during injection of air, failure to obtain wedge waveform, bleeding back into balloon port) the balloon port should no longer be used and be labeled appropriately.

Bundle branch block   Decreased cardiac output

Right bundle branch block may occur during manipulation of the catheter in the right ventricle. Generally this is not a problem unless the patient also has left bundle branch block, in which case complete heart block could result.

Postinsertion

A chest radiograph must be obtained to rule out pneumothorax and to verify correct placement. Fluids should not be infused directly into the distal lumen of the PA catheter.

Alarm parameters should be set and maintained at all times.

Obtaining accurate measurements

Zero and balance the transducer with the phlebostatic axis every 4 hours and each time the patient is repositioned. The head of the bed can be elevated up to 45 degrees for readings, but the patient should be supine.

Because the heart is subject to the same intrathoracic pressures as the lungs, there may be respiratory variation in the hemodynamic waveforms. When respiratory variation is present, there will be a decrease in the waveform during spontaneous inspiration and a rise in the waveform during expiration. The opposite occurs with positive-pressure ventilation—the waveform rises with inspiration and falls with expiration. When the patient is receiving intermittent mandatory ventilation, the waveform will peak and trough at different times during the respiratory cycle, depending on whether the breath is spontaneous or mechanically induced. Pressure readings should be taken at end-expiration because at this point the intrathoracic pressure is constant and the pressure waveform is most stable. The digital display is often inaccurate when respiratory variation is present, so the reading should be taken from a calibrated strip chart recording at end-expiration.

In patients receiving positive pressure ventilation or PEEP, the pressure reading should be taken without removing the ventilator so that the effects of positive pressure on the patient's hemodynamic status can be realized. In patients with normal lung compliance, the following equation can be used to estimate the effects of PEEP on PAWP:

$$\text{PAWP (corrected)} = \text{Measured PAWP} - 0.5 \,(\text{PEEP})$$

In patients with ARDS or other conditions that decrease lung compliance, the following equation can be used to estimate the effects of PEEP on PAWP:

$$\text{PAWP (corrected)} = \text{Measured PAWP} - 0.5 \,(\text{PEEP} - 10)$$

The balloon should be inflated slowly when PAWP readings are taken, and inflation should cease as soon as the PAWP waveform is displayed. When obtaining a PAWP reading, do not leave the balloon inflated for more than 15 seconds; inflation longer than this can result in ischemia of the lung segment distal to the catheter. *Never* use more than the balloon capacity indicated by the manufacturer on the shaft of the catheter. Be sure that the PA waveform returns following passive deflation of the balloon.

PAD can be used to estimate LVEDP if the difference between PAD and PAWP is less than 5 mm Hg, there is no pulmonary vascular obstruction, and the heart rate is less than 130 beats per minute.

When obtaining thermodilution cardiac output (CO) readings, it is important to use the correct computation constant (provided in the catheter package insert). If the wrong computation constant is inadvertently used, the following equation can be used to correct the obtained reading:

$$\text{Correct CO} = \text{Wrong CO} \times \frac{\text{Correct computation constant}}{\text{Wrong computation constant}}$$

Room temperature injectate solution has been found to correlate closely with iced injectate; therefore standard practice is with use of room temperature solution.

Waveform interpretation

The pulmonary artery waveform looks similar to that seen with arterial pressure monitoring. The systolic pressure is seen as a steep rise as blood is ejected from the right ventricle. The diastolic component of the waveform occurs after the closure of the pulmonic valve, seen as the dicrotic notch.

The PAWP waveform is similar in appearance to the CVP waveform. The *a* wave on the PAWP tracing indicates left atrial contraction; it is followed by the *x* descent, which indicates left atrial relaxation. The *c* wave is rarely seen in the PAWP tracing. The *v* wave signifies left ventricular contraction, and the *y* descent following it represents the opening of the mitral valve.

Elevated *a* waves on the PAWP tracing can be indicative of mitral stenosis or left ventricular failure. Elevated *v* waves, on the other hand, indicate mitral insufficiency. Elevation of both *a* and *v* waves simultaneously indicates severe left ventricular failure.

Troubleshooting

Table 3-2 offers suggestions for troubleshooting invasive hemodynamic lines.

Additional problems that may be encountered with the PA catheter are spontaneous wedging of the balloon, migration of the catheter tip to the right ventricle, and right bundle branch block (see Complications, pp. 96-97).

If the catheter does not wedge and balloon rupture is not the cause, then the catheter may need to be advanced by the physician. The chest radiograph should be used as a guide in determining correct placement.

Obtaining mixed-venous blood gases

The procedure for drawing mixed-venous blood gases is similar to that of drawing arterial blood gases (see Arterial pressure monitoring: obtaining a blood sample, p. 85). However, mixed-venous gases are drawn from the distal lumen of the PA catheter. It is important to be sure the balloon is deflated during the aspiration of the sample; otherwise, only highly oxygen-saturated blood from "downstream" of the catheter tip will be drawn, causing erroneous results. Similarly, it is important to draw the sample slowly (not faster than 1 ml/20 sec), or arterialized blood from the pulmonary capillaries that is highly oxygenated will be drawn into the syringe and cause erroneously high readings. Following completion of the procedure, ensure the return of the PA waveform.

Removal

Before removing the PA catheter, actively deflate the balloon. The procedure is similar to that of CVP catheter removal (see Central venous pressure monitoring: removal, p. 91), except that the catheter should be rapidly pulled back to decrease the risk of ventricular dysrhythmias. If at any time resistance is felt, do *not* continue pulling and notify the physician immediately. The site should be covered with a sterile dressing.

LEFT ATRIAL PRESSURE MONITORING

Clinical Brief

Left atrial pressure (LAP) is monitored to evaluate left-sided heart pressures (LVEDP) following open-heart surgery.

Indications

LAP monitoring can be used for the perioperative and postoperative assessment of left ventricular function and cardiovascular status and to assess the hemodynamic response to vasoactive drugs or fluids.

Description

The LAP catheter is inserted into the left atrium during cardiac surgery; it is threaded through the superior pulmonary vein into the left atrium and the external end is brought out through a small incision at the inferior end of the mediastinal incision. The catheter is connected to a pressure transducer setup, and the waveform is monitored continuously. No manipulation of the catheter is required to ascertain LVEDP.

Values

Normal

4-12 mm Hg

Significance of abnormal values

Since the LAP is positioned in the left heart, it indirectly reflects the LVEDP. Therefore, the same factors that cause an increase or decrease in PAD and PAWP will cause abnormal LAP values (see Pulmonary artery pressure monitoring: significance of abnormal values, pp. 94-95).

Patient Care Management

Preinsertion

The LAP catheter is inserted during open-heart surgery, and the line will be in place when the patient arrives in the critical care unit.

▶ Complications and related nursing diagnoses

The potential risks of LAP monitoring are the same as those listed for CVP monitoring: air embolus, clot formation, infection, cardiac tamponade, and electrical hazards (see Central venous pressure monitoring: complications and related nursing diagnoses, p. 89). However, since the LAP line provides direct access to the systemic circulation, the risk of air embolus is more threatening than with the CVP or PA lines. To decrease this risk, an in-line air filter should be used, and the line should never be irrigated or flushed.

Bleeding or pericardial tamponade following removal	Decreased cardiac output Fluid volume deficit

Bleeding and pericardial tamponade can occur following removal of the LAP catheter. The mediastinal tubes should be left in place for at least 2 hours after the removal of the LAP line so that blood does not collect in the mediastinum.

Postinsertion

The LAP line should *never* be irrigated or flushed. The remainder of the postinsertion care is the same as that described with the CVP and PA lines (see pp. 89, 97).

Obtaining accurate measurements

The air port of the pressure transducer must be leveled with the phlebostatic axis during pressure readings. Readings should be taken at end-expiration and obtained from a calibrated strip chart recording if respiratory variation is present. The transducer should be zeroed at least every 4 hours and each time the patient has been repositioned. The patient should not be removed from the ventilator or PEEP during readings.

Waveform interpretation

The LAP waveform closely resembles that of the PAWP, and the mean pressure is monitored (Figure 3-9). The waveform has *a* and *v* waves, as well as *x* and *y* descents; these correlate to the same mechanical events of the cardiac cycle

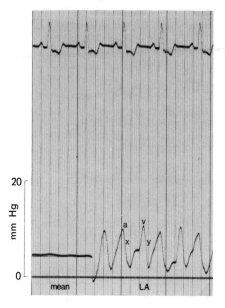

Figure 3-9 LAP waveform. (From Daily EK and Schroeder JS: Techniques in bedside hemodynamic monitoring, ed 4, St Louis, 1989, The CV Mosby Co.)

as the waves and descents of the PAWP waveform (see p. 99).

If large *a* and *v* waves appear on the waveform, it may be the result of catheter migration to the left ventricle; if this occurs, notify the physician at once and monitor the patient for ventricular dysrhythmias.

Troubleshooting

Basic troubleshooting of the LAP line is similar to that of other hemodynamic lines (see Table 3-2 on troubleshooting invasive hemodynamic monitoring lines), *except* that the LAP catheter is *never* flushed. If damping of the waveform occurs and clot formation is suspected as the cause, attempt to aspirate the clot. If the line cannot be aspirated or if the line remains damped, then the catheter needs to be discontinued.

Removal

The LAP catheter is removed by a physician or nurse, depending on the institutional protocol. It is usually removed after 24 to 48 hours because of the increased risk for air embolus. The procedure for removal is the same as that for a CVP catheter (see p. 91). The site is covered with a sterile occlusive dressing and must be observed frequently for bleeding. Following removal of the LAP catheter, the patient must be monitored closely for signs of pericardial tamponade (jugular vein distension; cyanosis; elevation of CVP, PAD, and PAWP; pulsus paradoxus; decreased systolic blood pressure).

Svo₂ MONITORING

Clinical Brief

Continuous monitoring of mixed-venous oxygen saturation (Svo₂) provides ongoing information about the balance between oxygen supply and demand. The blood in the pulmonary artery is a mixture of blood returned from the superior and inferior vena cavae, as well as the coronary sinus; the oxygen saturation of this blood returning from all perfused body parts indirectly reflects the amount of oxygen extracted systemically. The balance between oxygen supply and demand is affected by cardiac output, arterial oxygen saturation, amount of hemoglobin available to carry oxygen, and tissue oxygen consumption. When provided with an immediate warning that an imbalance exists, the clinician is able to determine the cause of the imbalance and intervene appropriately.

Indications

Svo₂ monitoring may be used in any of the following clinical situations: cardiogenic shock, following open-heart surgery, acute myocardial infarction, concomitant with IABP therapy, adult respiratory distress syndrome, cardiac tamponade, vasoactive drug therapy, and congestive heart failure. Additionally, Svo₂ monitoring is useful for early recognition of hemodynamic compromise, since a decrease in Svo₂ often occurs before changes in other parameters. Patients with an unstable hemodynamic or respiratory status may require fewer cardiac output or arterial blood gas measurements with the use of the Svo₂ monitor. Finally, the Svo₂ monitor is useful in assessing patient response to routine nursing interventions such as suctioning and repositioning.

Description

A thermodilution pulmonary artery catheter with a fiberoptic light is used. Reflection spectrophotometry is the technique by which oxygen saturation of venous blood is measured. The light reflected by the blood is transmitted to a photodetector, where it is converted to electrical signals and the oxygen saturation is computed and displayed. The Svo_2 is updated every second and is displayed on the digital screen as well as on a strip chart recording. The catheter has all other capabilities of the conventional PA catheter: right atrial, pulmonary artery, and pulmonary wedge pressure monitoring; thermodilution cardiac output; and infusion of intravenous fluids. Alarms can be set so that if the Svo_2 is outside the high and low limits the clinician is immediately alerted.

Values

Normal

60%-80%

Significance of abnormal values

A decreased (<60%) Svo_2 can be caused by (1) an increase in oxygen consumption (secondary to shivering, seizures, pain, activity, hyperthermia, or anxiety), or (2) a decrease in oxygen delivery (secondary to decreased cardiac output, dysrhythmias, hypoxemia, or anemia). An increased (80% to 95%) Svo_2 can be caused by (1) a decrease in oxygen consumption by the tissues (secondary to hypothermia, anesthesia, sepsis, or alkalosis) or (2) an increase in oxygen delivery (secondary to hyperoxia and left-to-right shunting).

Patient Care Management

Preinsertion

See Pulmonary artery pressure monitoring: preinsertion, p. 96.

▶ **Complications and related nursing diagnoses**

There are no complications associated with fiberoptic monitoring of mixed venous oxygen saturation. However, the same complications that are associated with the PA catheter pertain to the use of the Svo_2 catheter (see Pulmonary artery pressure monitoring: complications, pp. 96-97).

Postinsertion

See Pulmonary artery pressure monitoring: postinsertion, p. 97.

Obtaining accurate measurements

To maintain accuracy of the system, the oximeter should be calibrated daily to an in vivo measurement of mixed venous blood. The connection between the optical module and the catheter must remain intact; if for any reason the system becomes disconnected, an in vivo calibration should be performed. If fibrin develops on the tip of the catheter, it will interfere with the light intensity and accuracy of the readings; therefore, it is important to maintain patency of the catheter and to flush the line if there is a damped waveform or poor signal from the processor.

Changes of >10% in the Svo_2 reading or decreases in Svo_2 below 60% are significant and should be followed by examination of other variables (cardiac output, arterial blood gases, hemoglobin level) to determine the cause of the change.

PULSE OXIMETRY

Clinical Brief

Pulse oximetry (Spo_2) is a noninvasive method of monitoring arterial oxygen saturation. It provides an early and immediate warning of impending hypoxemia.

Indications

Pulse oximetry may be used in any of the following clinical situations: (1) recovery from anesthesia; (2) assessment of adequacy of oxygen therapy or ventilatory management; and (3) any patients who are at high risk for hypoventilation or respiratory arrest (such as those receiving epidural anesthesia, neurologically damaged patients, or those who are receiving high doses of narcotics).

Description

The pulse oximeter is a noninvasive optical method of measuring oxygen saturation of functional hemoglobin. The amount of arterial hemoglobin that is saturated with oxygen is determined by beams of light passing through the tissue. The sensor with the light source is placed on the finger or the bridge of the nose; the saturation is displayed on the monitor, and visual and audible alarms can be set to alert the clinician of changes in oxygenation.

Values

Normal

Spo_2 > 95%

Significance of abnormal values

When the arterial saturation falls below 95%, it could be the result of a variety of causes. It may signify that the respiratory effort or oxygen delivery system is inadequate to meet the tissue needs, or that CO is impaired resulting in tissue hypoxia. If arterial flow to the sensor is impaired for any reason, it could result in an erroneously low reading while tissue oxygenation is adequate; therefore, it is important to correlate the reading with other assessment parameters.

Patient Care Management

Obtaining accurate measurements

The sensor should be placed on clean, dry skin (finger or bridge of nose). If readings are consistently inaccurate, change the sensor or the site. The sensor should not be on the same extremity that has an automatic blood pressure cuff, since this reduces arterial blood flow distally and will alter readings. The patient and extremity should be kept as still as possible to reduce artifact and interference with the signal. If severe peripheral vasoconstriction interferes with measurements from a finger site, the sensor should be placed more centrally (e.g., the bridge of the nose).

CAPNOMETRY

Clinical Brief

Capnometry is a continuous, noninvasive method for evaluating the adequacy of CO_2 exchange in the lungs.

Indications

Capnometry is useful in the mechanically ventilated patient who requires frequent blood gas sampling or who has an unstable respiratory status where minute-to-minute assessment of gas exchange is necessary. Patient response to different modes of ventilation and tolerance to weaning can be assessed using capnometry.

Description

Capnometry is the measurement of CO_2 concentration in respired gas. This concentration varies with the respiratory cycle; the inspired concentration is lowest, whereas the end tidal (P_{ETCO_2}) concentration is highest and is assumed to represent alveolar gas. End-tidal CO_2 can be used to estimate the pressure of CO_2 in arterial blood (Pa_{CO_2}), thus allowing the clinician to evaluate adequacy of CO_2 exchange in the lung. Two methods frequently used to monitor CO_2 in critical care are infrared absorption spectrophotometry and mass spectroscopy. CO_2 concentration can be displayed digitally or as a capnogram (recorded tracing of the waveform).

Values

Normal

P_{ETCO_2} is usually 1 to 4 mm Hg below Pa_{CO_2} in normal individuals.

Significance of abnormal values

The gradient between $Paco_2$ and $Petco_2$ is increased in patients with ventilation-perfusion mismatching and chronic obstructive pulmonary disease. Increased $Petco_2$ suggests an increase in $Paco_2$, perhaps as a result of hypoventilation, while decreased $Petco_2$ suggests hyperventilation. Changes in $Petco_2$ should prompt the nurse to assess the patient and obtain arterial blood gases when a deterioration in respiratory status is suspected.

ARTERIAL BLOOD GAS ANALYSIS

Clinical Brief

Arterial blood gas analysis is done to assess the acid-base balance of the body, the adequacy of oxygenation and/or ventilation, and the adequacy of circulation, and to detect metabolic abnormalities.

Indications

Arterial blood gas analysis may be done in any of the following clinical situations: (1) serious respiratory problems or prolonged weaning from mechanical ventilation, (2) cardiac dysfunction associated with decreased CO, and (3) shock states.

Description

A sample of blood (1 to 3 ml) is drawn from an artery and analyzed; the partial pressures of oxygen (Pao_2) and carbon dioxide ($Paco_2$) are determined, as well as the pH and bicarbonate ion levels and oxygen saturation.

The pH measures hydrogen ion concentration, which is an indication of acid-base balance. The body maintains a normal pH by keeping bicarbonate ion (a function of the kidneys) and $Paco_2$ (a function of the lungs) in a constant ratio of 20:1. When there is a disturbance in acid-base balance, there will be compensation by the system (respiratory or renal) *not* primarily affected to return the pH to normal. If the disturbance is respiratory, the kidneys compensate by altering bicarbonate excretion in order to return the pH to normal; however, the kidneys are slow to respond to changes in pH and compensation may take days. If the disturbance is metabolic, the respiratory system will compensate by increasing or decreasing ventilation (and CO_2 removal) to return the pH to normal; the lungs respond to changes in pH within minutes.

The $Paco_2$ level is adjusted by the rate and depth of ventilation: hypoventilation results in *high* $Paco_2$ levels, whereas hyperventilation results in *low* $Paco_2$ levels.

The Pao_2 reflects the amount of oxygen dissolved in arterial blood. Pao_2 does not directly influence the acid-base balance, although hypoxemia with anaerobic metabolism can lead to lactic acidosis.

Oxygen saturation reflects the amount of oxygen combined with hemoglobin that is carried in arterial blood. The oxygen-hemoglobin dissociation curve demonstrates the relationship between Pao_2 and O_2 saturation. As tissues utilize the oxygen dissolved in arterial blood, oxygen dissociates from the hemoglobin, causing a decrease in saturation. Significant changes in oxygen saturation occur when the Pao_2 falls below 60 mm Hg. Various conditions can affect the oxygen-hemoglobin affinity and thus affect oxygen availability for tissues (see Figure 3-10).

The bicarbonate ion level represents the renal component of acid-base regulation. The kidneys adjust the level of bicarbonate ion by changes in the excretion rate.

Values
Normal
pH 7.35-7.45
$Paco_2$ 35-45 mm Hg

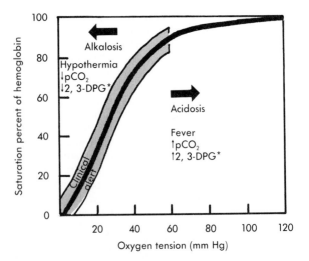

Figure 3-10 Oxyhemoglobin dissociation curve.

Pao$_2$ 80-100 mm Hg
O$_2$ saturation 95%-99%
Serum bicarbonate (HCO$_3$) 22-26 mEq/L
Significance of abnormal values
pH<7.35: acidosis, pH>7.45: alkalosis. It is impossible to determine the cause (respiratory or renal) of acidosis or alkalosis by looking at the pH alone.

Paco$_2$<35 mm Hg: respiratory alkalosis, caused by hyperventilation (may be secondary to ventilatory support, central nervous system disease, fever, liver disease, congestive heart failure, pulmonary embolism).

Paco$_2$>45 mm Hg: respiratory acidosis, caused by hypoventilation (may be secondary to impaired alveolar ventilation, respiratory depressants, intracranial tumors).

Pao$_2$<80 mm Hg: hypoxemia, with inadequate O$_2$ to meet tissue needs. If hypoxemia is left untreated, anaerobic metabolism and acidosis will result.

Pao$_2$>100 mm Hg: hyperoxemia, usually a result of excessive concentration of oxygen. Fio$_2$ should be lowered to produce Pao$_2$ > 60-70 mm Hg or O$_2$ saturation > 95%.

O$_2$ saturation <95%: hypoxemia.

HCO$_3$<22 mEq/L: metabolic acidosis (may be secondary to renal failure, lactic acidosis, diabetic ketoacidosis, diarrhea).

HCO$_3$>26 mEq/L: metabolic alkalosis (may be secondary to vomiting, ingestion of diuretics, nasogastric suction, steroid therapy, hyperaldosteronism, hyperadrenocorticism).
Steps to Interpret ABGs
1. Look at pH to determine whether imbalance is acidosis or alkalosis.
2. Look at Paco$_2$ and compare with pH; they are inversely proportional, so if the pH and Paco$_2$ are moving in opposite directions, the imbalance is the result of a respiratory problem.
3. Look at HCO$_3$ and compare with pH; they are directly proportional, so if the pH and HCO$_3$ are moving in the same direction, the imbalance is the result of a metabolic problem.
4. Compare Paco$_2$ and HCO$_3$ with each other; if they are moving in the same direction, one system is attempting to compensate for a disturbance in the opposite system. If they are moving in the opposite direction, a mixed imbalance is present. Usually the value that deviates most from normal is the primary disturbance.

5. Look at Pao_2 and O_2 saturation and determine whether they are decreased, normal, or increased; low values indicate the need for improved oxygenation and/or ventilation, and high values indicate the need to decrease the delivered concentration of oxygen.

Examples

1. pH 7.6 (increased)
   $Paco_2$ 25 mm Hg (decreased)
   HCO_3 24 mEq/L (normal)
   Disturbance: respiratory alkalosis, no compensation
2. pH 7.20 (decreased)
   $Paco_2$ 38 mm Hg (normal)
   HCO_3 15 mEq/L (decreased)
   Disturbance: metabolic acidosis, no compensation
3. pH 7.32 (decreased)
   $Paco_2$ 66 mm Hg (increased)
   HCO_3 28 mEq/L (increased)
   Disturbance: respiratory acidosis with kidneys trying to compensate (Note: Compensation is not complete until pH is within normal limits.)
4. pH 7.56 (increased)
   $Paco_2$ 32 mm Hg (decreased)
   HCO_3 38 mEq/L (increased)
   Disturbance: mixed metabolic and respiratory alkalosis

ECG MONITORING

Choosing a Lead

Three-lead system

1. Lead II (Figure 3-11): This is the most common lead used in cardiac monitoring. The advantage of this lead is that it allows observation of QRS axis changes associated with left anterior hemiblock.
2. Modified chest lead (MCL_1) (Figure 3-12): This lead is useful for differentiating left from right ectopic activity and ventricular tachycardia from supraventricular tachycardia. QRS complex is normally negative.
3. Lewis lead (Figure 3-13): This lead is useful for identification of atrial dysrhythmias.
4. MCL_6 lead (Figure 3-14): The use of this lead enables the clinician to switch from viewing MCL_1 to MCL_6 (V_6) by moving only the positive electrode. It is a useful lead in those patients with a median sternotomy.

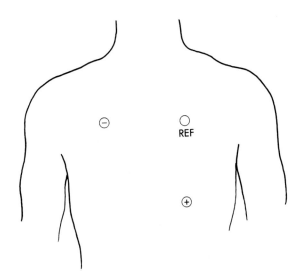

Figure 3-11 Lead II. Positive electrode—left leg; negative electrode—right arm.

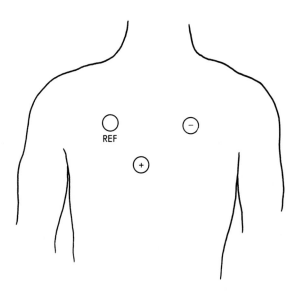

Figure 3-12 Lead MCL_1. Positive electrode—fourth intercostal space, right of sternum; negative electrode—beneath left midclavicle.

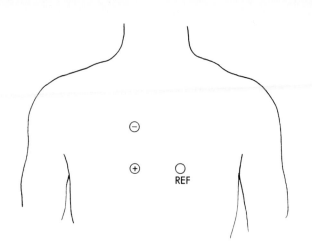

Figure 3-13 Lewis lead. Positive electrode—fourth intercostal space, right of sternum; negative electrode—second intercostal space, right of sternum.

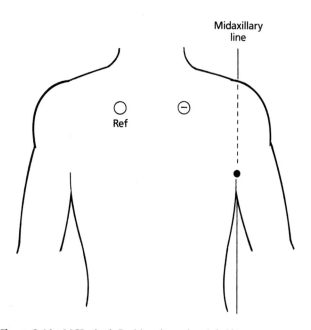

Figure 3-14 MCL$_6$ lead. Positive electrode—left fifth intercostal space, midaxillary line; negative electrode—below left clavicle.

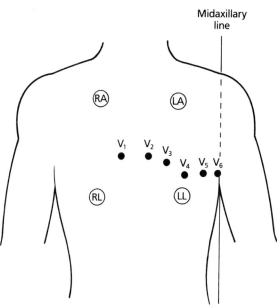

Figure 3-15 Five-lead system. RA electrode—below right clavicle, midclavicular line. LA electrode—below left clavicle, midclavicular line. RL electrode—sixth intercostal space, right midclavicular line. LL electrode—sixth intercostal space, left midclavicular line. Chest lead— place chest lead on V_1, V_2, V_3, V_4, V_5, or V_6 position.

Five-lead system (Figure 3-15)
This system allows the clinician to place the chest lead on se- lect sites on the chest for ECG monitoring.
Rhythm Strip Analysis
Heart rate determination
Standard ECG paper is made up of a series of 1 mm squares, with each millimeter equal to 0.04 seconds. Each group of 5 small squares is marked by a darker line, so that 1 large square (5 mm) equals 0.20 seconds (Figure 3-16).

See Figures 3-17 and 3-18 for determining heart rate.
Rhythm determination
To determine whether the rhythm is regular, measure the R- R or P-P intervals and determine whether the length is con- stant. The rhythm is regular if the length of the shortest and

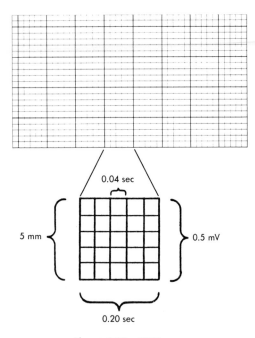

Figure 3-16 ECG paper.

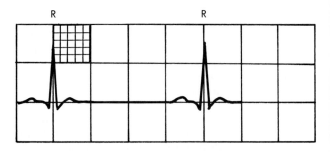

Figure 3-17 Heart rate determination with regular rhythm. Rate can be determined by dividing 300 by the number of large squares between cardiac cycles (300/4) or by dividing the number of small squares between cardiac cycles into 1500 (1500/20 = 75 beats/min).

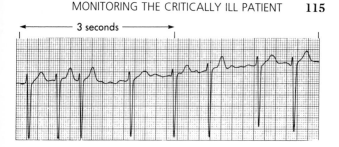

Figure 3-18   Heart rate determination with irregular rhythm. Heart rate can be approximated by multiplying the number of cardiac cycles in a 6-second period by 10; the heart rate is approximately 80.

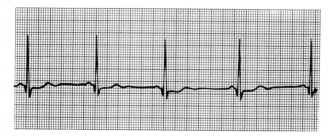

Figure 3-19   Sinus bradycardia. (From Conover M: Pocket guide to electrocardiography, ed 2, St Louis, 1990, The CV Mosby Co.)

longest interval varies by less than 0.16 seconds. If the rhythm is irregular, it should be determined whether there is any kind of pattern to the irregularity or if it is totally erratic.

In addition to the rate and regularity of the rhythm, the PR and QRS intervals must be determined, as well as the relationship of atrial activity (P waves) to ventricular activity (QRS complex) (see Table 2-3). Normal PR interval is 0.12-0.20 seconds in duration and normal QRS interval is 0.10 seconds in duration. QT interval is usually less than half the preceding R-R interval.

Dysrhythmias
Sinus bradycardia (Figure 3-19)
1. Determinants
   Rhythm: Regular
   Rate: Less than 60

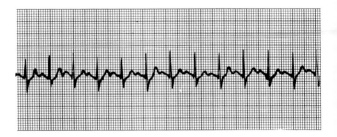

Figure 3-20 Sinus tachycardia. (From Conover M: Pocket guide to electrocardiography, ed 2, St Louis, 1990, The CV Mosby Co.)

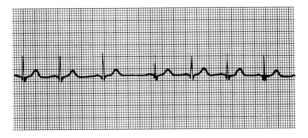

Figure 3-21 Sinus arrhythmia. (From Conover M: Pocket guide to electrocardiography, ed 2, St Louis, 1990, The CV Mosby Co.)

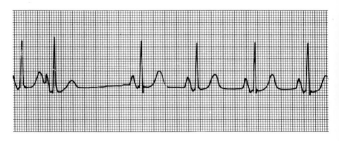

Figure 3-22 Premature atrial complex. (From Conover M: Pocket guide to electrocardiography, ed 2, St Louis, 1990, The CV Mosby Co.)

P waves: Present, same morphology
PR interval: 0.12-0.20 seconds
QRS: 0.10 seconds, same morphology
Ratio (P:QRS): 1:1

2. Treatment: If the patient is asymptomatic, none. If the patient is symptomatic (i.e., hypotensive, syncopal), the treatment is atropine, isoproterenol, pacemaker. (See Figure A-5, Appendix A.)

Sinus tachycardia (Figure 3-20)

1. Determinants
   Rhythm: Regular
   Rate: 100-160
   P waves: Present, same morphology
   PR interval: 0.12-0.20 seconds
   QRS: 0.10 seconds, same morphology
   Ratio: 1:1
2. Treatment: Treat the cause, e.g., stress/anxiety, fever, pain, hypoxia, hyperthyroidism. β Blockers may be necessary.

Sinus arrhythmia (Figure 3-21)

1. Determinants
   Rhythm: Irregular, varies by more than 0.16 seconds
   Rate: 60-100
   P waves: Present, same morphology
   PR interval: 0.12-0.20 seconds
   QRS: 0.10 seconds, same morphology
   Ratio: 1:1
2. Treatment: None

Premature atrial complex (Figure 3-22)

1. Determinants
   Rhythm: Regular except for ectopic beats
   Rate: 60-100
   P waves: Present, same morphology except for ectopic beat
   PR interval: 0.12-0.20 seconds (PR interval of the ectopic beat may vary from the others)
   QRS: 0.10 seconds, same morphology
   Ratio: 1:1
2. Treatment: Usually none

Atrial tachycardia with block (Figure 3-23)

1. Determinants
   Rhythm: Regular
   Rate: Atrial rate 150-250, ventricular rate less than atrial rate due to lack of conduction through the AV node

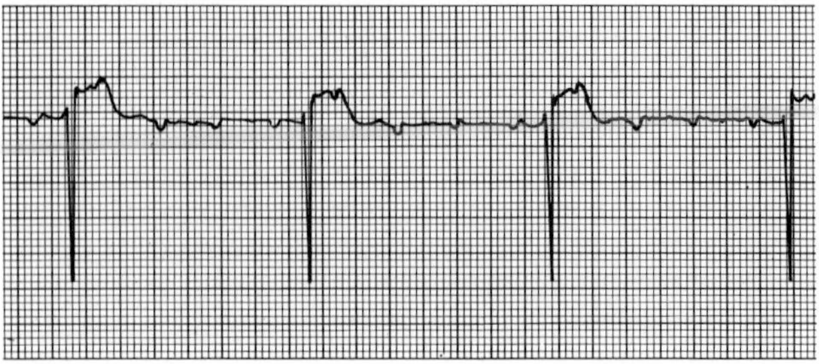

Figure 3-23 Atrial tachycardia with block. (From Conover M: Pocket guide to electrocardiography, ed 2, St Louis, 1990, The CV Mosby Co.)

P waves: Present, same morphology, may be hidden as a result of the extremely rapid rate
PR interval: 0.12-0.20 seconds
QRS: 0.10 seconds, same morphology
Ratio: 2:1 most common
2. Treatment: If symptomatic, carotid massage, Valsalva maneuver, verapamil, cardioversion

Atrial flutter (Figure 3-24)
1. Determinants
Rhythm: Atrial rhythm is regular; ventricular rhythm regular or irregular, depending on the degree of blocking
Rate: Atrial rate 250-400; ventricular rate usually less than 150 (depends on the degree of blocking)
P waves: Absent; replaced by flutter waves, which have a sawtooth appearance
PR interval: None
QRS: 0.10 seconds, same morphology
Ratio: 2:1 is most common in the untreated patient; 4:1 is most common in the treated patient; varying conduction may be present, which results in irregular rhythm
2. Treatment: For rapid and symptomatic rates, cardioversion; may also be treated with β blockers, calcium channel blockers, or digitalis

Atrial fibrillation (Figure 3-25)
1. Determinants
Rhythm: Irregular

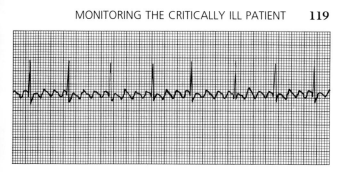

Figure 3-24   Atrial flutter. (From Conover M: Pocket guide to electrocardiography, ed 2, St Louis, 1990, The CV Mosby Co.)

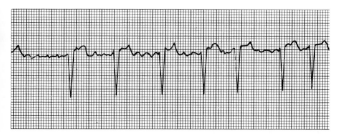

Figure 3-25   Atrial fibrillation. (From Conover M: Pocket guide to electrocardiography, ed 2, St Louis, 1990, The CV Mosby Co.)

Rate: Atrial rate greater than 350; ventricular rate is variable
P waves: None; fibrillatory waves create a wavy, undulating baseline
PR interval: None
QRS: 0.10 seconds, normal morphology
Ratio: None; many fibrillatory waves per QRS
2. Treatment: If symptomatic, immediate synchronized cardioversion; digitalis, verapamil, quinidine may be required

Accelerated idioventricular rhythm (Figure 3-26)
1. Determinants
Rhythm: Regular
Rate: 40-100 beats/min
P waves: Absent

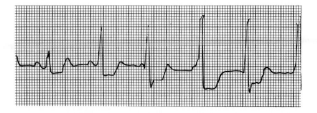

Figure 3-26 Accelerated idioventricular rhythm. (From Conover M: Pocket guide to electrocardiography, ed 2, St Louis, 1990, The CV Mosby Co.)

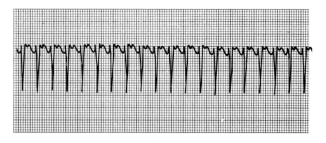

Figure 3-27 Paroxysmal supraventricular tachycardia. (From Conover M: Pocket guide to electrocardiography, ed 2, St Louis, 1990, The CV Mosby Co.)

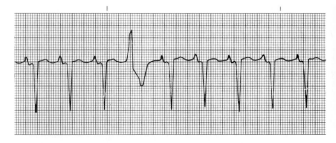

Figure 3-28 Premature ventricular complex. (From Conover M: Pocket guide to electrocardiography, ed 2, St Louis, 1990, The CV Mosby Co.)

PR interval: None
QRS: Wide (>0.12 seconds), bizarre appearance with same morphology
Ratio: None

2. Treatment: None unless hemodynamically unstable, then treat as with other bradydysrhythmias (atropine, isoproterenol, and/or pacemaker)

Paroxysmal supraventricular tachycardia (Figure 3-27)

1. Determinants

Rhythm: Regular; occurs in bursts that begin and end abruptly
Rate: 150-250
P waves: Cannot be clearly identified; may distort the preceding T wave
PR interval: None measurable
QRS: 0.10 seconds, same morphology
Ratio: Unable to determine

2. Treatment: If symptomatic, cardioversion. (See Figure A-7, Appendix A.)

Premature ventricular complex (Figure 3-28)

1. Determinants

Rhythm: Regular except for the ectopic beat(s)
Rate: 60-100, varies with the underlying rhythm
P waves: Present (except for the ectopic beat); same morphology
PR interval: 0.12-0.20 seconds
QRS: 0.10 seconds except for the ectopic beat (wide [>0.12 seconds] and bizarre morphology)
Ratio: 1:1 except for ectopic beat

2. Treatment: None if benign; if greater than 6/min, couplets, multifocal, or PVCs that fall on the preceding T wave, treat with lidocaine, procainamide, bretylium

Ventricular tachycardia (Figure 3-29)

1. Determinants

Rhythm: Regular or slightly irregular
Rate: 100-180
P waves: Usually not seen; if present, will be dissociated from ventricular rhythm
PR interval: None measurable
QRS: Wide (>0.12 seconds) and bizarre morphology
Ratio: None

2. Treatment: If conscious with a pulse: cardiovert if unstable or administer lidocaine if the patient is stable. (See

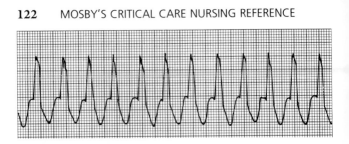

Figure 3-29 Ventricular tachycardia. (From Conover M: Pocket guide to electrocardiography, ed 2, St Louis, 1990, The CV Mosby Co.)

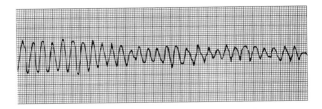

Figure 3-30 Ventricular fibrillation. (From Conover M: Pocket guide to electrocardiography, ed 2, St Louis, 1990, The CV Mosby Co.)

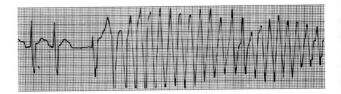

Figure 3-31 Torsade de pointes. (From Conover M: Pocket guide to electrocardiography, ed 2, St Louis, 1990, The CV Mosby Co.)

Figure A-3, Appendix A.) If the patient is unconscious without a pulse, defibrillate (see Figure A-3, Appendix A)

Ventricular fibrillation (Figure 3-30)
1. Determinants
   Rhythm: Irregular, chaotic baseline
   Rate: Unable to measure

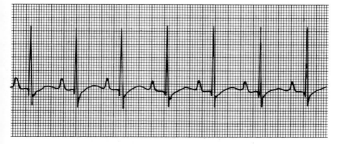

Figure 3-32   First-degree AV block. (From Conover M: Pocket guide to electrocardiography, ed 2, St Louis, 1990, The CV Mosby Co.)

    P waves: None
    PR interval: None
    QRS: None
    Ratio: None
2. Treatment: CPR until defibrillator available, then rapid defibrillation beginning at 200 joules; defibrillation may be repeated three times at successively higher levels if restoration of rhythm does not occur. (See Figure A-2, Appendix A.)

Torsade de pointes (Figure 3-31)

1. Determinants
    Rhythm: Regular or slightly irregular
    Rate: 150-250
    P waves: Usually not seen; if present, will be dissociated from ventricular rhythm
    PR interval: None measurable
    QRS: Wide (>0.12 seconds) and bizarre morphology; QRS complexes appear to be constantly changing and twist in a spiral pattern around the baseline
    Ratio: None
2. Treatment: IV magnesium sulfate or magnesium chloride; temporary overdrive pacing. Identify and treat cause: toxicity to type 1A antidysrhythmic agents; hypokalemia, digitalis toxicity, hypocalcemia, hypomagnesemia, coronary artery spasm

First-degree AV block (Figure 3-32)

1. Determinants
    Rhythm: Regular
    Rate: 60-100

P waves: Normal, same morphology
PR interval: Greater than 0.20 seconds
QRS: 0.10 seconds, same morphology
Ratio: 1:1

2. Treatment: Usually none unless associated with symptomatic bradycardia

Second-degree AV block (Type I) (Figure 3-33)

1. Determinants
Rhythm: Irregular
Rate: Atrial rate 60-100; ventricular rate is slower as a result of dropped beats
P waves: Normal, same morphology
PR interval: Progressive lengthening with each beat until a P wave is nonconducted; the PR interval is reset to normal with the dropped beat and the cycle of PR lengthening begins again
QRS: Normal, same morphology

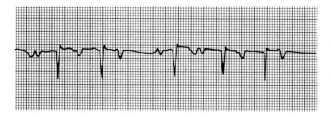

Figure 3-33 Second-degree AV block, type I. (From Conover M: Pocket guide to electrocardiography, ed 2, St Louis, 1990, The CV Mosby Co.)

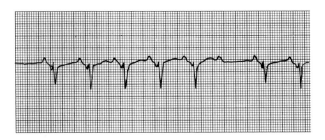

Figure 3-34 Second-degree AV block, type II. (From Conover M: Pocket guide to electrocardiography, ed 2, St Louis, 1990, The CV Mosby Co.)

Ratio: 1:1 until beat is nonconducted, then 2:1
2. Treatment: If symptomatic, treat as with bradydysrhythmias (atropine, isoproterenol, pacemaker).

Second-degree AV block (Type II) (Figure 3-34)

1. Determinants

   Rhythm: Regular except for dropped beats

   Rate: Atrial 60-100; ventricular rate is slower due to dropped beats

   P waves: Normal, same morphology

   PR interval: 0.12-0.20 seconds, except where beat is nonconducted

   QRS: Normal, same morphology

   Ratio: 1:1 except when P waves are nonconducted

2. Treatment: Careful monitoring; there is a high tendency to progress to complete heart block; if the patient is symptomatic: atropine, isoproterenol, pacemaker

Third-degree heart block (complete heart block) (Figure 3-35)

1. Determinants

   Rhythm: Regular

   Rate: Atrial 60-100; ventricular depends on site of escape rhythm, usually 20-60

   P waves: Normal, same morphology

   PR interval: Not measurable; no association between atrial rhythm and ventricular rhythm

   QRS: Normal (<0.12 seconds) if from AV junction; widened (>0.12 seconds) if from below bundle of His

   Ratio: Variable; atrial rate is greater than ventricular rate

2. Treatment: Atropine, isoproterenol, pacemaker

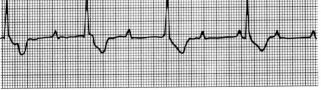

Figure 3-35 Third-degree AV block (complete heart block). (From Conover M: Pocket guide to electrocardiography, ed 2, St Louis, 1990, The CV Mosby Co.)

REFERENCES

1. Baele PL et al: Continuous monitoring of mixed venous oxygen saturation in critically ill patients, Anesth Analg 61(6):513, 1982.
2. Campbell ML and Greenberg CA: Reading pulmonary artery wedge pressure at end-expiration, Focus Crit Care 15(2):60, 1988.
3. Carlon CG et al: Capnography in mechanically ventilated patients, Crit Care Med 16:550, 1988.
4. Cengiz M, Crapo RO, and Gardner RM: The effect of ventilation on the accuracy of pulmonary artery and wedge pressure measurements, Crit Care Med 11(7):502, 1983.
5. Chulay M and Miller T: The effect of backrest elevation on pulmonary artery and pulmonary capillary wedge pressures in patients after cardiac surgery, Heart Lung 13(2):138, 1984.
6. Chyun D: A comparison of intra-arterial and auscultatory blood pressure readings, Heart Lung 14(3):223, 1985.
7. Civetta JM, Taylor RW, and Kirby RR: Textbook of critical care, Philadelphia, 1988, JB Lippincott Co.
8. Conover MB: Pocket guide to electrocardiography, ed 2, St Louis, 1990, The CV Mosby Co.
9. Cross JA and Vargo RL: Cardiac output: iced versus room temperature solution, DCCN 7(3):146, 1988.
10. Daily EK and Schroeder JS: Techniques in bedside hemodynamic monitoring, ed 4, St Louis, 1989, The CV Mosby Co.
11. Daily EK and Tilkian AG: Hemodynamic monitoring. In Tilkian AG and Daily (editors): Cardiovascular procedures, St Louis, 1986, The CV Mosby Co.
12. Darovic GO: Hemodynamic monitoring: invasive and noninvasive clinical application, Philadelphia, 1987, WB Saunders Co.
13. Divertie MB and McMichan JC: Continuous monitoring of mixed venous oxygen saturation, Chest 85(3):423, 1984.
14. Enger EL: Pulmonary artery wedge pressure: When it's valid, when it's not, Crit Care Nurs Clin North Am 1(3):603, 1989.
15. Fahey PJ, Harris K, and Vanderwarf C: Clinical experience with continuous monitoring of mixed venous oxygen saturation in respiratory failure, Chest 86(5):748, 1984.
16. Garnett AR et al: End-tidal carbon dioxide monitoring during cardiopulmonary resuscitation, JAMA 257:512, 1987.
17. Germon K: Interpretation of ICP pulse waves to determine intracerebral compliance, J Neurosci Nurs 20(6):344, 1988.
18. Gilliam EE: Intracranial hypertension: advances in intracranial pressure monitoring, Crit Care Nurs Clin North Am 2(1):21, 1990.

19. Groom L, Elliott M, and Frisch S: Injectate temperature: effects on thermodilution CO measurements, Crit Care Nurse 10(5):112, 1990.

20. Hickey JV: The clinical practice of neurological and neurosurgical nursing, ed 2, Philadelphia, 1986, JB Lippincott Co.

21. Hickman KM, Mayer BL, and Muwaswes M: Intracranial pressure monitoring: review of risk factors associated with infection, Heart Lung 19(1):84, 1990.

22. Hudson-Civetta J and Banner TE: Intravascular catheters: current guidelines for care and maintenance, Heart Lung 12(5):466, 1983.

23. Hurst JM: Invasive hemodynamic monitoring: an overview, J Emerg Nurs 10(1):11, 1984.

24. Jamieson WRE et al: Continuous monitoring of mixed venous oxygen saturation in cardiac surgery, Can J Surg 25(5):538, 1982.

25. Johnson KC: Hemodynamic monitoring. In Miller S (editor): AACN procedure manual for critical care, Philadelphia, 1985, WB Saunders Co.

26. Kaye W: Invasive monitoring techniques: arterial cannulation, bedside pulmonary artery catheterization, and arterial puncture, Heart Lung 12(4):395, 1983.

27. Lazarus M, Nolasco V, and Luckett C: Cardiac arrhythmias: diagnosis and treatment, Crit Care Nurse 8(7):57, 1988.

28. Lynch L: Torsade de pointes: a malignant arrhythmia, Am J Nurs 86(7):826, 1986.

29. North JB and Reilly PL: A comparison between three methods of ICP recording. In Miller JD et al (editors): Intracranial pressure VI, New York, 1986, Springer-Verlag.

30. Rudy EB: Advanced neurological and neurosurgical nursing, St Louis, 1984, The CV Mosby Co.

31. St. John RE: Exhaled gas analysis: technical and clinical aspects of capnography and oxygen consumption, Crit Care Nurs Clin North Am 1(4):669, 1990.

32. Schermer L: Physiologic and technical variables affecting hemodynamic measurements, Crit Care Nurse 8(2):33, 1988.

33. Taylor T: Monitoring left atrial pressures in the open-heart surgical patient, Crit Care Nurse 6(2):62, 1986.

34. Vennix CV, Nelson DH, and Pierpont GL: Thermodilution cardiac output in critically ill patients: comparison of room temperature and iced injectate, Heart Lung 13(5):574, 1984.

35. Woods SL and Mansfield LW: Effect of body position upon pulmonary artery and pulmonary capillary wedge pressures in noncritically ill patients, Heart Lung 5(1):83, 1976.

CHAPTER 4

Management of Behavioral Manifestations in the Critically Ill Patient

A patient may experience a myriad of fears and concerns when admitted to the technologically sophisticated world of critical care. The patient enters a complex setting where staff members converge with many procedures and devices in an attempt to strengthen or stabilize the physiological condition. The patient is immediately separated from significant others and surrounded by strangers who move about the critical care environment with familiarity and professional expertise. Although the patient may feel secure knowing that skilled and knowledgeable health care personnel are attending to the physiological crisis, feelings of anxiety, anger, depression, hopelessness, and powerlessness may also be experienced during the critical illness.

Anxiety occurs as a reaction to a threat to the person; the threat encompasses potential physiological loss, lifestyle changes, potential death, invasive procedures, or concerns about the unknown. The critically ill patient's biological integrity has been temporarily or permanently compromised, and the patient responds by becoming anxious.

As the patient's illness, injury, or disease begins to stabilize, anger may be manifested. Anger may be expressed verbally or turned inward in the form of blame or depression. The critically ill patient who has always enjoyed good health experiences tremendous stress when confronted with an illness that leads to limitations, disability, or disfigurement.

Depression can also result when feelings associated with a major loss have broken through an individual's defense. The patient's normal performance is decreased, leading to a perceived negative view of self, experiences, and the future. Depression is also a manifestation of felt hopelessness.

Hopelessness is associated with the patient's feeling of personal deficit and is an attempt to ward off feelings of despair. The critically ill patient may feel that a particular physiological alteration is irreversible and that there are no alternatives available. Generally, the patient is unable to cope and unable to mobilize energy on the patient's own behalf.

Powerlessness is a perceived lack of control. The patient feels unable to control the outcomes of the illness. In this instance, the critically ill patient feels physiological, cognitive, environmental, and decisional powerlessness.

Regardless of the specific behavioral manifestations, critical care nurses can reduce the patient's feelings of anxiety, direct anger to the appropriate source, and assist the patient in recognizing a positive view of self, experiences, and the future. The nurse can also provide a realistic sense of hope and can foster physiological, cognitive, environmental, and decisional control.

ANXIETY

Clinical Brief

Anxiety is a state of apprehension or tension within a person that occurs when an interpersonal need for security and/or freedom from tension is not met. Anxiety's origin is nonspecific or unknown to the individual.

Risk factors

Lack of control over events
Threats to self-control
Threat of illness or disease
Threat of hospital environment
Separation from others
Role changes
Sensorimotor loss
Financial problems
Threat of death
Divorce
Unemployment
Forced retirement
Threat of invasive procedures or supportive devices
Situational or maturational crisis
Loss of status
Unfamiliar environmental settings
Inability to comprehend the consequences of illness
Obstruction of goals
Dependence
Lack of knowledge
Loss of decision-making power

Presenting signs and symptoms

Regulatory	Cognitive
Palpitations	Apprehension
Nausea	Nervousness
Increased respiratory rate	Fear
Increased heart rate	Agitation
Diaphoresis	Irritability
Muscle tension	Withdrawal
Vertigo	Anger
Elevated blood pressure	Regression
Hand tremors	Inability to concentrate
Increased palmar sweating	Forgetfulness
Increased gastrointestinal activity	Lack of initiative or motivation
Insomnia	Escape behavior
Urinary frequency and urgency	Helplessness
Dilated pupils	Loss of control
Flushing	Thinking of past versus present
Faintness	Crying
Dry mouth	Loss of self-confidence
Paresthesia	Worry
Vomiting	Tension
Dilation of bronchioles	Overexcitement
Weakness	Reduced perceptual field
	Excessive verbalization

▶ **Nursing Diagnosis:** Anxiety
Patient outcomes
- The patient's agitation eases in response to specific therapeutic relaxation interventions.
- The patient recognizes the anxiety and verbalizes anxious feelings.
- The patient, family, or significant other exhibits a reduction in anxiety.
- The patient experiences an increase in physiological comfort.

- The patient initiates measures to decrease the onset of anxiety.
- The patient uses appropriate coping mechanisms in controlling anxiety.

Interventions

1. Provide information about threatening or stressful situations, including invasive procedures.
2. Orient patients to the environment, staff, and potentially threatening procedures so they know what to expect.
3. Encourage patients to acknowledge and verbalize their fears.
4. Minimize anxiety-provoking stimuli in the environment.
5. Provide accurate information regarding the current illness and care outcomes.
6. Help the patient establish goals, knowing that small accomplishments can promote feelings of independence and self-esteem.
7. Use distraction technique to focus the patient's attention on nonthreatening stimuli that counteract those eliciting anxiety.
8. Provide information regarding sensations that might be expected during potentially painful procedures.
9. Encourage the use of externally oriented relaxation techniques: progressive muscle relaxation, biofeedback, or hypnosis.
10. Encourage the use of internally oriented relaxation techniques: autogenic relaxation, meditation, or imagery.
11. Allow the patient a degree of control in personal self-care.
12. Explain the purpose of interventions and changes in care in brief, simple terms and at repetitive intervals.
13. Give the patient positive feedback when alternative coping strategies are used to counteract feelings of anxiety.
14. Use therapeutic touch to relax the patient before and during perceived stressful situations.
15. Clarify the patient's reaction to anxiety.
16. Establish a reassuring interpersonal relationship with the patient.

17. Plan the transfer out of critical care and discuss it with the patient.
18. Administer antianxiety agents and monitor the patient's response, noting potential side effects.

ANGER

Clinical Brief

Anger is an emotional defense that occurs in an attempt to protect the individual's integrity and does not involve a destructive element. Anger is a relatively automatic response that occurs when the individual is threatened and can be internalized or externalized.

Risk factors

Anger expression inhibited: Internalization
    Perceived threat involving:
        Blocked goal
        Failure of individuals to live up to the patient's expectations
        Disappointment
        Blow to self-concept
        Illness perceived to be life-threatening
        Physical dependence
        Altered social integrity
    Agent of harm located:
        Authoritative figure (health care giver) perceived to be threatening
        Family
        Self
Anger directly expressed: Externalization
    Perceived threat involving:
        Obstructed goal
        Role changes
        Financial dependence
    Agent of harm located:
        Environment
        Critical care team

Presenting signs and symptoms

Regulatory	Cognitive
Increased blood pressure	Clenched muscles or fists
Increased pulse rate	Turned away body
Increased respirations	Avoidance of eye contact
Muscle tension	Tardiness

Perspiration	Silence
Flushed skin	Sarcasm
Nausea	Insulting remarks
Dry mouth	Verbal abuse
	Argumentativeness
	Demanding attitude

▶ **Nursing Diagnosis: Coping, ineffective: anger**
Patient outcomes
- The patient is able to identify situations contributing to expressions of anger.
- The patient monitors behavior leading to internalization or externalization of anger.

Interventions
  1. Assist the patient to identify the prehospital situations contributing to the expression of anger.
  2. Teach the patient to evaluate feelings that lead to either internalization or externalization of anger.
  3. Assist the patient to identify situations in which anger is felt.
  4. Encourage the patient to acknowledge and express feelings of anger.
  5. Assist the patient to use alternative coping strategies.
  6. Teach the patient to use progressive relaxation technique, meditation, or guided imagery to reduce feelings of anger and hostility.
  7. Assist the patient to identify positive aspects of the illness or injury.
  8. Encourage the family to accept the patient's behavior without judgment.
  9. Encourage the patient to participate in decision making and self-care.
  10. Provide diversional activities as a way to reduce stress.
  11. Explore with the patient reasons behind angry feelings.
  12. Explore ways in which the patient's behavior can change.
  13. Establish a reassuring interpersonal relationship so that the patient can express angry feelings.

DEPRESSION
Clinical Brief
Depression is any decrease in normal performance, such as slowing of psychomotor activity or reduction of intellectual

functioning. It covers a wide range of changes in the affective state, ranging in severity from normal, everyday moods of sadness or despondency to psychotic episodes with risk of suicide.

Risk factors

PHYSIOLOGICAL CAUSES

Cardiac and vascular disease:
  Arteriosclerosis
  Congestive heart failure
  Hypertension
  Postmyocardial infarction
Drugs:
  Sedatives
  Tranquilizers
  Antihypertensive medications
    Clonidine
    Methyldopa
    Propranolol
    Reserpine
  Corticosteroids
Electrolyte imbalance:
  Bicarbonate excess
  Hypercalcemia
  Hypomagnesemia
  Hyperkalemia (uremic patient)
  Hypokalemia (vomiting, diarrhea, steroids)
  Hyponatremia

PSYCHOSOCIAL CAUSES

Financial loss
Feeling of powerlessness
Guilt
Role changes
Lifestyle changes
Separation from significant others
Threat to body integrity
Loss of control

Presenting signs and symptoms

Regulatory	Cognitive
Constipation	Agitation
Diarrhea	Anger
Headaches	Anxiety

Indigestion
Insomnia
Menstrual changes
Muscle aches
Nausea
Tachycardia
Ulcers
Weight loss or gain
Anorexia

Avoidance
Boredom
Careless appearance
Confusion
Crying
Denial
Dependence
Emptiness
Fatigue
Fearfulness
Feeling of worthlessness
Guilt
Hopelessness
Indecisiveness
Indifference
Irritability
Loss of interest
Loss of feeling
Low self-esteem
Poor communication skills
Sadness
Self-criticism
Sleep disturbance
Slow thinking
Social withdrawal
Submissiveness
Tension
Tiredness

Nursing Diagnosis: Coping, ineffective: depression
Patient outcomes
- The patient will be able to verbalize when feeling depressed.
- The patient initiates measures to decrease feelings of depression.
- The patient uses appropriate coping mechanisms in controlling depression.

Interventions

1. Assist the patient to achieve a positive view of self by facilitating accurate perception of the illness, disease, or injury.
2. Assist the patient to facilitate realistic appraisal of role changes.
3. Encourage the patient to assume decision-making control in the care.
4. Give the patient positive feedback when the patient accomplishes specific tasks.
5. Provide the patient with personal space in the technical environment.
6. Encourage the patient to participate in self-care.
7. Encourage the patient to discuss the illness, treatment, or prognosis.
8. Assist the patient in identifying situations contributing to feelings of depression.
9. Assist the patient to establish realistic goals, knowing that small accomplishments can enhance positive feelings of the future.
10. Administer antidepressive agents and monitor the patient's response, noting any potential side effects.

HOPELESSNESS

Clinical Brief

Hopelessness is an emotional state displaying the sense of impossibility, the feeling that life is too much to handle. It is a subjective state in which an individual sees limited or no alternatives or personal choices available and is unable to mobilize energy in own behalf.

Risk factors

Threats to internal resources:
> Autonomy
> Self-esteem
> Independence
> Strength
> Integrity
> Biological security

Threats to perceptions of external resources:
> Environment
> Staff
> Family

Abandonment

Failing or deteriorating condition
Long-term stress

Presenting signs and symptoms

Regulatory	Cognitive
Weight loss	Reduced activity
Appetite loss	Lack of initiative
Weakness	Decreased response to stimuli
Sleep disorder	Decreased affect
	Passivity
	Interference with learning
	Muteness
	Closing eyes
	Saddened expression
	Noncompliance with treatment regimen

▶ **Nursing Diagnosis: Hopelessness**
Patient outcomes
- The patient will maintain adequate self-care.
- The patient will assess situations causing feelings of hopelessness.
- The patient will identify feelings of hopelessness and goals for self.
- The patient maintains relationships with significant others.

Interventions
1. Provide an atmosphere of realistic hope.
2. Inform the patient of progress with the illness, disease, or injury.
3. Create the environment to facilitate the patient's active participation in self-care.
4. Teach the patient how to identify feelings of hopelessness.
5. Provide the patient with positive feedback for successful attempts at becoming involved in self-care.
6. Encourage the patient to express feelings about self and illness by active listening and asking open-ended questions.
7. Motivate the patient to begin participating in the care.
8. Encourage physical activities that give the patient a feeling of progress and hope.

9. Evaluate whether physical discomfort is causing the patient's feeling of hopelessness.
10. Encourage the patient to accept help from others.
11. Assist the patient to identify and use alternative coping mechanisms.

POWERLESSNESS

Clinical Brief

Powerlessness is the perceived lack of control over current and future physiological, psychological, and environmental situations.

Risk factors

Sensorimotor loss
Inability to communicate
Inability to perform roles
Lack of knowledge
Lack of privacy
Social isolation
Inability to control personal care
Separation from significant others
Loss of control to others
Lack of decision-making control
Fear of pain

Presenting signs and symptoms

Regulatory	Cognitive
Tiredness	Apathy
Fatigue	Withdrawal
Dizziness	Resignation
Headache	Empty feeling
Nausea	Feeling of lack of control
	Fatalism
	Malleability
	Lack of knowledge of illness
	Anxiety
	Uneasiness
	Acting out of behavior
	Restlessness
	Sleeplessness
	Aimlessness

Lack of decision making

Aggression

Anger

Expression of doubt about role performance

Dependence on others

Passivity

▶ **Nursing Diagnosis: Powerlessness**
Patient outcomes
- The patient is able to identify situations causing feelings of powerlessness.
- The patient exhibits control over the illness and care.
- The patient experiences an increase in physiological control.
- The patient engages in problem-solving and decision-making behaviors.
- The patient seeks information about the illness, treatment, and prognosis.
- The patient establishes realistic goals that foster an increased sense of control.

Interventions
1. Encourage the patient to identify situations in which powerlessness is felt.
2. Enhance effective communication between the patient, family, and health care team.
3. Provide information regarding the illness, treatment, and prognosis.
4. Encourage the patient to express feelings about self and illness.
5. Organize care so that the patient has consistent health care providers.
6. Encourage the patient to participate in making decisions pertaining to self-care.
7. Encourage the patient to ask questions and seek information.
8. Accept the patient's feelings of anger caused by a loss of control.
9. Provide the opportunity for control in establishing privacy.
10. Teach the patient about sensory changes associated with invasive procedures.

11. Teach the patient how to document progress through maintaining a journal.
12. Teach the patient how to accept the illness and potential changes in lifestyle.
13. Encourage the use of progressive relaxation, meditation, and guided imagery techniques to achieve a sense of acceptance or uncontrol (letting go).
14. Provide the patient with relevant educational information.
15. Provide the patient with decisional options.
16. Encourage the use of appropriate diversional activity such as play.
17. Assist the patient in redefining the illness situation to identify positive aspects.
18. Listen to the patient's discussion regarding possible role changes and financial concerns.

REFERENCES

1. Averill J: Anger and aggression: an essay on emotion, New York, 1982, Springer-Verlag.
2. Biaggio MK: Therapeutic management of anger, Clin Psychol Rev 7:663-675, 1987.
3. Carpenito LJ: Anxiety. Nursing Diagnosis Application to Clinical Practice New York, 1983, J.B. Lippincott, pp. 78-87.
4. Carpenito LJ: Powerlessness. Nursing Diagnosis Application to Clinical Practice New York, 1983, J.B. Lippincott, pp. 332-337.
5. Field N: Physical causes of depression, J Psychosoc Nurs Mental Health Serv 23:7-11, 1985.
6. Kendell PC, Watson D. Anxiety and Depression Distinctive and Overlapping Features. New York, 1989. Academic Press, Inc.
7. Light RW et al: Prevalence of depression and anxiety in patients in COPD, Chest 87:35-38, 1985.
8. McFarland GK and McFarlane EA: Anxiety, Nursing diagnosis and interventions: planning for patient care, St Louis, 1989, The CV Mosby Co.

9. McFarland GK and McFarlane EA: Hopelessness, Nursing diagnosis and interventions: planning for patient care, St Louis, 1989, The CV Mosby Co.

10. Moch SD: Towards a personal control/uncontrol balance, J Adv Nurs 13:119-123, 1988.

11. North American Nursing Diagnosis Association: Classification of nursing diagnosis: proceedings of the ninth national conference, St Louis, 1990, Mosby–Year Book, Inc.

12. Noyes R, Roth M and Burrows GD: Handbook of anxiety, New York, 1988, Elsevier Publishing.

13. Roberts SL: Anxiety, Nursing diagnosis and the critically ill patient, Norwalk, Conn, 1987, Appleton & Lange.

14. Roberts SL: Anger, Nursing diagnosis and the critically ill patient, Norwalk, Conn, 1987, Appleton & Lange.

15. Roberts SL: Depression, Nursing diagnosis and the critically ill patient, Norwalk, Conn, 1987, Appleton & Lange.

16. Roberts SL: Hopelessness, Nursing diagnosis and the critically ill patient, Norwalk, Conn, 1987, Appleton & Lange.

17. Roberts SL: Powerlessness, Nursing diagnosis and the critically ill patient, Norwalk, Conn, 1987, Appleton & Lange.

18. Roberts SL: Anger and hostility, Behavioral concepts and the critically ill patient, ed 2, Norwalk, Conn, 1986, Appleton-Century-Crofts.

19. Roberts SL: Depression, Behavioral concepts and the critically ill patient, ed 2, Englewood Cliffs, NJ, 1985, Prentice-Hall, Inc.

20. Roberts SL: Hopelessness, Behavioral concepts and the critically ill patient, ed 2, Englewood Cliffs, NJ, 1985, Prentice-Hall, Inc.

21. Roberts SL: Powerlessness, Behavioral concepts and the critically ill patient, ed 2, Englewood Cliffs, NJ, 1985, Prentice-Hall, Inc.

22. Roberts SL: Cognitive model of depression and the myocardial infarction patient, Prog Cardiovasc Nurs 4:61-70, 1989.

23. Rubin J: The emotion of anger: some conceptual and theoretical issues, Prof Psychol Res Pract 17:115-124, 1986.

24. Schneider J: Hopelessness and helplessness, J Psychosoc Nurs Mental Health Serv 23:12-21, 1985.

The Critically Ill Patient

Aspects of Nursing Common to All Critically Ill Patients

ELECTRICAL SAFETY

In the critical care environment, the increased complexity of the technology has also increased the potential for patient injury from electrical shock. Electrical systems should be designed to provide a grounding system that protects the patient and staff from becoming part of an electrical circuit and to protect critical care patients, who are electrically sensitive, from current leakage that may disrupt the electrical conduction system of the heart.

Conductors of electricity include all metals (for example, copper, silver, and iron) and ionic fluids. Insulators, which are highly resistant to the flow of electricity, include such items as rubber, glass, plastic, cotton, and intact dry skin. A ground is a low-resistance electrical pathway that is used to return stray current to the ground and is an important concept in electrical safety.

Nursing diagnosis: High risk for injury: Electrical shock

PATIENT OUTCOME

• Patient will not experience electrical shock.

INTERVENTIONS

1. Wear rubber gloves when handling uninsulated pacemaker wires or when adjusting pacemaker settings.
2. Place plastic caps or rubber sleeving over uninsulated wires and terminals.
3. Cover external pacemaker battery with a rubber glove.
4. Examine patient-owned equipment. Only battery-powered appliances should be allowed.
5. Inspect metal beds for adequate grounding.
6. Keep wet items (drinking water, saline, ice chips) off monitors and other electrical equipment.

7. Change wet bed linens and wipe up spills immediately.
8. Do not touch the patient and an electrical device simultaneously; touch the bed rails before touching the patient.
9. Observe the ECG tracing for 60-cycle interference, an indicator of current leakage. Replace patient cable or electrode pads. If these measures do not relieve the problem, identify and remove the offending equipment for repair.
10. Check all electrical equipment for a current safety inspection tag.
11. Inspect the plugs and cords of electrical devices, because these parts are the most susceptible to damage. Plugs should be three prong and damage free; cord line should be free from frayed wires or cracked insulation. Remove a plug from an outlet by grasping the plug, not pulling on the cord.
12. Turn equipment off before unplugging it.
13. Avoid using extension cords and connectors that allow three-prong plugs to be used in two-prong outlets.
14. Report malfunctioning or damaged equipment to the biomedical engineering department. Dropped equipment should be serviced by the biomedical engineering department before use, since the equipment may malfunction without visible signs of damage.

INFECTION CONTROL

Critically ill patients are exposed to many factors in addition to their underlying illness that depress the immune system and lower the body's defenses. The patient's own organisms, as well as environmental sources of organisms or cross-contamination can cause infection. The first, second, and third lines of defense can be adversely affected by therapeutic interventions, thus placing the patient at risk for infection.

The patient's first line of defense includes epithelial surfaces and secretions that provide a barrier between the internal and external environments. Table 5-1 lists a patient's first line of defense and examples that interrupt the system.

The patient's second line of defense involves the inflammatory response, which occurs when the first line of defense fails, or as a result of the patient's condition (for example, cancer, myocardial infarction). The response can be localized (red, edematous, warm, painful) or systemic (fever, malaise,

TABLE 5-1 First Line of Defense

Body system	Protective barrier	Conditions disrupting protective barriers
Integument	Skin	Pressure ulcers Surgical incisions Invasive lines Invasive procedures Burns Steroids
Pulmonary	Mucociliary escalator Reflexes: sneeze, cough, gag Normal flora	Intubation Endoscopic procedures Sedation Cranial nerve impairment Antibiotics
Gastrointestinal	Gastric pH Motility Intact mucosal epithelium Normal flora	NG/NI intubation H_2 antagonists Antacids Endoscopic procedures Antibiotics Electrolyte imbalance
Genitourinary	Micturation Urine pH Bladder mucosa Vaginal pH Normal flora	Urinary catheterization Incontinence Glycosuria Antibiotics

leukocytosis, neutrophilia). The inflammatory response always accompanies an infection; however, it can also occur without an infection. Factors that impair the inflammatory response include stress and pharmacological agents such as corticosteroids, immunosuppressants, and aspirin.

The patient's third line of defense involves acquired immunity. Malnutrition, age, anesthesia, radiation, and chemotherapy can adversely affect the third line of defense.

Nursing diagnosis: High risk for altered protection

PATIENT OUTCOMES

- Temperature 36.5° C-38.9° C (97.7° F-102° F)
- Absence of chills, diaphoresis
- Skin without redness and exudate
- Mucous membranes intact
- Clear breath sounds

- Absence of dysuria
- Urine clear yellow
- WBC 5-10 × $10^3/\mu l$

INTERVENTIONS

1. Avoid cross-contamination: wash hands, avoid sharing equipment, use sterile equipment, avoid "dirty" to "clean" activities.
2. Obtain temperature q4h and assess for diaphoresis and chills. Monitor serial WBC counts.
3. Maintain ICU environmental temperature ~75° F (23.8° C).

INTEGUMENT

1. Provide meticulous skin care:
   a. Assess pressure points (see Figure 5-1). Red areas that do not disappear in 15″ after the pressure is removed are the first sign of a pressure ulcer.
   b. Turn and reposition the patient at least q2h; provide ROM q2-4h to increase circulation.
   c. Use pressure-relieving or pressure-reducing devices, such as eggcrate or air mattress or specialty beds. Avoid "doughnuts," since these devices may increase pressure.

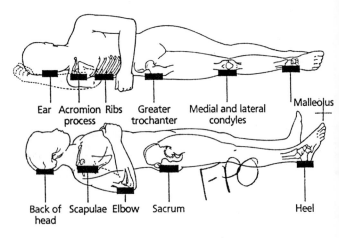

Figure 5-1 Pressure points.

    d. Moisturize skin sparingly, because too much moisture can macerate skin. Avoid vigorous massaging, since further damage to underlying tissue can occur.

    e. Clean skin of feces or urine immediately. Apply petrolatum ointment or a spray that protects against moisture to perianal area.

    f. Avoid skin stripping by using gauze or a stockinette to secure dressings if at all possible or Montgomery straps to avoid multiple tape applications.

2. Consult with nutritionist regarding the dietary needs of the patient. Patient should be hydrated and in positive nitrogen balance.

3. Avoid shearing forces by limiting HOB to no greater than 30 degrees. Use sheepskin elbow and heel protectors to prevent friction; however, pressure-reducing devices may be required.

4. Assess nares for pressure areas associated with NG or ET tubes; assess periostomal skin for chemical irritation; assess mouth and lips for dryness associated with NPO status.

5. Closely monitor patient receiving vasopressors for tissue ischemia.

6. Use sterile technique with invasive lines, incisions, tubings, drains, and so on. Keep stopcocks covered with sterile caps. Change wet or soiled dressings immediately.

7. Follow infection control protocol for changing IV sites, dressings, tubing, and solutions.

PULMONARY

1. Assess cough and gag reflexes to evaluate presence of protective reflexes.

2. Assess lungs for adventitious sounds.

3. Provide pulmonary hygiene: C & DB, chest physiotherapy, incentive spirometry.

4. Position the patient to facilitate chest excursion. Mobilize patient as soon as possible.

5. Keep HOB elevated or place the patient in sidelying position if LOC is decreased or the patient is receiving tube feedings. Turn tube feedings off during chest physiotherapy and bedscale weighing to prevent aspiration.

6. If the patient is intubated, check cuff pressure to prevent mucosal injury; drain respiratory circuit of water accumulation.

7. Use sterile technique when suctioning.
8. Ensure that respiratory equipment is replaced periodically, generally q24h.

GASTROINTESTINAL

1. Assess the patient's abdomen for distention or change in
   bowel sounds.
2. Prevent GI contamination by changing tube feeding
   containers q24h. Rinse container before adding new
   feeding to the bag. Fill container with enough tube
   feeding for 4 hours. Refrigerate unused feeding.
3. Assess for tube feeding residual q4h.

GENITOURINARY

1. Inspect urinary meatus for any drainage.
2. Assess urine for cloudiness, presence of glucose, or foul
   odor.
3. If the patient is incontinent of stool, clean the patient
   and the catheter tubing; avoid a back-and-forth motion
   on tubing, which could lead to fecal contamination of
   the urinary meatus.
4. Check catheter tubing for any kinks that may obstruct
   urine flow. Do not irrigate the catheter unless an obstruction is suspected. Keep the drainage bag lower than
   the patient's bladder. Secure the catheter to the patient's
   leg and avoid excessive manipulation of the catheter.
   Provide each patient with a container for emptying the
   drainage bag.
5. Remove the catheter as soon as possible.
6. When the catheter is removed, assess the patient for dysuria, frequency, urgency, and flank or labial pain.

NUTRITION

Adequate nutrition is essential in critically ill persons to decrease the risks of malnutrition-associated complications. Patients with fevers, burns, or trauma may require as much as
8000 to 10,000 kcal a day to meet their metabolic needs. Inability to ingest food orally because of unconsciousness,
weakness, dysphagia, intubation, vomiting, or trauma rapidly results in muscle catabolism. Not only can fluid and
electrolyte imbalance cause severe cardiopulmonary problems, but protein and mineral loss can also delay healing and
recovery, as well as lead to shock.

   To supply the calories needed for seriously ill persons to
regain their strength, most patients in the intensive care unit

receive nutritional support either by enteral or parenteral routes. Enteral nutrition is considered superior to parenteral nutrition, since it is physiological and maintains the integrity of the GI tract. (Disruption of intestinal mucosa may lead to hypermetabolism and multiple organ failure.) Parenteral nutrition is instituted when the GI tract is not functioning properly. Ongoing nutritional assessments are required and adjustments made based on the patient's response and changing caloric needs.

Nursing diagnosis: Altered nutrition: less than body requirements

PATIENT OUTCOMES

- Stabilized target weight
- Serum albumin 3.5-5 g/dl
- Serum transferrin >200
- Lymphocytes >1500 cells/mm^3
- Positive nitrogen balance

INTERVENTIONS

1. Conduct calorie counts to provide information about the adequacy of intake required to meet metabolic needs.
2. Compare serial weights; rapid (0.5-1.0 kg/day) changes indicate fluid imbalance and not an imbalance between nutritional needs and intake.
3. Assess GI status: bowel sounds, vomiting, diarrhea, or abdominal pain may interfere with nutritional absorption.
4. Review nutritional profile to evaluate patient response to therapy.
5. Consult with the nutritionist for formal nutritional evaluation.
6. Provide mouth care to prevent stomatitis, which can adversely affect the patient's ability to eat.
7. Create a pleasing environment; avoid offensive sights at the bedside; prepare the patient by making certain that hands and face have been washed.
8. Assist the patient as necessary, since fatigue and weakness or the presence of invasive equipment may discourage the patient from feeding self.
9. Administer enteral nutrition as prescribed. (See Chapter 6 for more information on nutrition.)
10. Administer parenteral nutrition as prescribed. (See Chapter 6 for more information on nutrition.)

FAMILY

The hospitalization of a family member can be very stressful and create specific needs for the family. If these needs go unmet, tension may mount, leading to major disorganization and ineffective coping. Although the critical care nurse intervenes to resolve life-threatening problems, a holistic approach to the patient, which includes the family, is essential to the well-being of the patient.

▶ **Nursing diagnosis:**   High risk for altered family process

FAMILY OUTCOMES

• Family will state that their needs are met.
• Family will demonstrate adequate coping behaviors.

INTERVENTIONS

1. Introduce yourself to the family. Display competence in caring for their relative.
2. Provide continuity of care givers whenever possible.
3. Approach the family with a relaxed and humanistic attitude and volunteer information frequently without waiting to be asked. Listen to their expressions of fear, anger, or anxiety. Provide the family a time away from the bedside to ventilate their concerns. Answer questions honestly and provide facts frequently regarding their relative's condition. Anticipate repeating information and allowing time for them to digest the information during this crisis period.
4. Provide the family with written information about the unit policies and services available. Information should include the phone number of the unit as well as location of the waiting room.
5. Obtain the family contact phone number and contact the family spokesperson at least daily with information about the patient's condition and any changes in medical or nursing care.
6. Clarify the family's perception of their relative's illness and validate their understanding of the situation. Let them know the staff cares for their relative and that the best care is being given. Allow family to "hope" as long as it does not interfere with the patient's care.
7. Individualize visiting hours; explain the equipment being used and why things are being done; assess family members' need to participate in their relative's care and allow as much participation as is reasonably possible. Be sensitive to the family's need to be left alone with

their relative. Arrange equipment so that family members can touch their relative.

8. Reassure the family that they will be contacted if the relative's condition worsens.

9. Offer the family an opportunity to meet with the hospital chaplain or social worker.

10. Encourage the family to meet their own physical and personal needs, such as eating and sleeping.

TEACHING-LEARNING

The critically ill patient requires constant intensive nursing care of life-threatening physiological problems. However, critical care nursing also focuses on supporting psychological and social integrity and restoring health. Teaching is an independent nursing activity that can assist the patient and family to understand the disease process and prescribed therapies so that the patient and family are provided the necessary information and resources to maintain optimal health.

Questions should be answered honestly and procedures explained; however, teaching should not be initiated when the patient and family are feeling the impact of the illness and expressing feelings of dying, loss of control, and hopelessness. Once the patient and family express the need for explanations or discuss the events that led to the ICU hospitalization, the patient and family may be ready to learn. Learning everything one needs to know will not occur in one ICU hospitalization; however, the process can be initiated in the ICU.

▶ **Nursing diagnosis:**   Knowledge deficit

PATIENT OUTCOMES

• Patient will verbalize accurate understanding of illness and treatment plan.

• Patient will demonstrate self management skills.

INTERVENTIONS

1. Assess the patient's and family's perception of the illness. Be sensitive to questions asked about the illness or a demonstrated interest in what is being done for them. Validate the learning need.

2. Provide information by answering questions immediately or if possible schedule a time to include the family and discuss the disease process, medications, dietary restrictions, activity level, signs and symptoms to report to a health care professional, or any procedure or therapeu-

tic measure the patient is interested in. Include other health care team members as needed to meet the learning needs of the patient and family.

3. Tailor the teaching to the patient's strengths. Take into account that fever, pain, fatigue, lack of sleep, fear, and some medications may interfere with the patient's learning. "Teaching sessions" may be incidental, but an overall plan should be developed based on the assessed needs. The plan should include patient outcomes, content to be learned, and strategies to facilitate learning.

4. Provide printed materials and written information as appropriate. Allow opportunities for answering questions and clarifying misconceptions.

5. Discuss available support services and resources; offer to contact the service if the patient or family request it (for example, social worker, dietician).

6. Forward a copy of the teaching-learning plan to the nursing staff when the patient is transferred from the ICU. Communicate the degree of learning (patient outcome achievement) to the staff and document the information in the chart.

7. If the patient is undergoing surgery, provide information about the surgical experience: preoperative expectations, including NPO status, breathing exercises, surgical preparation, and preoperative medications. Include specifics regarding the surgical procedure. Discuss the postoperative experience: nurse availability, pain control, ET tube and communication, IV lines, tubes and equipment, C & DB and early mobilization, as well as any specifics on the surgical procedure.

TRANSFER

When the critically ill patient is physiologically stable and is to be transferred, anxiety similar to separation anxiety may be experienced. Physically the patient is ready to transfer but psychologically may not feel secure about the move to the new environment. New nurse-patient relationships must be developed as trusting ICU nurse-patient relationships are terminated and family members decide to terminate their all night vigils, thinking their relative is "out of danger." Thus the patient's anxiety may be heightened during a time when support systems are needed yet less available.

▶ **Nursing diagnosis:**   Anxiety related to transfer

PATIENT OUTCOMES

- Patient will recognize own anxiety and verbalize anxious feelings.
- Patient will use appropriate coping mechanisms in controlling anxiety.

INTERVENTIONS

1. Discuss transfer plans early in an ICU hospitalization.
2. Keep the patient and family informed of any improvement and present the transfer in a positive manner; emphasize the recovery and not the need for a bed.
3. Explain what is expected of the patient and family in the new environment, such as what is restricted and what is not and the floor routine.
4. During the ICU stay, identify patient and family learning needs about the illness, medications, and signs and symptoms to report.
5. Allow the patient and family to verbalize their feelings and acknowledge these feelings.
6. Ideally, have the patient meet the new staff members before the actual transfer. Acknowledge the skill and expertise of the nurses on the unit to which the patient is to be transferred.
7. Transfer the patient during the day if at all possible so that the patient has time to become oriented to the new environment.
8. If the family is not present during the transfer, contact the family and inform them that their relative has been transferred.

Neurological Disorders

ACUTE SPINAL CORD INJURY (ASCI)
Clinical Brief

Most injuries to the spinal cord result from trauma and are usually associated with complete loss of function below the level of injury. Risk factors include lack of safety practices in driving, diving in shallow water, and other sports activities. Damage to the cord may also be related to tumors, abscesses, or other pathological conditions of the spine, such as congenital malformations or arthritis.

A *complete* spinal cord injury implies transection of the cord either in the form of a shearing injury, hemorrhagic contusion, or actual tear of the cord parenchyma. Complete injuries are associated with total loss of all motor and sensory functions below the level of the injury and represent irreversible spinal cord damage. Cervical cord injury is associated with a loss of motor function in the upper and lower extremities (quadriplegia), whereas injuries below the cervicothoracic junction affect only the lower extremities (paraplegia).

Incomplete spinal cord injuries are manifested by varying degrees of motor and sensory loss. The box on pp. 156-157 lists various syndromes associated with incomplete injuries.

Spinal shock is a state characterized by areflexia and flaccid paralysis that occurs immediately after the injury. The loss of reflexes and sensorimotor and autonomic function below the level of injury is temporary and may last a few hours to several weeks. The appearance of involuntary spastic movement indicates that spinal shock has ended.

Neurogenic shock is a syndrome characterized by hypotension and bradycardia; it can occur in patients with cervical cord injuries. The hemodynamic changes result from a disruption in the autonomic nervous system in which there is a loss of sympathetic outflow. The terms *spinal shock* and *neurogenic shock* tend to be used interchangeably with reference to acute spinal cord injury; however, spinal shock is more appropriate when referring to the sequelae of ASCI.

Incomplete Spinal Cord Lesion and Corresponding Acute Functional Loss

Anterior cord syndrome

Anterior cord syndrome is caused by damage to or an infarction of the anterior two thirds of the spinal cord. A hyperflexion injury of the cervical spine may cause bone fragments or disk material to collapse or press on the anterior spinal artery, which supplies two thirds of the anterior cord, while the posterior portion of the spinal cord is spared.

Patient presentation

- Loss of spinothalamic function (pain and temperature) below the level of the lesion
- Complete paralysis below the level of the lesion
- Spared posterior column function (position, pressure, vibration and light touch sensations)
- Hyperesthesia (unusual sensitivity to sensory stimuli) and hypalgesia (lessened sensitivity to pain) below the level of the lesion

Central cord syndrome

This syndrome is caused by damage or edema to the center portion of the spinal cord in the cervical region. There is central squeezing of the cord, while the periphery of the cord is spared. This pattern is usually associated with degenerative arthritis or osteophytic changes in the cervical vertebrae. A hyperextension injury can cause buckling of the ligamentum flavum, which in turn puts a "squeeze" on the cord as the column bends, interrupting the blood supply.

Patient presentation

- Motor loss in the upper extremities is greater than in the lower extremities, more profound in hands and fingers
- Leg function is usually intact but may be weak
- Sensory loss in upper extremities is greater than lower extremities and more profound in hands and fingers
- Bowel and bladder problems may or may not be present; some saddle sensation is retained

Posterior cord syndrome

Posterior cord syndrome is a very rare condition in which the posterior third of the spinal cord is affected. It is usually caused by a hyperextension injury or a direct penetrating mechanism, such as a knife wound.

Patient presentation

- Loss of positional sense, vibration, and light touch below the level of the lesion
- Motor function, pain, and temperature sense are usually intact

Brown-Sequard syndrome

Brown-Sequard syndrome is usually caused by a transverse hemisection of the cord. Damage is to one side of the cord only and is usually associated with a penetrating injury, herniated disk, or bone fragment.

Patient presentation

- Loss of position, vibration, and light touch sensation on the same side of the body (ipsilateral) below the level of the lesion
- Loss of motor function on the same side of the body (ipsilateral) below the level of the lesion
- Loss of pain and temperature sensation on the opposite side of the body (contralateral) below the level of the lesion

Horner's syndrome

This syndrome is caused by a partial cord transection at T1 or above. A lesion of either the preganglionic sympathetic trunk or the postganglionic sympathetic neurons of the superior cervical ganglion will result in this syndrome.

Patient presentation

- The pupil on the same side (ipsilateral) of the injury is smaller (miosis) than the opposite pupil
- The ipsilateral eyeball sinks (enophthalmus) and the affected eyelid droops (ptosis)
- The ipsilateral side of the face does not sweat (anhidrosis)
- Difficulty in speaking or hoarseness (dysphonia) may occur with hyperextension sprains that also cause injury to the laryngeal nerve

Presenting signs and symptoms

The signs and symptoms depend on the level and degree of injury (see the box on p. 156-157 and Table 5-2).

Physical examination

The box on p. 156-157 and Table 5-2 describe spinal cord injuries and corresponding functional losses.

VITAL SIGNS

Neurogenic shock

    BP: Hypotension

    HR: Bradycardia

    Temperature: Hypothermia—96° F-98° F (35.5° C-36.6° C)

Diagnostic findings

No one diagnostic test is used; a combination of tests and clinical presentation confirms the diagnosis of vertebral and/or spinal cord injury.

SPINAL RADIOGRAPHY

- Multiple spinal radiographs confirm the type and location of vertebral fracture.
- Fractures and/or dislocations can occur in different segments in 20% of severe trauma patients.
- Tumors, arthritic changes, and congenital abnormalities may also be visualized.

COMPUTED TOMOGRAPHY (CT SCAN)

- Visualizes fractures not detected on radiographs.
- Reflects compromise of the spinal canal or nerve roots by bony fragments or extensive fractures.

MAGNETIC RESONANCE IMAGING (MRI)

- Identifies extent of spinal cord damage, degree of cord contusion.
- Demonstrates presence of blood, edema, necrotic tissue, disc herniation, or tumor growth.

Acute Care Patient Management

Goals of treatment

Stabilize the spine and prevent secondary injury to the cord

    Cervical collar or brace

    Cervical traction with tongs

    Halo brace

    Kinetic bed

    Corticosteroids, such as methylprednisolone (controversial)

    Osmotic diuretics, such as mannitol (controversial)

    Surgery: decompression laminectomy, closed or open reduction of fracture, or spinal fusion

TABLE 5-2 Complete Spinal Cord Segmental Lesion and Corresponding Acute Functional Loss

Spinal level	Muscles	Dermatome	Acute dysfunction	At risk for
C1-C2	All muscles below trapezius, sternocleidomastoid	Back of head	Quadriplegia (complete); total loss of independent respiratory function; total loss of motor and sensory function from neck down	Death, hypotension, bradycardia, dysrhythmias, hypothermia, ileus, atonic bladder, skin breakdown
C3-C5 C5	Diaphragm Trapezius	Ear, neckline from clavicle to wrist	Quadriplegia (complete); minimal or absent diaphragmatic function; absent intercostal respiratory effort; loss of all motor function below shoulders and sensation below clavicles	Hypotension, bradycardia, dysrhythmias, hypothermia, ileus, atonic bladder, skin breakdown
C6	Deltoid, biceps	Lateral third of arm, shoulder to thumb and index finger	Quadriplegia (complete); decreased respiratory function: absent intercostal respiratory effort (diaphragm intact); can move head, shoulders, with some gross arm flexion	Same as above

Continued.

NEURO

TABLE 5-2 Complete Spinal Cord Segmental Lesion and Corresponding Acute Functional Loss—cont'd

Spinal level	Muscles	Dermatome	Acute dysfunction	At risk for
C7	Latissimus, serratus, pectoralis, radial wrist extensors	Dorsal and palmar midarm to first two digits	Quadriplegia (incomplete); decreased respiratory function: absent intercostal effort (diaphragm intact); can flex and extend elbow	Same as above
C8	Triceps, finger extensors and flexors	Medial third of arm, including digits three and four	Quadriplegia (incomplete); decreased respiratory function: decreased intercostal effort (diaphragm intact); some intrinsic hand function, thumb and index pincher movement present	Same as above
T1	Hand intrinsics, ulnar, wrist, and fingers	Medial arm, axilla	Paraplegia; decreased respiratory function with diaphragmatic breathing; arm function intact; finger spreading, grip and wrist flexion present	Same as above
T2-T6	Upper intercostals, upper back	T4 is at nipple line	Paraplegia; some use of intercostal muscles; good upper body strength; loss of bowel and bladder function; loss of leg function; can stand with	Ileus, atonic bladder, skin breakdown

T6-T12	Abdominals, thoracic extensors	T10 is at umbilicus; T12 is at groin	Paraplegia; no interference with respiratory function; loss of bowel and bladder function; spastic paralysis of legs; can ambulate with braces
L1-L4	Iliopsoas	Groin, upper thigh and knee	With injuries below L2, a loss in sensorimotor, bowel, bladder, and sexual function may result, depending on nerve root damage in the acute phase
L2-L4	Quadriceps	Anterior thigh, knee and lower leg	
L5-S2	Hamstrings, extensor digitorum, gluteus maximus, gastrocnemius	Great toe, lateral foot, sole, achilles, posterior thigh	Injuries above the sacrum convert to reflex, and bowel and bladder are uninhibited when reflexes return; with sacral injuries they are likely to retain atonic bowel and bladder secondary to absent reflexes
S3, S4, S5	Bowel and bladder sphincters	Genitals, saddle area	Atonic bladder, fecal retention

TABLE 5-3 Clinical Sequelae of Acute Spinal Cord Injuries*

Complication	Signs and symptoms
Respiratory insufficiency or arrest	Increasing work of breathing, NIF >−30, VC <15ml/kg, shallow and rapid respirations, cessation of breathing
Neurogenic pulmonary edema	Severe restlessness, anxiety, confusion, diaphoresis, cyanosis, distended neck veins, moist rapid and shallow respirations, crackles, rhonchi, elevated BP, thready pulse, frothy and bloody sputum
Cardiac dysrhythmias/arrest	Irregular heart rhythm, pulselessness
Spinal shock	Flaccid, total paralysis of all skeletal muscles, loss of spinal reflexes, loss of sensation (pain, proprioception, touch, temperature, and pressure) below the level of injury; bowel and bladder dysfunction and possible priapism
Neurogenic shock	Unstable hypotension: SBP <90 mm Hg Bradycardia: HR <50 beats/min Hypothermia: Temperature <37° C (<98.6° F)
Autonomic dysreflexia (hyperreflexia)	Occurs only in patients with injuries above the T6 level once recovered from spinal shock and reflex activity has returned; paroxysmal hypertension (SBP 240 to 300 mm Hg), with bradycardia, pounding headache, blurred vision, vasodilation, flushing, profuse sweating, piloerection (gooseflesh) above the level of lesion, nasal congestion, nausea, possible chest pain; if not controlled, status epilepticus, stroke, and death are possible
Orthostatic hypotension	Dizziness, lightheadedness, loss of consciousness, drop in SBP when assuming an upright position
Immobility	Contractures, skin impairment, deep-vein thrombosis, emboli, pneumonia, atelectasis

*Above T6 level.

Support cardiopulmonary function
    Supplemental oxygen
    Intubation and mechanical ventilation
    Kinetic bed
    Crystalloid infusions
    Inotropic and/or vasopressor agents
    Atropine for bradycardia
Decrease/alleviate pain and muscle spasms
    Analgesics (e.g., acetaminophen, codeine, morphine)
    Muscle relaxants (e.g., diazepam, baclofen)
Detect/prevent clinical sequelae (Table 5-3)

Priority nursing diagnoses
High risk for injury
Impaired gas exchange
High risk for decreased cardiac output
Ineffective breathing pattern
Ineffective airway clearance
High risk for altered protection (see p. 145)
Altered nutrition: less than body requirements (see p. 149)
High risk for altered family process (see p. 150)

▶ **High risk for injury** related to displacement of fracture, spinal shock, or ascending cord edema

PATIENT OUTCOMES
• Absence of progressive neurological dysfunction
• Improved sensory, motor, and reflex functions

PATIENT MONITORING
1. CVP and PA pressures may be used to evaluate fluid volume status; both overhydration and dehydration can adversely affect spinal cord circulation.

PHYSICAL ASSESSMENT
1. Determine baseline motor function (strength and tone) and conduct ongoing assessments for changes that may indicate increasing cord edema (see the box on p. 156-157 and Table 5-2).
2. Assess baseline sensory level (pain, light touch, and positional sense) and mark level of sensation on the patient's body (see Figure 1-4). Conduct ongoing assessments to determine improvement or deterioration. Also note the patient's reports of paresthesia (numbness or tingling) in his extremities.
3. Observe for priapsim, assess rectal tone, and note reflexive activity to evaluate course of spinal shock and/or return of neurological function.

4. Assess the patient for development of clinical sequelae (see Table 5-3).

DIAGNOSTICS ASSESSMENT

1. Review serial radiographs for proper spinal alignment.

PATIENT MANAGEMENT

1. Maintain the patient's neck in alignment until tongs or a halo ring is applied; avoid neck flexion, extension, or rotation.

2. Record the amount of weights necessary to achieve re-alignment. Ensure that the weights hang free and that the body is in proper alignment for optimal traction. If vertebral alignment of the neck is incorrect, additional weights will be applied to the tongs and follow-up lateral cervical radiographs will be taken until realignment is reached. Proper body alignment should be ensured, especially if a kinetic bed is used.

3. Corticosteroids, e.g., methylprednisolone (controversial), may be ordered. Generally, a bolus loading dose is given over 1 hour, followed by a constant infusion for 23 hours. An osmotic diuretic, e.g., mannitol, may be ordered to decrease edema at the site of injury. Muscle relaxants, e.g., diazepam, baclofen, and analgesics, e.g., acetaminophen, codeine, or morphine, may be ordered to decrease pain and/or muscle spasms to facilitate spinal realignment.

4. Anticipate surgical decompression and open reduction if alignment is not achieved by closed reduction.

▶ **Impaired gas exchange** related to alveolar hypoventilation secondary to paresis or paralysis of respiratory muscles **(Ineffective breathing pattern);** and bronchial secretions and impaired cough **(Ineffective airway clearance)**

PATIENT OUTCOMES

- Alert and oriented
- O_2 sat >95%
- Pao_2 80-100 mm Hg
- $Paco_2$ 35-45 mm Hg
- Vital capacity 15 ml/kg
- NIF >−30 cm H_2O
- V_T >5 ml/kg
- RR 12-20, eupnea
- HR 60-100 beats/min
- SBP 90-140 mm Hg
- Lungs clear to auscultation

PATIENT MONITORING

1. Continuously monitor ECG, since hypoxemia is a risk factor for dysrhythmias.
2. Continuously monitor oxygen saturation with pulse oximetry (SpO_2). Monitor interventions and patient activities that may adversely affect oxygen saturation.
3. Monitor spontaneous ventilation, negative inspiratory force, tidal volume, and vital capacity every 4 to 8 hours. Decreasing values suggest loss of intercostal and abdominal muscle motion and strength and are parameters for predicting impending respiratory failure requiring intubation and mechanical ventilation. (Hypoxemia and hypercapnia may be late findings.)

PHYSICAL ASSESSMENT

1. Assess respiratory rate, pattern, use of accessory muscles, and the ability to and strength of cough hourly (or more frequently if indicated) for the first 24 to 48 hours then every 4 hours if the patient's condition remains stable. Inspect chest expansion for symmetry and to assess intercostal muscle strength and observe epigastric area to assess diaphragmatic function. Increasing difficulty swallowing or coughing may indicate ascending cord edema. If halo traction has been placed, check to see that the fiberglass vest does not restrict ventilatory efforts.
2. Auscultate all lung fields and record breath sounds every 2 to 4 hours. Be alert to areas of absent or decreasing breath sounds or the development of adventitious sounds (i.e., crackles, rhonchi). Hypoventilation is common and leads to accumulation of secretions, atelectasis, and possible pneumonia.
3. Assess for signs of respiratory distress, e.g., patient's complaints of SOB, shallow and rapid respirations, vital capacity <15 ml/kg, and changes in sensorium.
4. Auscultate abdomen in all four quadrants for the presence of bowel sounds. Measure and record abdominal girth every 4 to 8 hours, since paralytic ileus and abdominal distention can interfere with respirations and potentiate the risk for aspiration.
5. Assess the patient for development of clinical sequelae (see Table 5-3).

DIAGNOSTICS ASSESSMENT

1. Review serial ABGs for adequacy of gas exchange.
2. Review serial chest radiographs to evaluate pulmonary

NEURO

congestion and possible development of atelectasis, consolidation, or pneumonia.

3. Review a flat plate of the abdomen (as available) if distension persists.

4. Review serial Hgb and Hct levels to detect possible blood loss from internal bleeding. Oxygen-carrying capability can be adversely affected with blood loss.

PATIENT MANAGEMENT

1. Decrease factors that increase oxygen demands, such as fever and anxiety.

2. If cervical injury is present, or has not been ruled out, *do not hyperextend* the patient's neck for oral intubation—use the jaw-thrust method to prevent further cervical injury.

3. Once the spinal cord injury is stabilized, promote pulmonary hygiene: incentive spirometry, C & DB, chest physiotherapy, and position changes every 2 hours. Position the patient for effective chest excursion. A kinetic bed may be used to promote mobilization of secretions. If the patient is unable to cough effectively, manually assist by placing the palm of the hand under the diaphragm (between the xiphoid and umbilicus) and push up on the abdominal muscles as the patient exhales.

4. Administer oxygen as ordered. Mechanical ventilation may be required. (See Chapter 6, Therapeutic Modalities, for information on mechanical ventilation.)

5. Suction the patient's secretions if needed. Hyperoxygenate the patient's lungs before suctioning and limit passes of the suction catheter to 15 seconds or less to avoid periods of desaturation and bradycardia. Document the quality and quantity of secretions.

6. Check patency and functioning of the nasogastric tube every 2 to 4 hours, since abdominal distention can impair diaphragmatic breathing.

7. Conduct passive range of motion exercises and apply antiembolism stockings to promote venous return and decrease the risk for deep-vein thrombosis (DVT) and pulmonary embolus. Sequential compression devices may be used. Measure thigh and calf circumference to detect any increase in size that may suggest DVT. Heparin therapy (controversial) may also be used.

▶ **High risk for decreased cardiac output** related to relative hypovolemia and bradycardia secondary to neurogenic/spinal shock

PATIENT OUTCOMES
- Alert and oriented
- SBP 90-140 mm Hg
- HR 60-100 beats/min
- CVP 2-6 mm Hg
- PAP$\frac{15\text{-}30}{5\text{-}15}$ mm Hg
- PAWP 4-12 mm Hg
- CI 2.4-4.0 L/min/m^2
- SVR 900-1200 dynes/sec/cm^{-5}
- Peripheral pulses strong and equal
- u/o 30 ml/hr or 0.5-1.0 ml/kg/hr

PATIENT MONITORING
1. Monitor ECG rhythm and rate for dysrhythmia development. Bradycardia and sinus pauses are common complications in acute cervical injuries. Hypothermia may aggravate bradycardia.
2. Continuously monitor blood pressure (via arterial catheter if possible) since spinal shock or autonomic dysreflexia can cause fluctuations in BP. Note adverse changes in blood pressure that may be related to patient position.
3. CVP and PA pressure monitoring may be used to evaluate fluid volume status. Fluid volume overload may lead to pulmonary edema. Obtain CO and calculate CI; calculate SVR.
4. Measure intake and output hourly and determine fluid volume balance every shift. Urinary output <30 ml/hr for 2 consecutive hours may signal decreased renal perfusion secondary to decreased CO.

PHYSICAL ASSESSMENT
1. Assess skin temperature and color, capillary refill, and peripheral pulses as indicators of CO.
2. Assess LOC to evaluate cerebral perfusion; lightheadedness, fainting, or dizziness may occur with a change in patient position (orthostatic hypotension).
3. Observe for the appearance of involuntary spastic movement, which indicates spinal shock has ended and the potential for autonomic dysreflexia exists.
4. Assess patient for development of clinical sequelae (see Table 5-3).

DIAGNOSTICS ASSESSMENT
None

NEURO

PATIENT MANAGEMENT

1. Optimize venous return or decrease risk of hypotension by changing patient's position slowly and performing passive range of motion exercises every 2 hours. If necessary, elevate lower extremities to support blood pressure. Use antiembolism hose, ace wraps to legs, and/or abdominal binder when getting the patient out of bed.

2. Administer intravenous crystalloids (lactated Ringer's, $D_5\frac{1}{2}$ normal saline) as ordered to maintain hydration and circulatory volume and to control mild hypotension. Monitor for mild dehydration or overhydration, since both conditions can compromise spinal circulation.

3. Dopamine or dobutamine may be ordered to support BP related to compromised sympathetic outflow. Titrate infusions to desired effect. (See Chapter 7, Pharmacology, for additional drug information.)

4. Administer atropine as ordered to treat bradydysrhythmias.

ARTERIOVENOUS MALFORMATION (AVM)

Clinical Brief

AVMs are congenital malformations of the cerebral vascular system in which a portion of the brain retains an embryonic type of circulation. Tortuous, tangled, and malformed arterial channels drain directly into the venous system without an intervening capillary bed. Because there is a direct communication of arteries to veins, the blood in the veins is under a higher pressure than normal.

The arteries supplying the AVM tend to dilate with time as a result of increased flow through the lesion. Likewise, the veins enlarge as the flow increases, creating a vicious cycle that can make these lesions increase in size. This large flow or shunting of blood through the AVM can render adjacent areas (and sometimes distal areas) of the brain ischemic.

Presenting signs and symptoms

Headache, seizures, syncope, and progressive neurological deficits may be present. A devastating hemorrhage can result in a comatose, moribund state.

Physical examination

BP: Normotensive or hypertensive

HR: Mild tachycardia may be present

RR: Eupnea

Neurological: Depending on the area of the brain in which the AVM is located, there may be speech, motor, or sensory deficits. There also may be problems with vision, memory, and coordination.

Diagnostic findings

Skull films: Calcified deposits common in AVMs may appear on radiographs, requiring further investigation.

CT scan without contrast: Identifies the location of the AVM and presence of hemorrhage or hydrocephalus.

CT scan with contrast: Visualizes the extent and location of the AVM, and possible feeding arteries.

MRI: Confirms relationship of the vascular channels to the surrounding brain and the degree of surrounding hemorrhage or edema. Aids in the planning of the surgical approach.

Cerebral angiography: Essential in planning for resection of AVM. Will include the carotid and vertebral circulations to assess all possible areas of vascular supply. Essential for determining the flow dynamics of the AVM and possibility for embolization.

Acute Care Patient Management

Goals of treatment

Obliterate/excise malformation

Embolization: Silastic beads, balloons, or gluing for thrombosis and destruction of lesions

Surgical: Craniotomy for complete removal, clipping, or ligation of feeding vessels

Radiotherapy: Proton-beam radiation, laser therapy

Prevent cerebral vascular bleed

Subarachnoid precautions

Antihypertensives, e.g., labetalol, hydralazine hydrochloride, methyldopa, propranolol, sodium nitroprusside

Stool softeners or mild laxatives

Sedatives, e.g., phenobarbital

Control symptoms

Antipyretics, e.g., acetaminophen

Anticonvulsants, e.g., phenytoin, phenobarbital

Analgesics, e.g., acetaminophen, Tylenol with codeine

Detect/prevent clinical sequelae (Table 5-4)

Priority nursing diagnoses

Altered tissue perfusion: cerebral

High risk for injury

High risk for altered protection (see p. 145)

TABLE 5-4 Clinical Sequelae of AVM

Complication	Signs and symptoms
Intracerebral bleeding	Clinical signs vary, depending on the area involved. In general there is deterioration in consciousness, worsening headache, unilateral motor weakness, decreased EOMs, visual deficits, and changes in vital signs, particularly the respiratory pattern. There may be speech deficits (e.g., slurring or receptive or expressive aphasia).
	Meningeal signs may be present (e.g., severe headache, nuchal rigidity, fever, photophobia, lethargy, nausea, and vomiting).
Increased intracranial pressure (IICP)	Sudden severe headache, decreasing LOC, nausea, pupillary abnormalities, motor dysfunction, papilledema, and seizures may occur.
Herniation	Alterations in LOC may occur, ranging from alert to profoundly comatose, with no response to any stimuli; VS changes (vary with level of ICP); bradycardia; increasing systolic BP with a widening pulse pressure; irregular respiratory pattern (e.g., Cheyne-Stokes, central neurogenic hyperventilation, ataxic, apneustic); motor/sensory changes on one side, pupillary dilation (initially on the side of the edema, may later involve both pupils), dysconjugate gaze, and other indicators of cranial nerve involvement, depending on severity.

Altered nutrition: less than body requirements (see p. 149)
High risk for altered family process (see p. 150)
See also CVA (p. 186)
▶ **Altered tissue perfusion: cerebral** related to shunting of blood from cerebral tissue and/or intracerebral hemorrhage
PATIENT OUTCOMES
• Awake, alert, and oriented to person, place, and time
• Pupils equal and normoreactive

- SBP 90-140 mm Hg
- HR 60-100 beats/min
- RR 12-20, eupnea
- Motor function equal bilaterally
- Absence of headache, nystagmus, and nausea
- ICP <15 mm Hg
- CPP 60-100 mm Hg

PATIENT MONITORING

1. Monitor ECG continuously, since hypoxemia and cerebral bleeding are risk factors for pronounced ST segment and T wave changes and life-threatening dysrhythmias.
2. Monitor ICP, analyze the ICP waveform, and calculate cerebral perfusion pressure (CPP) every hour. (See Chapter 3 for ICP monitoring.)
3. Monitor BP, P every 15-30″ initially; obtain CVP and/or PA pressures every hour or more frequently if indicated.

PHYSICAL ASSESSMENT

1. Assess neurological status using Glasgow coma scale and assess for changes suggesting IICP and herniation. Be alert for subtle changes and new focal deficits.
2. Assess for factors that can cause IICP; evaluate patient for restlessness, distended bladder, constipation, hypoxemia, headache, fear, or anxiety.
3. Assess patient for development of clinical sequelae.

DIAGNOSTICS ASSESSMENT

1. Review serial ABGs for decreasing Pao_2 (<60 mm Hg) or increasing $Paco_2$ (<45 mm Hg) because these disturbances can increase ICP.

PATIENT MANAGEMENT

1. Maintain patient airway and administer oxygen as ordered to prevent hypoxemia
2. Institute measures to minimize external stimuli and maintain BP (see the box on p. 174).
3. Administer antihypertensives as ordered, e.g., labetalol hydrochloride (Trandate), hydralazine hydrochloride (Apresoline), methyldopa (Aldomet), propranolol (Inderal), or sodium nitroprusside (Nipride) to control blood pressure. Monitor drug's effect on MAP and CPP.
4. If vasospasm is suspected, hypertension/hypervolemic therapy and calcium channel blockers may be ordered. Monitor PAWP, BP, and CPP closely.

5. Sedatives and stool softeners may be ordered to reduce agitation and straining.
6. Anticipate surgical intervention for embolization, clipping, or ligation of feeding vessels.

▶ **High risk for injury:** seizure

PATIENT OUTCOMES
• Patient will be seizure free
• Patient will not injure self

PATIENT MONITORING
None

PHYSICAL ASSESSMENT
1. Observe clinical presentation during seizure activity. Note time of onset, body parts involved, and characteristics of movement; observe respiratory pattern; note pupil size, deviation, and nystagmus; and note duration of seizure activity.
2. Evaluate neurological status during postictal state and examine patient for any injuries.

DIAGNOSTICS ASSESSMENT
1. Review serum anticonvulsant drug levels (if available) for therapeutic range.

PATIENT MANAGEMENT
1. Institute seizure precautions: pad side rails, maintain the bed in low position; keep an airway at bedside. Have suction and oxygen available.
2. Protect the patient during seizure activity: protect head from injury, avoid restraining the patient; and do not force an airway into the mouth once a seizure has begun.
3. Suction the patient's secretions if necessary and maintain an adequate airway during postictal state.
4. Administer anticonvulsant medications as prescribed.

CEREBRAL ANEURYSM AND SUBARACHNOID HEMORRHAGE

Clinical Brief

An aneurysm is a thin-walled, round or saccular dilation arising from a cerebral artery. The most common site is at the bifurcation of the main cerebral vessels that make up the circle of Willis. Large aneurysms may produce focal neurological deficits from compressing brain tissue or lead to a stroke secondary to thrombus formation and embolization. Aneurysms can rupture, sending blood into the subarachnoid space, ventricular system, and surrounding brain tissue. Aneurysmal subarachnoid hemorrhage is the most frequently seen cerebral aneurysm.

Presenting signs and symptoms

Often the patient will report the sudden onset of a violent headache—"the worst headache of my life"—at the time of bleeding. This usually continues as a severe headache accompanied by nausea and vomiting, photophobia, and nuchal rigidity. Specific neurological deficits are related to the site and extent of the hemorrhage and may include a deteriorating level of consciousness, oculomotor nerve dysfunction, paralysis of extraocular muscles, and sensorimotor deficits in the patient.

Physical examination

BP: Generally hypertensive or very labile, depending on extent of hemorrhage and level of ICP

HR: Mild tachycardia, dysrhythmias

RR: Tachypnea

Temperature: Low-grade fever 24 hours after initial rupture as a result of meningeal irritation

Pulmonary: Respiratory pattern changes may be present, depending on the level of ICP and area of hemorrhage (see Table 1-7)

Neurological: As the severity of the hemorrhage increases, the level of consciousness generally decreases with corresponding severity of neurological deficits; signs of meningeal irritation: stiff neck, and positive Kernig's and Brudzinski's signs may be present (see Table 5-5 for a classification of cerebral aneurysm hemorrhage)

Diagnostic findings

COMPUTED TOMOGRAPHY (CT SCAN)

- Identifies the aneurysm and the size, location, and extent of subarachnoid or intracerebral hemorrhage.
- Detects the presence of hydrocephalus.

CEREBRAL ANGIOGRAPHY

- Anterior and posterior circulations are studied to document presence of aneurysm(s) and possible vasospasm.

MAGNETIC RESONANCE IMAGING (MRI)

- Reveals small aneurysms not visualized with CT scan or angiography.

TRANSCRANIAL DOPPLER (TCD)

- Noninvasive cerebral blood flow studies to aid in diagnosing vasospasm.

TABLE 5-5 Classification of Cerebral Aneurysm
Hemorrhage

Category	Criteria
Grade I	Asymptomatic or minimal headache and slight nuchal rigidity
Grade II	Moderate to severe headache
	Nuchal rigidity, no neurological deficit other than cranial nerve palsy
Grade III	Drowsiness, confusion or mild focal deficit
Grade IV	Stupor, moderate to severe hemiparesis, possibly early decerebrate rigidity and vegetative disturbances
Grade V	Deep coma, decerebrate rigidity, moribund appearance

From Hunt W and Hess R: Surgical risk as related to time of intervention in the repair of intracranial aneurysms, J Neurosurg 14:28, 1968.

Subarachnoid Precautions

- Place the patient in a quiet, dimly lit private room. Television, telephone, radio, and reading may be restricted.
- Complete bed rest is required, and the patient should be positioned with the HOB elevated 30 to 40 degrees.
- Instruct the patient to avoid a Valsalva maneuver or straining of any kind, since these activities can increase ICP. Have the patient exhale while being turned. Caution the patient against coughing and sneezing.
- Obtain BP, P, RR, and assess neurological signs at least every 30″ initially (may be as frequently as every 5″ to 15″). This schedule may be altered, depending on patient condition.
- Perform activities for the patient, e.g., feeding, bathing, or shaving, that could cause the patient to overexert and raise the blood pressure. Keep activities at a minimum, pace interventions, and provide uninterrupted rest periods.
- Caution visitors against upsetting the patient in any way, because excitement or anger could increase blood pressure and intracranial pressure. The number of visitors as well as the duration of their visits may need to be limited.
- Provide analgesics for headache, since pain can cause restlessness and elevated BP. Sedatives and stool softeners may also be required.

CSF STUDIES
- Confirms blood in CSF.
- Reflects elevated pressure, which can be as high as 250 cm H_2O (normal is 90-180 cm H_2O) and elevated protein of 80-200 mg/dl (normal is 15-45 mg/dl).

Acute Care Patient Management
Goals of treatment
Secure the aneurysm
  Surgery: aneurysm clipping or ligation
Prevent rebleeding
  Subarachnoid precautions (see the box on p. 174)
  Antihypertensives, e.g., labetalol, hydralazine hydrochloride, methyldopa, propranolol, sodium nitroprusside
  Stool softeners
  Anticonvulsants, e.g., phenytoin, phenobarbital
Control cerebral vasospasm
  Ensure hydration and normalize BP (hypervolemic/hypertension therapy)
  Calcium channel blocking agents, e.g., nimodipine
Detect/prevent clinical sequelae (Table 5-6)
Priority nursing diagnoses
Altered tissue perfusion: cerebral
High risk for altered protection (see p. 145)
Altered nutrition: less than body requirements (see p. 149)
High risk for altered family process (see p. 150)
See also CVA (p. 186)

▶ **Altered tissue perfusion: cerebral** related to bleeding and cerebral vasospasm

PATIENT OUTCOMES
- Patient will be awake, alert, and oriented to person, place, and time
- Pupils equal and normoreactive
- SBP 90-140 mm Hg
- HR 60-100 beats/min
- RR 12-20, eupnea
- Motor function equal bilaterally
- Absence of headache, papilledema, nystagmus, nausea, and seizures
- ICP <15 mm Hg
- CPP 60-100 mm Hg

PATIENT MONITORING
1. Continuously monitor BP to evaluate patient response to antihypertensive agents. Fluctuations in BP may increase risk of aneurysm rebleeding.

TABLE 5-6 Clinical Sequelae of Cerebral Aneurysm Rupture

Complication	Signs and symptoms
Intracerebral bleeding	Lethargy, nausea, vomiting, focal neurological deficits
Cerebral vasospasm	In general there is progressive deterioration in consciousness, mental confusion, motor weakness, and sensory deficits; visual and speech deficits may also be present
Increased intracranial pressure (IICP)	Sudden severe headache, decreasing LOC, nausea, pupillary abnormalities, motor dysfunction, seizures
Herniation	Alterations in LOC ranging from alert to profoundly comatose, with no response to any stimuli; VS changes (vary with level of ICP); bradycardia; increasing systolic BP with a widening pulse pressure; irregular respiratory pattern (e.g., Cheyne-Stokes, central neurogenic hyperventilation, ataxia, apneusis); contralateral sensorimotor changes; ipsilateral pupillary dilation, dysconjugate gaze, and other indicators of cranial nerve involvement, depending on severity

2. Continuously monitor ECG, since hypoxemia and cerebral bleeding are risk factors for pronounced ST segment and T wave changes and life-threatening dysrhythmias.
3. Monitor ICP; analyze ICP waveform and calculate cerebral perfusion pressure (CPP) every hour (see Chapter 3 for ICP monitoring).
4. Monitor vital signs q15-30″ initially and evaluate patient response to therapy.
5. Monitor intake and output hourly and calculate hourly running totals to determine fluid volume balance.

PHYSICAL ASSESSMENT
1. Assess neurological status for signs/symptoms of IICP and cerebral vasospasm (see Table 5-6). Be alert for sub-

tle changes and new focal deficits. Cerebral vasospasms generally affect the major vessels near the site of the ruptured aneurysm and can cause focal neurological deficits with or without a major or sudden loss of consciousness.

2. Assess temperature every 2-4 hours. Because of the concern of possible seizure activity, avoid oral temperature taking.

3. Assess for factors that can cause IICP: distended bladder, constipation, hypoxemia, hypercapnia, headache, fear, or anxiety.

4. Assess patient for development of clinical sequelae (see Table 5-6).

DIAGNOSTICS ASSESSMENT

1. Review serial ABGs for decreasing Pao_2 (<60 mm Hg) or increasing $Paco_2$ (>45 mm Hg), since these disturbances can increase ICP.

2. Review serial electrolytes for hyponatremia, which may contribute to an altered mental state.

3. Note trends on transcranial Doppler (TCD) studies; an increasing mean value may reflect vasospasm.

PATIENT MANAGEMENT

1. Maintain patent airway and administer oxygen as ordered. If patient is intubated and mechanically ventilated, see Chapter 6 for more information on mechanical ventilation.

2. Institute subarachnoid precautions (see the box on p. 174).

3. Administer antihypertensives as ordered to control sustained elevated BP, e.g., labetalol, hydralazine hydrochloride, methyldopa, propranolol, or sodium nitroprusside. Monitor MAP and CPP closely.

4. IV fluids (D_5NS) and pharmacological agents such as phenylephrine, dopamine, or dobutamine may be ordered to improve CPP (maintain SBP no greater than 160 mm Hg). Monitor BP and CPP closely.

5. Calcium channel blocking agents may be ordered to control cerebral vasospasm. Monitor the drug's effect on BP and HR.

6. Other pharmacological agents to prevent rebleeding and increased ICP include antipyretics, e.g., acetaminophen, to keep patient normothermic; anticonvulsants, e.g., phenytoin; phenobarbital, to prevent or control seizures; analgesics, e.g., acetaminophen or Tylenol with codeine,

for headaches; stool softeners or mild laxatives, to prevent constipation and straining; and sedatives, e.g., phenobarbital, to decrease agitation.

7. Anticipate early surgical intervention for clipping or ligation of the aneurysm. (See Chapter 6, Therapeutic Modalities, for information on craniotomy.)

SEIZURES—STATUS EPILEPTICUS

Clinical Brief

Seizures represent intermittent, sudden, massive discharge of abnormal activity from a group of neurons within the brain. The electrical discharges may remain localized within one area of the brain, spread to involve adjacent areas in the same hemisphere, or spread across the midline to affect the contralateral hemisphere. Depending on the area of the brain involved and the pattern of spread, seizures may be generalized: tonic-clonic (grand mal), absence (petite mal), and bilateral myoclonus; or partial: focal motor, focal sensory, or complex.

Status epilepticus (convulsive status) represents a neurological emergency in which recurrent abnormal discharges occur without allowing the brain time to recover between seizures.

Causes of status epilepticus include sudden and total suppression of anticonvulsants (withdrawal), subtherapeutic levels of anticonvulsants, meningitis, encephalitis, cortical brain tumors, metabolic and toxic encephalopathies, subarachnoid and intracerebral hemorrhage, and severe head injury. Drug overdoses, hypoxia (e.g., carbon monoxide poisoning, drowning), and withdrawal from alcohol use may also potentiate status epilepticus.

Presenting signs and symptoms

The patient is comatose, and motor activity is divided between the repetitive tonic and clonic phases of the seizure.

Physical examination

BP: Mild hypertension initially; hypotension with circulatory collapse

HR: Tachycardia

RR: Apnea during tonic phase; irregular gasping respiration during clonic phase

Temperature: Mild to moderately elevated

Pulmonary: Hypoxia and cyanosis during seizure activity

CV: With sustained seizure activity, cardiovascular collapse possible

Neurological: Recurring, generalized tonic-clonic movements without the patient regaining consciousness; incontinence, perspiration, salivation, and emesis may occur; pupils are often fixed and dilated; eyes may be deviated or dysconjugate

Diagnostic findings

Clinical manifestations are the basis for diagnosis. Diagnostic tests are performed to identify the cause of the seizure.

Acute Care Patient Management

Goals of treatment

Maintain oxygenation
   Establishment of an airway
   Supplemental oxygen
   Intubation
   Mechanical ventilation
Maintain hemodynamic stability
   IV fluids
   Vasopressor or vasodilator agents
Control seizure activity
   Fast-acting anticonvulsant therapy, e.g., intravenous
      lorazepam or diazepam (Valium)
   Long-acting anticonvulsant therapy, e.g., intravenous
      phenytoin, phenobarbital
   Neuromuscular blockade, e.g., paraldehyde, lidocaine,
      general anesthesia
Identify and treat cause
   Implementation of appropriate therapy

Priority nursing diagnoses

High risk for injury
High risk for altered protection (see p. 145)
Altered nutrition: less than body requirements (see p.
   149)
High risk for altered family process (see p. 150)
High risk for injury related to increased metabolic demand
secondary to continuous seizure activity
PATIENT OUTCOMES
• Patient will be alert and oriented
• Pupils equal, round, and normoreactive
• Motor strength equal in all extremities
• SBP 90-140 mm Hg
• HR 60-100 beats/min
• RR 12-20, eupnea
• Normothermic

NEURO

- Pao_2 80-100 mm Hg
- $Paco_2$ 35-45 mm Hg
- O_2 sat >95%
- pH 7.35-7.45
- Hco_3 22-25 mEq/L
- Absence of musculoskeletal trauma
- u/o 30 ml/hr or 0.5-1.0 ml/kg/hr

PATIENT MONITORING

1. Continuously monitor for cardiac dysrhythmias, which may occur as a result of hypoxemia, acidosis, or anticonvulsant drug administration.
2. Continuously monitor oxygen saturation with pulse oximetry (Spo_2).
3. Monitor CPP if ICP monitoring is available.
4. Monitor the compressed spectral analysis (CSA), if available, for continued EEG trends and effectiveness of medications.
5. Monitor intake and output; myoglobinuria may occur with prolonged seizure activity and lead to renal failure.

PHYSICAL ASSESSMENT

1. Assess and document information detailing seizure activity: length of tonic and clonic phases, motor characteristics and body involvement, and deviation of eyes and pupil reaction. NOTE: Use room light to assess pupils, since a direct flashing light may elicit or cause progression of seizure. Note any automatic behavior (e.g., lip smacking, chewing), incontinence, or cyanosis.
2. Assess respiratory status, including airway patency; rate, depth, and rhythm of respirations; breath sounds; use of accessory muscles; and color of skin, lips, and nailbeds. Monitor ability to handle secretions, and assess gag, cough, and swallow reflexes.
3. Assess peripheral pulses, skin, and urinary output at least every hour to evaluate tissue perfusion.
4. During seizure activity and during the administration of anticonvulsant drugs, monitor VS. Respiratory depression, decreased BP, and dysrhythmias can occur with rapid infusion of diazepam, phenytoin, and phenobarbital.
5. Perform baseline and serial neurological assessments after status is interrupted. During the postictal phase of the seizure, assessment should include LOC (confusion), motor response to stimuli (lethargy and weakness), and

speech every 15″ ×4 then every 30″ min ×4. Patient responses should improve with each assessment. Be alert to the presence of focal findings suggestive of an expanding lesion and signs of IICP.
6. After the seizure, assess skin integrity for bruises, lacerations, or shearing injuries. Assess tongue, lips, and mouth for evidence of bite injuries.
7. Assess IV insertion sites for patency and extravasation of anticonvulsants.

NEURO

DIAGNOSTICS ASSESSMENT
1. Review EEG recording and maintain communication with the physician regarding the results.
2. Review electrolyte and blood glucose levels, since electrolyte imbalance and hypoglycemia may precipitate seizures or occur as a result of prolonged seizure activity.
3. Review serum anticonvulsant drug levels for therapeutic ranges.
4. Review ABGs for hypoxemia and acidosis; both abnormalities can precipitate seizures or can occur as a result of prolonged seizure activity.
5. Review lumbar puncture (LP) results if available.
6. Review chest radiographs for indications of pulmonary complications, e.g., infiltrates, aspiration.

PATIENT MANAGEMENT
1. Pad side rails and keep them up at all times; maintain the bed in its lowest position.
2. Keep an oral airway at the bedside with suction equipment.
3. Protect the patient during the seizure, e.g., do not restrain the patient, and guide extremity movement during the seizure to prevent injury and protect the patient's head.
4. Maintain airway and ventilation to ensure maximum delivery of oxygen to the brain cells. Administer Fio_2 100% during seizure activity. An oral airway may help to maintain airway patency, but *do not force an airway* during seizure activity.
5. Position the patient on one side to facilitate drainage of oral secretions and suction as necessary. *Do not* simply turn the patient's head to the side; this position promotes aspiration of emesis or secretions, occludes the airway, and interferes with venous return, which increases ICP. Maintain a suction setup at all times.

6. Be prepared to assist with intubation and mechanical ventilation if necessary. (See Chapter 6, Therapeutic Modalities, for information on mechanical ventilation.)
7. An NG tube may be required to prevent vomiting and the risk of aspiration.
8. Maintain a large-bore IV line for fluids and medication administration. Assess IV insertion sites for patency, especially after seizure activity, and be particularly careful to avoid extravasation of anticonvulsants.
9. Administer anticonvulsants as ordered:
   - Lorazepam can be administered 1-2 mg slow IVP while monitoring blood pressure.
   - Diazepam can be administered 2 mg/min slow IVP. If seizure continues, diazepam per continuous drip may be required—usual dosage is 100 mg in 500 ml D_5W at 10-15 mg/hr. Monitor patient continuously for respiratory depression and hypotension.
   - Phenobarbital 500-1000 mg (10-20 mg/kg) IV and/or phenytoin 500-1000 mg (18 mg/kg) IV may be ordered. IV line must be flushed with NS before and after administration. No other medications may be infused in the same line at the same time. Monitor LOC, BP, RR.
   - Other pharmacological therapy may include paraldehyde, lidocaine, general anesthesia, or neuromuscular blockade to stop the seizure activity. If neuromuscular blocking agents are used, the tonic-clonic motor activity will stop but *not* the abnormal cerebral electrical activity. (See Chapter 7, Pharmacology.)
10. After the seizure, stay with the patient, reassuring and reorienting the patient as necessary. Keep the patient in a side-lying position to facilitate drainage of oral secretions; suction the secretions as needed.

CEREBROVASCULAR ACCIDENT (CVA) OR STROKE
Clinical Brief
A CVA is an interruption of blood supply to brain tissue causing ischemia or infarction, resulting in temporary or permanent focal neurological deficits. The neurological deficits exhibited depend on the severity of the interruption and the cerebral artery involved. Temporary deficits or transient ischemic attacks (TIAs) produce slight symptoms that disap-

pear in a few minutes to hours; these may be a warning sign of an impending stroke, whereas a major stroke is more severe, symptoms persist longer than 24 hours, and permanent deficits occur. CVAs are classified as thrombotic, embolic, and hemorrhagic.

Thrombotic stroke

A thrombotic stroke, the most common type, is associated with atherosclerosis and narrowing of the lumen of the cerebral artery. The progression of occlusion may take several hours or days, and the evolution of symptoms are referred to as a "stroke in evolution." A stroke is complete when symptoms have stabilized and the neurological deficits are permanent.

Embolic stroke

An embolic stroke is most often associated with heart disease (e.g., rheumatic heart disease with mitral stenosis, subacute bacterial endocarditis), atrial fibrillation, and cardiac or vascular surgery. Embolic strokes evolve rapidly over a few seconds or minutes and are usually without warning signs.

Hemorrhagic stroke

A hemorrhagic stroke is most commonly associated with severe hypertension, ruptured cerebral aneurysm, or AVM, or it is precipitated by bleeding disorders that result in intracerebral hemorrhage. The onset of symptoms develops suddenly, with rapid progression of neurological deficits.

Risk factors for stroke are many and varied but include a history of hypertension, heart disease (especially valvular), cardiac dysrhythmias, cigarette smoking, diabetes mellitus, and obesity. In addition, patients with a strong family history of ischemic heart disease and stroke, as well as those with hyperlipidemia, appear at greatest risk. Medications such as oral contraceptives, aspirin, and anticoagulants may also place patients at risk.

Presenting signs and symptoms

Signs and symptoms are directly related to the cerebral artery affected and the function of the portion of the brain that it supplies. A list of major cerebral vessels and their common correlating manifestations are listed in the box.

Physical examination

Vital signs may be normal, or the following may be found:
BP: With preexisting hypertension, BP may exceed 200/ 100 mm Hg

NEURO

Correlation of Cerebral Artery Involvement and Common Manifestations

Internal carotid artery

Contralateral paresthesia (abnormal sensations) and hemiparesis (weakness) of arm, face, and leg

Eventually complete contralateral hemiplegia (paralysis) and hemianesthesia (loss of sensation)

Visual blurring or changes, hemianopsia (loss of half of visual field), repeated attacks of blindness in the ipsilateral eye

Dysphasia with dominant hemisphere involvement

Anterior cerebral artery

Mental impairment such as perseveration, confusion, amnesia, and personality changes

Contralateral hemiparesis or hemiplegia with leg loss > than arm

Sensory loss over toes, foot, and leg

Ataxia (motor incoordination), impaired gait, incontinence, and akinetic mutism

Middle cerebral artery

LOC varies from confusion to coma

Contralateral hemiparesis or hemiplegia with face and arm loss > than leg

Sensory impairment over same areas of hemiplegia

Aphasia (inability to express or interpret speech) or dysphasia (impaired speech) with dominant hemisphere involvement

Homonymous hemianopsia (loss of vision on the same side of both visual fields), inability to turn eyes toward the paralyzed side

Posterior cerebral artery

Contralateral hemiplegia with sensory loss

Confusion, memory involvement, and receptive speech deficits with dominant hemisphere involvement

Homonymous hemianopsia

Vertebrobasilar artery

Dizziness, vertigo, nausea, ataxia, and syncope

Visual disturbances, nystagmus, diplopia, field deficits, and blindness

Numbness and paresis (face, tongue, mouth, one or more limbs), dysphagia (inability to swallow), and dysarthria (difficulty in articulation)

Correlation of Cerebral Artery Involvement and Common Manifestations—cont'd

Symptoms related to left versus right hemisphere involvement

Left hemisphere	*Right hemisphere*
Right-sided hemiplegia or hemiparesis	Left-sided hemiplegia or hemiparesis
Expressive, receptive, or global aphasia	Spatial, perceptual deficits
Decreased performance on verbal and math testing	Denial of the disability on affected side
Slow and cautious behavior	Distractibility, impulsive behavior and poor judgment
Defects in right visual field	Defects in left visual field
Difficulty in distinguishing left from right	

HR: Mild tachycardia may be present or the rhythm irregular if associated with atrial fibrillation

RR: Eupnea or Cheyne-Stokes respirations may be present

Temperature: Afebrile, or elevated if the thermoregulation center is involved

CV: Peripheral pulses may be diminished or weak in the presence of atrial fibrillation; jugular bruits may be present with atherosclerosis

Pulmonary: Chest is clear to auscultation; some rhonchi may be present if there is a history of smoking

Neurological: See the box.

Diagnostic findings

CT SCAN

• Visualizes areas of ischemia or infarction.

CEREBRAL ANGIOGRAM

• Usually postponed until patient's condition is stabilized; evaluates and identifies areas of ulceration, stenosis, thrombus, and occlusion and patterns of collateral flow.

• Demonstrates presence of an aneurysm or AVM and any avascular zones and displaced arteries and veins from hemorrhage.

• Areas studied include aortic arch, carotids, and cerebral blood vessels.

LUMBAR PUNCTURE

- Normal pressure will be seen in cerebral thrombosis, embolus, and TIA; fluid is usually clear.
- In subarachnoid and intracerebral hemorrhage, the pressure is usually elevated and fluid is grossly bloody.
- Total protein level may be elevated in cases of thrombosis as a result of the inflammatory process.

ECHOCARDIOGRAM

- Rules out a cardiac source of emboli.

ECG

- Rules out the presence of a silent myocardial infarction.
- Determines the presence of dysrhythmias as a source of emboli.

MRI

- Reflects areas of infarction as early as 8 hours after the ischemic insult.

Acute Care Patient Management

Goals of treatment

Prevent further thrombotic events
  Cerebral vasodilators
  Possible anticoagulation therapy
  Low-cholesterol, low-fat diet
  For TIAs, possible carotid endarterectomy or extracranial graft
  Thrombectomy
Prevent further embolic events
  Treat the source of the embolus
  Anticoagulation therapy
  Embolectomy
Prevent further hemorrhagic events
  Treat the cause: AVM, cerebral aneurysm, or hypertension
Reduce increased intracranial pressure (IICP)
  Ventriculostomy for ICP monitoring and CSF drainage
  Corticosteroids, e.g., dexamethasone (Decadron)
  Osmotic diuretics, e.g., mannitol, urea
  Loop diuretics, e.g., furosemide (Lasix)

Priority nursing diagnoses

Altered tissue perfusion: cerebral
Ineffective airway clearance
High risk for aspiration
Impaired communication

High risk for altered protection (see p. 145)
Altered nutrition: less than body requirements (see p. 149)
High risk for altered family process (see p. 150)
▶ **Altered tissue perfusion: cerebral** related to increased intracranial pressure secondary to cerebral ischemia, edema, or hemorrhage

(see p. 145)
(see p. 149)
(see p. 150)

PATIENT OUTCOMES
* Patient will remain awake, alert, and oriented
* Pupils equal and normoreactive
* Improvement in presenting neurological deficits and/or the absence of any new focal deficits
* ICP <15 mm Hg
* CPP 60-100 mm Hg

PATIENT MONITORING
1. Continuously monitor ECG, since a dysrhythmia, e.g., atrial fibrillation, is a risk factor for cerebral emboli.
2. Continuously monitor oxygen saturation with pulse oximetry (Spo_2). Monitor interventions and patient activities that may adversely affect oxygen saturation.
3. If ICP monitoring is being used, calculate CPP to evaluate the patient's response to therapy (see Chapter 3 for ICP monitoring).
4. Monitor blood pressure q15-30″ initially and if titrating vasoactive agents.
5. Monitor CVP and PA pressures (as appropriate to patient's clinical condition). Increasing pressures may signal the onset of fluid overload, which may increase cerebral edema.
6. Monitor intake and output hourly and calculate fluid balance every shift to evaluate fluid volume status. Fluid overload can increase cerebral edema and further increase ICP.

PHYSICAL ASSESSMENT
1. Establish a neurological baseline with the Glasgow coma scale and perform ongoing assessments. Assess for signs and symptoms of IICP: headache, nausea, vomiting, altered LOC, pupillary changes, visual defects, and sensorimotor dysfunction. Test protective reflexes, e.g., cough, gag, corneal.
2. Assess for factors that can increase ICP: hypoxemia, hypercapnia, fever, anxiety, constipation, and bladder distension.

NEURO

DIAGNOSTICS ASSESSMENT

1. Review serial PT and PTT for therapeutic levels if the patient is receiving anticoagulant therapy. Generally $1.5\times$ control PT is the goal of therapy.
2. Review serial electrolytes levels, especially if diuretic therapy is employed.
3. Review serial ABGs to identify hypoxemia (Pao_2 <60 mm Hg) and hypercapnia ($Paco_2$ >45 mm Hg), since these disturbances can cause IICP.

PATIENT MANAGEMENT

1. Maintain the head of the bed at 30 degrees or as ordered. Keep the patient's head in straight alignment and prevent extreme hip flexion. Pace nursing activities to allow the patient uninterrupted rest periods. Assist the patient with positioning and turning and instruct the patient to exhale while being turned or repositioned.
2. Prevent constipation by establishing a bowel regimen as individually warranted. Provide the patient and family with realistic information and a rationale for frequent assessments, the relationship between the patient's condition and clinical symptoms, and the treatment/care plan.
3. Osmotic diuretics, e.g., mannitol or urea, may be ordered to decrease cerebral edema. Carefully monitor CPP, ICP, urine output, and blood pressure.
4. Vasodilator or vasopressor drugs may be ordered. Maintain BP within the parameters ordered and avoid rapid changes in BP, which may precipitate another stroke. Hypertension should be lowered gradually and only as far as cerebral perfusion is maintained (e.g., no further neurological deterioration is noted as the BP is lowered).
5. Anticoagulation medications e.g., heparin, coumadin, may be ordered for patients who have had an embolic stroke. Antiplatelet drugs, e.g., aspirin and dipyridamole, may also be ordered. Monitor for bruising and guaiac-test urine, stool, and NG aspirate for occult blood. Protect the patient from injury, e.g., use soft toothbrush for oral hygiene and use electric razor.
6. Prepare the patient for possible thrombectomy, embolectomy, or surgery, e.g., carotid endarterectomy; or for an extracranial or intracranial graft.
7. Maintain ventriculostomy (if present) and drain CSF according to established parameters.

▶ **Ineffective airway clearance** and **High risk for aspiration** related to altered consciousness or cough reflex dysfunction

PATIENT OUTCOMES
- Patient will maintain a patent airway
- Absence of aspiration
- RR 12-20, eupnea
- Lungs clear to auscultation
- O_2 sat >95%
- Pao_2 80-100 mm Hg
- $Paco_2$ 35-45 mm Hg
- pH 7.35-7.45

PATIENT MONITORING
1. Continuously monitor oxygen saturation with pulse oximetry (Spo_2). Monitor interventions and patient activities that may adversely affect oxygen saturation.

PHYSICAL ASSESSMENT
1. Ongoing assessment of respiratory status should be done. Note the rate, quality, and pattern; the patency of the upper airway and the patient's ability to handle oral secretions; skin color, nail beds, peripheral pulses, and skin temperature; and the presence and strength of gag, cough, and swallow reflexes.
2. Assess the lungs and note the presence of adventitious sounds. Note any restlessness or change in LOC that may suggest hypoxia.

DIAGNOSTICS ASSESSMENT
1. Review serial ABGs for hypoxemia and hypercapnia, since these disturbances can increase ICP.
2. Review serial chest radiographs to evaluate for possible aspiration or pulmonary congestion.

PATIENT MANAGEMENT
1. Maintain a patent airway by turning and positioning the patient to facilitate drainage of oropharyngeal secretions, providing an oral airway if necessary and suctioning secretions.
2. Once the patient's breathing is stabilized, provide pulmonary hygiene: C & DB therapy every hour and prn; provide chest physiotherapy and postural drainage if warranted and not contraindicated by IICP.
3. Administer oxygen as ordered. (See Chapter 6 for further information on mechanical ventilation.)
4. An NG tube may be required to prevent gastric distention and potential aspiration; check placement and patency.

5. Assist the patient with feedings if the gag and cough reflexes are intact; place the patient in an upright position and offer semisoft foods to avoid the risk of aspiration. Contact the speech therapist for swallowing evaluation if necessary.

▶ **Impaired communication:** dysarthria (impaired muscle involvement), expressive aphasia (inability to express thoughts verbally or in writing), receptive aphasia (inability to understand the spoken or written word), or dysphasia (impaired speech) related to cerebral ischemia or injury

PATIENT OUTCOME
• Patient will be able to communicate needs

PATIENT MONITORING
None

PHYSICAL ASSESSMENT
1. Assess for any deficits/decreases in communication skills/ ability, articulation, comprehension/verbalization.
2. Record the following characteristics of the patient's speech: spontaneity, fluency, and context.
3. Examine the muscles used for speech, testing cranial nerves VII, IX, X, and XII (see Table 1-2).
4. Ask the patient to follow verbal, then demonstrated commands.
5. Ask the patient to repeat simple phrases and sentences; test the patient for the ability to follow written commands.
6. Ask the patient to identify common objects, such as pen, scissors, pin.

DIAGNOSTICS ASSESSMENT
None

PATIENT MANAGEMENT
1. Limit the amount of environmental stimuli to decrease distractions and reduce confusion for the patient.
2. Encourage the patient to focus on one task at a time; speak in a clear, calm voice. Focus on simple, basic words and short sentences, allowing time for the patient to respond. Repeat or rephrase sentences as necessary.
3. Avoid appearing rushed; anticipate the patient's needs and encourage patience when the patient is frustrated by attempts at communication.
4. Try to assign consistent caregivers.
5. Instruct the family about limiting stimuli to prevent confusion for the patient. Keep the family informed and involved in the plan of care.

6. For expressive aphasia, encourage the patient's present speech and encourage spontaneous attempts at speech; allow sufficient time for the patient to respond to questions and words; cue with the first syllable or give a choice of words; provide alternate means, such as picture cards, word cards, or writing table.

7. For receptive aphasia, use concrete words to communicate nouns and verbs; use gestures and pictures and write messages; use word and phrase cards. Begin introducing words to the patient in the following order: noun, verb, pronoun.

8. Refer the patient to a speech therapist or pathologist for formal evaluation.

HEAD INJURY

Clinical Brief

Head injury involves trauma to the scalp, skull (cranium and facial bones), or brain. The severity of the injury is related to the degree of initial brain damage and associated secondary changes.

Primary injury occurs with an impact from an acceleration-deceleration or rotational force, and includes fracture, concussion, contusion, and laceration. The effects of injury on cerebral tissue can be focal or diffuse. Secondary injuries such as hematomas, intracranial hypertension, CNS infections, hypotension, hypoxemia, and hypercapnia often follow the primary injury. The clinician has no control over the primary injury; however, every attempt must be made to prevent or control secondary injuries, which can increase morbidity and mortality.

Classification of head injuries according to location and effect on the brain, as well as presenting signs and symptoms and diagnostic tests, are covered in Table 5-7.

Presenting signs and symptoms

Depending on the extent, degree, and location of brain injury, patients may have varying levels of consciousness and neurological deficits (see Table 5-7).

Physical examination

BP: Wide fluctuations may be seen; commonly patient is hypertensive, which may reflect IICP or may also be a preexisting condition

When hypertension is present with bradycardia, a wid-

Text continued on p. 197.

TABLE 5-7 Classification of Head Injury According to Location and Effect on the Brain

Location	Description and presenting signs and symptoms	Diagnostic findings
Scalp injuries		
Contusion	Bruise injury to the tissue of the scalp, with possible effusion of blood into the subcutaneous space without a break in the skin	Objective observation
Abrasion	Scraping away of part of the top layer of skin on the scalp	
Laceration	Wound or tear in the tissue of the scalp that tends to bleed profusely	
Skull fracture injuries		Diagnosis is primarily based on skull radiographs; these are viewed carefully to note air in the paranasal sinuses or other areas that may indicate a basilar skull fracture
Linear	Nondisplaced fracture of the skull at point of injury; swelling, ecchymosis, or tenderness is noted on the scalp; scalp contusion or laceration may also be present	
Comminuted	Multiple fragmented linear fractures	
Depressed	Displacement of comminuted fragments, associated with dural laceration and brain injury; look for cerebrospinal fluid leakage from the ear (otorrhea) or nose (rhinorrhea); swelling, ecchymosis, and other scalp injuries are common	

Compound	May be linear, comminuted, or depressed; external opening through scalp, mucous membranes of sinuses, or the tympanum (also see S&S for depressed fracture)	
Basilar skull	Linear fracture from base of temporal or frontal bone extending into the anterior, middle, or posterior fossa; produces characteristic clinical features, depending on site of fracture, e.g., raccoon's eyes (periorbital ecchymosis), Battle's sign (mastoidal ecchymosis), otorrhea, rhinorrhea, and anosmia (impairment of the sense of smell)	Radiograph may or may not reveal basilar fracture; CT scan and/or clinical features confirm the diagnosis; skull radiographs and CT scan confirm location and extent
Facial	Fractures of the facial bones produce disfigurement and facial motor and sensory dysfunction	
Meningeal tears	Dural laceration from compound or depressed fractures or from penetrating objects; S&S of meningitis (elevated temperature, stiff neck, pain on flexion of neck, deterioration of neurological signs, elevated WBC)	Leakage of CSF may be observed and will test positive for glucose; blood with CSF produces halo sign; CSF leak confirmed by cisternography

Continued.

TABLE 5-7 Classification of Head Injury According to Location and Effect on the Brain—cont'd

Location	Description and presenting signs and symptoms	Diagnostic findings
Cerebral injuries Concussion	Violent jarring or shaking of the brain; transient loss of consciousness, memory loss, nausea, vomiting, dizziness, unsteady gait, headache	Diagnosis made by clinical findings in the absence of focal lesion on CT; CT scan without contrast or MRI detects presence of contusion, hematoma, hemorrhage, hydrocephalus, edema, or midline shift; echo shows size of hematoma judged by midline shift
Contusion	Bruising of the brain with perivascular hemorrhage; loss of consciousness, speech, sensory or motor disturbances, depending on site involved; anterograde or retrograde memory loss	
Laceration	Tearing of brain tissue accompanied by focal swelling; can lead to intracranial bleeding, brain displacement, and death Decreased LOC, sensorimotor dysfunction, abnormal size and reaction in pupils, extraocular paralysis, other cranial nerve dysfunctions, seizures, and aphasia	

Brainstem injury	Primary—results from direct trauma, fracture, or torsion injury; secondary—may occur as a result of compression from IICP and herniation of temporal lobe; decreased LOC, abnormal breathing patterns, abnormal size and reaction in pupils, abnormal eye movement, motor deficits, and abnormal reflexes	Same as above
Hemorrhage Subdural hematoma	Bleeding occurs into the subdural space (between the dura mater and above the arachnoid layer); hematoma caused by slow bleeding usually from venous vessels; S&S usually slower than epidural hematoma; altered LOC, headache, personality changes, ipsilateral dilated pupil, and contralateral weakness	Same as cerebral injuries
Intracerebral hematoma	Bleeding is located within the brain tissue and may involve small arteries or veins; mortality is high; S&S depend on the location and size and are frequently indistinguishable from those of contusion; sudden onset of headache may be accompanied with nausea and vomiting; rapid deterioration with respiratory distress and coma	Same as cerebral injuries; CT with contrast will demonstrate presence of aneurysm, AVM, or tumor

Continued.

TABLE 5-7 Classification of Head Injury According to Location and Effect on the Brain—cont'd

Location	Description and presenting signs and symptoms	Diagnostic findings
Hemorrhage—cont'd Epidural hematoma	Extradural bleeding above the dura mater (between the periosteal lining of the skull and dura mater); usually caused by arterial bleeding from a torn middle meningeal artery and often associated with a fracture of the temporal bone; clot presses on brain and can cause rapid herniation and death; brief loss of consciousness followed by lucid period; severe vomiting, headache, rapid deterioration with decreased LOC, ipsilateral dilated pupil, contralateral hemiparesis, and seizures may occur	Same as cerebral injuries; brain scan is helpful with isodense hematomas; MRI may differentiate hemorrhages that occurred at different times
Subarachnoid hemorrhage and intraventricular hemorrhage	Bleeding is usually associated with ruptured aneurysm or AVM; S&S of restlessness, severe headache, nuchal rigidity, elevated temperature, positive Kernig's sign (loss of ability to extend leg when thigh is flexed on abdomen)	Same as cerebral injuries; CSF studies will reflect blood and elevated protein and pressure

ened pulse pressure, and irregular respirations (Cushing's triad), it reflects a late and possibly terminal sign of IICP indicative of loss of autoregulation

Hypotension from head injury alone is rare but may also indicate a terminal event

HR: Bradycardia, associated with IICP

Tachycardia, seen with occult hemorrhage or as a terminal event

RR: Pathological respiratory pattern will roughly correlate with the level of neurological injury, ranging from Cheyne-Stokes, central neurogenic hyperventilation, apneustic to ataxic breathing (see Table 1-7)

Temperature: Will vary widely with hypothalamic injuries

Hyperthermic with subarachnoid hemorrhage or infections

Pulmonary: Adventitious sounds may be present

CV: Cardiac dysrhythmias are not uncommon and may be life threatening

Neurological: See Table 5-7

Diagnostic findings

See Table 5-7.

Acute Care Patient Management

Goals of treatment

Optimize oxygenation

Ensuring of patent airway

Supplemental oxygen

Intubation and mechanical ventilation

IV fluids, blood replacement

Vasopressor, antihypertensive, and vasodilator agents

Control and/or reduce increased ICP

CSF drainage

Osmotic diuretics

Glucocorticoids (controversial)

Evacuation of hematoma via burr hole or craniotomy

Hyperventilation therapy

Barbiturate coma

Priority nursing diagnoses

Impaired gas exchange

Altered tissue perfusion: cerebral

High risk for altered protection (see p. 145)

Altered nutrition: less than body requirements (see p. 149)

High risk for altered family process (see p. 150)

▶ **Impaired gas exchange** related to hypoventilation secondary to altered level of consciousness or interstitial fluid secondary to neurogenic pulmonary edema and **Ineffective breathing pattern** secondary to injury to respiratory center

PATIENT OUTCOMES
- Patient will be alert and oriented
- Pao_2 80-100 mm Hg
- O_2 sat >95%
- $Paco_2$ in low limits of normal range (35-40 mm Hg)
- pH 7.35-7.45
- RR 12-20, eupnea
- Absence of adventitious breath sounds
- PAWP 4-12 mm Hg

PATIENT MONITORING
1. Continuously monitor oxygen saturation with pulse oximetry (Spo_2). Monitor interventions and patient activities that may adversely affect oxygen saturation.
2. Monitor CVP and PA pressures, including PAWP as appropriate to patient's clinical condition, to monitor fluid volume status. Increasing wedge pressure may indicate development of neurogenic pulmonary edema. Calculate PVR; hypoxemia can increase sympathetic tone and increase pulmonary vasoconstriction.

PHYSICAL ASSESSMENT
1. Assess the patient's ability to handle oral secretions. Assess respiratory rate, depth, and rhythm frequently. Auscultate breath sounds q1-2h and prn.
2. Assess for signs and symptoms of hypoxia: change in LOC, increased restlessness, and irritability. Assess nailbeds, capillary refill, and skin temperature. Cyanosis is a late sign.
3. Assess integrity of the gag and cough reflexes; the patient may need to be intubated if reflexes are not intact.

DIAGNOSTICS ASSESSMENT
1. Review serial ABGs for hypoxemia (Pao_2 <60 mm Hg) and hypercapnia ($Paco_2$ >45 mm Hg); these disturbances can increase ICP.
2. Review serial chest radiographs for pulmonary congestion.

PATIENT MANAGEMENT
1. Administer oxygen as ordered. Ensure airway patency by proper positioning of the head and neck. Keep HOB elevated at 30 degrees to enhance chest excursion. If cer-

vical injury has not been ruled out, *do not hyperextend the neck* for oral intubation; use the jaw-thrust method. Because of the risk of direct brain trauma or infection during insertion, nasopharyngeal airways should be avoided in the presence of rhinorrhea (a sign that may reflect a break in the integrity of the skull). An oral airway or bite block can prevent the patient from biting an endotracheal tube if orally intubated.

2. Provide pulmonary hygiene to reduce the risk of pulmonary complications, e.g., pneumonia, atelectasis. Initiate C & DB therapy and reposition the patient to mobilize secretions, carefully monitoring for IICP. *Avoid* coughing exercises for a patient at risk of IICP.

3. Suction secretions only as needed. Hyperoxygenate before and after suctioning and limit passes of suction catheter to 15 seconds or less to avoid hypoxia. Document quality and quantity of secretions. *Never* use nasotracheal suctioning in the presence of rhinorrhea because of the risk of direct brain trauma or infection.

▶ **Altered tissue perfusion: cerebral** related to IICP secondary to space-occupying lesion or cerebral edema

PATIENT OUTCOMES

- Patient will be alert and oriented
- Pupils equal and normoreactive
- Motor strength equal bilaterally
- RR 12-20, eupnea
- HR 60-100 beats/min
- ICP 0-15 mm Hg
- CPP 60-100 mm Hg
- Absence of headache, vomiting, seizures

PATIENT MONITORING

1. Continuously monitor ECG for changes in rate and rhythm (most often bradycardia) and nonspecific ST and T-wave changes.

2. Monitor ICP trends every hour or more often if patient's condition warrants. Analyze the ICP waveform and calculate cerebral perfusion pressure (CPP) q30-60″. CPP less than 60 mm Hg leads to decreased cerebral blood flow (CBF), resulting in cerebral ischemia (see Chapter 3 for ICP monitoring).

3. Monitor blood pressure frequently, since hypotension and hypertension can increase ICP and vasopressor or vasodilator therapy may be used.

TABLE 5-8 Cranial Nerve Functions and Clinical Correlations

Nerve	Function	Clinical correlation
I Olfactory	Smell	Anterior fossa or cribiform plate fracture, frontal lobe or pituitary lesion, tumor, or meningitis
II Optic	Vision	Anterior fossa or orbital plate fracture, direct eye trauma, vascular disruption via carotid system and cerebral lesion
III Oculomotor	Elevates lid, moves eyeball, constricts pupil	Orbital plate fracture, temporal lobe swelling, IICP, aneurysm compression, or damage to midbrain
IV Trochlear	Moves eyeball	Inflammation or aneurysm
V Trigeminal	Muscles of mastication, facial sensation	Fractures of skull/face, pontine tumors, trauma
VI Abducens	Moves eyeball	Trauma, IICP, aneurysms, inflammation
VII Facial	Muscles of facial movement and taste	Temporal bone or middle fossa fracture, tumors, stroke, Bell's palsy, pons and medulla damage
VIII Acoustic	Hearing and balance	Temporal bone or middle fossa fractures, tumors, infection
IX Glossopharyngeal	Sensation for gag, swallow	Dysfunction usually seen with vagus nerve
X Vagus	Innervation of pharynx and thoracic/abdominal viscera	Surgery, e.g., endarterectomy; unopposed action with cervical spine injuries, medulla damage
XI Accessory	Turns head	Neck surgery or trauma
XII Hypoglossal	Tongue movement	Brainstem involvement or higher

Modified from Plum F and Posner J, 1980; Hickey J, 1986; and Kenney M, Packa D, and Dunbar S, 1988.

4. Monitor CVP and/or PA pressure (as appropriate to patient's clinical condition) every hour, since both parameters reflect the capacity of the vascular system to accept volume and can be used to monitor for imbalances that can compromise CPP.
5. Monitor I & O hourly and calculate hourly running totals. Polyuria (5-10 L/day) or oliguria (400-500 ml/day) may signal onset of diabetes insipidus or SIADH.

PHYSICAL ASSESSMENT

1. Assess neurological status for signs and symptoms of herniation: progressive deterioration in LOC and motor function; changes in respiratory patterns (deep sighing and yawning may signal impending herniation); ipsilateral pupil dilation, pupils sluggish or nonreactive to light (see Table 1-7).
2. Assess for factors that can cause IICP, such as a distended bladder, hypoxemia, hypercapnia, headache, fear, or anxiety.
3. Assess temperature; fever may reflect damage to the hypothalamus and increase metabolic demands and oxygen consumption. Because of the concern of possible seizure activity, avoid oral temperature taking.
4. Test cranial nerve function, since nerve damage can result from craniocerebral trauma (see Table 1-2). Table 5-8 identifies conditions that may have cranial nerve involvement.

DIAGNOSTICS ASSESSMENT

1. Review serial ABGs for hypoxemia (Pao_2 <60 mm Hg) and hypercapnia ($Paco_2$ >45 mm Hg); these disturbances can increase ICP.
2. Review serial electrolyte studies, serum and urine osmolality, and specific gravity for imbalances secondary to diuretic use and/or development of diabetes insipidus (DI) or SIADH. Urine specific gravity will be increased in SIADH and decreased with diuretic administration; urine specific gravity will be decreased with the diuresis associated with DI.
3. Review serial Hgb and Hct levels for anemic states; WBC counts to evaluate the inflammatory process; FDP, PT, and PTT to identify coagulation deficiencies; and glucose levels for hyperglycemia from steroid use.
4. Review findings of lumbar puncture for indications of meningitis.
5. Review baseline and serial CT or MRI reports.

PATIENT MANAGEMENT

1. Administer oxygen as ordered to maximize cerebral perfusion.
2. Reduce or minimize fluctuations in ICP by maintaining the patient's head and neck in neutral position, elevating the HOB to 30 degrees to promote cerebral venous drainage, and avoiding extreme flexion of hips. Avoid taping the endotracheal tube around the patient's neck and avoid restraining the patient unless there is a danger of extubation.
3. Space nursing activities and allow the patient to rest between activities to decrease possible IICP. If an increase in ICP is observed, stop the activity and allow the patient to rest until the ICP returns to the previous reading.
4. Administer intravenous fluids carefully to minimize fluctuations in vascular load and ICP. Hypotonic fluids (D_5W) are usually avoided to reduce the risk of cerebral edema.
5. Antihypertensive agents and vasopressor agents may be ordered to maintain BP. Monitor BP and CPP carefully.
6. Osmotic diuretics, e.g., mannitol, may be used to reduce edema. Monitor serum osmolality closely; an increased osmolality (greater than 310 mOsm/kg) may disrupt the blood brain barrier and actually increase edema. Monitor for hypotension, which decreases CPP, and observe for increased ICP, which may occur 8 to 12 hours after osmotic diuresis. If loop diuretics are used, monitor urine output and electrolytes.
7. Corticosteroids, e.g., dexamethasone, methylprednisolone, may be ordered. Monitor electrolytes and glucose levels.
8. Other pharmacological agents to reduce ICP may include phenytoin (Dilantin), to treat or prevent seizure activity; acetaminophen, to maintain normothermia, since hyperthermia increases metabolic needs; and pancuronium bromide, to reduce intracranial hypertension associated with agitation and posturing.
9. Hyperventilation therapy and barbiturate coma may be employed (see Chapter 6, Therapeutic Modalities).
10. Surgical intervention may be required to evacuate the hematoma (see Chapter 6, Craniotomy).

INTRACEREBRAL HEMORRHAGE (ICH)

Clinical Brief

Bleeding into the brain tissue is frequently the result of sudden rupture of a blood vessel within the brain. The effects depend on the location of the rupture and actual size of the clot. Brain tissue adjacent to the clot is displaced and produces focal neurological signs. The most common site for this type of hematoma is in the basal ganglia, followed by the thalamic region.

The usual precipitating factor of a cerebral hemorrhage is hypertension. Other possible causes may include an aneurysm, AVM, tumors, trauma, or hemorrhagic disorders. In addition, illicit use of cocaine or crack may result in an intracerebral hemorrhage.

Presenting signs and symptoms

A headache of sudden onset, occasionally accompanied by nausea and vomiting, may accompany intracerebral hemorrhage. The neurological deficits that are initially seen will reflect the anatomical location of the hemorrhage. As the intracranial pressure increases there is evidence of developing uncal or central herniation with accompanying changes in pupils, respirations, and vital signs.

Acute Care Patient Management

The management of intracerebral hemorrhage secondary to hypertension is similar to hemorrhage associated with head trauma. Treatment is aimed toward reducing the severely elevated BP and normalizing ICP (see Acute head injury, p. 191).

NEURO

Pulmonary Disorders

ADULT RESPIRATORY DISTRESS SYNDROME (ARDS)
Clinical Brief
ARDS is a syndrome that results from an acute injury. Causes are multifactorial and may include trauma, sepsis, aspiration, shock, or any condition that causes a direct or indirect lung injury. Noncardiogenic pulmonary edema, decreased lung compliance, and hypoxemia refractory to supplemental oxygen characterize ARDS.

Presenting signs and symptoms
The patient may have acute respiratory distress, dyspnea, tachypnea, tachycardia, restlessness, and anxiety.

Physical examination
BP: May be ↑ in response to hypoxemia or ↓ in response to hemodynamic compromise

HR: ↑ or ↓ in response to hypoxemia

RR: >30/min

Neurological: Restlessness, agitation, decrease in sensorium

Pulmonary: Cough, fine inspiratory crackles, use of accessory muscles

Diagnostic findings
ARTERIAL BLOOD GASES
Pao_2 <50 mm Hg on Fio_2 60%

CHEST RADIOGRAPH
May be normal for the first 12 to 24 hours after the respiratory distress occurs. The earliest abnormalities seen are patchy, bilateral, interstitial, and alveolar infiltrates. If the patient improves, the radiographic appearance may return to normal. When the disease progresses, the alveolar infiltrates advance to a diffuse consolidation (see Figure 2-3).

PULMONARY FUNCTION
- Compliance <50 ml/cm H_2O
- Decreased FRC
- Shunt fraction (Qs/Qt) >5%
- Deadspace ventilation (V_D/V_T) >0.45

- Alveolar-arterial gradient $(P[A-a]o_2)$ >15 mm Hg on room air or >50 mm Hg on Fio_2 100%
- PAWP <18 mm Hg

Acute Care Patient Management

Goals of treatment

Optimize tissue oxygenation
    Intubation/mechanical ventilation
    PEEP
    High-frequency ventilation
    Inverse ratio ventilation
    Extracorporeal membrane oxygenation (ECMO)
    Ensure adequate CO and Hgb
    Treat underlying cause
Maintain hemodynamic stability
    Crystalloid or colloid infusion
    Diuretic agents
    Inotropic agents
    Prostaglandin E_1
    Nonsteroidal antiinflammatory agents
    Corticosteroids (controversial)
Detect/prevent clinical sequelae (Table 5-9)

Priority nursing diagnoses

Impaired gas exchange
Altered tissue perfusion
High risk for altered protection (see p. 145)
Altered nutrition: less than body requirements (see p. 149)
High risk for altered family process (see p. 150)

TABLE 5-9 Clinical Sequelae of Adult Respiratory Distress Syndrome

Complication	Signs and symptoms
Dysrhythmias	Changes in rate, rhythm
	Change in LOC or syncope
Pneumonia	Purulent sputum, fever
GI bleeding	Coffee-ground emesis, guaiac-positive emesis and stool
DIC	Bleeding from any orifice, mucous membranes, petechiae, hematuria, hematemesis; prolonged PT/PTT; ↑ fibrin split products; ↓ platelets
Renal failure	Decreased u/o; ↑ BUN and Cr
Respiratory arrest	Cessation of breathing

► Impaired gas exchange related to interstitial and alveolar fluid accumulation; and **Ineffective breathing pattern** (decreased compliance)

PATIENT OUTCOMES

- Patient will be alert and oriented to person, place, and time
- O_2 sat >90%
- Svo_2 60%-80%
- VC 10-15 ml/kg
- RR 12-20/min
- Eupnea
- Lung sounds clear to auscultation
- HR 60-100 beats/min
- $P(a/A)o_2$ ratio >0.60

PULM

PATIENT MONITORING

1. Continuously monitor ECG for dysrhythmias that may be related to hypoxemia or acid-base imbalances.
2. Continuously monitor oxygen saturation with pulse oximetry (Spo_2). Carefully monitor interventions and patient activities that may adversely affect oxygen saturation.
3. Continuously monitor Svo_2 (as appropriate to patient's clinical condition); carefully monitor interventions and patient activities that may adversely affect oxygenation.
4. Monitor pulmonary function by evaluating serial vital capacities and tidal volumes. Calculate compliance q8h. (See pulmonary function tests in Chapter 2.)
5. Monitor PA systolic, since hypoxia can increase sympathetic tone and increase pulmonary vasoconstriction. Calculate PVR.
6. Obtain CO readings, since oxygen delivery depends on adequate cardiac output.
7. Calculate $P(a/A)o_2$ ratio to evaluate intrapulmonary shunt.
8. Monitor fluid volume status: measure I & O q1h, determine fluid balance q8h. Compare serial weights for changes (1 kg ~ 1000 ml of fluid). Fluid excess may cause cardiogenic pulmonary edema.
9. If the patient's lungs are mechanically ventilated, see Mechanical ventilation in Chapter 6.

PHYSICAL ASSESSMENT

1. Assess respiratory status q2h or more often, depending on patient condition. Note respiratory rate, rhythm, depth, and use of accessory muscles. Observe for para-

doxical breathing pattern, increased restlessness, increased complaints of dyspnea, and changes in level of consciousness. Cyanosis is a late sign of respiratory distress.

2. Assess the patient for development of clinical sequelae (see Table 5-9).

DIAGNOSTICS ASSESSMENT

1. Review serial ABGs to evaluate oxygenation and acid-base balance.
2. Review serial chest radiographs to evaluate improvement or worsening condition. Chest radiographs can provide a rough estimate of extravascular lung water.
3. Review serial Hgb and Hct levels; a reduced Hgb can adversely affect oxygen-carrying capacity.

PATIENT MANAGEMENT

1. Administer oxygen as ordered; intubation and mechanical ventilation are usually required (see Chapter 6 for information on mechanical ventilation).
2. Reposition the patient to improve oxygenation and mobilize secretions. Evaluate the patient's response to position changes with ABGs to determine the best position for oxygenation.
3. Provide chest physiotherapy and postural drainage to mobilize secretions; follow with deep breathing and coughing or suctioning. Preoxygenate the patient's lungs with Fio_2 100% to prevent a decrease in oxygen saturation. Note the characteristics of the sputum.
4. Administer antibiotics as ordered to treat the identified organism.
5. Anticipate diuretic therapy to keep the patient "dry" without adversely affecting intravascular volume and cardiac output.
6. Decrease oxygen consumption by limiting and pacing activities, providing uninterrupted rest, limiting visitors if necessary, decreasing anxiety with distraction or relaxation therapy, and decreasing fever.
7. High-frequency ventilation, inverse-ratio ventilation, or ECMO may be used to improve gas exchange (see Chapter 6, Therapeutic Modalities).
8. Anticipate volume therapy, inotropic agents, vasodilators, prostaglandin E_1, and steroids to decrease pulmonary vasoconstriction.

9. NG intubation may be required to decompress the stomach and decrease the risk of aspiration.

10. Nutritional support will be required to prevent respiratory muscle dysfunction and to maintain immunological defense mechanisms.

▶ **Altered tissue perfusion** related to hypoxia and/or **decreased cardiac output** secondary to decreased venous return with PEEP and diuretic therapy

PATIENT OUTCOMES

- Patient will be alert and oriented to person, place, and time
- SBP 90-140 mm Hg
- MAP 70-105 mm Hg
- CVP 2-6 mm Hg
- HR 60-100 beats/min
- SV 50-100 ml
- CO 4-8 L/min
- CI 2.4-4 L/min/m^2
- u/o 30 ml/hr or 0.5-1.0 ml/kg/hr
- Peripheral pulses strong
- PAWP 4-12 mm Hg
- SVR 900-1400 dynes/sec/cm^{-5}
- PVR 100-250 dynes/sec/cm^{-5}

PATIENT MONITORING

1. Obtain PA, arterial BP, and CVP readings q1h or more often if titrating pharmacological agents or increasing PEEP levels. Calculate MAP; a MAP <60 can adversely affect cerebral and renal perfusion. Obtain CO and calculate CI and SV; pulse pressure is also an indicator of stroke volume. Calculate SVR and PVR.

2. Monitor fluid volume status: measure I & O hourly; determine fluid balance every 8 hours. Compare serial weights for changes (1 kg ~1000 ml of fluid). Decrease in urinary output may be related to decreased renal perfusion secondary to decreased CO or development of SIADH in the patient undergoing mechanical ventilation therapy.

3. Continuously monitor ECG for signs of myocardial ischemia or the onset of dysrhythmias.

PHYSICAL ASSESSMENT

1. Assess LOC, skin, peripheral pulses, and capillary refill as indicators of cardiac output and tissue perfusion.

PULM

2. Assess the patient for development of clinical sequelae (see Table 5-9).

DIAGNOSTICS ASSESSMENT

1. Review serial ABGs; hypoxemia and acidosis can adversely affect myocardial contractility and contribute to decreasing CO.

2. Review serial Hgb and Hct levels; adequate hemoglobin is necessary to maintain normal oxygen transport.

3. Review lactate levels, which are an indicator of anaerobic metabolism. Increased levels may signal decreased O_2 delivery.

PATIENT MANAGEMENT

1. Administer crystalloids or colloids as ordered to maintain adequate preload. Monitor fluid status carefully, since excessive fluid can increase hydrostatic pressure and worsen pulmonary edema.

2. Titrate positive inotropic agents to improve myocardial contractility and increase CO. Vasopressor agents may be required to maintain SBP >90 mm Hg.

PULMONARY EMBOLI

Clinical Brief

A pulmonary embolus is an occlusion in pulmonary vasculature that occurs from a fibrin or blood clot. Most commonly emboli are detached from the deep veins of the legs. Predisposing factors include Virchow's triad: acute injury to blood vessel walls, venous stasis, and hypercoagulable states. Air emboli usually result from air entering the circulatory system through intravascular catheters. Fat emboli occur with long-bone fractures.

Presenting signs and symptoms

The patient may be apprehensive and have dyspnea, pleuritic pain, hemoptysis, tachycardia, tachypnea, and crackles.

Physical examination

Appearance: restlessness, anxiety, petechiae if fat emboli are present

BP: Normal or ↑ BP as a result of anxiety

HR: Normal or ↑ HR >100 beats/min

RR: ↑ rate

CV: Increased intensity of pulmonic S_2, S_3, S_4 gallop

Pulmonary: SOB, crackles (localized)

Massive PE: Cyanosis, altered LOC, sudden shock

DVT symptoms: Calf swelling, warmth, and tenderness

Diagnostic findings
HISTORY OF RISK FACTORS
Immobility, traumatic injury, pregnancy, use of oral contraceptives, atrial fibrillation, or mitral stenosis
ARTERIAL BLOOD GASES
Pao_2 <60 mm Hg, $Paco_2$ <35 mm Hg, and pH >7.45
Increased alveolar-arterial oxygen tension gradient
CHEST RADIOGRAPH
Initially normal; later findings include pleural effusions, wedge collapse, focal oligemic lung.
ECG
Usually nonspecific; right-axis deviation, ST-segment depression in V_1-V_4, new right bundle branch block, and tachycardic rhythms all are suggestive.
VENTILATION-PERFUSION LUNG SCAN
Results are suggestive of PE if a perfusion defect is found with normal ventilation.
PULMONARY ANGIOGRAPHY
Pulmonary angiography is the most definitive test for PE, showing an abrupt cutoff of a vessel or a filling defect. PA pressures may be elevated; PVR may be increased.

Acute Care Patient Management
Goals of treatment
Optimize tissue oxygenation
  Oxygen therapy
  Pulmonary embolectomy
  Thrombolytic therapy
  Analgesia
Prevent embolic phenomenon
  Sequential compression devices
  Antithromboemboli stockings
  Anticoagulation
  Filter or ligation of vena cava
Detect/prevent clinical sequelae (Table 5-10)
Priority nursing diagnoses
Impaired gas exchange
Altered tissue perfusion: cardiopulmonary
High risk for injury
High risk for altered protection (see p. 145)
Altered nutrition: less than body requirements (see p. 149)
High risk for altered family process (see p. 150)
▶ Impaired gas exchange related to ventilation-perfusion mismatch; hypoventilation secondary to pain

TABLE 5-10 Clinical Sequelae of Pulmonary Emboli

Complication	Signs and symptoms
Pulmonary infarction	Pleuritic pain, friction rub, hemoptysis, elevated temperature, cyanosis, shock, death
Pleural effusions	On affected side: decreased respiratory excursion and breath sounds, dullness on percussion
Right ventricular failure	Jugular venous distention; increased CVP, RAP, and RV pressure; Kussmaul's sign

PATIENT OUTCOMES
- Patient will be alert and oriented to person, place, and time
- Pao_2 60-100 mm Hg
- O_2 sat >90%
- RR 12-20
- Eupnea
- Absence of adventitious breath sounds
- $P(a/A)o_2$ ratio >0.60

PATIENT MONITORING
1. Continuously monitor oxygen saturation with pulse oximetry (Spo_2). Carefully monitor patient activities and interventions that may adversely affect oxygen saturation.
2. Continuously monitor ECG for dysrhythmias or ischemic changes.
3. Calculate $P(a/A)o_2$ ratio to evaluate intrapulmonary shunt.

PHYSICAL ASSESSMENT
1. Assess respiratory status: note rate and depth of respirations; observe for dyspnea and restlessness. Hypoxia may be manifested as increased restlessness or change in level of consciousness and respiratory rate >30/min. Auscultate breath sounds; crackles and pleuritic rub may be present.
2. Assess pain using a visual analogue scale (see Figure 1-1).
3. Assess the patient for development of clinical sequelae (see Table 5-10).

DIAGNOSTICS ASSESSMENT

1. Review ABGs for changes in Sao_2 and Pao_2 to evaluate improvement or deterioration in the patient's pulmonary status.

PATIENT MANAGEMENT

1. Place patient on bed rest initially and assist patient to assume a comfortable position.
2. Administer supplemental oxygen as ordered.
3. Pace activities to decrease the patient's oxygen demand, allowing adequate time for patient recovery.
4. Turn, C & DB the patient q4h; note the color and character of sputum.
5. Administer analgesics as ordered to prevent splinting and improve chest excursion.

▸ **Altered tissue perfusion: cardiopulmonary** related to embolic phenomenon

PATIENT OUTCOMES

- Patient will be alert and oriented to person, place, and time
- RR 12-20
- Eupnea
- Pao_2 60-100 mm Hg
- O_2 sat >90%
- Lungs clear to auscultation
- SBP 90-140 mm Hg
- HR 60-100 beats/min
- Peripheral pulses strong
- Skin pink, warm, and dry
- Absence of jugular venous distension (JVD)

PATIENT MONITORING

1. Continuously monitor oxygen saturation with pulse oximetry (Spo_2). Carefully monitor patient activities and interventions that may adversely affect oxygen saturation.
2. Continuously monitor ECG for dysrhythmias and ischemic changes.
3. Monitor PAP, CVP, and arterial BP (as appropriate to patient's clinical condition) and calculate PVR. Increases in PVR may lead to right ventricular failure.

PHYSICAL ASSESSMENT

1. Assess for thrombophlebitis: warmth, redness, tenderness, and swelling of lower extremity.
2. Assess the patient for manifestations of right ventricular failure: JVD, peripheral edema.

PULM

3. Assess respiratory status: auscultate breath sounds, note increased work of breathing, e.g., increased respiratory rate, use of accessory muscles, and dyspnea.
4. Be alert for emboli in other body systems. Assess level of consciousness and muscle strength to monitor for cerebral infarction; note any abdominal pain, nausea or vomiting, decreased or absent bowel sounds to monitor for GI infarction; check for decreased urinary output and hematuria to monitor for renal infarction.
5. Assess the patient for development of clinical sequelae.

DIAGNOSTICS ASSESSMENT
1. Review serial ABGs to evaluate oxygenation status.
2. Review cardiac profile (if available) for evidence of myocardial infarction.
3. Review serial BUN and creatinine studies to evaluate renal function.

PATIENT MANAGEMENT
1. Assist the patient to a position that will promote chest excursion and ease of breathing.
2. Administer oxygen therapy as ordered.
3. Administer anticoagulants as ordered. An initial bolus of 5000-10,000 units of heparin may be required, followed by a continuous infusion at a rate of approximately 1000 U/hr. Monitor PTT results; if greater than two times the control, consult with the physician.
4. Reduce risk factors: conduct range-of-motion exercises to extremities; avoid sharp flexion at knees and groin; apply antithromboembolism stockings and sequential compression devices on admission. Remove devices every shift to assess skin and prevent skin breakdown. Mobilize the patient as soon as possible.
5. See Chapter 6, Thrombolytic therapy.

▶ **High risk for injury:** bleeding related to anticoagulant or thrombolytic agents

PATIENT OUTCOMES
- Absence of bleeding
- Hct: 40%-54% (males)
  37%-47% (females)
- Hgb: 14-18 g/dl (males)
  12-16 g/dl (females)
- PT/PTT within therapeutic range
- SBP 90-140 mm Hg
- HR 60-100 beats/min

PATIENT MONITORING
None specific

PHYSICAL ASSESSMENT

1. Assess the patient for bleeding from puncture sites, wounds, gums, or any body orifice. Note any altered level of consciousness or abdominal pain that may indicate internal bleeding.

2. Test NG aspirate, emesis, urine, stool, and sputum for occult blood.

DIAGNOSTICS ASSESSMENT

1. Review serial Hgb and Hct levels for decreasing trend that may suggest bleeding.

2. Review serial PTT results. If results are greater than two times the control, consult with the physician.

3. Review serial platelet counts to monitor for thrombocytopenia.

PATIENT MANAGEMENT

1. Reposition the patient at least q2h to prevent high pressure areas. Handle the patient gently to prevent bruising.

2. An arterial line should be used to obtain specimens when at all possible. If venipuncture becomes necessary, apply direct pressure to the puncture site for 10 to 15 minutes and then apply a pressure dressing. When discontinuing intravenous or arterial catheters apply pressure for 20 to 30 minutes, then apply a pressure dressing to assure hemostasis. Reassess sites within 30 minutes for further bleeding or hematoma formation.

3. Antacids and/or H_2 antagonists may be ordered to prevent gastric bleeding. Monitor gastric pH (if equipment is available).

4. Stool softeners should be administered to prevent straining and rectal bleeding.

5. Avoid aspirin or aspirin-containing products, which may contribute to bleeding.

CHEST TRAUMA

Clinical Brief

Injuries to the structures of the thorax can be caused by blunt or penetrating injuries, e.g., motor vehicle accidents, falls, gunshot wounds, and stab wounds. Tissue hypoxia is a major concern, since the intrathoracic organs are highly vascular and hemorrhagic shock is common. Pleural pressures

PULM

can change, leading to collapsed lungs or mediastinal shift; ventilation-perfusion mismatch can also occur as a result of the injury. Dysrhythmias can occur with myocardial injury secondary to trauma to the sternum. According to the American College of Surgeons, approximately 25% of all trauma deaths are a result of chest injuries. (See Table 5-11 for a summary of chest injuries.)

Acute Care Patient Management

Goals of treatment

Improve ventilation and gas exchange
  Oxygen therapy
  Intubation and mechanical ventilation
  Chest tube insertion
  Flail chest: stabilize chest wall (PEEP, PSV)
  Hemothorax: CT, thoracotomy
  Pulmonary contusion: diuretics, methylprednisone (controversial), unilateral lung ventilation, ECMO
  Tracheobronchial tear: thoracotomy: HFJV
  Esophageal rupture: NG intubation, surgical repair
Maintain hemodynamic stability
  Crystalloid infusion
  Blood products
  Autotransfusion
  Inotropic agents
  Needle decompression for tension pneumothorax
  Myocardial contusion: antidysrhythmic agents
Decrease/alleviate pain
  Narcotics
  Patient-controlled analgesia (PCA)
  Intercostal nerve block
  Epidural analgesia
Detect/prevent clinical sequelae (Table 5-12)

Priority nursing diagnoses

Impaired gas exchange
Altered tissue perfusion
Pain
High risk for altered protection (see p. 145)
Altered nutrition: less than body requirements (see p. 149)
High risk for altered family process (see p. 150)

▶ **Impaired gas exchange** related to ventilation-perfusion mismatch, decreased compliance, inadequate ventilation
PATIENT OUTCOMES
• Patient will be alert and oriented to person, place, and time

TABLE 5-11 Summary of Chest Injuries

Injury	Clinical brief	Signs and symptoms
Flail chest	Instability of chest wall as a result of multiple rib or sternal fractures Diagnostic findings: chest radiograph confirms fractures; abnormal respiratory motion and crepitus aids diagnosis	Paradoxical chest motion, labored shallow respirations, subcutaneous emphysema
Pneumothorax	Accumulation of air in the pleural space; partial or total lung collapse Diagnostic findings: chest radiograph visualizes air between visceral and parietal pleura	Dyspnea, decreased or absent breath sounds Open pneumothorax: wound present, often sucking in nature Closed pneumothorax: no opening to external environment
Tension pneumothorax	Accumulation of air without a means of escape, causing complete collapse of the lung and mediastinal shift; immediate decompression necessary Diagnostic findings: clinical findings are the basis for diagnosis	Severe dyspnea, cyanosis, restlessness, distended neck veins, tracheal shift to the unaffected side, hypotension, distant heart sounds, tachycardia, subcutaneous emphysema
Hemothorax	Accumulation of blood in the pleural space Diagnostic findings: chest radiograph visualizes blood accumulation	Cool, clammy skin; hypotension, decreased capillary refill, tachycardia, absent breath sounds on affected side

Continued.

PULM

TABLE 5-11 Summary of Chest Injuries—cont'd

Injury	Clinical brief	Signs and symptoms
Pulmonary contusion	Injury to lung tissue that can cause respiratory failure, potentially lethal Diagnostic findings: chest radiograph shows local or diffuse patchy, poorly outlined densities, or irregular linear infiltrates; ABGs: hypoxemia and hypercarbia	Dyspnea, restlessness, hemoptysis, tachycardia, ineffective cough, crackles, decreased lung compliance
Tracheobronchial tear	Injury to tracheobronchial tree that can result in airway obstruction and tension pneumothorax Diagnostic findings: clinical findings are the basis of diagnosis; bronchoscopy confirms tear	Noisy breathing, hemoptysis, subcutaneous emphysema, possible s/s of tension pneumothorax
Myocardial contusion	Injury to cardiac muscle that may result in dysrhythmias, muscle damage, cardiac rupture Diagnostic findings: no one diagnostic test is used, ECHO is helpful to evaluate abnormal wall motion; serial CKs may be used to evaluate myocardial damage	Chest discomfort, tachycardia, ST-T wave changes evidence of sternal injury

| Diaphragm rupture | Tear in the diaphragm that may allow abdominal contents to herniate into thorax Diagnostic findings: chest radiograph with contrast confirms tear; NG tube may be observed curled in lower left chest; appearance of peritoneal lavage fluid in chest tube drainage confirms the diagnosis | Chest pain referred to shoulder, dyspnea, decreased breath sounds, bowel sounds auscultated in chest, possible rhonchi |
| Esophageal rupture | Perforation of the esophagus that allows gastric and esophageal contents to contaminate the mediastinum and pleura Diagnostic findings: chest radiograph visualizes mediastinal air on the left side, pleural effusion, pneumothorax; esophagogram or endoscopy confirms tear | Pain correlates to location of tear; hoarseness, dysphagia, bloody emesis/NG aspirate, subcutaneous emphysema |

TABLE 5-12 Clinical Sequelae of Chest Trauma

Complication	Signs and symptoms
Hypoxemia	Restlessness, RR >30/min, HR >120 beats/min, labored breathing, increase in PAP
Infection	Temperature >38.5° C (> 101.3° F), purulent secretions
	Ineffective cough, diminished breath sounds
Tension pneumothorax	Severe dyspnea, tracheal deviation toward unaffected side, absence of breath sounds, distended neck veins, unequal chest symmetry (chest is larger on side of pneumothorax), cyanosis, hypotension
ARDS	Dyspnea, RR >30, labored breathing, tachycardia, decreased compliance (30-40 cm H_2O), PAWP <18 mm Hg, hypoxemia refractory to increase in Fio_2
Hemothorax	
Shock	Decrease in sensorium; cool, clammy skin; HR >120 beats/min, SBP <90 mm Hg; u/o <0.5 ml/kg/hr
Pulmonary contusion	
Pulmonary edema	Tachypnea, cough, frothy sputum, crackles

- Pao_2 60-100 mm Hg
- pH 7.35-7.45
- $Paco_2$ 35-45 mm Hg
- RR 12-20, eupnea
- $P(a/A)o_2$: 0.75-0.90
- Qs/Q_T <5%
- Minute ventilation <10 L/min

PATIENT MONITORING
1. Continuously monitor ECG, since hypoxemia is a risk factor for dysrhythmias.
2. Continuously monitor oxygen saturation with pulse oximetry (Spo_2). Be alert for interventions and patient activities that may adversely affect oxygen saturation.

3. Continuously monitor end-tidal CO_2 with capnography (as appropriate to patient's clinical condition) to evaluate adequacy of ventilation (can also be used to select ventilator settings and calculate various oxygenation parameters).
4. Monitor pulmonary function by reviewing serial minute ventilation, calculating physiologic shunt (Qs/Qt), or calculating arterial-alveolar oxygen tension ratio $P(a/A)o_2$.
5. Monitor PA systolic (as appropriate to patient's clinical condition), since hypoxemia can increase sympathetic tone and increase pulmonary vasoconstriction. Calculate PVR.
6. Monitor the chest drainage system, which is used to drain air or fluid from the pleural space. Record drainage hourly; consult with physician if drainage >200 ml/hr. If drainage suddenly ceases, check the patient and system—a tension pneumothorax can develop. (See Chest drainage in Chapter 6 for more information.)
7. If the patient is undergoing mechanical ventilation therapy, see Chapter 6, Mechanical ventilation, for more information.

PHYSICAL ASSESSMENT

1. Assess respiratory status and observe for respiratory distress and increased patient effort: RR >30; paradoxical motion of the ribcage and abdomen; and presence of intercostal and supraclavicular retraction. Auscultate lungs and note any adventitious sounds.
2. Assess for signs and symptoms of hypoxia: increased restlessness, increased complaints of dyspnea, and changes in LOC. Cyanosis is a late sign.
3. Assess the patient for development of clinical sequelae (see Table 5-12).

DIAGNOSTICS ASSESSMENT

1. Review ABGs for decreasing trend in Pao_2, despite increasing Fio_2, which may suggest ARDS; ARDS can develop with lung injury, e.g., flail chest, pulmonary contusion.
2. Review serial chest radiographs to evaluate patient progress or worsening lung condition and to verify the placement of CT and other invasive catheters.
3. Review Hgb and Hct levels, since oxygen-carrying capacity can be adversely affected with decreased Hgb.

PATIENT MANAGEMENT

1. Promote pulmonary hygiene with incentive spirometry, chest physiotherapy, postural drainage, C & DB therapy, and position changes q2h. Note sputum color and consistency. Patients with impaired breathing patterns who are immobilized and have an ineffective cough are at risk for atelectasis and secretion retention. Anticipate antibiotic therapy for pulmonary infections.

2. If the patient develops respiratory distress, be prepared for intubation and mechanical ventilation. Nonconventional modes of ventilation may be employed if ventilation and gas exchange do not improve. (See Chapter 6, Therapeutic Modalities, for information on mechanical ventilation.)

3. Flail chest: Stabilization of chest wall is controversial. Sandbags placed on the chest may cause hypoventilation or complications resulting from perforation of underlying structures. Positive pressure ventilation with PEEP or pressure support ventilation may be required to splint the chest wall internally.

4. Open pneumothorax: Place a sterile dressing on the wound, taping only three sides; this type of dressing will allow air to escape but not reenter the pleural space. Continue to assess the patient for tension pneumothorax.

5. Pulmonary contusion: Methylprednisone (controversial) may be ordered to reduce inflammation.

6. Diaphragmatic and esophageal rupture: Anticipate NG insertion to decompress the stomach and reduce the risk of contaminating the thorax. Anticipate antibiotic therapy.

7. Prepare the patient for surgical repair of the injured structures.

▶ Altered tissue perfusion related to Decreased cardiac output secondary to blood loss, development of tension pneumothorax, dysrhythmias

PATIENT OUTCOMES

- Patient will be alert and oriented to person, place, and time
- Skin warm and dry
- Peripheral pulses strong
- HR 60-100 beats/min
- Absence of life-threatening dysrhythmias

- SBP 90-140 mm Hg
- MAP 70-105 mm Hg
- RR 12-20, eupnea
- u/o 30 ml/hr or 0.5-1.0 ml/kg/hr
- O_2 sat >90%
- Hgb 13-18 g/dl (males)
       12-16 g/dl (females)
- CVP 2-6 mm Hg
- CI 2.8-4.2 L/min/m^2
- DO_2 900-1200 ml/min
- VO_2 200-250 ml/min

PATIENT MONITORING

1. Measure hemodynamic pressures (as appropriate to patient's clinical condition). Obtain PAP and CVP hourly or more frequently if the patient's condition is unstable. Obtain CO and calculate CI, and note trends or the patient's response to therapy.
2. Calculate arterial oxygen delivery (DO_2) and consumption (VO_2) to monitor indicators of tissue perfusion.
3. Obtain BP hourly or more frequently if the patient's condition is unstable, calculate MAP and pulse pressure, note trends and patient response to therapy.
4. Monitor hourly urine output to evaluate effects of decreased CO and/or pharmacological intervention. Determine fluid volume balance q8h (1kg ~ 1000 ml of fluid).
5. Continuously monitor ECG for dysrhythmia development, which may further compromise cardiac output and tissue perfusion.
6. Continuously monitor oxygen saturation with pulse oximetry (Spo_2). Carefully monitor patient activities and nursing interventions that may adversely affect oxygen saturation.
7. Monitor the chest drainage system, which is used to drain air or fluid from the pleural space. Record drainage hourly; consult with the physician if drainage >200 ml/hr. If drainage suddenly ceases, check the patient and the system; a tension pneumothorax can develop. (See Chapter 6, Therapeutic Modalities, for more information on chest drainage.)
8. If patient's lungs are being mechanically ventilated, see Chapter 6, Therapeutic Modalities, for more information on mechanical ventilation.

PULM

PHYSICAL ASSESSMENT

1. Assess the patient's mentation, peripheral pulses, and skin, and note urine output at least hourly as indicators of tissue perfusion.
2. Obtain BP, HR, and RR q1h or more frequently if the patient's condition is unstable.
3. Check the patient for a deviated trachea; tracheal deviation, severe dyspnea, unilateral absence of breath sounds, and distended neck veins are highly suggestive of tension pneumothorax and must be treated immediately with CT insertion or needle decompression.
4. Assess the patient for development of clinical sequelae.

DIAGNOSTICS ASSESSMENT

1. Review ABGs (if available) for hypoxemia (Pao_2 <60 mm Hg) and acidosis (pH <7.35), since both conditions compromise CO and tissue perfusion.
2. Review Hgb and Hct levels to evaluate blood loss. Oxygen-carrying capacity can be adversely affected with blood loss.

PATIENT MANAGEMENT

1. Insert large-bore IV catheters to administer crystalloids and blood products as ordered to maintain intravascular volume and replace blood loss. Autotransfusion may be performed in patients with bleeding into the thorax. Measure PAP, CVP (if available), and BP to evaluate effectiveness of fluid resuscitation.
2. Pulmonary contusion: Limit IV fluids unless patient is in shock. Rapid fluid administration can increase hydrostatic pressure and cause pulmonary edema. Blood products and albumin may be given to replace blood loss and maintain oncotic pressure.
3. If tension pneumothorax is suspected, immediate treatment is required with needle decompression and CT insertion.
4. Be alert for dysrhythmia risk factors: anemia, hypovolemia, hypotension, hypokalemia, hyperkalemia, hypomagnesemia, acidosis, and decreased coronary perfusion pressure. Treat life-threatening dysrhythmias according to ACLS algorithms (see Appendix A).

▶ **Pain** related to injured body structures

PATIENT OUTCOME

- Patient verbalizes decreased pain

PATIENT MONITORING
None
PHYSICAL ASSESSMENT
1. Use a visual analogue scale or rating scale to assess pain and evaluate effectiveness of analgesia (see Figure 1-1).
2. Assess respirations before administering medications. Do not administer CNS depressants if RR <12.
DIAGNOSTICS ASSESSMENT
None
PATIENT MANAGEMENT
1. Anticipate analgesia administration if the patient exhibits restlessness, increased HR, and increased BP and if hypoxemia is not the cause.
2. Administer medication as ordered, evaluating its effects on respiration and pain control.
3. Administer medication before initiating pulmonary hygiene; patients with chest trauma are reluctant to participate because of the pain.
4. Epidural analgesia (see Chapter 6, Therapeutic Modalities), intercostal nerve blocks, or patient-controlled analgesia may be used to control pain.
5. Consult with the physician if the medication proves ineffective.

PNEUMONIA

Clinical Brief
Pneumonia is an inflammation of the lung parenchyma caused by infectious agents or toxins via aspiration, inhalation, or translocation of organisms. Critically ill patients are at increased risk for nosocomial pneumonia because normal defense mechanisms are disrupted. Table 5-13 summarizes pathogens and risk factors for pneumonia.

Presenting signs and symptoms
The patient may have fever, chills, cough with purulent or rust-colored sputum, recent influenza, and shortness of breath.

Physical examination
HR: >100 beats/min
RR: >24
Temperature: >38.5° C (>101.3° F) rectally
Pulmonary: Tachypnea, crackles or bronchial breath sounds, nasal flaring or intercostal retractions may be

PULM

TABLE 5-13 Pathogens and Risk Factors Associated with Pneumonia

Type	Pathogens	Risk factors
Bacteria	*Streptococcus pneumoniae*	COPD, alcoholism, advanced age, multiple myeloma, recent influenza
	Staphylococcus aureus	Alcoholism, DM
	Haemophilus influenzae	COPD, alcoholism
	Pseudomonas aeruginosa	Mechanical ventilation
	Escherichia coli	Mechanical ventilation
	Klebsiella pneumonia	Advanced age, nosocominal infection
	Legionella pneumophila	Immunodeficiency
Viral	Cytomegalovirus	AIDS, lymphomas, organ transplantation
Fungal	*Candida species*	AIDS, immunosuppression
Protozoa	*Pneumocystis carinii*	AIDS, immunosuppression

present; dullness to percussion over the affected area may also be present

Diagnostic findings

SPUTUM SPECIMEN

Characteristics: purulent or rust-colored. Gram stain is used to rapidly identify the pathogen. Specialized testing techniques are available for tuberculosis, fungi, and protozoa identification. Electron microscopes can be helpful to identify viruses. Cultures for precise identification take approximately 2 to 3 days.

CHEST RADIOGRAPH

"Silhouette sign" will be present on the radiograph. There will be loss of distinct outlines of the heart, aorta, or diaphragm when pneumonia is present in a portion of the lung. Diffuse pulmonary infiltrates may also be present in pneumonia.

Acute Care Patient Management

Goals of treatment

Optimize oxygenation
  Oxygen therapy
  Hydration with 3 L/day

TABLE 5-14 Clinical Sequelae of Pneumonia

Complications	Signs and symptoms
Respiratory failure	Restlessness, increased RR, Pao_2 <50 mm Hg, $Paco_2$ >50 mm Hg, pH <7.35
Septic shock	SBP <90 mm Hg, HR >90 beats/min, RR >20, altered mental status, plasma lactate >2 mmol/L, u/o <0.5 ml/kg/hr

Treat infectious process
  Antibiotics
Detect/prevent clinical sequelae (Table 5-14)
Priority nursing diagnoses
Impaired gas exchange
Altered body temperature: hyperthermia
Altered protection (see p. 145)
Altered nutrition: less than body requirements (see p. 149)
High risk for altered family process (see p. 150)
Impaired gas exchange related to ventilation-perfusion mismatch
PATIENT OUTCOMES
• Patient will be alert and oriented to person, place, and time
• pH 7.35-7.45
• Pao_2 60-100 mm Hg
• $Paco_2$ 35-45 mm Hg
• O_2 sat >90%
• Lungs clear to auscultation
• RR 12-20, eupnea
PATIENT MONITORING
1. Continuously monitor oxygen saturation with pulse oximetry (Spo_2). Carefully monitor patient activities and nursing interventions that may adversely affect oxygen saturation.
2. Continuously monitor ECG, since hypoxemia is a risk factor for dysrhythmia development.
3. Monitor PA systolic pressure (as appropriate to patient's clinical condition), since hypoxemia can increase sympathetic tone and increase pulmonary vasoconstriction.
PHYSICAL ASSESSMENT
1. Assess respiratory status: auscultate breath sounds; note rate, rhythm, depth, and use of accessory muscles. Ob-

serve for paradoxical breathing, increased restlessness, increased complaints of dyspnea, respiratory rate >30/min, and changes in LOC.

2. Assess for the presence of protective reflexes, e.g., gag and cough, since a loss of these reflexes increases the risk for aspiration.

3. Assess the patient for development of clinical sequelae (see Table 5-14).

DIAGNOSTICS ASSESSMENT

1. Review ABGs to evaluate oxygenation status and acid-base balance.

2. Review serial chest radiographs to evaluate improvement or worsening condition.

PATIENT MANAGEMENT

1. Administer oxygen therapy as ordered and assist the patient to a position of comfort.

2. Reposition the patient to improve oxygenation and mobilize secretions. Evaluate the patient's response to position changes with ABGs to determine the best position for oxygenation.

3. Provide chest physiotherapy and postural drainage to mobilize secretions, followed by deep breathing and coughing or suctioning. Perform endotracheal suctioning when rhonchi are present in the intubated patient, nasopharyngeal suctioning in patients unable to expectorate secretions. Document the color and consistency of sputum.

4. If the patient's lungs are mechanically ventilated, see Chapter 6, Therapeutic Modalities, for more information on mechanical ventilation.

5. Maintain endotracheal cuff pressure between 15-25 cm H_2O or maximal occlusive volume. However, even properly inflated cuffs do not prevent aspiration. Carefully monitor patients receiving tube feedings.

6. Reduce oxygen demand: pace patient activities, relieve anxiety and pain, and decrease fever.

▶ **Altered body temperature: hyperthermia**

PATIENT OUTCOME

• Temperature: 36.5° C-38.3° C (97.7° F-100.9° F)

PATIENT MONITORING

1. Monitor temperature q4h; obtain temperature 1 hour after antipyretics have been administered. If a hypothermia blanket is being used, continuously monitor core

temperature. (See Chapter 6, Therapeutic Modalities, for more information on thermal regulation.)
2. Monitor BP, CO, and PAP (as appropriate to patient's clinical condition). Calculate CI, PVR, SVR, pulse pressure, and MAP, since hemodynamic changes occur in the presence of sepsis.

PHYSICAL ASSESSMENT
1. Assess for chills, rigors, diaphoresis.
2. Assess the patient for development of clinical sequelae (see Table 5-14).

DIAGNOSTICS ASSESSMENT
1. Review culture reports for identification of the infecting pathogen.
2. Review serial WBC count for leukocytosis as the body attempts to fight infection.

PATIENT MANAGEMENT
1. Consult with the physician when temperature >38.5° C (>101.3° F). Obtain cultures before initiating antibiotics whenever possible.
2. Administer acetaminophen as ordered and monitor patient response. A hypothermia blanket may be required to decrease temperature (See Chapter 6, Therapeutic Modalities, for more information on thermal regulation).
3. Prevent the patient from shivering by covering the patient with a light blanket or using pharmacological agents if necessary, since shivering can cause an increase in oxygen demand.

ACUTE RESPIRATORY FAILURE (ARF)

Clinical Brief

Respiratory failure results from the inability of the lungs to adequately oxygenate the blood to meet the metabolic needs of the body. The impaired gas exchange results in hypoxemia with or without hypoventilation. Causes of ARF (Table 5-15) involve four mechanisms.

Alveolar hypoventilation occurs in disorders of the CNS or neuromuscular system, causing less oxygen to be supplied and less carbon dioxide to be removed.

Intrapulmonary shunting occurs when oxygenated blood is shunted past the alveoli; e.g., the alveolus is fluid filled or collapsed, and the shunted blood, which is poorly oxygenated, mixes with oxygenated blood, lowering the Pao_2.

TABLE 5-15 Causes of Respiratory Failure

System	Disorder	Example
Central nervous	Overdose	Narcotics, sedatives, anesthetics, barbiturates
	Head trauma	Brainstem injury
	Infections	Meningitis, encephalitis
Neuromuscular	Infections	Polio
	Trauma	Spinal cord injury
	Neurological condition	Myasthenia gravis Guillain-Barré syndrome
Respiratory	Airway obstruction	Epiglottitis, fractured trachea, laryngeal edema, laryngospasm, asthma
	Pulmonary	Flail chest, pneumothorax, hemothorax, COPD exacerbation, pneumonia, pulmonary edema, ARDS

Ventilation-perfusion mismatch occurs when there is blood flow to the underventilated areas of the lung or when there is adequate ventilation but blood flow is decreased or absent in that area.

Diffusion abnormalities occur when gas exchange across the alveolar capillary membrane is disrupted, such as in pulmonary edema or pulmonary fibrosis.

Presenting signs and symptoms
The patient may have an increased respiratory rate, shallow respirations, use of accessory muscles, and altered level of consciousness. COPD patients may exhibit increased cough and dyspnea.

Physical examination
Diaphoretic, agitated, restless

BP ↑ due to hypoxemia or ↓ in sepsis

HR: Tachycardia

RR: >30

Temperature: normal or ↑ with infectious process

Skin: Cool and dry to diaphoretic

Neurological: Restlessness, anxiety to confusion and coma

TABLE 5-16 Clinical Sequelae of Respiratory Failure

Complication	Signs and symptoms
Tissue hypoxia	Restlessness, decreased level of consciousness, dysrhythmias, angina, myocardial infarction, right-sided heart failure
Cardiopulmonary arrest	Absence of palpable pulses, no spontaneous respirations (nonventilated patients)

Pulmonary: Shallow breathing, use of accessory muscles
Tachypnea, progressing to respiratory arrest
Diagnostic findings
Room air arterial blood gases: Pao_2 <50 mm Hg, usually with an increased $Paco_2$ and decreased pH.
The development of ARF in COPD patients reveals a low to normal pH, elevated bicarbonate level, and decreased serum chloride level.

Acute Care Patient Management
Goals of treatment
Optimize oxygenation
  Oxygen therapy
  Mechanical ventilation
  Bronchodilator therapy
  Treatment of underlying problem
Detect/prevent clinical sequelae (Table 5-16)
Priority nursing diagnoses
Impaired gas exchange
Altered protection (see p. 145)
Altered nutrition: less than body requirements (see p. 149)
High risk for altered family process (see p. 150)
▶ **Impaired gas exchange** related to hypoventilation, increased pulmonary shunt, ventilation-perfusion mismatch, and diffusion disturbances
PATIENT OUTCOMES
• Patient will be alert and oriented to person, place, and time
• Lungs clear to auscultation
• Pao_2 60-100 mm Hg (50-55 mm Hg in a COPD patient)

PULM

- pH 7.35-7.45
- $Paco_2$ 35-45 mm Hg
- O_2 sat >90%
- Svo_2 60%-80%
- SBP 90-140 mm Hg
- MAP 70-105 mm Hg
- HR 60-100 beats/min
- RR 12-20, eupnea

PATIENT MONITORING

1. Continuously monitor oxygen saturation with pulse oximetry (Spo_2). If Svo_2 monitoring is available, continuously monitor readings. Carefully monitor nursing interventions and patient activities that may adversely affect oxygenation status.

2. Monitor PA systolic pressure (as appropriate to patient's clinical condition) since hypoxemia can increase sympathetic tone and increase pulmonary vasoconstriction.

3. Continuously monitor ECG for changes in HR, ischemic changes, and development of dysrhythmias.

4. Continuously monitor arterial BP, PA pressures, CO, and CVP (as appropriate to patient's clinical condition), since hypoxemia can produce deleterious effects on the cardiovascular system.

PHYSICAL ASSESSMENT

1. Assess LOC: If the patient becomes restless or agitated or complains of a headache, these signs may signal decreased cerebral oxygenation.

2. Assess for signs of respiratory distress, signaling the need for mechanical ventilation: intercostal retractions, RR >30/min, and paradoxical breathing.

3. Assess lung sounds: wheezes indicate bronchospasm, which may require bronchodilator treatment.

4. Assess the patient for signs of heart failure: JVD, peripheral edema, cough, crackles, S_3, tachycardia.

5. Assess the patient for development of clinical sequelae (see Table 5-16).

DIAGNOSTICS ASSESSMENT

1. Review ABGs for decreasing Pao_2 and acidosis. In COPD patients, $Paco_2$ levels are normally high and are not the sole factor on which to base the decision to intubate and mechanically ventilate the patient's lungs.

2. Review Hgb and Hct levels, since inadequate hemoglobin adversely affects oxygen-carrying capacity.

Patient Management

1. Administer oxygen therapy as ordered; generally the patient with COPD will require nasal prongs or a Venturi-type mask.
2. Assist the patient to assume a position that improves chest excursion. Correlate the effects of position changes on oxygen saturation to determine which position improves oxygenation.
3. If the patient's lungs are mechanically ventilated, see Chapter 6, Therapeutic Modalities, for more information on mechanical ventilation.
4. β Agonists (metaproterenol) may be prescribed to relieve bronchoconstriction; intravenous theophylline may be required to decrease airway reactivity, improve diaphragmatic muscle contractility, and reverse muscle fatigue.
5. Anticholinergic agents (atropine, ipratropium) may be administered by inhalation to relieve bronchoconstriction.
6. Proceed in a calm manner and reassure the anxious and fearful patient, since anxiety and fear may increase feelings of dyspnea.
7. Reduce oxygen demands by pacing activities and scheduling rest periods for the patient, relieving anxiety and fever, and sedating the patient as needed, closely monitoring respiratory function.
8. Provide pulmonary hygiene: chest physiotherapy, postural drainage, deep breathing and coughing. Suction secretions if the patient's cough is ineffective.

PULM

Cardiovascular Disorders

ANGINA
Clinical Brief
Angina is a subjective experience of chest discomfort resulting from an imbalance in myocardial oxygen supply and demand. Etiological factors in angina are usually related to the atherosclerotic disease process, whereby the coronary arteries lose their ability to dilate and increase blood flow in the presence of increased oxygen consumption. Angina may be classified as (1) stable angina, which typically results from atherosclerotic vessel changes, (2) unstable angina, which usually results from accelerated or multivessel disease, and (3) Prinzmetal's angina, which usually results from coronary artery vasospasm. Prolonged myocardial ischemia may ultimately result in a myocardial infarction.

Risk factors mirror the risk factors for coronary artery disease: cigarette smoking, hyperlipidemia, hypertension, diabetes, obesity, and stress; angina occurs most frequently in men, especially those over 50 years of age, or in postmenopausal women. A positive family history of cardiovascular disease predisposes an individual to angina.

Presenting signs and symptoms
Stable angina: chest discomfort that is predictable to the patient; usually follows exertion, meals or increased activity levels; is relieved by rest and/or nitroglycerin; and manifests as ST-T segment depression (subendocardial ischemia) on ECG.

Unstable angina (crescendo or preinfarction angina): chest discomfort that has changed in character and is now more severe, lasts longer, is more difficult to relieve and occurs with less exertion than previously.

Prinzmetal's angina (variant angina): chest discomfort that is nontypical; occurs with rest, not relieved with nitroglycerin or rest, manifests as ST-T segment elevation on ECG during an episode and subsides to baseline with pain relief.

Physical examination
Appearance: Anxious

BP may be elevated or decreased
HR may be elevated secondary to pain
Cardiovascular: S_4 may be present
Pulmonary: Dyspnea, tachypnea may be present
Diagnostic findings
ECG changes: ST-T segment depression (classic and unstable) or ST-T segment elevation (Prinzmetal)
Acute Care Patient Management
Goals of treatment
Improve myocardial oxygen supply
    Supplemental oxygen
    Nitroglycerin
    Calcium channel blockers
    Possible PTCA or CABG
Decrease myocardial oxygen demand
    Bed rest
    Nitroglycerin
    β-Adrenergic blockers
    Calcium channel blockers
Priority nursing diagnoses
Pain
High risk for altered family process (see p. 150)
Knowledge deficit (see p. 151)
▶ Pain related to impaired myocardial oxygenation
PATIENT OUTCOMES
- Patient verbalizes pain relief
- Absence of ST-T wave changes
PATIENT MONITORING
1. Continuous ECG monitoring to evaluate ST, T wave changes, which may indicate ischemia, injury, or infarction, and to detect dysrhythmia development.
PHYSICAL ASSESSMENT
1. Assess pain to validate ischemic origin (see Table 5-17). Use a visual analogue scale (see Figure 1-1) to evaluate the severity of the pain.
2. Check VS frequently during anginal episode and with administration of antianginal agents. Hypotension can occur with these agents.
DIAGNOSTICS ASSESSMENT
1. Review serial 12-lead ECGs to evaluate patterns of ischemia, injury, and infarction.
2. Review cardiac enzyme laboratory results (if available) for characteristic signs of myocardial infarction.

TABLE 5-17 Differentiating Chest Pain

Type	Symptoms	Signs	Pain relief
Cardiac			
Ischemic	Substernal "crushing" chest pain; may radiate to LUE and/or jaw (common), or RUE and/or back (less common)	Anxiety; skin: pale/cyanotic, diaphoretic	Depends on specific ischemic condition
Stable angina	Predictable: follows exertion, meals, or increased activity	ECG: ST-T seg $\downarrow$	Rest, NTG, $\uparrow O_2$
Unstable or crescendo or preinfarction angina	Less predictable: occurs with less exertion than before	ECG: ST-T seg $\downarrow$	Rest, NTG, $\uparrow O_2$
Prinzmetal's or variant	Unpredictable: may occur at rest	ECG: ST-T seg $\uparrow$	Not relieved by NTG or rest
AMI	May not differ from angina; SOB, crackles, S_3, S_4, nausea	ECG: new Q waves ST-T seg $\uparrow$ or ST-T seg $\downarrow$, cardiac enzymes $\uparrow$	Thrombolytic therapy Rest, O_2, and NTG may not relieve pain; MSO_4 may or may not relieve pain

Continued.

CV

TABLE 5-17 Differentiating Chest Pain—cont'd

Type	Symptoms	Signs	Pain relief
Cardiac—cont'd			
Nonischemic Pericarditis	Severe, sharp, precordial pain that may radiate to LUE	Pt appears restless; friction rub, pulsus paradoxus, ↑ RR dyspnea, ECG: diffuse ST-T seg ↑	Leaning forward Drugs: indomethacin, ibuprofen
Gastrointestinal			
Gastric reflux	"Burning" pain, midepigastric area; nonradiating	Anxiety Skin: diaphoretic/pale Hx PUD	Antacids, cimetidine/ranitidine, viscous lidocaine
Musculoskeletal			
Costochondritis	Chest pain that may/may not be discrete; ↑ when ribs/sternum palpated and on deep inspiration	Anxiety Skin: diaphoretic/pale Shallow respirations ↑ ESR, ↑ WBCs	Position changes, ibuprofen, indomethacin

Chest wall trauma	Chest pain that may/may not be discrete; ↑ on deep inspiration	Anxiety Skin: diaphoretic/pale May see bruises/lacerations/distortions/crepitus/subcutaneous emphysema Hx of trauma	Position changes, depends on cause
Pulmonary			
Pulmonary embolism	Severe, sharp chest pain that is usually diffuse; "breathlessness"	Anxiety Skin: pale/diaphoretic Dyspnea/tachypnea, hyperpnea ABG: ↓ O_2 sat, ↓ PaO_2, ↓ $PaCO_2$ May see hemoptysis	Analgesic support may provide some relief; narcotics are usually contraindicated or used with caution
Pleurisy	Sudden onset Stabbing chest pain that may/may not be discrete; ↑ with deep inspiration	Anxiety Rapid, shallow respirations	ASA/ibuprofen; position changes; codeine may be used with caution

CV

3. Review result of cardiac catheterization (if available) for degree of coronary artery disease involvement.

PATIENT MANAGEMENT

1. Stay with the patient, providing a calm, quiet environment. Assess level of anxiety and other factors that increase myocardial oxygen demand, such as fever, dysrhythmias, anger, hypertension, and hypoxemia.

2. Provide oxygen at 2 to 4 L/min to maintain or improve oxygenation.

3. Initiate and maintain IV line(s) for emergent drug and fluid resuscitation.

4. Administer nitroglycerin as indicated to decrease afterload, decrease myocardial oxygen demand, and increase myocardial oxygen supply: sublingual, 1 tablet q5min × 3; intravenous, start with an infusion of 5 μg/min; titrate to desired response or to maintain SBP >90 mm Hg. Increase dosage q5-10min by 5-10 μg/min. If hypotension occurs, raise the patient's legs and stop infusion. (See Chapter 7 for more information.)

5. Administer morphine sulfate as ordered. Give IVP in 2 mg increments q5min to relieve chest discomfort. Dilute with 5 ml NS and administer over 4 to 5 minutes. Monitor the patient's respirations, because narcotics are respiratory depressants. Notify the physician if pain is not relieved despite pharmacological intervention or if pain has subsided but recurs.

6. Administer calcium channel blockers such as diltiazem or nifedipine as ordered to decrease myocardial oxygen demand, increase myocardial oxygen supply, and decrease coronary artery vasospasm. Monitor drug effects on HR and BP.

7. Administer β blockers such as propranolol as ordered to decrease myocardial oxygen demand. Monitor drug effects on HR and BP.

8. Prepare patient for possible angioplasty or revascularization surgery. (See Chapter 6, Therapeutic Modalities, for further information.)

ACUTE MYOCARDIAL INFARCTION (MI)

Clinical Brief

The death of myocardial tissue is a result of decreased blood supply to the myocardium. A myocardial infarction can go unnoticed (silent MI) or produce major hemodynamic consequences and death. It may result from arteriosclerosis, coronary artery spasm, or coronary thrombosis.

Risk factors

Risk factors mirror the risk factors for coronary artery disease: cigarette smoking, hyperlipidemia, hypertension, diabetes, obesity, and stress. Men, especially if over 50 years of age, are predisposed to MI, as are postmenopausal women. A positive family history of cardiovascular disease is also a predisposing factor.

Presenting signs and symptoms

Chest discomfort >20-30 min unrelieved by NTG (see Table 5-17), anxiety, feeling of impending doom; nausea/vomiting, dyspnea, weakness, diaphoresis, palpitations.

Physical examination

Appearance: Anxious, pale

Vital signs: BP may be ↑ in response to pain, or ↓ secondary to hemodynamic compromise

HR may be ↑ in response to pain or ↓ secondary to ischemia and/or pharmacological therapy; may be irregular secondary to dysrhythmias

Cardiovascular: S_3, S_4, murmur, and/or rubs may be present

Pulmonary: SOB, tachypnea crackles

RV Infarction

Cardiovascular: Distended jugular veins, hypotension, Kussmaul's sign, heart block may be present

Pulmonary: Clear lungs

Diagnostic findings

Cardiac enzymes: Characteristic changes are evident (see Table 5-18).

TABLE 5-18 Cardiac Enzymes

Laboratory study	Onset	Peak	Return to normal
CK	2-5 hr	~24 hr	2-3 days
CK-MB	4-8 hr	16-24 hr	2-3 days
AST (SGOT)	6-8 hr	24-48 hr	4-8 days
LDH	6-12 hr	48-72 hr	7-10 days
LDH_1	6-12 hr	24-48 hr	3-4 days

TABLE 5-19 Types of Myocardial Infarction and Related ECG Leads

Type	Indicative changes	Reciprocal changes
Anterior	V_2-V_4	II, III, aV_F
Anteroseptal	V_1-V_4	
Anterolateral	I, aV_L, V_3-V_6	
Lateral	I, aV_L, V_5-V_6	II, III, aV_F
Inferior	II, III, aV_F	I, aV_L, V_1-V_4
Posterior		V_1-V_3

NOTE: Right ventricular infarction demonstrates ST segment elevation in V_{3R}, V_{4R}.

Isoenzymes: CK-MB are cardiac specific, positive MB are diagnostic for MI; LDH_1 and LDH_2 are cardiac specific, an LDH "flip" ($LDH_1 > LDH_2$) is diagnostic for MI.

ECG changes: Usually occur from hours to within 7 days (see Table 5-19).

Q wave infarctions: Pathological Q waves (>0.04 sec or ⅓ the amplitude of the QRS complex), ST segment elevation with reciprocal ST depression in opposite leads; T wave changes are initially positive, then become negative in leads facing the infarcted area.

Non-Q-wave infarctions: ST depression and inverted T waves in leads facing the epicardial surface overlying the infarction; ST elevation and upright T waves in opposite leads.

Acute Care Patient Management

Goals of treatment

Salvage myocardium/limit infarction size
  Thrombolytic therapy
  Counterpulsation
  Percutaneous transluminal coronary angioplasty (PTCA)
Improve myocardial oxygen supply
  Supplemental oxygen
  Heparin
  Calcium channel-blocking agents
  Antiplatelet agents
Decrease myocardial oxygen demand
  Mechanical assist devices
  Bed rest
  NPO, liquid/soft diet
  β-Adrenergic blocking agents

Decrease preload
  Morphine sulfate
  Nitroglycerin
  Diuretic agents
Decrease afterload
  Morphine sulfate
  Nitroglycerin
  Calcium channel-blocking agents
  Diuretic agents
  Antihypertensive agents
Increase contractility
  Dobutamine
Maintain electrophysiological stability
  Lidocaine
  β-Adrenergic blocking agents
  Calcium channel blocking agents
Maintain hemodynamic stability
  Volume loading to provide adequate filling pressure
Detect/prevent clinical sequelae
  See Table 5-20

Priority nursing diagnoses
Pain
Decreased cardiac output
Altered tissue perfusion
High risk for altered protection (see p. 145)
High risk for altered family process (see p. 150)
▶ **Pain** related to impaired myocardial oxygenation

PATIENT OUTCOMES
• Verbalizes pain relief
• Absence of ST-T wave changes

PATIENT MONITORING
1. Continuous ECG monitoring to evaluate ST, T wave changes, which may indicate ischemia, injury, or infarction (extension or new onset) and to detect dysrhythmia development.

PHYSICAL ASSESSMENT
1. Assess pain to validate ischemic origin (see Table 5-17). Use a visual analogue scale (see Figure 1-1) to evaluate the severity of the pain.
2. Check VS frequently during anginal episode and with administration of antianginal agents. Hypotension can occur with these agents.
3. Assess patient for development of clinical sequelae (see Table 5-20).

CV

TABLE 5-20 Clinical Sequelae Associated with Myocardial Infarction

Complications	Signs and symptoms
Congestive heart failure	Sustained elevated HR, dry cough, S_3, crackles, PAWP >20 mm Hg
Pulmonary edema	Worsening CHF, breathlessness, moist cough, frothy sputum, diaphoresis, cyanosis
Reinfarction/extension of infarction	Recurrence of chest pain, ST-T wave changes, hemodynamic changes
Cardiogenic shock	↓ Mentation, ↑ ↓ HR, SBP <90 mm Hg, CI <2.0, u/o <20 ml/hr, cool, clammy, mottled skin
Dysrhythmias	Change in rate or rhythm, change in LOC, syncope, chest discomfort, possible ↓ in BP
Pericarditis	Chest discomfort aggravated by supine position or on deep inspiration, intermittent friction rub may be present, fever
Papillary muscle rupture	Abrupt onset holosystolic murmur, sudden left ventricular failure, S_3, S_4, midsystolic ejection click, crackles
Ventricular aneurysm	Paradoxical pulse, ventricular ectopy, MAP <80 mm Hg, possible atrial fibrillation with BP changes, change in HR, outward bulging of precordium
Ventricular septal rupture	Sudden onset of palpable thrill, holosystolic murmur at LSB, SOB, cough

DIAGNOSTICS ASSESSMENT
1. Obtain 12-lead ECG and compare with previous ECGs to evaluate effects of ischemic episode.
2. Review cardiac enzyme laboratory results, if ordered, with ischemic episode.

PATIENT MANAGEMENT
1. Stay with the patient, providing a calm, quiet environment.

2. Maintain O_2 therapy and assist the patient to a position of comfort.
3. Administer NTG: sublingual, 1 tablet q5min × 3; as an infusion, start at 5 μg/min; titrate to desired response or SBP >90 mm Hg. Increase dosage q5-10 min by 5-10 μg/min. If hypotension occurs, raise legs and stop infusion. (See Chapter 7 for further drug information.)
4. Administer morphine sulfate as ordered. Give IVP in 2 mg increments q5min to relieve chest discomfort. Dilute with 5 ml NS and administer over 4-5 minutes. Monitor respirations.
5. Administer β-adrenergic blocking agents such as propranolol or esmolol as ordered. These pharmacological agents decrease SNS tone, reduce cardiac demand, and have been shown to prevent myocardial reinfarction. Monitor drug's effect on HR and BP.
6. Administer a calcium channel-blocking agent such as nifedipine as ordered to reduce coronary vasospasm; these agents can also reduce afterload and control dysrhythmias. Monitor drug's effect on HR and BP.
7. Administer antiplatelet agents to prevent platelet adherence in coronary arteries.
8. Administer an anticoagulant such as heparin as ordered. This agent may be given prophylactically or with thrombolytic therapy to prevent further clot formation. Monitor patient for overt and covert bleeding and check daily PTT for therapeutic anticoagulation (1.5-2.5 times normal).
9. IABP insertion may be required (see Chapter 6, Therapeutic Modalities).
10. Thrombolytic therapy may be required (see Chapter 6, Therapeutic Modalities).

▶ **Decreased cardiac output** related to electrophysiological instability and impaired inotropic state

PATIENT OUTCOMES
• Patient will be alert and oriented to person, place, and time
• Skin w/d
• Pulses strong, equal bilaterally
• Capillary refill <3 sec
• SBP 90-140 mm Hg
• MAP 70-105 mm Hg

CV

- Pulse pressure 30-40 mm Hg
- HR 60-100 beats/min
- Absence of life-threatening dysrhythmias
- u/o 30 ml/hr or 0.5-1 ml/kg/hr
- CVP 2-6 mm Hg
- PAS 15-30 mm Hg
- PAD 5-15 mm Hg
- PAWP 4-12 mm Hg
- CI 2.5-4.0 L/min/m^2
- SVR 900-1600 dynes sec/cm^{-5}
- PVR 100-250 dynes sec/cm^{-5}
- Svo_2 60%-80%
- DO_2 900-1200 ml/min
- VO_2 200-250 ml/min

PATIENT MONITORING

1. Monitor in the lead appropriate for ischemia or dysrhythmia identification. Place in lead II to monitor for SVT and axis deviation. Place in lead MCL_1 to differentiate between ventricular ectopy and aberrantly conducted beats, to determine types of BBB, or to verify RV pacemaker beats (paced QRS beat should be negative). (See Table 5-21 for dysrhythmias and related site of infarction.)

TABLE 5-21 Dysrhythmias and Related Site of Infarction

Site	Dysrhythmia
Anterior MI	BBB as a result of septal involvement; check widened QRS
	RBBB = rSR′ in V_1, Rs in V_6
	LBBB = rS in V_1, large monophasic R wave in V_6
	Left anterior hemiblock: LAD >−45; negative QRS in I, III; AV block
Inferior MI	Bradycardia, second-degree AV block
Posterior MI	See Inferior MI
Right ventricular infarction	Second degree AV block

2. Analyze ECG rhythm strip at least q4h and note rate, rhythm, PR, QRS, and QT intervals (prolonged QT is associated with torsade de pointes). Note ST, T wave changes, which may indicate ischemia, injury, or infarction. Note occurrence of PACs or PVCs, since premature beats are frequently the forerunner of more serious dysrhythmias. Mobitz type II heart block may progress to complete heart block. (See Chapter 3, Monitoring the Critically Ill Patient, for dysrhythmia interpretation.)

3. Obtain PA pressures and CVP (RA) hourly (if available) or more frequently if titrating pharmacological agents. Obtain CO as patient condition indicates; note trends and patient response to therapy. Calculate CI, PVR, and SVR and note trends and patient response to therapy. Calculate LVSWI, RVSWI to evaluate contractility.

4. Calculate arterial oxygen delivery (DO_2) and oxygen consumption (VO_2) to monitor indicators of tissue perfusion.

5. Obtain BP hourly; calculate MAP and pulse pressure, note trends and patient response to therapy.

6. Monitor hourly u/o to evaluate effects of decreased CO and/or pharmacological intervention. Determine fluid balance each shift. Compare serial weights for rapid changes (0.5-1.0 kg/day) suggesting fluid gain or loss.

7. Continuously monitor Svo_2 (if available) to evaluate oxygen supply and demand; a downward trend can indicate decreased supply or increased demand.

PHYSICAL ASSESSMENT

1. Obtain HR, RR, BP q15min during acute phase and when titrating vasoactive drugs. Obtain T q4h.

2. Assess patient's mentation, skin color and temperature, capillary refill, and peripheral pulses at least hourly to monitor adequacy of CO.

3. Assess patient for development of clinical sequelae (see Table 5-20).

DIAGNOSTICS ASSESSMENT

1. Review serial 12-lead ECGs to determine location and extension of MI.

2. Review serial electrolyte levels, since a disturbance in potassium is a risk factor for dysrhythmia development.

3. Review serial ABGs for hypoxemia and acidosis, since these conditions increase the risk for dysrhythmias and decreased contractility.

CV

Patient Management

1. Provide oxygen at 2-4 L/min to maintain or improve oxygenation.

2. Minimize oxygen demand: decrease anxiety, keep the patient NPO or provide a liquid diet in the acute phase, decrease pain.

3. Maintain patient on bed rest to decrease myocardial oxygen demand during the acute phase.

4. Initiate IV to ensure emergency vascular access.

5. Administer IV fluids as ordered to provide adequate filling pressures that maintain CO. A PAD ~ 15 to 20 mm Hg may be required.

6. Be alert for dysrhythmia risk factors: anemia, hypovolemia, hypokalemia, acidosis, decreased coronary perfusion pressure, administration of digitalis and other antidysrhythmic agents, pain, or CVP/PA or pacemaker catheter misplacement. Treat life-threatening dysrhythmias according to ACLS algorithms (see Appendix B).

7. Lidocaine may be used prophylactically to prevent ventricular dysrhythmias. The patient may be given a bolus dose of 2 mg/kg, followed with infusion: 1-4 mg/min. Do not exceed 4 mg/min. (See Chapter 7, Pharmacology, for more information.)

8. If the patient is bradycardic, be prepared to administer atropine 0.5 mg IV if the patient manifests the following s/s: SBP <90 mm Hg, decreased mentation, PVCs, chest discomfort, or dyspnea. Pacemaker insertion may be required.

9. If the patient is tachycardic, check BP and mentation. Drug therapy depends on the tachydysrhythmia. (See ACLS algorithms, Appendix A.) Be prepared to countershock/defibrillate.

10. Administer nitroglycerin and calcium channel-blocking agents as ordered to reduce preload and afterload. Monitor drug effects on BP and HR.

11. Administer furosemide as ordered to rid the body of excess fluid. Monitor urine output and electrolytes.

12. Dobutamine may be required to enhance contractility. Dopamine may be ordered to increase renal blood flow. (See Chapter 7, Pharmacology, for drug administration information.)

13. Invasive therapeutic modalities may be required: counterpulsation (IABP), percutaneous transluminal coronary angioplasty (PTCA), thrombolytic therapy; or

revascularization surgery. (See Chapter 6, Therapeutic Modalities.)

Altered tissue perfusion related to inadequate cardiac output

PATIENT OUTCOMES

- Patient will be alert and oriented to person, place, and time
- Skin w/d
- Pulses strong, equal bilaterally
- Capillary refill <3 sec
- u/o 30 ml/hr or 0.5-1 ml/kg/hr
- HR 60-100 beats/min
- Absence of life-threatening dysrhythmias
- SBP 90-140 mm Hg
- Pulse pressure 30-40 mm Hg
- MAP 70-105 mm Hg
- CI 2.4-4.0 L/min/m^2
- DO_2 900-1200 ml/min
- VO_2 200-250 ml/min
- Svo_2 60%-80%
- O_2 sat >95%

PATIENT MONITORING

1. Obtain PA pressures and CVP (RA) hourly (if available) or more frequently if titrating pharmacological agents. Obtain CO and calculate CI as patient condition indicates; note trends and the patient's response to therapy.
2. Calculate arterial oxygen delivery (DO_2) and oxygen consumption (VO_2) to monitor indicators of tissue perfusion.
3. Obtain BP hourly or more frequently if the patient's condition is unstable; calculate MAP and pulse pressure; note trends and patient response to therapy.
4. Monitor hourly urine output to evaluate effects of decreased CO and/or pharmacological intervention.
5. Continuously monitor oxygen status with pulse oximetry (Spo_2) or Svo_2 (if available) and monitor patient activities and nursing interventions that may adversely affect oxygenation.

PHYSICAL ASSESSMENT

1. Obtain HR, RR, BP q15min during acute phase and when titrating vasoactive drugs.
2. Assess mentation, skin temperature and color, capillary refill, and peripheral pulses as indicators of tissue perfusion.

3. Assess chest discomfort to validate ischemic origin (see Table 5-17). Use a visual analogue to evaluate severity of pain (Figure 1-1).
4. Assess the patient for development of clinical sequelae (see Table 5-20).

DIAGNOSTICS ASSESSMENT

1. Review serial ABGs for hypoxemia (<60 mm Hg) and acidosis (pH <7.35), which may further compromise tissue perfusion.
2. Review lactate levels, an indicator of anaerobic metabolism.
3. Review serial BUN and Cr levels to evaluate renal function; BUN >20 and Cr >1.5 suggest renal impairment, which may be a result of decreased renal perfusion.
4. Review echocardiography or cardiac catheterization results (if available) to assess ventricular function (ejection fraction and wall motion).

PATIENT MANAGEMENT

A progressive reduction in cardiac output leading to decreased tissue perfusion in the MI patient may be a result of congestive heart failure (see p. 254), cardiogenic pulmonary edema (p. 262), or cardiogenic shock (p. 410).

SUDDEN CARDIAC DEATH

Clinical Brief

Sudden cardiac death is the unexpected collapse and cardiopulmonary arrest of a previously well-appearing individual within minutes to 1 hour after the collapse occurs. Sudden cardiac death occurs as a primary manifestation of ischemic heart disease with victims usually suffering from multivessel coronary artery atherosclerosis.

Risk factors mirror the risk factors for coronary artery disease: cigarette smoking, hyperlipidemia, hypertension, diabetes, obesity, stress, and a positive family history of cardiovascular disease; men, especially those over 50 years of age, are susceptible, as are postmenopausal women. In addition, patients who (1) are known sudden cardiac death survivors, (2) have had an acute MI within the last 6 months and evidenced early dysrhythmias and/or who had demonstrated left ventricular ejection fractions <40%, and (3) had QT intervals that were prolonged and who had a history of syncopal episodes are particularly at risk for sudden cardiac death.

Presenting signs and symptoms

A previously normal-appearing adult will suddenly collapse with cardiopulmonary arrest, not associated with accidental or traumatic causes. There may be a brief period of chest discomfort just before the arrest; however, most commonly there are no prodromal symptoms.

Physical examination

Full cardiopulmonary arrest

Pulselessness

No respirations

Monitor may depict VT/VF

Diagnostic findings

Clinical findings are the basis for diagnosis of sudden cardiac death.

Acute Care Patient Management

Goals of treatment

Salvage the victim
   CPR and ACLS protocols
   Supplemental oxygen
Salvage myocardium at risk
   Supplemental oxygen
   Morphine sulfate
   Antidysrhythmic agents
   Automatic implantable cardiac defibrillator (AICD)
Detect/prevent clinical sequelae
   See Table 5-22

Priority nursing diagnoses

Decreased cardiac output

High risk for altered family process (see p. 150)

Decreased cardiac output related to electrophysiological instability.

PATIENT OUTCOMES

- Patient will be alert and awake
- Skin w/d
- HR 60-100 beats/min
- Absence of lethal dysrhythmias
- SBP 90-140 mm Hg
- MAP 70-105 mm Hg
- u/o 30 ml/hr or 0.5-1 ml/kg/hr
- CI 2.5-4.0 L/min/m^2

PATIENT MONITORING

1. Monitor in the lead appropriate for ischemia or dysrhythmia identification. Place in lead II to monitor for

TABLE 5-22 Clinical Sequelae Associated with Sudden Cardiac Death

Complications	Signs and symptoms
CP arrest	Recurrent CP arrest following sudden death is common; pulselessness
Acute myocardial infarction	ECG and cardiac enzyme changes indicative of AMI (See Tables 5-18 and 5-19); dysrhythmias, ↓ BP, tachycardia (>100 beats/min)
Dysrhythmias	Change in rate and rhythm, change in LOC, syncope, chest discomfort, ↓ SBP (<90 mm Hg)
CHF	Tachycardia (>100 beats/min), cough, S_3, S_4, PAWP >20 mm Hg
Pulmonary edema	Worsening CHF, moist cough, frothy sputum, ↓ Pao_2, ↑ RR, ↓ SBP (<90 mm Hg)

SVT and axis deviation. Place in lead MCL_1 to differentiate between ventricular ectopy and aberrantly conducted beats, to determine types of BBB, or to verify RV pacemaker beats (paced QRS beat should be negative). Recurrence of dysrhythmias is most common within the first 72 hours.

2. Analyze ECG rhythm strip at least q4h and note rate, rhythm, PR, QRS, and QT intervals (prolonged QT is associated with torsade de pointes). Note ST, T wave changes, which may indicate ischemia, injury, or infarction. Note occurrence of PACs or PVCs, since premature beats are frequently the forerunner of more serious dysrhythmias. Mobitz type II heart block may progress to complete heart block. (See Chapter 3, Monitoring the Critically Ill Patient, for dysrhythmia interpretation.)

3. Obtain PA pressures and CVP (RA) hourly (if available) or more frequently if titrating pharmacological agents. Obtain CO as patient condition indicates; note trends and patient response to therapy. Calculate CI, PVR, and SVR and note trends and patient response to therapy. Calculate LVSWI, RVSWI to evaluate contractility.

4. Calculate arterial oxygen delivery (DO_2) and oxygen consumption (VO_2) to monitor indicators of tissue perfusion.
5. Obtain BP hourly; calculate MAP and pulse pressure; note trends and patient response to therapy.
6. Monitor hourly urine output to evaluate effects of decreased CO and/or pharmacological intervention. Determine fluid volume balance each shift. Compare serial weights. A rapid (0.5-1.0 kg/day) change in weight suggests fluid gain or loss (1 kg ~ 1 L fluid).
7. Continuously monitor Svo_2 (if available) to evaluate oxygen supply and demand; a downward trend can indicate decreased supply or increased demand.

PHYSICAL ASSESSMENT
1. Obtain HR, RR, BP q15min during acute phase and when titrating vasoactive drugs. Obtain T q4h.
2. Assess patient's mentation, skin temperature and color, and peripheral pulses at least hourly to monitor adequacy of CO.
3. Be alert to the formation of dysrhythmias, i.e., change in rate or rhythm, change in LOC, syncope, chest discomfort, hypotension, and/or pulselessness.
4. Assess patient for development of clinical sequelae (Table 5-22).

DIAGNOSTICS ASSESSMENT
1. Review serial 12-lead ECGs and cardiac enzymes to determine whether MI has occurred.
2. Review serial electrolyte levels, since a disturbance in potassium is a risk factor for dysrhythmia development.
3. Review ABGs for hypoxemia and acidosis, since these conditions increase the risk for dysrhythmias and decreased contractility.

PATIENT MANAGEMENT
1. Provide supplemental oxygen to maintain or improve oxygenation. Patient may be intubated and mechanically ventilated.
2. Minimize oxygen demand: decrease anxiety, keep the patient NPO or provide a liquid diet in the acute phase, decrease pain.
3. Maintain patient on bed rest to decrease myocardial oxygen demand during the acute phase.
4. Initiate and maintain IV line(s) for emergent drug and fluid resuscitation.
5. Be alert for dysrhythmia risk factors: anemia, hypovole-

CV

mia, hypokalemia, acidosis, decreased coronary perfusion pressure, administration of digitalis and other antidys-rhythmic agents, pain, or CVP/PA or pacemaker cathe-ter misplacement. Treat life-threatening dysrhythmias according to ACLS algorithms (see Appendix A). Be prepared to countershock/defibrillate the patient.

6. Lidocaine may be used prophylactically to prevent ven-tricular dysrhythmias. Administer a bolus dose 2 mg/kg, follow with infusion: 1-4 mg/min. Do not exceed 4 mg/min. (See Chapter 7, Pharmacology, for drug informa-tion.)

7. Since most sudden cardiac death occurrences are second-ary to a lethal dysrhythmia, 24-hour Holter monitoring and possible electrophysiological study (EPS) may be done to determine the effectiveness of a pharmacological regimen. Cardiac catheterization may be indicated to determine underlying disease.

8. Anticipate AICD insertion. (See Chapter 6, Therapeutic Modalities.)

CONGESTIVE HEART FAILURE (CHF)

Clinical Brief

CHF is the inability of the heart to maintain adequate car-diac output sufficient to meet the metabolic and oxygen de-mands of the tissues despite adequate venous return. Condi-tions that produce abnormal cardiac muscle contraction or relaxation or both (cardiomyopathies), conditions that lead to pressure or volume overload (increased preload or in-creased afterload), and conditions or diseases that greatly in-crease demands on the heart (anemia, thyrotoxicosis) are as-sociated with the development of CHF.

Risk factors

Risk factors for CHF include ischemic heart disease, valvular disease, cardiomyopathies, high cardiac output.

Presenting signs and symptoms

Left-sided heart failure	Right-sided heart failure
Signs	Signs
Cardiomegaly	RV heave
LV heave	JVD
S_3, S_4	Ascites
Crackles	Right pleural effusion

Symptoms

Dyspnea

Orthopnea

Fatigue

Nocturia and night cough

Both right- and left-sided failure include:

Increased RR, HR

Decreased pulses

Pulsus alternans

S_3

Cheynes-Stokes respirations
(associated with advanced
failure)

Symptoms

Fatigue

Dependent edema

RUQ pain

Anorexia and bloating

Physical examination
See Presenting signs and symptoms.

Diagnostic findings
ECG: May have evidence of LV hypertrophy and/or strain pattern, evidence of RV hypertrophy and/or strain pattern

CXR: Heart shadow may be enlarged
Redistribution of fluid to upper lobes
Kerley B lines
Pleural effusion
Dilated aorta
Left atrial enlargement

CXR findings may lag clinical presentation by 24 hours.

Acute Care Patient Management

Goals of treatment
Improve myocardial function
Supplemental oxygen
Inotropes: digoxin, dobutamine, amrinone

Reduce myocardial work
Bed rest
Vasodilators: nitroglycerin, captopril, hydralazine, prazosin

Reduce circulating volume
Diuretics: furosemide, bumetanide
Vasodilators: nitroglycerin, captopril, hydralazine, prazosin

TABLE 5-23 Clinical Sequelae Associated with Congestive Heart Failure

Complications	Signs and symptoms
Pulmonary edema	Worsening CHF, ↑ RR, ↓ BP, moist cough, frothy sputum, ↓ Pao$_2$
Acute myocardial infarction	ECG changes consistent with AMI, dysrhythmias, ↓ BP, hemodynamic compromise
Cardiogenic shock	↓ Mentation, ↑ HR, SBP <90 mm Hg, CI <2.0, u/o <20 ml/hr
Embolic events	
Spleen	Sharp LUQ pain, splenomegaly, local tenderness, abdominal rigidity
Kidneys	Flank pain, hematuria
Small, peripheral vessels	Mottled, cool skin; peripheral pain
CNS	Change in LOC, focal signs, loss of vision
Lungs	↑ RR, SOB, ↓ Pao$_2$

Detect/prevent clinical sequelae
    See Table 5-23
Priority nursing diagnoses
Decreased cardiac output
Impaired gas exchange
Fluid volume excess
High risk for altered protection (see p. 145)
High risk for altered family process (see p. 150)
▶ **Decreased cardiac output** related to impaired inotropic state of the myocardium
PATIENT OUTCOMES
• Patient will be alert and oriented to person, place, and time
• Skin w/d
• Pulses strong, equal bilaterally
• Capillary refill <3 sec
• SBP 90-140 mm Hg
• MAP 70-105 mm Hg

- Pulse pressure 30-40 mm Hg
- HR 60-100 beats/min
- Absence of life-threatening dysrhythmias
- u/o 30 ml/hr or 0.5-1 ml/kg/hr
- CVP 2-6 mm Hg
- PAS 15-30 mm Hg
- PAD 5-15 mm Hg
- PAWP 4-12 mm Hg
- SVR 900-1600 dynes sec/cm^{-5}
- PVR 100-250 dynes sec/cm^{-5}
- CI 2.4-4.0 L/min/m^2

PATIENT MONITORING

1. Obtain PA pressures and CVP (RA) hourly (if available) or more frequently if titrating pharmacological agents. Obtain CO as patient condition indicates and calculate CI. Note trends or the patient's response to therapy.
2. Obtain BP hourly or more frequently if the patient is unstable; calculate MAP and pulse pressure; note trends and the patient's response to therapy.
3. Monitor hourly urine output to evaluate effects of decreased CO and/or pharmacological intervention.
4. Analyze ECG rhythm strip at least q4h and note rate, rhythm, PR, QRS, and QT intervals. Note ST, T wave changes, which may indicate ischemia.

PHYSICAL ASSESSMENT

1. Obtain HR, RR, BP q15min during acute phase and when titrating vasoactive drugs.
2. Assess for changes in neurological function hourly and as clinically indicated; note orientation to person, place, and time, arousability to verbal and/or tactile stimuli, and bilateral motor and sensory responses.
3. Assess skin for warmth and uniform color. Assess briskness of capillary refill. Assess distal pulses bilaterally for strength, regularity, and symmetry.
4. Assess for chest discomfort, because myocardial ischemia may be the net result of poor perfusion secondary to decreased cardiac output.
5. Assess heart sounds q4h and as clinically indicated. S$_3$ is a hallmark of congestive heart failure. Note degree of jugular vein distention and presence of peripheral edema.
6. Assess the patient for development of clinical sequelae (see Table 5-23).

CV

DIAGNOSTICS ASSESSMENT

1. Review serial BUN and Cr levels to evaluate renal function. BUN >20 and Cr >1.5 suggest renal impairment that may be a result of decreased renal perfusion.
2. Review echocardiography or cardiac catheterization results (if available) to assess ventricular function (ejection fraction and wall motion).

PATIENT MANAGEMENT

1. Provide supplemental oxygen at 2-4 L/min to maintain or improve oxygenation.
2. Minimize oxygen demand: decrease anxiety, keep the patient NPO or provide liquid diet in the acute phase, decrease pain.
3. Maintain the patient on bed rest to decrease myocardial oxygen demand during the acute phase.
4. Initiate and maintain IV line(s) for emergent drug and/or fluid resuscitation.
5. Administer pharmacological agents as ordered to reduce preload and afterload (i.e., diuretics such as furosemide or bumetanide). Administer furosemide IVP as ordered at the rate of 10 mg/min. Doses as high as 120 mg may be required. Administer bumetanide IVP at the rate of 0.5 mg/min. Doses may be repeated as indicated q2h not to exceed 10 mg in 24 hours. A common effect of furosemide and bumetanide administration is potassium (K^+) depletion; therefore monitor serum K^+ before and after administration of furosemide and administer K^+ supplements orally and/or intravenously as ordered. Serum K^+ levels should range from 3.5-5.0. Signs and symptoms of hypokalemia (K^+ <3.5) include muscle weakness, tetany, and dysrhythmia formation.
6. Administer vasodilators (e.g., captopril, hydralazine, prazosin) to reduce preload and afterload. Nitroglycerin may be administered emergently: sublingual, 1 tablet q5min × 3; IV, start with an infusion of 5 μg/min; titrate to desired response or to maintain SBP >90 mm Hg. Increase dosage q5-10 min by 5-10 μg/min. If hypotension occurs, raise the patient's legs and stop the infusion. (See Chapter 7, Pharmacology, for drug information.)
7. Titrate pharmacological agents as ordered to enhance contractility (e.g., digoxin, dopamine, dobutamine, and amrinone). Monitor drug effects on hemodynamic sta-

tus. Calculate CI, SVR, PVR, PP, and MAP. Patients may require digitalization. Monitor serum digoxin levels for efficacy within the first 24 hours of administration. Assess for signs and symptoms of digitalis toxicity: dysrhythmia formation, AV nodal dissociation, PSVT, nausea, vomiting, diarrhea, blurred or yellow vision. Monitor serum K^+ levels closely, especially if digoxin is given concomitantly with furosemide or bumetanide, since hypokalemia increases the risk for digitalis toxicity. Dobutamine may be required; initiate the infusion at 0.5 μg/kg/min. Amrinone may be required. It is typically administered via initial IV bolus, followed by a maintenance drip. Initial IV bolus should be given as 0.75 mg/kg over 2-3 min. Follow this with an infusion, titrating the dose at 5-10 μg/kg/min to the desired effects. Total 24-hour dose should not exceed 10 mg/kg. (See Chapter 7, Pharmacology.)

8. Prophylactic heparin may be ordered to prevent thromboembolus formation secondary to venous pooling. Generally 5000 U are given subcutaneously bid.

▶ **Impaired gas exchange** related to increased pulmonary congestion secondary to increased left ventricular end diastolic pressure (LVEDP)

PATIENT OUTCOMES
- Pao_2 60-100 mm Hg
- pH 7.35-7.45
- $Paco_2$ 35-45 mm Hg
- O_2 sat >95%
- Svo_2 60%-80%
- RR 12-20/min
- Lungs clear to auscultation
- PAWP 4-12 mm Hg
- $P(a/A)O_2$ ratio 0.75-0.90

PATIENT MONITORING
1. Obtain PA pressures, including PAWP; increasing PAWP may signal development of pulmonary edema. Increasing PA systolic pressure may signal hypoxia. Calculate PVR. (See Chapter 3 for information on pulmonary artery catheterization.)

2. Continuously monitor oxygenation status with pulse oximetry (Spo_2) or Svo_2 monitoring. Note patient activities and nursing interventions that may adversely affect oxygen saturation.

CV

3. Continuously monitor ECG for dysrhythmia development that may be related to hypoxemia or acid-base imbalance.
4. Calculate arterial-alveolar oxygen tension ratio ($P(a/A)o_2$ ratio) as an index of gas exchange efficiency.
5. Monitor fluid volume status, since excess fluid can further compromise myocardial functioning. Measure I & O hourly. Determine fluid balance each shift. Compare serial weights. Rapid (0.5-1.0 kg/day) changes in weight suggest fluid gain or loss.

PHYSICAL ASSESSMENT
1. Assess respiratory status frequently during the acute phase. RR >30, increasing complaints of dyspnea, increasing restlessness, and use of accessory muscles indicate respiratory distress and increased patient effort. Cyanosis is a late sign.
2. Assess lung sounds for adventitious sounds and to evaluate the course of pulmonary congestion.
3. Assess the patient for the development of clinical sequelae (see Table 5-23).

DIAGNOSTICS ASSESSMENT
1. Review serial ABGs for hypoxemia (Pao_2 <60 mm Hg) and acidosis (pH <7.35), which may further compromise tissue perfusion.
2. Review lactate levels, an indicator of anaerobic metabolism.
3. Review serial chest radiographs for pulmonary congestion.

PATIENT MANAGEMENT
1. Provide supplemental oxygen as ordered to maintain or improve oxygenation. If patient develops respiratory distress, be prepared for intubation and mechanical ventilation.
2. Minimize oxygen demand: decrease anxiety, keep the patient NPO or provide liquid diet in the acute phase, decrease pain, limit patient activities, pace activities and nursing interventions, and provide uninterrupted rest periods.
3. Maintain the patient on bed rest to decrease myocardial oxygen demand during the acute phase.
4. Position the patient to maximize chest excursion. Evaluate patient response to position changes with Spo_2 or Svo_2 monitoring.

5. Promote pulmonary hygiene to reduce risk of pneumonia and atelectasis; C & DB the patient, encourage incentive spirometry, and reposition the patient frequently.
6. Low-dose morphine sulfate may be ordered to promote venous pooling and decrease dyspnea.
7. Diurectic agents may be ordered to reduce circulating volume. Monitor urine output and electrolytes.

▶ **Fluid volume excess** related to fluid retention secondary to decreased renal perfusion

PATIENT OUTCOMES
- Absence of peripheral edema
- Lungs will be clear to auscultation
- PAWP 4-12 mm Hg or not to exceed 18 mm Hg
- PAP 15-30/5-15 mm Hg
- CVP 2-6 mm Hg
- u/o 30 ml/hr or 0.5-1.0 ml/kg/hr

PATIENT MONITORING
1. Obtain PA pressures and CVP readings hourly or more frequently, depending on patient condition. Both parameters reflect the capacity of the vascular system to accept volume and can be used to monitor for fluid overload.
2. Monitor fluid volume status; measure I & O hourly and determine fluid balance each shift. Compare serial weights. Rapid (0.5-1.0 kg/day) changes in weight suggest fluid gain or loss (NOTE: 1 kg ~ 1000 ml fluid).

PHYSICAL ASSESSMENT
1. Assess fluid volume status: note increase in JVP, peripheral edema, tachycardia, S_3, adventitious breath sounds.
2. Assess the patient for development of clinical sequelae (see Table 5-23).

DIAGNOSTICS ASSESSMENT
1. Review serial BUN and Cr levels to evaluate renal function. BUN >20 and Cr >1.5 suggest renal impairment.

PATIENT MANAGEMENT
1. Administer diuretic agents as ordered and monitor urine output and electrolytes. Monitor for s/s hypovolemia, dehydration.
2. Provide meticulous skin care and reposition the patient frequently.
3. Titrate pharmacological agents (e.g., dopamine, dobutamine) as ordered to improve cardiac output to kidneys. (See Chapter 7 for drug information.)

CV

CARDIOGENIC PULMONARY EDEMA

Clinical Brief

Pulmonary edema is an abnormal accumulation of extravascular fluid in the lung parenchyma that interferes with adequate gas exchange. This is a life-threatening situation that needs immediate treatment. The most common cause of cardiogenic pulmonary edema is left ventricular failure. Risk factors include ischemic heart disease and valvular disease.

Presenting signs and symptoms

Signs and symptoms include shortness of breath, orthopnea, moist cough with pink frothy sputum, chest discomfort, and palpitations.

Physical examination

Appearance: Anxious

HR sustained tachycardia

SBP <90 mm Hg

RR >30/min

Cardiovascular: Alteration in rhythm with ectopy

  Murmur

  Rub

  S_3 with possible S_4

Pulmonary: Respiratory distress

  Orthopnea

  Coarse bilateral crackles

  Frothy sputum

Diagnostic findings

ABGs: Acidosis (pH <7.35) with hypoxia (Pao_2 <60)

CXR: Increased heart shadow

  Kerley B lines

  ↑ Distribution of fluid to upper lobes

  Intraalveolar fluid

PAP: PAWP >20 mm Hg

Acute Care Patient Management

Goals of treatment

Reduce extravascular fluid in lung

  Diuretics: furosemide, bumetanide

Improve LV function

  Bed rest

  Diuretics: furosemide, bumetanide

  Inotropes: digoxin, dobutamine, amrinone, dopamine

  Vasodilators: morphine sulfate, nitroglycerin, nitroprusside

  Rotating tourniquets

Improve oxygenation/ventilation
   Bed rest
   Supplemental oxygen
   Diuretics: furosemide, bumetanide
   Endotracheal intubation and mechanical ventilation
Priority nursing diagnoses
Impaired gas exchange
Decreased cardiac output
High risk for altered protection (see p. 145)
High risk for altered family process (see p. 150)

▶ **Impaired gas exchange** related to increased pulmonary congestion secondary to increased LVEDP

PATIENT OUTCOMES
- RR 12-20/min
- Eupnea
- Lungs clear to auscultation
- pH 7.35-7.45
- Pao_2 60-100 mm Hg
- $Paco_2$ 35-45 mm Hg
- O_2 sat >95%
- Svo_2 60%-80%
- $P(a/A)O_2$ ratio 0.75-0.95

PATIENT MONITORING
1. Obtain PA pressures, including PAWP, to evaluate course of pulmonary edema and/or patient response to therapy.
2. Continuously monitor oxygenation status with pulse oximetry (Spo_2) or Svo_2 monitoring. Note patient activities and nursing interventions that may adversely affect oxygen saturation.
3. Continuously monitor ECG for dysrhythmia development that may be related to hypoxemia or acid-base imbalance.
4. Calculate arterial-alveolar oxygen tension ratio ($P(a/A)o_2$) as an index of gas exchange efficiency.
5. Monitor fluid volume status, since excess fluid can further compromise myocardial functioning. Measure I & O hourly; determine fluid balance each shift. Compare serial weights. Rapid (0.5-1.0 kg/day) changes in weight suggest fluid gain or loss.

PHYSICAL ASSESSMENT
1. Measure HR, RR, BP q15min to evaluate patient response to therapy and detect cardiopulmonary deterioration.

CV

2. Assess the patient for changes that may indicate respiratory compromise, necessitating intubation and mechanical ventilation: air hunger, acute onset of production of pink, frothy sputum, diaphoresis, and cyanosis. (See Chapter 6, Therapeutic Modalities, for information on mechanical ventilation.)

DIAGNOSTICS ASSESSMENT

1. Review ABGs for hypoxemia (Pao_2 <60 mm Hg) and acidosis (pH <7.35), which may further compromise tissue perfusion.
2. Review lactate levels, an indicator of anaerobic metabolism.
3. Review serial chest radiographs for worsening or resolving pulmonary congestion.

PATIENT MANAGEMENT

1. Be prepared to provide assisted ventilation; PEEP will most likely be employed to improve gas exchange. (See information on mechanical ventilation in Chapter 6.)
2. Minimize oxygen demand: decrease anxiety, keep the patient NPO in the acute phase, pace nursing interventions, and provide uninterrupted rest periods.
3. Position the patient to maximize chest excursion; evaluate patient response to position changes with Spo_2 or Svo_2 monitoring.
4. Once the patient's condition is stabilized, promote pulmonary hygiene to reduce risk of pneumonia and atelectasis: C & DB the patient, encourage incentive spirometry, and reposition the patient frequently.
5. Low-dose morphine sulfate may be ordered to promote venous pooling, decrease anxiety, and decrease dyspnea.
6. Diuretic agents may be ordered to reduce circulating volume. Monitor urine output and electrolytes.
7. Rotating tourniquets may be required if pharmacological agents fail (see box).

▶ **Decreased cardiac output** related to impaired LV function

PATIENT OUTCOMES

- Patient will be alert and oriented to person, place, and time
- Skin w/d
- Pulses strong, equal bilaterally
- Capillary refill <3 sec
- SBP 90-140 mm Hg
- MAP 70-105 mm Hg
- Pulse pressure 30-40 mm Hg

Rotating Tourniquets

Principles

- Apply tourniquets to three extremities; set pressure midway between systolic blood pressure and diastolic blood pressure.
- Check peripheral pulses, temperature, and color of extremities (maintain a palpable pulse). Note any pain, edema, or loss of function of extremities.
- Tourniquets should be rotated q15min.
- Remove tourniquet by rotating off one at a time q15min.

- HR 60-100 beats/min
- Absence of life-threatening dysrhythmias
- u/o 30 ml/hr or 0.5-1 ml/kg/hr
- CVP 2-6 mm Hg
- PAS 15-30 mm Hg
- PAD 5-15 mm Hg
- PAWP 4-12 mm Hg
- SVR 900-1600 dynes sec/cm^{-5}
- PVR 100-250 dynes sec/cm^{-5}
- CI 2.4-4.0 L/min/m^2
- SvO_2 60%-80%

PATIENT MONITORING

1. Obtain PA pressures and CVP (RA) hourly (if available) or more frequently if titrating pharmacological agents. Obtain CO as patient condition indicates and calculate CI. Note trends or the patient's response to therapy.
2. Obtain BP hourly or more frequently if the patient's condition is unstable. Calculate MAP and pulse pressure; note trends and the patient's response to therapy.
3. Monitor hourly urine output to evaluate effects of decreased CO and/or pharmacological intervention.
4. Analyze ECG rhythm strip at least q4h and note rate, rhythm, PR, QRS, and QT intervals. Note ST, T wave changes, which may indicate ischemia.

PHYSICAL ASSESSMENT

1. Obtain HR, RR, BP q15min during acute phase and when titrating vasoactive drugs.
2. Assess for changes in neurological function hourly and as clinically indicated; note orientation to person, place,

CV

and time, arousability to verbal and/or tactile stimuli, and bilateral motor and sensory responses.
3. Assess skin for warmth and uniform color. Assess briskness of capillary refill. Assess distal pulses bilaterally for strength, regularity, and symmetry.
4. Assess for chest discomfort, because myocardial ischemia may be the result of hypoxemia and decreased CO.
5. Assess heart and lung sounds q4h and as clinically indicated to evaluate the course of pulmonary edema.
6. Assess the patient for development of clinical sequelae (see Table 5-23).

DIAGNOSTICS ASSESSMENT
1. Review serial BUN and Cr levels to evaluate renal function; BUN >20 and Cr >1.5 suggest renal impairment, which may be a result of decreased renal perfusion.
2. Review echocardiography or cardiac catheterization results (if available) to assess ventricular function (ejection fraction and wall motion).

PATIENT MANAGEMENT
1. Mechanical ventilation with adjunctive PEEP therapy may be required. (See Chapter 6, Therapeutic Modalities, for information on mechanical ventilation.)
2. Minimize oxygen demand: decrease anxiety, keep the patient NPO or provide liquid diet in the acute phase, decrease pain.
3. Initiate an IV line to ensure emergency vascular access. Multiple IV sites may be necessary to maintain multiple vasopressor drips. Verify drug compatibilities should IV sites need to be shared by more than one IV drug.
4. Administer pharmacological agents as ordered to reduce preload and afterload (e.g., diuretics such as furosemide or bumetanide). Administer furosemide IVP as ordered at the rate of 10 mg/min. Doses as high as 120 mg may be required. Administer bumetanide 0.5-1.0 mg IVP at the rate of 0.5 mg/min. Doses may be repeated as indicated q2h, not to exceed 10 mg in 24 hours. A common effect of furosemide and bumetanide administration is potassium (K^+) depletion; therefore monitor serum K^+ before and after administration of furosemide and administer K^+ supplements orally and/or intravenously as ordered. Serum K^+ levels should range from 3.5 to 5.0. Signs and symptoms of hypokalemia (K^+ <3.5) include muscle weakness, tetany, and dysrhythmia formation.
5. Administer vasodilators as ordered to reduce preload

and afterload. Administer morphine sulfate as ordered. Give IVP in 2 mg increments q5min to relieve symptoms. Dilute with 5 ml NS and administer over 4-5 min. Nitroglycerin may be administered emergently: sublingual, 1 tablet q5min × 3; IV, start with an infusion of 5 μg/min; titrate to desired response or to maintain SBP >90 mm Hg. Increase dosage q5-10 min by 5-10 μg/min. If hypotension occurs, raise the patient's legs and stop the infusion. Sodium nitroprusside may be administered continuously via intravenous drip emergently in patients whose SBP is >100 mm Hg. Do not administer more than 10 μg/kg/min, or patient may exhibit signs and symptoms of cyanide toxicity: tinnitus, blurred vision, delirium, and muscle spasm. (See Chapter 7, Pharmacology, for specific drug information.)

6. Titrate pharmacological agents as ordered to enhance contractility (e.g., digoxin, dopamine, dobutamine, and amrinone). Monitor serum digoxin levels within the first 24 hours of administration for efficacy. Note for signs and symptoms of digitalis toxicity, which may include dysrhythmia formation, AV nodal dissociation, PSVT, nausea, vomiting, diarrhea, and blurred or yellow vision. Monitor serum K^+ levels closely, especially if digoxin is given concomitantly with furosemide or bumetanide. Signs and symptoms of digitalis toxicity will be exhibited earlier if the patient is hypokalemic. Dobutamine can be initiated at 0.5 mg/kg/min. Amrinone is typically administered via initial IV bolus, followed by a maintenance drip. An initial IV bolus should be given as 0.75 mg/kg over 2-3 min. Follow this with an infusion, titrating the dose at 5-10 μg/kg/min to the desired effects. Total 24-hour dose should not exceed 10 mg/kg. Dopamine administered at low dose (1-2 μg/kg/min) increases renal blood flow; at moderate doses (2-10 μg/kg/min), contractility is enhanced. (See Chapter 7 for further information on pharmacological agents.)

7. Apply rotating tourniquets as ordered (see the box on p. 265).

PERICARDITIS

Clinical Brief

Pericarditis is an inflammation of the pericardium, the sac that contains the heart. The inflammation may spread to the epicardium or pleurae. Atrial and ventricular dysrhythmias

CV

may result. Resulting fibrosis and/or pericardial fluid accumulation may limit the cardiac chambers to fill, affecting cardiac output.

Risk factors include infections, vasculitis–connective tissue disease, myocardial infarction, uremia, neoplasms, and trauma; iatrogenic (after cardiac surgery, drugs, cardiac resuscitation) and idiopathic pericarditis may also occur.

Presenting signs and symptoms

Chest pain is the most common manifestation. A pericardial friction rub is a clinical hallmark sign. Typically, the pain begins suddenly, is severe and sharp, and is aggravated by inspiration and deep breathing. Pain is usually anterior to the precordium and radiates to the left shoulder and is generally relieved by sitting up and leaning forward.

Physical examination

Appearance: Restlessness
            Irritability
            Weakness
VS: ↑ HR
     ↑ Temperature
Cardiovascular: Friction rub
                Pulsus paradoxus
Pulmonary: Dyspnea
            Tachypnea

Diagnostic findings

ECG: Early phase—diffuse ST-T segment elevation with concave curvature representing injury caused by inflammation, present in all leads except aV_L and V_1; several days later—ST segments return to normal; T wave inversion may be apparent

Cardiac enzymes: Normal, but are increased with underlying acute myocardial infarction

Echocardiogram: May indicate presence of pericardial effusion

Acute Care Patient Management

Goals of treatment

Treat underlying disease and relieve pain
    Antibiotic therapy
    Surgery
    Supplemental oxygen
    Antiinflammatory agents: indomethacin, ibuprofen, ASA, and prednisone
Detect/prevent clinical sequelae
    See Table 5-24

TABLE 5-24 Clinical Sequelae Associated
with Pericarditis

Complication	Signs and symptoms
Cardiac tamponade	↓ SBP, narrowed pulse pressure, pulsus paradoxus, ↑ CVP, ↑ JVP, ↑ HR, ↑ RR, possible friction rub, muffled heart sounds, low-voltage ECG, electrical alternans, rapidly enlarging cardiac silhouette on CXR, peripheral cyanosis, anxiety, chest pain

Priority nursing diagnoses

Pain

High risk for altered protection (see p. 145)

High risk for altered family process (see p. 150)

▶ **Pain** related to inflammation and aggravated by position and inspiration

PATIENT OUTCOMES

• Patient verbalizes pain relief

• Patient breathes with comfort

• O_2 sat >95%

PATIENT MONITORING

1. Check temperature q4h to evaluate course of inflammatory process.

PHYSICAL ASSESSMENT

1. Assess pain to validate inflammation-type chest pain versus ischemic pain (see Table 5-17). Use a visual analogue scale to evaluate severity of pain (see Figure 1-1).

2. Auscultate the anterior chest to determine the quality of the friction rub.

3. Assess respiratory status, since the patient may hypoventilate as a result of pain. Note respiratory rate and depth and ease of breathing.

4. Assess the patient for development of clinical sequelae (see Table 5-24).

DIAGNOSTICS ASSESSMENT

1. Review ABGs to evaluate oxygenation and acid-base status.

2. Review results of echocardiogram, if available. Pleural effusion can be identified with echocardiography.

CV

3. Review serial ECGs for changes. ST segments generally return to baseline within 7 days, followed by T wave inversion within 1 to 2 weeks from the onset of pain.

PATIENT MANAGEMENT

1. Administer pharmacological agents, such as ibuprofen and indomethacin as ordered to reduce inflammation and pain. Other agents may be ordered for pain relief; note patient response to therapy.
2. Stay with the patient, providing a calm, quiet environment.
3. Assist the patient to maintain a position of comfort (leaning forward may help).
4. Ensure activity restrictions while the patient is symptomatic, febrile, or if a friction rub is present.
5. Promote pulmonary hygiene to prevent risk of atelectasis; C & DB the patient and encourage incentive spirometry.

CARDIOMYOPATHY

Clinical Brief

Cardiomyopathy is a dysfunction of cardiac muscle not associated with coronary artery disease (CAD), hypertension (HTN), or valvular, vascular, or pulmonary disease. Cardiomyopathies are classified into three groups:

- Dilated or congestive cardiomyopathy is characterized by ventricular dilation and impaired systolic function. Emboli may occur because of blood stasis in the dilated ventricles.
- Restrictive cardiomyopathy is characterized by a decreased diastolic compliance. The ventricular cavity is decreased, and clinical manifestations are similar to chronic constrictive pericarditis.
- Hypertrophic cardiomyopathy is characterized by inappropriate myocardial hypertrophy without ventricular dilation. Obstruction to left ventricular outflow may or may not be present. Ventricular compliance is decreased and diastolic filling is impaired.

Presenting signs and symptoms

Signs and symptoms of cardiomyopathy include manifestations of heart failure, dysrhythmias, or conduction disturbances. Sudden death may result from cardiomyopathy.

Physical examination

HR tachycardia

BP hypotension or hypertension, depending on underlying
    disease or degree of heart failure
RR may be ↑, depending on degree of heart failure
Cardiovascular: Murmurs
                 Rubs
                 S_3 and/or S_4
                 Ectopy
                 ↑ JVP
Pulmonary: Crackles
            Dry cough
Diagnostic findings
ECG: Indicative of LV hypertrophy and/or strain or indic-
      ative of RV hypertrophy and/or strain
CXR: Evidence of congestive heart failure, enlarged heart
      silhouette
Echocardiogram: LV hypertrophy
                 RV hypertrophy
                 ↓ EF
                 ↓ CO
                 Possible area of hypokinesia
Hemodynamics: ↑ PAWP
               ↑ SVR

Acute Care Patient Management
Goals of treatment
DILATED CARDIOMYOPATHY
Maximize cardiac output
    Bed rest
    Inotropic drugs: digoxin, dobutamine, amrinone
    Antidysrhythmic agents
    β Blockers: propranolol
Decrease myocardial work
    Supplemental oxygen
    Diuretics: furosemide, bumetanide
    Vasodilators: nitroglycerin, nitroprusside
    β Blockers: propranolol
Detect/prevent clinical sequelae
    See Table 5-25
NOTE: Inotropic and vasodilator agents are contraindicated
    in hypertrophic cardiomyopathy.
Priority nursing diagnoses
Decreased cardiac output
Pain
Impaired gas exchange

TABLE 5-25 Clinical Sequelae Associated with Cardiomyopathy

Complications	Signs and symptoms
Pulmonary edema	Worsening CHF: SOB, moist cough, frothy sputum, ↓ Pao$_2$, ↑ HR
Cardiogenic shock	↓ Mentation, ↑ or ↓ HR, SBP <90 mm Hg, CI <2.0 L/min/m^2, u/o <0.5 ml/kg/hr, cool, clammy, mottled skin
Dysrhythmias/sudden death	Change in rate and/or rhythm, change in LOC, syncope, chest discomfort
Thrombus with embolic event	Change in LOC, ECG changes indicative of ischemia, dysrhythmias, renal failure, GI ileus, abdominal pain, SOB, ↓ Pao$_2$, crackles

Fluid volume excess
High risk for altered protection (see p. 145)
High risk for altered family process (see p. 150)
Altered nutrition: less than body requirements (see p. 149)
▶ **Decreased cardiac output** related to dysrhythmias and left ventricular dysfunction
PATIENT OUTCOMES
• Patient will be alert and oriented to person, place, and time
• Skin w/d
• Pulses strong, equal bilaterally
• Capillary refill <3 sec
• SBP 90-140 mm Hg
• MAP 70-105 mm Hg
• Pulse pressure 30-40 mm Hg
• HR 60-100 beats/min
• Absence of life-threatening dysrhythmias
• u/o 30 ml/hr or 0.5-1 ml/kg/hr
• CVP 2-6 mm Hg
• PAS 15-30 mm Hg
• PAD 5-15 mm Hg

- PAWP 4-12 mm Hg
- SVR 900-1600 dynes sec/cm^{-5}
- PVR 100-250 dynes sec/cm^{-5}
- CI 2.4-4.0 L/min/m^2

PATIENT MONITORING

1. Obtain PA pressures and CVP (RA) hourly (if available) or more frequently if titrating pharmacological agents. Obtain CO as patient condition indicates and calculate CI. Note trends or patient's response to therapy.
2. Obtain BP hourly or more frequently if the patient's condition is unstable. Calculate MAP and pulse pressure; note trends and patient's response to therapy.
3. Monitor hourly urine output to evaluate effects of decreased CO and/or pharmacological intervention.
4. Analyze ECG rhythm strip at least q4h and note rate, rhythm, PR, QRS, and QT intervals. Note ST, T wave changes, which may indicate ischemia.

PHYSICAL ASSESSMENT

1. Obtain HR, RR, BP q15min during acute phase and when titrating vasoactive drugs.
2. Assess for changes in neurological function hourly and as clinically indicated; note orientation to person, place, and time, arousability to verbal and/or tactile stimuli, and bilateral motor and sensory responses.
3. Assess skin for warmth and uniform color. Assess briskness of capillary refill. Assess distal pulses bilaterally for strength, regularity, and symmetry.
4. Assess for chest discomfort, because myocardial ischemia may be the net result of poor perfusion secondary to decreased cardiac output.
5. Assess heart and lung sounds to evaluate course of heart failure.
6. Assess the patient for development of clinical sequelae (see Table 5-25).

DIAGNOSTICS ASSESSMENT

1. Review echocardiography or cardiac catheterization results (if available) and note ventricular function (ejection fraction and wall motion).

PATIENT MANAGEMENT

1. Provide O$_2$ at 2-4 L/min to maintain or improve oxygenation.
2. Minimize oxygen demand: decrease anxiety, keep the patient NPO or provide a liquid diet in acute phase.

CV

3. Maintain the patient on bed rest to decrease myocardial oxygen demand during the acute phase.
4. Initiate and maintain IV line(s) for emergent drug and/ or fluid resuscitation.
5. Administer pharmacological agents as ordered to reduce preload and afterload (e.g., diuretics such as furosemide or bumetanide). Administer furosemide IVP as ordered at the rate of 10 mg/min. Doses as high as 120 mg may be required. Administer bumetanide IVP at the rate of 0.5 mg/min. Doses may be repeated as indicated q2h not to exceed 10 mg in 24 hours. A common effect of furosemide and bumetanide administration is potassium (K^+) depletion; therefore monitor serum K^+ before and after administration of furosemide and administer K^+ supplements orally and/or intravenously as ordered. Serum K^+ levels should range from 3.5 to 5.0. Signs and symptoms of hypokalemia $(K^+ <3.5)$ include muscle weakness, tetany, and dysrhythmia formation.
6. Administer vasodilators to reduce preload and afterload in patients with dilated cardiomyopathy. Vasodilators are contraindicated in hypertrophic cardiomyopathy. If nitroglycerin is ordered, start the infusion at 5 µg/min; titrate to desired response or to maintain SBP >90 mm Hg. Increase dosage q5-10 min by 5-10 µg/min. If hypotension occurs, raise the patient's legs and stop the infusion. If nitroprusside is ordered, titrate the infusion to maintain systolic BP at 100-120 mm Hg. Dose may range from 0.5-10 µg/kg/min. Do not administer more than 10 µg/kg/min or patient may exhibit signs and symptoms of cyanide toxicity: tinnitus, blurred vision, delirium, and muscle spasm. (See Chapter 7, Pharmacology, for specific drug information.)
7. Titrate pharmacological agents as ordered if necessary to enhance contractility (e.g., digoxin, dobutamine, and amrinone). Monitor drug effects on hemodynamic states. Calculate CI, SVR, PVR, PP, MAP. Patients may require digitalization. Monitor serum digoxin levels within the first 24 hours of administration for efficacy. Assess for signs and symptoms of digitalis toxicity: dysrhythmia formation, AV nodal dissociation, PSVT, nausea, vomiting, diarrhea, blurred or yellow vision. Monitor serum K^+ levels closely, especially if digoxin is given concomitantly with furosemide or bumetanide, since

hypokalemia increases the risk for toxicity. Dobutamine may be required; initiate the infusion at 0.5 µg/kg/min. Amrinone may be required. It is typically administered via initial IV bolus, followed by a maintenance drip. An initial IV bolus should be given as 0.75 mg/kg over 2-3 min. Follow this with an infusion, titrating the dose at 5-10 µg/kg/min to the desired effects. Total 24-hour dose should not exceed 10 mg/kg. (See Chapter 7, Pharmacology, for specific drug information.)

8. Prophylactic heparin may be ordered to prevent thromboembolus formation secondary to venous pooling. Generally, 5000 U are given subcutaneously bid.

▶ **Pain** related to decreased oxygen supply secondary to outflow tract obstruction (hypertrophic cardiomyopathy) or impaired systolic function (dilated cardiomyopathy)

PATIENT OUTCOMES
• Patient verbalizes pain relief
• Absence of ST-T wave changes

PATIENT MONITORING
1. Continuously monitor ECG to evaluate ST, T wave changes, which may indicate ischemia, injury, or infarction and to detect dysrhythmia development.

PHYSICAL ASSESSMENT
1. Assess pain to validate ischemic origin (see Table 5-17). Use a visual analogue scale to evaluate severity of pain (see Figure 1-1).
2. Check VS frequently during anginal episode and with administration of antianginal agents. Hypotension can occur with these agents.
3. Assess patient for development of clinical sequelae (see Table 5-25).

DIAGNOSTICS ASSESSMENT
1. Review serial 12-lead ECGs to evaluate effects of the ischemic episode.

PATIENT MANAGEMENT
1. Stay with the patient, providing a calm, quiet environment. Assess the level of anxiety and other factors that increase myocardial oxygen demand, such as fever, dysrhythmias, anger, hypertension, and hypoxemia.
2. Provide supplemental oxygen at 2-4 L/min to maintain or improve oxygenation.
3. Initiate and maintain IV line(s) for emergent drug and fluid resuscitation.

CV

4. Administer NTG to patients with dilated cardiomyopathy as indicated to decrease afterload, decrease myocardial oxygen demand, and increase myocardial oxygen supply: sublingual, 1 tablet q5min × 3; IV, start with an infusion of 5 μg/min; titrate to desired response or to maintain SBP >90 mm Hg. Increase dosage q5-10min by 5-10 μg/min. If hypotension occurs, raise the patient's legs and stop the infusion. Nitroglycerin may aggravate angina in patients with hypertrophic cardiomyopathy.

5. Administer morphine sulfate as ordered. Give IVP in 2 mg increments q5min to relieve chest discomfort. Dilute with 5 ml NS and administer over 4-5 min. Monitor respirations, because narcotics are respiratory depressants.

6. Notify the physician if pain is not relieved despite pharmacological intervention or if pain has subsided but recurs.

7. Administer β blockers such as propranolol as ordered to decrease myocardial oxygen demand. Monitor drug effects on HR and BP.

8. Avoid drugs that may increase outflow obstruction in patients with hypertrophic cardiomyopathy (e.g., digitalis, β-adrenergic agents, and vasodilators).

▶ **Impaired gas exchange** related to increased pulmonary congestion secondary to increased left ventricular end diastolic pressure associated with ventricular failure

PATIENT OUTCOMES
- Pao_2 60-100 mm Hg
- pH 7.35-7.45
- $Paco_2$ 35-45 mm Hg
- O_2 sat >95%
- RR 12-20/min, eupnea
- Lungs clear to auscultation

PATIENT MONITORING
1. Obtain PA pressures, including PAWP; increasing PAWP may signal development of pulmonary edema. Increasing PA systolic pressure may signal hypoxia. Calculate PVR.

2. Continuously monitor oxygenation status with pulse oximetry (Spo_2) or Svo_2 monitoring. Note patient activities and nursing interventions that may adversely affect oxygen saturation.

3. Continuously monitor ECG for dysrhythmia development that may be related to hypoxemia or acid-base imbalance.
4. Calculate arterial-alveolar oxygen tension ratio ($P(a/A)o_2$ ratio) as an index of gas exchange efficiency.
5. Monitor fluid volume status, since excess fluid can further compromise myocardial functioning. Measure I & O hourly. Determine fluid balance each shift. Compare serial weights. Rapid (0.5-1.0 kg/day) changes in weight suggest fluid gain or loss.

PHYSICAL ASSESSMENT

1. Assess respiratory status frequently during the acute phase. RR >30/min, increasing complaints of dyspnea, increasing restlessness, and use of accessory muscles indicate respiratory distress and increased patient effort. Cyanosis is a late sign.
2. Assess lung sounds for adventitious sounds and to evaluate the course of pulmonary congestion.
3. Assess the patient for the development of clinical sequelae (see Table 5-25).

DIAGNOSTICS ASSESSMENT

1. Review serial ABGs for hypoxemia (Pao_2 <60 mm Hg) and acidosis (pH <7.35), which may further compromise tissue perfusion.
2. Review lactate levels, an indicator of anaerobic metabolism.
3. Review serial chest radiographs for pulmonary congestion.

PATIENT MANAGEMENT

1. Provide supplemental oxygen as ordered to maintain or improve oxygenation. If patient develops respiratory distress, be prepared for intubation and mechanical ventilation.
2. Minimize oxygen demand: decrease anxiety, keep the patient NPO or provide a liquid diet in the acute phase, decrease pain, limit patient activities, pace activities and nursing interventions, and provide uninterrupted rest periods.
3. Maintain the patient on bed rest to decrease myocardial oxygen demand during the acute phase.
4. Position the patient to maximize chest excursion; evaluate patient response to position changes with Spo_2 or Svo_2 monitoring.

CV

5. Promote pulmonary hygiene to reduce the risk of pneumonia and atelectasis; C & DB the patient, encourage incentive spirometry, and reposition the patient frequently.
6. Low-dose morphine sulfate may be ordered to promote venous pooling and decrease dyspnea.
7. Diurectic agents may be ordered to reduce circulating volume. Monitor urine output and electrolytes.

▶ **Fluid volume excess** related to fluid retention secondary to decreased renal perfusion

PATIENT OUTCOMES
• Absence of peripheral edema
• Lungs clear to auscultation
• PAWP 4-12 mm Hg or not to exceed 18 mm Hg
• PAP $\dfrac{15\text{-}30}{5\text{-}15}$ mm Hg
• CVP 2-6 mm Hg
• u/o 30 ml/hr or 0.5-1.0 ml/kg/hr

PATIENT MONITORING
1. Obtain PA pressures and CVP readings hourly or more frequently, depending on patient condition. Both parameters reflect the capacity of the vascular system to accept volume and can be used to monitor for fluid overload.
2. Monitor fluid volume status; measure I & O hourly and determine fluid balance each shift. Compare serial weights. Rapid (0.5-1.0 kg/day) changes in weight suggest fluid gain or loss (NOTE: 1 kg ~ 1000 ml fluid).

PHYSICAL ASSESSMENT
1. Assess fluid volume status: note increase in JVP, peripheral edema, tachycardia, S_3, adventitious breath sounds.
2. Assess the patient for development of clinical sequelae (see Table 5-25).

DIAGNOSTICS ASSESSMENT
1. Review serial BUN and Cr levels to evaluate renal function. BUN >20 and Cr >1.5 suggest renal impairment.

PATIENT MANAGEMENT
1. Administer diuretic agents as ordered and monitor urine output and electrolytes.
2. Provide meticulous skin care and reposition the patient frequently.
3. Titrate pharmacological agents as ordered to improve cardiac output to kidneys. (See Chapter 7, Pharmacology, for specific drug information.)

ENDOCARDITIS
Clinical Brief

Endocarditis is an inflammation of the endocardium; it is usually limited to the membrane lining the valves. The cause of endocarditis may be viral, fungal, or, most commonly, bacterial; the most common agent is *Streptococcus viridans*. Vegetations (growths or lesions) may cause valvular dysfunction.

Risk factors include any high-risk individual (such as a patient with valvular disease or mitral valve prolapse) undergoing any type of invasive procedure, especially dental surgery; any chronically ill individual, especially one who is immunosuppressed; any individual with previously damaged or congenitally malformed valves or who has prosthetic valves; and illicit drug abusers.

Presenting signs and symptoms

Signs and symptoms may be nonspecific. Fever is the most common early manifestation.

Physical examination

Physical findings are nonspecific. A new murmur may be auscultated. Signs/symptoms of heart failure may be present.

Diagnostic findings

History and physical examination: High index of suspicion in individuals with fever of unknown origin, who are anemic, and who have the presence of a new murmur

Blood cultures and sensitivity, aerobic and anaerobic, may isolate the offending organism

CXR: Findings consistent with CHF:
    Possible enlargement of heart shadow
    Redistribution of fluid to upper lobes
    Kerley B lines
    Pleural effusion
    Dilated aorta
    Left atrial enlargement

Echocardiogram: Valve disease or vegetations may be seen

Acute Care Patient Management
Goals of treatment

Eliminate infection
    Antibiotic therapy

Maintain valvular integrity or improve myocardial function
    Surgical valve repair and/or replacement
    Supplemental oxygen
    Inotropic drugs: digoxin, dobutamine, amrinone
    Vasodilators: nitroglycerin

CV

Reduce myocardial work
    Bed rest
    Vasodilators: nitroglycerin
Reduce circulating volume
    Diuretics: furosemide, bumetanide
    Vasodilators: nitroglycerin
Priority nursing diagnoses
Decreased cardiac output
Altered tissue perfusion
High risk for altered protection (see p. 145)
High risk for altered family process (see p. 150)
Altered nutrition: less than body requirements (see p. 149)

▶ **Decreased cardiac output** secondary to valvular dysfunction from infective process
PATIENT OUTCOMES
- Patient will be alert and oriented to person, place, and time
- Skin w/d
- Pulses strong, equal bilaterally
- Capillary refill <3 sec
- SBP 90-140 mm Hg
- MAP 70-105 mm Hg
- Pulse pressure 30-40 mm Hg
- HR 60-100 beats/min
- Absence of life-threatening dysrhythmias
- u/o 30 ml/hr or 0.5-1 ml/kg/hr
- CVP 2-6 mm Hg
- PAS 15-30 mm Hg
- PAD 5-15 mm Hg
- PAWP 4-12 mm Hg
- CI 2.5-4.0 L/min/m²
- SVR 900-1600 dynes sec/cm^{-5}
- PVR 100-250 dynes sec/cm^{-5}

PATIENT MONITORING
1. Measure hemodynamic pressures if PA catheter is utilized: obtain PA pressure and CVP (RA) hourly or more frequently if titrating pharmacological agents. Obtain CO as patient condition indicates and calculate CI. Note trends or patient's response to therapy.
2. Obtain BP hourly or more frequently if the patient's condition is unstable. Calculate MAP and pulse pressure; note trends and patient response to therapy.
3. Monitor hourly urine output to evaluate effects of decreased CO and/or pharmacological intervention.

4. Analyze ECG rhythm strip at least q4h and note rate, rhythm, PR, QRS, and QT intervals. Note ST, T wave changes, which may indicate ischemia.
5. Continuously monitor Svo_2 (if available) to evaluate oxygen supply and demand; a downward trend can indicate decreased supply or increased demand.

PHYSICAL ASSESSMENT

1. Obtain HR, RR, BP q15min if the patient is exhibiting signs and symptoms of congestive heart failure and vasoactive drugs are being administered. If the patient is stable and not in CHF, vital signs may be obtained hourly or less frequently, depending on patient condition.
2. Assess for changes in neurological function hourly and as clinically indicated; note orientation to person, place, and time, arousability to verbal and/or tactile stimuli, and bilateral motor and sensory responses.
3. Assess skin for warmth and uniform color. Assess briskness of capillary refill. Assess distal pulses bilaterally for strength, regularity, and symmetry.
4. Assess for chest discomfort, because myocardial ischemia may be the net result of poor perfusion secondary to decreased cardiac output.
5. Assess heart and lung sounds q4h and as clinically indicated for signs of progressive valvular dysfunction. Note the degree of jugular venous distention, dyspnea, sustained tachycardia, and crackles.

DIAGNOSTICS ASSESSMENT

1. Review BUN and Cr levels to evaluate renal function; BUN >20 and Cr >1.5 suggest renal impairment, which may be a result of decreased renal perfusion.
2. Review echocardiography findings (if available) for valvular and ventricular function (ejection fraction and wall motion) and presence of vegetations.
3. Review WBC counts to evaluate course of infection.

PATIENT MANAGEMENT

1. Provide supplemental oxygen at 2-4 L/min to maintain or improve oxygenation.
2. Minimize oxygen demand: decrease anxiety and maintain the patient on bed rest if in acute CHF and keep NPO or on a clear liquid diet as tolerated during the acute phase.
3. Initiate and maintain IV line(s) for emergent drug and fluid resuscitation.
4. Administer IV antibiotics as ordered and obtain serum

CV

antibiotic peak and trough levels as ordered to determine efficacy.

5. Monitor temperature hourly. Administer antipyretics as ordered and monitor patient's temperature.

6. Administer pharmacological agents as ordered if the patient is in acute CHF to reduce preload and afterload (diuretics such as furosemide or bumetanide). Administer furosemide IVP as ordered at the rate of 10 mg/min. Administer bumetanide IVP at the rate of 0.5 mg/min. Doses may be repeated as indicated q2h, not to exceed 10 mg in 24 hours. A common effect of furosemide and bumetanide administration is potassium (K^+) depletion; therefore monitor serum K^+ before and after administration of furosemide and administer K^+ supplements orally and/or intravenously as ordered. Serum K^+ levels should range from 3.5 to 5.0. Signs and symptoms of hypokalemia (K^+ <3.5) include muscle weakness, tetany, and dysrhythmia formation. Nitroglycerin may be administered to decrease preload. Start the infusion at 5 μg/min; titrate to desired response or to maintain SBP >90 mm Hg. Increase dosage q5-10min by 5-10 μg/min. If hypotension occurs, raise the patient's legs and stop the infusion. (See Chapter 7, Pharmacology, for specific drug information.)

7. Titrate pharmacological agents as ordered to enhance contractility (e.g., digoxin, dopamine, dobutamine, and amrinone). Monitor drug effects on hemodynamic status. Calculate CI, SVR, PVR, PP, and MAP if a PA catheter is utilized, and note patient response to pharmacological therapy. Patients may require digitalization. Monitor serum digoxin levels within the first 24 hours of administration for efficacy. Assess for signs and symptoms of digitalis toxicity: dysrhythmia formation, AV nodal dissociation, PSVT, nausea, vomiting, diarrhea, blurred or yellow vision. Monitor serum K^+ levels closely, especially if digoxin is given concomitantly with furosemide or bumetanide, since hypokalemia increases the risk for digitalis toxicity. Dobutamine may be required; initiate the infusion at 0.5 μg/kg/min. Amrinone may be required. It is typically administered via an initial IV bolus, followed by a maintenance drip. The initial IV bolus should be given as 0.75 mg/kg over 2-3 min. Follow this with an infusion, titrating the dose at

5-10 μg/kg/min to the desired effects. Total 24-hour dose should not exceed 10 mg/kg. Dopamine at low doses (1-2 μg/kg/min) increases renal blood flow and enhances contractility at moderate doses (2-10 μg/kg/min). (See Chapter 7, Pharmacology, for specific drug information.)

8. Prepare the patient for anticipated surgical intervention to repair/replace affected valve(s). In stable patients, this will usually occur 6 weeks after the completion of antibiotic therapy. In patients with acute CHF, this surgery may be performed emergently.

▶ **Altered tissue perfusion** secondary to embolic event

PATIENT OUTCOMES
- Patient will be alert and oriented to person, place, and time
- Vision unchanged
- RR 12-20/min, regular and nonlabored
- u/o 30 ml/hr or 0.5 ml/kg/hr and clear yellow
- Skin w/d
- No c/o pain to either flank, LUQ, or periphery

PATIENT MONITORING
1. Monitor urine output for volume and clarity hourly. Check for hematuria.

PHYSICAL ASSESSMENT
1. Assess neurological status: note any change in LOC or change in motor or sensory responses.
2. Assess for chest discomfort that may signal myocardial infarction.
3. Note skin color and temperature of extremities. Check pulses and capillary refill for development of peripheral emboli.
4. Assess respiratory status for increasing dyspnea, restlessness, tachypnea, pleuritic chest pain, and tachycardia suggesting a pulmonary embolus.
5. Investigate complaints of LUQ pain or flank pain, which may suggest decreased perfusion to the spleen or kidney.

DIAGNOSTICS ASSESSMENT
1. Review results of echocardiogram for presence of vegetations and extent of myocardial compromise.
2. Review ABGs to evaluate oxygenation and acid-base status.
3. Monitor serial BUN and Cr levels to evaluate renal

CV

function; BUN >20 and Cr >1.5 suggest renal impairment, which may be a result of decreased renal perfusion.

4. Review results of blood cultures to determine the infecting organism.

PATIENT MANAGEMENT

1. Administer antibiotics as ordered in a timely fashion.
2. Protect IV site, since antibiotic therapy may be required over several weeks. Observe the site for redness, tenderness, or infiltration.
3. Provide pulmonary hygiene to decrease the risk of atelectasis and pneumonia during the acute phase when the patient is maintained on bed rest. C & DB the patient, encourage incentive spirometry, and reposition the patient frequently.
4. Assist with ROM exercises while the patient is maintained on bed rest.

VALVULAR DISORDERS

Clinical Brief

Valvular disorders may be congenital or acquired. Common causes of acquired valvular heart disease include rheumatic heart disease (which is declining in incidence), infective endocarditis, ischemia (which usually affects the mitral valve), traumatic damage (commonly caused by blunt chest trauma), and syphilitic disease (aortic valvular disease). When valve leaflets fail to close properly, blood leaks from one chamber back into another; this is called a *regurgitant valve*. When the valve orifice is restricted and is not allowed to open properly, forward blood flow is obstructed and the valve is described as *stenotic*. All valves can be diseased; however, the mitral and aortic valves are most commonly affected. Murmurs and related valvular disorders are listed in Table 5-26.

Presenting signs and symptoms

Symptoms reflect left ventricular or biventricular failure (see Congestive heart failure, p. 254). Atrial dysrhythmias can also be present (see Table 5-26).

Diagnostic findings

See Table 5-26

Acute Care Patient Management

See Cardiac surgery, p. 501, and Congestive heart failure, p. 254.

TABLE 5-26 Valvular Disorders

Type	Physical examination	Diagnostic study findings
Mitral stenosis	Diastolic heart murmur Dyspnea on exertion (DOE) Weakness Fatigue Predisposition to respiratory infections Orthopnea Paroxysmal nocturnal dyspnea Palpitations (from atrial fibrillation) Hemoptysis	ECG: Left atrial enlargement Prolonged, notched P waves (P mitrale) Right ventricular hypertrophy Chest radiograph: Left atrial enlargement Pulmonary venous congestion Interstitial pulmonary edema Right ventricular enlargement Cardiac catheterization: ↑ Pressure across mitral valve ↑ Left atrial pressure ↑ PAWP ↓ CO Echocardiogram: ↓ Excursion of leaflets Diminished E-F slope

Continued.

CV

TABLE 5-26 Valvular Disorders—cont'd

Type	Physical examination	Diagnostic study findings
Mitral regurgitation	Murmur throughout systole Weakness Fatigue DOE Palpitations	ECG: Left atrial enlargement (P mitrale) Left ventricular hypertrophy Atrial fibrillation Chest radiograph: Left atrial enlargement Left ventricular enlargement Pulmonary vascular congestion Cardiac catheterization: Angiography and contrast medium used to iden- tify and quantify regurgitation Echocardiogram: Left atrial enlargement Hyperdynamic left ventricle

Aortic stenosis	Systolic murmur	ECG:
	Syncope (especially on exertion)	Left ventricular hypertrophy
	Angina pectoris	Chest radiographs:
	Left ventricular failure	Poststenotic aortic dilation
	Fatigue	Aortic valve calcification
	Dyspnea	Cardiac catheterization:
		Pressure gradient in systole between left ventricle and aorta (across aortic valve)
		↑ Diastolic ventricular pressure
		Normal left atrial and pulmonary pressures
		Echocardiogram:
		Restricted movement of aortic valve
		Increased echoes
		Thickening of left ventricular wall
Aortic regurgitation	Diastolic and systolic murmurs	ECG:
	Water-hammer pulse	Left ventricular hypertrophy
	Palpitations	Chest radiograph:
	Syncope	Aortic valve calcification
	DOE	Left ventricular enlargement
	Chest pain	Dilation of ascending aorta
	CHF	Cardiac catheterization:
		↑ Pulse pressure
		↑ Diastolic pulse slope

CV

HYPERTENSIVE CRISIS
Clinical Brief
Hypertensive crisis is an emergent situation in which a marked elevation in diastolic BP can cause end organ damage. Severe hypertension (usually a diastolic reading above 130 mm Hg) can cause irreversible injury to the brain, heart, and kidneys and can rapidly lead to death. Hypertensive crisis can occur in patients with either essential hypertension, which has no known cause, or secondary hypertension, which can be a result of renal or endocrine disease. Emergencies include hypertension in association with encephalopathy, acute aortic dissection, pulmonary edema, pheochromocytoma crisis, intracranial bleeding, and eclampsia.
Presenting signs and symptoms
Signs and symptoms depend on the underlying disease and end-organ damage. Headache, nausea, dizziness, and visual disturbances may be present.
Physical examination
DBP >130 mm Hg (see Presenting signs and symptoms). Other findings may be the result of damage to end-organs (see Table 5-27).
Diagnostic findings
Diagnostic tests are used to evaluate the effects of ↑ BP on target organs or to determine the cause of secondary hypertension.
Acute Care Patient Management
Goals of treatment
Reduce BP
    Vasodilators: nitroprusside, diazoxide
    Sympatholytics: labetalol
    Calcium channel-blocking agents: nifedipine
    Ganglionic blockers: trimethaphan
    Surgical intervention
Detect/prevent clinical sequelae
    See Table 5-27
Priority nursing diagnosis
High risk for injury
High risk for altered protection (see p. 145)
High risk for altered family process (see p. 150)
Altered nutrition: less than body requirements (see p. 149)
▶ **High risk for injury:** end-organ damage secondary to severe hypertension
PATIENT OUTCOMES
• Patient will be alert and oriented

- Skin w/d
- Pulses strong, equal bilaterally
- Capillary refill <3 sec
- MAP 70-120 mm Hg
- HR 60-100 beats/min
- Absence of life-threatening dysrhythmias
- u/o 30 ml/hr or 0.5-1 ml/kg/hr
- BUN <20 mg/dl, Cr <1.5 mg/dl

PATIENT MONITORING

1. Monitor arterial BP continuously and note sudden increases or decreases in readings. A precipitous drop in blood pressure can cause reflex ischemia to the heart, brain, kidneys, and/or the GI tract. Calculate MAP and note trends and the patient's response to therapy.
2. Monitor hourly urine output and note any presence of blood in the urine.
3. Continuously monitor the ECG for dysrhythmias or ST, T wave changes associated with ischemia.

PHYSICAL ASSESSMENT

1. Assess the patient for development of clinical sequelae.

CV

TABLE 5-27 Clinical Sequelae Associated with Hypertensive Crisis

Complications	Signs and symptoms
CHF	Sustained elevated HR, cough, S_3, crackles, PAWP >20 mm Hg
Pulmonary edema	Worsening CHF, SOB, ↑ RR, ↑ HR, moist cough, frothy sputum, PAWP >22 mm Hg
Acute myocardial infarction	Chest pain, ECG changes indicative of ischemia, hemodynamic compromise
CVA	Change in LOC, change in focal neurological signs, pupil changes
Renal failure	u/o <0.5 ml/kg/hr, edema
Aortic dissection	Severe pain to chest, abdomen, or lumbar area; pulse and BP differentials between RUE and LUE; murmur; initial ↑ BP followed by drop in BP and tachycardia
Hypertensive encephalopathy	Change in LOC, ↑ ICP, retinopathy with papilledema, seizures

DIAGNOSTICS ASSESSMENT

1. Review BUN and Cr to evaluate the effect of BP on kidneys. BUN >20 and Cr >1.5 suggest renal impairment.
2. Review serial chest radiographs for pulmonary congestion.
3. Review serial 12-lead ECGs for patterns of injury, ischemia, and infarction.

PATIENT MANAGEMENT

1. Provide oxygen at 2-4 L/min to maintain or improve oxygenation.
2. Minimize oxygen demand: decrease anxiety and keep the patient NPO or provide a liquid diet in the acute phase.
3. Maintain the patient on bed rest to decrease myocardial oxygen demand during the acute phase.
4. Vasodilators such as nitroprusside or diazoxide may be ordered. Nitroprusside can be initiated with an infusion at a rate 0.5 μg/kg/min, not to exceed 10 μg/kg/min. Diazoxide can be given as miniboluses or as an infusion. If hypotension occurs, raise the patient's legs and stop the infusion. (See Chapter 7 for drug information.)
5. Labetalol may be given intravenously, usually 1-2 mg/kg over 10 min to rapidly lower BP. Miniboluses or an infusion may be ordered.
6. A ganglionic blocking agent such as trimethaphan camsylate may be ordered to emergently lower BP. Begin continuous IV infusion and titrate to the desired BP response. The usual dosage range may be 0.3 mg/min to 6 mg/min. If hypotension occurs, raise the patient's legs and stop the infusion (see Chapter 7).
7. Prepare the patient and family for surgical intervention to correct the underlying cause, if this is indicated.

CARDIAC TAMPONADE

Clinical Brief

Cardiac tamponade is the accumulation of excess fluid within the pericardial space, resulting in impaired cardiac filling, reduction in stroke volume, and epicardial coronary artery compression with resultant myocardial ischemia. Clinical signs of cardiac tamponade depend on the rapidity of fluid accumulation as well as fluid volume. The acute accumulation of 200 ml of blood within the pericardium as a result of blunt or penetrating trauma to the thorax will result in rapid evidence of decompensation, whereas an insidious effusion may not evidence decompensation until as much as 2000 ml of fluid have slowly accumulated.

Risk factors include recent cardiac trauma such as open trauma to the thorax (gunshot wounds and stabs), closed trauma to the thorax (impact of the chest on a steering wheel from a motor vehicle accident), cardiac surgery, cardiac catheterization, or pacemaker electrode perforation; nontraumatic factors include metastatic neoplasm, tuberculosis, acute viral or idiopathic pericarditis, renal failure, and hemopericardium from anticoagulant therapy.

Presenting signs and symptoms
Symptoms are highly variable and depend on the cause. However, decreased cardiac output and poor tissue perfusion are the net result.

Physical examination
Pulsus paradoxus >10 mm Hg (hallmark)
Narrowed pulse pressure (<30 mm Hg)
Hypotension
Neurological: Anxiety, confusion, obtunded if decompensation is advanced
Cardiovascular: Jugular venous distension
    Kussmaul's sign (rise in venous pressure with inspiration) may be present
    Muffled, distant heart sounds
    Pericardial rub may be present
Skin: Cool, pale, may be clammy

Diagnostic findings
Cardiac tamponade should be suspected if there is a rise in CVP, fall in arterial pressure, and a "quiet" heart.

OTHER
ECG: Usually nonspecific; may note electrical alternans
CXR: In acute cases, is rarely diagnostic. Chronic effusions may result in a "water bottle" appearance of the cardiac silhouette.
Echocardiography: Usually reveals widespread compression of the heart as well as inferior and superior vena cava congestion
Hemodynamics: As cardiac tamponade progresses, RA pressure begins to approximate PAWP (pressure plateau), ↑SVR

Acute Care Patient Management
Goals of treatment
Maintain hemodynamic stability
   Supplemental oxygen

CV

Crystalloids
Vasodilators: nitroprusside
β-Adrenergic agents: isoproterenol
Relieve cardiac compression
Pericardiocentesis/pericardiectomy
Possible thoracotomy

Priority nursing diagnoses
Decreased cardiac output
High risk for altered protection (see p. 145)
High risk for altered family process (see p. 150)

▶ **Decreased cardiac output** related to reduced ventricular filling secondary to increased intrapericardial pressure
PATIENT OUTCOMES
• Patient will be alert and oriented to person, place, and time
• Skin w/d
• Pulses strong, equal bilaterally
• Capillary refill <3 sec
• HR 60-100 beats/min
• Systolic BP 90-140 mm Hg
• Pulse pressure 30-40 mm Hg
• MAP 70-105 mm Hg
• CVP 2-6 mm Hg
• PAWP 4-12 mm Hg
• CO 4-8 L/min
• CI 2.4-4.0 L/min/m^2
• SVR 900-1600 dynes sec/cm^{-5}
• u/o 30 ml/hr or 1 ml/kg/hr

PATIENT MONITORING
1. Continuously monitor ECG for dysrhythmia formation, which may be a result of myocardial ischemia secondary to epicardial coronary artery compression. Electrical alternans, a waxing and waning of the R wave, may be evident.
2. Monitor the BP q5-15min during the acute phase. Monitor for pulsus paradoxus via arterial tracing or during manual BP reading. A drop in SBP >10 mm Hg during the inspiratory phase of a normal respiratory cycle confirms the presence of pulsus paradoxus.
3. Monitor PA pressures and CVP for pressure plateau. Right atrial and wedge pressures will equalize as fluid accumulates in the pericardial space.
4. Calculate MAP, SVR, and PP to evaluate patient response to intrapericardial pressure and/or therapy. As

the pressure increases, MAP will fall, PP will narrow, and SVR will increase.

5. Monitor urine output hourly; a drop in urine output may indicate decreased renal perfusion as a result of decreased stroke volume secondary to cardiac compression.

PHYSICAL ASSESSMENT

1. Assess cardiovascular status: determine jugular venous pressure and presence of Kussmaul's sign. Note skin temperature and color and capillary refill. Assess amplitude of femoral pulse during quiet breathing. Pulse amplitude that decreases or disappears may indicate pulsus paradoxus. Auscultate the anterior chest for muffled or distant heart sounds.

2. Assess LOC for changes that may indicate decreased cerebral perfusion.

DIAGNOSTICS ASSESSMENT

None specific

PATIENT MANAGEMENT

1. Provide supplemental oxygen as ordered.

2. Initiate two large-bore IVs for fluid administration to maintain filling pressure.

3. Pharmacological therapy may include nitroprusside to decrease afterload and isoproterenol to enhance myocardial contractility and decrease peripheral vascular resistance. These interventions are temporary measures to maintain CO and tissue perfusion. Nitroprusside infusion can be initiated at 0.5 μg/kg/min. Do not administer more than 10 μg/kg/min or patient may become toxic. Signs and symptoms of cyanide toxicity may include tinnitus, blurred vision, delirium, and muscle spasm. Isoproterenol infusion can be initiated at 1 μg/min. Monitor for cardiac dysrhythmias and hypotension. (See Chapter 7 for specific drug information.)

4. Pericardiocentesis may be performed. Monitor the patient for dysrhythmias, coronary artery laceration (chest discomfort suggestive of ischemia), or hemopneumothorax (dyspnea, decreased or absent ipsilateral breath sounds, contralateral tracheal shift).

5. Surgical resection of the pericardium may be required.

AORTIC DISSECTION

Clinical Brief

Aortic dissection involves a tear in the intimal layer of the aortic wall, causing blood to extravasate into the media and thus compromising blood flow to the brain, heart, and other organs. Usually the causative factor is an underlying disease of the media. Dissection can be classified by the site(s) involved: (1) DeBakey type I—classified by a tear antegrade around the aortic arch and into the descending aorta, (2) DeBakey type II—classified by a tear of the ascending aorta, and (3) DeBakey type III—classified by a tear of the descending aorta distal to the origin of the subclavian artery.

Demographic risk factors include being male, black, and in the fifth to seventh decade of life. Medical risk factors include having hypertension, aortic valve disease, coarctation of the aorta, patent foramen ovale, Marfan's syndrome, and/or a recent deceleration injury.

Presenting signs and symptoms

The patient experiences severe, "tearing" pain that may be localized in the anterior chest, abdomen, or lumbar area. The pain is usually nonprogressive and most intense at its onset.

Physical examination

Appearance: anxiety, paleness

↑ BP, diastolic BP may be greater than 150 mm Hg

↓ BP, if hypovolemic (aortic rupture) or cardiac tamponade develops

Neurological: May have intermittent episodes of lightheadedness, clouded mentation

Cardiovascular: Pericardial friction rubs or murmurs may be present

Pulse deficits and BP differences between right and left limbs may be noted

Diagnostic findings

Chest radiographs: Changes seen may include a widened mediastinum, enlarged ascending aorta, blurring of the aortic knob and/or a left-sided effusion.

Aortography: Confirms presence and location of tear

Acute Care Patient Management

Goals of treatment

Reduce BP to prevent further dissection of aorta and relieve pain

Antihypertensive agents

Propranolol

Relief of stress/anxiety

Correct problem

Aortic resection

Priority nursing diagnoses

Altered tissue perfusion

Pain

High risk for altered protection (see p. 145)

High risk for altered family process (see p. 150)

▶ **Altered tissue perfusion** related to compromised arterial blood flow secondary to blood extravasation via aortic dissection

PATIENT OUTCOMES

- Patient will be alert and oriented
- Skin w/d
- SBP 100-120 mm Hg or as low as can possibly maintain systemic perfusion
- u/o 30 ml/hr or 0.5-1.0 ml/kg/hr
- Pulses strong, equal bilaterally
- Capillary refill <3 sec
- Pupils equal and normoreactive
- Extremities strong, equal bilaterally

PATIENT MONITORING

1. Continuously monitor arterial BP during acute phase to evaluate the patient's response to therapy.
2. Monitor hourly urine output, since a drop in output may indicate renal artery dissection or a decrease in arterial blood flow.
3. Continuously monitor ECG for dysrhythmia formation or ST, T wave changes suggesting coronary artery involvement or a decrease in arterial blood flow.

PHYSICAL ASSESSMENT

1. Assess neurological status to evaluate the course of dissection. Confusion or changes in sensation and motor strength may indicate compromised cerebral blood flow.
2. Assess cardiovascular status for signs and symptoms of heart failure (e.g., sustained tachycardia, S_3, crackles), which may indicate that the dissection involves the aortic valve.
3. Compare BP from both arms to determine differences. Assess pulses for differences in quality.

DIAGNOSTICS ASSESSMENT

1. Review serial BUN and Cr levels to evaluate renal function.
2. Review cardiac enzymes, since a dissection involving coronary arteries may result in MI.
3. Review the ECG for patterns of ischemia, injury, and infarction.

CV

PATIENT MANAGEMENT

1. Administer oxygen therapy as ordered.
2. Keep patient on bed rest to prevent further dissection.
3. Nitroprusside may be ordered to lower BP. Titrate the infusion to desired BP. Dose may range from 0.5-10 μg/kg/min. Do not administer more than 10 μg/kg/min, or the patient may exhibit signs and symptoms of cyanide toxicity: tinnitus, blurred vision, delirium, and muscle spasm. (See Chapter 7, Pharmacology.)
4. A β-blocking agent such as propranolol may be ordered to reduce stress on the aortic wall.
5. Nifedipine may be given sublingually in an emergent situation to rapidly lower BP. Administer 10-20 mg as directed by the physician by expelling the contents of the capsule under the patient's tongue.
6. Anticipate surgical intervention. Surgery typically consists of resection of the torn portion of the aorta and replacement with a prosthetic graft. With severe aortic regurgitation, valve replacement may also be indicated.

▶ **Pain** related to aortic dissection

PATIENT OUTCOMES

• Patient verbalizes that pain is reduced or tolerable

PATIENT MONITORING

1. Monitor vital signs for evidence of pain and anxiety, e.g., increased HR, SBP, and RR. Be sure to differentiate these signs of pain from signs of hypovolemic shock.

PHYSICAL ASSESSMENT

1. Note facial expression and evidence of guarding. Use a visual analogue to evaluate course of pain (see Figure 1-1). Increased severity may indicate increasing dissection. Note BP, since an increased BP can cause further dissection and increase pain.

DIAGNOSTICS ASSESSMENT

None specific

PATIENT MANAGEMENT

1. Assure the patient that the pain has probably peaked.
2. Pharmacological analgesics are usually contraindicated, since they mask the progression of the dissection. Inform the patient of the necessity of these being withheld. If analgesics are ordered, use them with caution.
3. Alleviate anxieties by providing realistic assurances and providing family support as indicated. Administer anti-anxiety agents as ordered.
4. Administer antihypertensive agents to control BP.

Gastrointestinal Disorders

ACUTE PANCREATITIS
Clinical Brief
Acute pancreatitis is an inflammation of the pancreas that results in autodigestion of the pancreas by its enzymes. Alcoholism and biliary tract disease are commonly associated with acute pancreatitis. The inflammatory process is thought to be precipitated by an obstruction of a pancreatic duct. Other causes include trauma to the pancreas, pharmacological agents (thiazide diuretics, furosemide), hyperlipidemia, and infection. Acute pancreatitis ranges from glandular swelling to hemorrhagic necrosis. Systemic effects depend on the severity of the inflammatory process. Hypoxemia is common, as is metabolic alterations, including hypocalcemia, hyperglycemia, hypertriglyceridemia, and acidosis. Hypotension and shock can also occur.

Presenting signs and symptoms
Signs and symptoms include persistent and unrelenting abdominal pain that is midepigastric and often radiates to the back. Nausea and vomiting generally accompany the pain. Patient may be in respiratory distress and complain of thirst.

Physical examination
BP and HR may be elevated as a result of pain or reduced as a result of the septic shock

T is elevated

RR tachypnea

Neurological: Restlessness

Pulmonary: Dyspnea

Crackles may be present

Abdominal: Distended, ascites may be present

Cullen's sign (bluish-brown discoloration periumbilically)

Bowel sounds decreased or absent

Upper left quadrant (interstitial) or epigastric rebound tenderness with guarding (hemorrhagic)

Skin: Grey-Turner's sign (bluish-brown discoloration)

Jaundice may be present

Decreased turgor

Diagnostic findings

Diagnostic findings are dependent on the clinical examination: acute noncolicky epigastric pain, history of risk factors, serum amylase >200 U/dl, serum calcium <8 mg/dl, serum glucose may be >200 mg/dl, decreasing trend in Hct.

Acute Care Patient Management

Goals of treatment

Restore fluid and electrolyte balance

Crystalloids, colloids

Electrolyte replacement

Maintain adequate oxygenation

Supplemental oxygen

Intubation/mechanical ventilation

Alleviate the pain

Meperidine

Rest the pancreas

NPO, NG intubation

Antacids, parenteral nutrition

Treat the cause

Appropriate therapy

Detect/prevent clinical sequelae

See Table 5-28

Priority nursing diagnoses

Fluid volume deficit

Impaired gas exchange

Pain

Altered nutrition: less than body requirements

High risk for altered protection (see p. 145)

High risk for altered family process (see p. 150)

▶ **Fluid volume deficit** related to fluid sequestration to retroperitoneum and interstitium, intraperitoneal bleed, vomiting, or NG suction

PATIENT OUTCOMES

- CVP 2-6 mmHg
- PAP $\frac{15\text{-}30}{5\text{-}15}$ mm Hg
- SBP 90-140 mm Hg
- MAP 70-105 mm Hg
- Serum protein 6-8 g/dl
- Serum sodium 135-145 mEq/L
- Serum potassium 3.5-4.5 mEq/L
- Serum calcium 8.5-10.5 mg/dl

TABLE 5-28 Clinical Sequelae Associated
with Acute Pancreatitis

Complications	Signs and symptoms
Shock	Tachycardia, hypotension, altered mentation, cool clammy skin
Respiratory insufficiency	Dyspnea, hypoxemia, tachypnea, use of accessory muscles
Acute tubular necrosis	Oliguria, increased BUN and creatinine levels
Sepsis	SBP <90 mm Hg, decreased sensorium, oliguria, hypoxemia, elevated serum lactate
Coagulopathies	Thrombocytopenia, delayed thrombin time, decreased fibrinogen, elevated fibrin degradation products
Diabetes	Elevated serum glucose, glycosuria
Pancreatic abscess	Increasing temperature, elevated WBC count, abdominal distention, pain
Pancreatic cutaneous fistula	Drainage through skin tract
Pseudocysts	Seen on CT, ultrasound evaluation

GI

- HR 60-100 beats/min
- Hgb >10 g/dl
- Hct >30%
- Moist mucous membranes
- Elastic skin turgor
- u/o 30 ml/hr or 0.5-1.0 ml/kg/hr

PATIENT MONITORING

1. Obtain CVP, PA pressures, and BP q1h or more frequently during rapid fluid resuscitation. Calculate MAP, an indicator of tissue perfusion. MAP <60 mm Hg adversely affects renal perfusion.
2. Monitor fluid volume status: measure urine output hourly, determine fluid balance q8h, and include other bodily drainage. Compare serial weights for rapid (0.5-1.0 kg/day) changes that suggest fluid imbalances (1 kg ~ 1000 ml fluid)
3. Continuously monitor ECG for dysrhythmias secondary to electrolyte imbalance associated with NG suction.

PHYSICAL ASSESSMENT

1. Assess tissue perfusion: note level of mentation, skin color and temperature, peripheral pulses, and capillary refill.
2. Assess hydration status: note skin turgor on inner thigh or forehead, condition of buccal membranes, development of edema or crackles. Fever increases fluid loss.
3. Assess abdomen: measure abdominal girth once each shift to determine the degree of ascites.
4. Assess for signs and symptoms of electrolyte imbalance.
5. Assess the patient for development of clinical sequelae (see Table 5-28).

DIAGNOSTICS ASSESSMENT

1. Review serial serum electrolytes to evaluate degree of imbalance or the patient's response to therapy.
2. Review serial serum hemoglobin and hematocrit, since intraperitoneal bleeding may occur.

PATIENT MANAGEMENT

1. Administer crystalloids for fluid resuscitation as ordered. Albumin may be required in hypoproteinemic patients to pull fluid back into the intravascular space. Blood or blood products may be required in case of bleeding or coagulopathies.
2. Calcium, magnesium, or potassium supplements may be needed to restore serum levels.
3. Sympathomimetic agents, such as dopamine, may be necessary if hypotension persists despite fluid resuscitation (see Hypovolemic shock, p. 406).

▶ **Impaired gas exchange** related to pulmonary complications: infiltrates, atelectasis, diaphragmatic elevation, pleural effusion secondary to toxic effects of pancreatic enzymes on pulmonary membranes

PATIENT OUTCOMES

- RR 12-20/min, eupnea
- Pa_{O_2} 60-100 mm Hg
- Pa_{CO_2} 35-45 mm Hg
- pH 7.35-7.45
- O_2 sat >90%
- Lungs clear to auscultation
- HR 60-100 beats/min

PATIENT MONITORING

1. Continuously monitor ECG for dysrhythmias and ischemic changes (ST, T wave changes) secondary to hypoxemia.

2. Continuously monitor oxygen saturation with pulse oximetry (SpO_2). Monitor interventions and patient activities that may adversely affect oxygen saturation.
3. Continuously monitor PA systolic pressure (if available), since hypoxia can increase sympathetic tone and increase pulmonary vasoconstriction.

PHYSICAL ASSESSMENT

1. Assess respiratory status: note respiratory rate and depth; auscultate breath sounds and note onset of adventitious sounds. Signs of hypoxemia include restlessness, RR >30/min, and altered mental status. ARDS may develop.
2. Assess the patient for development of clinical sequelae (see Table 5-28).

DIAGNOSTICS ASSESSMENT

1. Review serial ABGs; note trends of PaO_2, since pulmonary complications are associated with pancreatitis, and abdominal pain and distention may compromise ventilation. A decreasing trend in PaO_2, despite increases in FiO_2 administration, is indicative of ARDS.
2. Review serial chest radiographs for development or resolution of pleural effusions (left side most common), infiltrates, and atelectasis.
3. Review serum calcium and magnesium levels as well as triglycerides. Hypocalcemia and hypertriglyceridemia (>1000 mg/dl) are risk factors for ARDS in patients with pancreatitis.
4. Review serum amylase levels to evaluate pancreatic function.
5. Review serial serum glucose levels; hyperglycemia is often present in pancreatitis.

PATIENT MANAGEMENT

1. Administer supplemental oxygen; anticipate intubation and mechanical ventilation. (For patient care management of the mechanically ventilated, see Chapter 6, Therapeutic Modalities.)
2. Elevate HOB if at all possible to improve chest excursion.
3. Reposition patient q2h; C & DB the patient hourly to prevent atelectasis.
4. Administer meperidine (Demerol) for pain, since morphine may cause spasms of the sphincter of Oddi and increase pancreatic pain.

GI

5. Assist the patient in assuming a position of comfort; provide a calm environment and explore alternate means of pain control (e.g., distraction, imagery).

6. A peritoneal lavage may be performed to remove toxic substances and fluid and to decrease the pressure on the diaphragm.

▶ **Pain** related to the disease process

PATIENT OUTCOMES
• Patient will be pain free
• Eupnea

PATIENT MONITORING
1. Monitor pain using a visual analogue scale or any pain rating scale (see Figure 1-1).

PHYSICAL ASSESSMENT
1. Assess for anxiety and fear, which may increase the release of enzymes and increase pain.

DIAGNOSTICS ASSESSMENT
None specific

PATIENT MANAGEMENT
1. Keep the patient NPO to rest the GI tract and stop pancreatic enzyme excretion.

2. Connect the NG tube to suction to decompress the stomach and prevent gastric stimulation of the pancreatic enzymes.

3. Ensure bed rest and limit activities to decrease the metabolic rate and the production of pancreatic enzymes.

4. Assist the patient to assume a position of comfort; provide a restful environment and explore alternate means of pain relief (e.g., distraction, imagery).

5. Administer meperidine as ordered, since morphine intensifies spasms at the sphincter of Oddi.

▶ **Altered nutrition:** less than body requirements related to nausea, vomiting, hypermetabolic state, and NPO status

PATIENT OUTCOMES
• Absence of nausea and vomiting
• Positive nitrogen balance
• Serum albumin 3.5-5.0 g/dl
• Transferrin >230 mg/dl

PATIENT MONITORING
1. Monitor I & O and caloric intake when the patient is ingesting food and fluids.

2. Compare serial weights to determine whether the target weight is being achieved.

PHYSICAL ASSESSMENT

1. Assess GI status: auscultate bowel sounds and evaluate abdominal distention; assess for nausea, vomiting, and anorexia.
2. Assess the patient for development of clinical sequelae (see Table 5-28).

DIAGNOSTICS ASSESSMENT

1. Review serum glucose levels, since pancreatitis-associated hyperglycemia can be aggravated once enteral or parenteral nutrition is initiated.
2. Review nutritional panel (e.g., albumin, serum transferrin, total lymphocytes, and creatinine-height index) to evaluate nutritional status.
3. Review results of 24-hour urine urea nitrogen; increased levels indicate protein loss is taking place.

PATIENT MANAGEMENT

1. An NG tube will be required to reduce vomiting and abdominal distention.
2. Consult with a dietitian for a formal nutritional workup.
3. Administer parenteral nutrition and supplements (e.g., vitamins, fats) as ordered during the acute phase. Insulin may be required to control glucose levels.
4. Administer antacids and anticholinergic agents as ordered to reduce gastric acidity and pancreatic juices.
5. Oral feedings may be instituted once GI function returns. Note patient tolerance (i.e., absence of vomiting and abdominal distention).
6. Administer antiemetic as ordered and before meals if necessary. Small, frequent feedings and supplemental nourishment may be needed. Provide good mouth care to enhance appetite.
7. Decrease metabolic demands: allow rest periods between nursing activities, reduce anxiety, control fever and pain.

PERITONITIS

Clinical Brief

Acute peritonitis is an inflammation of the peritoneal cavity caused by chemical irritation or an infective organism. Causative factors can include leakage of contents from the GI tract; entry of a foreign object such as a bullet, knife or indwelling abdominal catheter or tube; and contaminated peritoneal dialysate. The inflammatory response causes an increased vascular permeability; thus hypovolemic shock may

GI

result as fluid shifts from the intravascular space to the interstitium. Septic shock may also develop in response to the infecting organism. At risk for developing peritonitis is any patient with recent abdominal surgery, penetrating or blunt trauma to the abdomen, or a history of GI disorders (Crohn's disease, ischemic colitis).

Presenting signs and symptoms
Signs and symptoms include an ill patient assuming a knees-flexed position; complaining of severe localized (parietal) or generalized (visceral) abdominal pain, nausea, vomiting, anorexia, and diarrhea.

Physical examination
HR tachycardia

BP hypotension

RR increased and shallow

T elevated

Neurological: Normal to decreased mentation

Skin: Pale, flushed, or diaphoretic

Cardiovascular: Pulse thready, weak, or may be bounding in presence of fever

Capillary refill <3 sec

Pulmonary: Breath sounds may be diminished secondary to shallow breathing

Abdominal: Rebound tenderness with guarding

May have referred pain to the shoulder

Rigid, distended abdomen

Bowel sounds decreased to absent

Diagnostic findings
Diagnostic findings are based on clinical manifestations of fever, abdominal pain, and rebound tenderness along with a history of precipitating factors. Cultures of peritoneal fluid will yield positive results.

In addition, the following may be found:

WBC >10 × $10^3/\mu l$

Serum protein <6 g/dl

Serum amylase >160 SU/dl

UA may show WBCs

Acute Care Patient Management
Goals of treatment
Restore fluid and electrolyte balance

Crystalloid, colloid, blood, and blood products

Electrolyte replacement

Eradicate infection

Antibiotic therapy

Control pain
  Analgesics
Rest GI tract
  NPO, NG intubation
Correct the underlying problem
  Surgery
Detect/prevent clinical sequelae
  See Table 5-29
Priority nursing diagnoses
Fluid volume deficit
Pain
Ineffective breathing pattern
High risk for altered protection (see p. 145)
High risk for altered family process (see p. 150)
Altered nutrition: less than body requirements (see p. 149)
▶ **Fluid volume deficit** related to intravascular fluid shift to
the peritoneal space and inability to ingest oral fluids
PATIENT OUTCOMES
• CVP 2-6 mm Hg
• SBP 90-140 mm Hg
• MAP 70-105 mm Hg
• PAP $\frac{15\text{-}30}{5\text{-}15}$ mm Hg
• HR 60-100 beats/min
• u/o 30 ml/hr or 0.5-1.0 ml/kg/hr

GI

TABLE 5-29 Clinical Sequelae Associated
with Pancreatitis

Complications	Signs and symptoms
Septic or hypovolemic shock	SBP <90 mm Hg, HR >120 beats/min, fever
Paralytic ileus	Absent bowel sounds, abdominal distention
Respiratory failure	Restlessness, RR >30/min, labored breathing, Pao$_2$ <60 mm Hg
Renal failure	Urinary output <30 ml/hr after fluid replacement, increasing BUN and creatinine
Liver failure	Jaundice, elevated AST (SGOT)
Dysrhythmias	Irregular rhythm, decreased mentation

PATIENT MONITORING

1. Obtain PA pressures and CVP if available and calculate MAP hourly or more frequently if the patient's hemodynamic status is unstable. Note the patient's response to therapy.
2. Monitor fluid volume status: measure urine output hourly and determine fluid balance q8h—include NG and other bodily drainage; urine output <0.5 ml/kg/hr may indicate renal insufficiency. Compare serial weights (1 kg ~ 1000 ml fluid) to evaluate for rapid (0.5-1.0 kg/day) changes, suggesting fluid imbalance.
3. Continuously monitor ECG for dysrhythmias resulting from electrolyte disturbances.

PHYSICAL ASSESSMENT

1. Assess tissue perfusion: note level of consciousness, skin color and temperature, pulses, and capillary refill.
2. Assess hydration status: note skin turgor on inner thigh or forehead, buccal membranes, development of edema or crackles.
3. Assess abdomen: note resolution of rigidity, rebound tenderness, and distension; auscultate bowel sounds.
4. Assess the patient for development of clinical sequelae (see Table 5-29).

DIAGNOSTICS ASSESSMENT

1. Review serum Na^+ and K^+ levels, which may become depleted with nasogastric suctioning, or fluid shifts.
2. Review serial WBC count to evaluate the course of infection.

PATIENT MANAGEMENT

1. Administer crystalloid or colloid solutions to improve intravascular volume. CVP and PA pressures reflect the capacity of the vascular system to accept volume and can be used to monitor fluid volume status.
2. Replace potassium as ordered; validate adequate urine output before administration.
3. Keep the patient NPO if the patient is nauseated and vomiting. NG intubation with suction may be required to decompress the stomach and prevent aspiration. When vomiting and ileus resolve, provide the patient with oral fluids as tolerated.
4. Parenteral nutritional support may be required to provide nutrients while the patient is NPO.
5. Administer antibiotics as prescribed. Most patients will require surgery to treat the cause of peritonitis.

▶ **Pain** related to inflammation of the peritoneal cavity

PATIENT OUTCOMES
• Patient will be pain free

PATIENT MONITORING
1. Monitor the patient's level and location of pain using a visual analogue scale or rating scale (see Figure 1-1).

PHYSICAL ASSESSMENT
1. Observe for nonverbal cues of pain intolerance.
2. Assess abdomen for increasing girth or rigidity.
3. Obtain BP, HR; elevated values may reflect the presence of pain.

DIAGNOSTICS ASSESSMENT
None specific

PATIENT MANAGEMENT
1. Administer pain medication as ordered and evaluate its effectiveness. Assess respiratory status before administering analgesics that depress the central nervous system.
2. Administer antibiotics as ordered to eradicate the infecting organism.
3. Provide a relaxed environment to alleviate anxiety.
4. Place the patient in a position of comfort. Elevating the HOB will help to localize the infection and enhance chest excursion.
5. Instruct the patient to request pain medication before the pain is out of control.
6. Explore alternate methods of pain relief with patient (e.g., distraction, imagery).

Ineffective breathing pattern related to abdominal distention and pain

PATIENT OUTCOMES
• RR 12-20/min, eupnea
• Pao_2 60-100 mm Hg
• $Paco_2$ 35-45 mm Hg
• pH 7.35-7.45
• Lungs clear to auscultation

PATIENT MONITORING
1. Continuously monitor oxygen saturation with pulse oximetry (Spo_2). Monitor interventions and patient activities that can adversely affect oxygen saturation.
2. Monitor PA systolic pressure, since hypoxia can increase sympathetic tone and pulmonary vasoconstriction.

PHYSICAL ASSESSMENT
1. Assess respiratory status: note rate and depth of respirations. Rate >30, labored breathing, and restlessness sug-

GI

gest respiratory distress. Auscultate lungs; the onset of crackles may suggest fluid volume overload. Diminished lung sounds may be associated with shallow breathing, atelectasis, or pleural effusion.

DIAGNOSTICS ASSESSMENT

1. Review serial ABGs to identify decreasing trends in Pao_2 (hypoxemia), pH (acidosis), and Sao_2.
2. Review serial chest radiographs to identify improvement or worsening of the condition.

PATIENT MANAGEMENT

1. Administer supplemental oxygen as ordered. If the patient's lungs are being mechanically ventilated, see Chapter 6, Therapeutic Modalities.
2. Elevate HOB to enhance chest excursion. C & DB the patient hourly to prevent atelectasis. Encourage slow, deep inspirations, since patients have a tendency to take short, shallow breaths.
3. Ensure NG tube patency to prevent gastric secretion accumulation, which might increase the risk for aspiration or increase abdominal distention and interfere with diaphragmatic motion.
4. Administer pain medication to promote pain-free respirations and deep breathing. Note the respiratory rate before and after pain-medication administration. Narcotics should not be given if respiratory rate <12/min.

HEPATIC FAILURE

Clinical Brief

Hepatic failure results from acute liver injury or chronic liver disease (e.g., cirrhosis). An alteration in hepatocyte functioning affects liver metabolism, detoxification processes, and protein synthesis. In fulminant hepatic failure, there is a rapid cessation of liver function that often leads to death. Causes include viral hepatitis, ingestion of toxic substances, acetaminophen overdose, severe ischemic insult (shock), and acute fatty liver of pregnancy. Common causes of cirrhosis include alcohol ingestion, viral hepatitis, and primary biliary cirrhosis. Patients experiencing major life-threatening complications of acute or chronic liver disease are hospitalized in the ICU. Patients may be at risk for development of hepatorenal syndrome, a form of oliguric renal failure observed in severe liver disease in the absence of other known causes of renal failure. This condition is almost always fatal.

Presenting signs and symptoms

Manifestations depend on the complications associated with the liver dysfunction. Patient behavior may range from agitation to frank coma. Evidence of GI bleeding, renal failure, or respiratory distress may also be present.

Physical examination

SBP <90 mm Hg (with shock)

HR >120 beats/min (with shock)

T may be elevated

RR tachypnea initially progressing to respiratory depression associated with encephalopathy

Neurological: Mildly confused to coma

Personality changes

Asterixis

Pulmonary: Crackles

Labored respirations

GI: Hematemesis, melena

Ascites

Hepatomegaly may be present

Fetor hepaticus

Skin: Jaundice, spider nevi may be present

Ecchymosis

Diagnostic findings

The following laboratory findings reflect hepatocellular dysfunction:

Serum bilirubin >1.2 mg/dl

Prolonged prothrombin time; 10 sec >normal suggests massive liver necrosis

AST >40 U/ml

ALT >40 U/ml

Other laboratory findings vary, depending on the severity of the disease and its impact on other bodily functions.

Acute Care Patient Management

Goals of treatment

Restore fluid volume and electrolyte balance

Crystalloids, colloids

Electrolyte therapy

Shunting procedures

Diuretic therapy

Maintain adequate oxygenation

Supplemental oxygen or intubation/mechanical ventilation

Blood products

Decrease circulating ammonia and toxins
   Bowel evacuations
   Neomycin
   Lactulose
   Protein-restricted diet
Detect/prevent clinical sequelae
   See Table 5-30
Priority nursing diagnoses
Fluid volume deficit
Impaired gas exchange
Altered thought process
High risk for altered protection (see p. 145)
High risk for altered family process (see p. 150)
Altered nutrition: less than body requirements (see p. 149)
▶ **Fluid volume deficit** related to fluid sequestration second-
ary to hypoalbuminemia, bleeding secondary to abnormal
clotting factors or variceal hemorrhage, and diuretic therapy
PATIENT OUTCOMES
• SBP 90-140 mm Hg
• MAP 70-105 mm Hg
• CVP 2-6 mm Hg

TABLE 5-30 Clinical Sequelae Associated
with Hepatic Failure

Complications	Signs and symptoms
Hepatorenal syndrome	Renal insufficiency, oliguria, azotemia, high urine osmolality, ↓ urinary Na
Gastrointestinal hemor-rhage	Bleeding from the upper or lower GI tract
Hepatic encephalopathy	Alterations in mentation advancing to coma
DIC	Prolonged bleeding from all sites, skin bruising, intracerebral bleed-ing
Septic shock	BP <90 mm Hg, organ failure
Hypoglycemia	Headache, impaired mentation, hunger, irritability, lethargy
Pulmonary edema	Tachypnea, dyspnea, cough, rest-lessness, frothy pink-tinged spu-tum

- PAP $\frac{15\text{-}30}{5\text{-}15}$ mm Hg
- PAWP 4-12 mm Hg
- Serum albumin 3.5-5.0 mg/dl
- Hgb >12 g/dl
- Hct >35%
- Palpable pulses
- u/o 30 ml/hr or 0.5-1.0 ml/kg/hr
- Serum sodium 135-145 mEq/L
- Serum potassium 3.5-5.0 mEq/L
- Intake approximates output

PATIENT MONITORING

1. Obtain PA, CVP, BP continuously until the patient's condition is stable, then hourly. Obtain PAWP and CO. Calculate pulse pressure and MAP to evaluate effectiveness of fluid resuscitation. Increased abdominal pressure secondary to fluid sequestration on the inferior vena cava can decrease venous return and consequently affect CO.
2. Continuously monitor ECG for lethal dysrhythmias that may result from electrolyte imbalances.
3. Monitor fluid volume status: measure urine output hourly; determine fluid balance q8h; compare serial weights to determine rapid (0.5-1.0 kg/day) changes indicating fluid imbalances.

PHYSICAL ASSESSMENT

1. Assess hydration status: note skin turgor on inner thigh or forehead, condition of buccal membranes, development of edema or crackles.
2. Assess for signs of bleeding: bleeding from gums or puncture sites, bruising or petechiae; test urine, stool, and gastric aspirate for occult blood.
3. Measure abdominal girth once each shift to determine progression of ascites. Percuss and palpate abdomen, since dullness is representative of fluid accumulation.
4. Assess respiratory status: note rate and depth of respirations; ascites may impair ventilation. Auscultate lungs for adventitious sounds.
5. Assess the patient for development of clinical sequelae (see Table 5-30).

DIAGNOSTICS ASSESSMENT

1. Review serial serum ammonia, albumin, bilirubin, AST (SGOT), ALT (SGPT), LDH, PT, and PTT results to evaluate hepatic function.

GI

2. Review serial serum electrolytes. Hypokalemia and other electrolyte imbalances can precipitate hepatic encephalopathy.
3. Review serial serum Hgb and Hct for decreasing values suggesting blood loss.
4. Review urine electrolytes, BUN, creatinine to evaluate renal function.

PATIENT MANAGEMENT

1. Administer intravenous crystalloids as ordered; dextrose solutions will be needed in acute fulminant hepatic failure, since the patient is at risk for hypoglycemia; colloids may be given to increase oncotic pressure and pull ascitic fluid into intravascular space. Blood and blood products may be required to replace RBCs and clotting factors. Carefully monitor the patient for fluid volume overload during fluid resuscitation.
2. Administer potassium as ordered. Validate adequate u/o before administration of potassium supplement.
3. Sodium restriction of 0.5 g/day and fluid restriction to 1000 ml/day may be ordered.
4. Vitamin K may be required to promote clotting process. Protect the patient from injury; pad side rails, keep the bed in low position, and minimize handling; avoid injections or invasive procedures if at all possible if results of clotting studies are abnormal.
5. Institute bleeding precautions: avoid razor blades and use soft-bristled toothbrushes.
6. In patients with ascites, diuretic agents may be required. Carefully monitor the patient for diuresis, hypovolemia, and electrolyte imbalances.
7. A peritoneovenous (LeVeen or Denver) shunt may be implanted to return ascitic fluid to the superior vena cava in patients who are refractory to medical therapy.
8. Paracentesis may be performed if abdominal distention is severe. Monitor the patient for shock and hepatorenal syndrome.
9. See Hypovolemic shock, p. 406.

▶ Impaired gas exchange related to intrapulmonary and portopulmonary shunt, hypoventilation secondary to ascites, pulmonary edema secondary to circulating toxic substances, or respiratory depression secondary to encephalopathy

PATIENT OUTCOMES

• Pao$_2$ 80-100 mm Hg
• Paco$_2$ 35-45 mm Hg

- pH 7.35-7.45
- O_2 sat >95%
- RR 12-20/min, eupnea
- Lungs clear to auscultation

PATIENT MONITORING

1. Continuously monitor of oxygen saturation with pulse oximetry (SpO_2). Monitor interventions and patient activities that may adversely affect oxygen saturation.
2. Continuously monitor ECG for dysrhythmias: hypoxia is a risk factor for dysrhythmias.

PHYSICAL ASSESSMENT

1. Assess respiratory status: note respiratory rate and depth; RR >30/min or <12/min suggests impending respiratory dysfunction. Auscultate breath sounds q2h or more frequently during fluid resuscitation; note development of crackles or other adventitious sounds suggesting pulmonary congestion. Note dyspnea and cough, which may suggest pulmonary edema. Cyanosis is a late sign.
2. Assess the patient for development of clinical sequelae.

DIAGNOSTICS ASSESSMENT

1. Review ABGs for decreasing trend in PaO_2 (hypoxemia) or pH (acidosis).
2. Review serial chest radiographs to evaluate a worsening lung condition. Right-sided pleural effusions are common in chronic liver disease.

PATIENT MANAGEMENT

1. Administer supplemental oxygen as ordered to prevent hypoxemia. Anticipate intubation and mechanical ventilation.
2. Turn, reposition C & DB patient q2h to prevent atelectasis. If necessary, suction secretions gently, being careful to avoid trauma to the mucosa, which can increase the risk for bleeding.
3. Elevate HOB to promote adequate chest excursion. A paracentesis may be performed to remove excess fluid from the abdomen and ease the work of breathing.

Altered thought process related to brain exposure to toxic substances (hepatic encephalopathy)

PATIENT OUTCOMES

- Patient will be alert and oriented, cooperative
- Serum ammonia 12-55 μmol/L
- Patient will not injure self

PATIENT MONITORING

1. Monitor LOC using Glasgow coma scale.

GI

PHYSICAL ASSESSMENT

1. Assess the patient's LOC at least hourly. A decreased awareness of the environment is an early manifestation of encephalopathy. Note any personality changes, slurred or slow speech. In acute liver failure, the mental impairment progresses to coma rapidly and includes a period of agitation, whereas the encephalopathy in chronic liver disease progresses gradually to coma without a phase of agitation.
2. Assess patient for asterixis (flapping tremors of the wrist when extended), an early manifestation of encephalopathy.
3. Assess sleep pattern, since a reversal of day-night sleep pattern is an early indicator of encephalopathy.
4. Assess the patient for development of clinical sequelae (see Table 5-30).

DIAGNOSTICS ASSESSMENT

1. Monitor serum ammonia levels, since ammonia is thought to be a factor contributing to encephalopathy.
2. Monitor serum glucose levels; hypoglycemia is a common finding in acute liver failure and may further impair cerebral functioning.

PATIENT MANAGEMENT

1. Administer ammonia-reducing medications as ordered (e.g., lactulose 10-30 ml or neomycin 1 g). Magnesium sulfate and lactulose enemas can be prescribed to cleanse the bowel of ammonia and prevent absorption of protein-breakdown products. The goal of therapy is 3 to 4 soft stools per day. If diarrhea occurs, hypovolemia and electrolyte imbalances may ensue.
2. Maintain a safe environment; restrain the patient only if necessary for safety.
3. Restrict dietary protein until normal mentation returns. Protein can be reinstituted at 10-20 g/day. If the patient is receiving TPN or enteral feedings, see the patient care management guidelines in Chapter 6, Therapeutic Modalities.
4. NG intubation may be required to decompress the stomach, reduce absorption of protein breakdown products, and reduce the risk of aspiration in an unconscious patient.
5. Avoid sedatives if at all possible or use with extreme caution, since respiratory depression and circulatory collapse can result.

UPPER GASTROINTESTINAL BLEEDING

Clinical Brief

Upper GI bleeding is characterized by the sudden onset of severe bleeding from an intestinal source proximal to the ligament of Treitz. Most upper GI bleeds are a direct result of peptic ulceration, erosive gastritis (resulting from alcohol or aspirin ingestion or stress), or esophageal varices (alcoholic cirrhosis, liver disease, and schistosomiasis). Mallory-Weiss tears can cause gastroesophageal bleeding as a result of severe wretching and vomiting. Hospitalized critically ill patients are also at risk for GI bleeding.

Mortality is highest among the elderly and in patients who have sustained multiple-organ hypoperfusion secondary to reduced blood volume.

Presenting signs and symptoms

Signs and symptoms depend on the extent of the bleeding; however, melena and hematemesis are usually present. Pain may be present with peptic ulcer disease, whereas the patient will be pain free if esophageal varices are the source of bleeding. Patients may have signs and symptoms of hypovolemic shock: cool clammy skin, pallor, apprehension to unresponsiveness, weak thready pulse, and hypotension.

Physical examination

BP <90 mm Hg or orthostatic BP
HR >100 beats/min
RR tachypnea
T may be elevated
Other: Obvious blood: hematemesis, melena, bloody stool
      with a fetid odor, coffee ground gastric aspirate
Neurological: Altered mentation, apprehension
Skin: Pale, diaphoretic
      Cool, clammy skin
      Jaundice, petechiae, or hematomas may be present
      with liver disease
Cardiovascular: Weak, thready pulse
         Capillary refill >3 sec (shock)
Abdominal: May be tender with guarding
      Bowel sounds hyperactive or absent

Diagnostic findings

BUN >20 mg/dl (newly elevated)
Emesis and/or stool positive for occult blood
Decreasing trend in Hgb and Hct
Endoscopy and angiography may be used to diagnose the site of bleeding

GI

Acute Care Patient Management
Goals of treatment
Optimize tissue oxygenation
   Supplemental oxygenation
   Intubation/mechanical ventilation
   Blood transfusion therapy
Stabilize the hemodynamic status
   Crystalloids, colloids, blood administration
Arrest/prevent bleeding and locate the source
   Gastric lavage
   Vasopressin therapy
   Esophageal tamponade (varices)
   Sclerotherapy (varices)
   Electrocoagulation
   Surgical intervention
   H_2 receptor antagonists
   Antacids
   Cytoprotection
Detect/prevent clinical sequelae
   See Table 5-31
Priority nursing diagnoses
Fluid volume deficit
Altered tissue perfusion
High risk for aspiration
Altered nutrition: less than body requirements (see p. 149)
High risk for altered protection (see p. 145)
High risk for altered family process (see p. 150)
▶ **Fluid volume deficit** related to blood loss from hemorrhage
PATIENT OUTCOMES
- Patient will be alert and oriented to person, place, and time
- Skin w/d, pink
- CVP 2-6 mm Hg
- PAP $\dfrac{15\text{-}30}{5\text{-}15}$ mm Hg
- SBP 90-140 mm Hg
- MAP 70-105 mm Hg
- HR 60-100 beats/min
- u/o 30 ml/hr or 0.5-1.0 ml/kg/hr
- Hgb 12-16 g/dl
- Hct >35%
PATIENT MONITORING
1. Obtain PA pressures, CVP, and BP q15min during acute episode to evaluate fluid needs and patient re-

TABLE 5-31 Clinical Sequelae Associated
with Gastrointestinal Bleeding

Complications	Signs and symptoms
General	
Hypovolemic shock	BP <90 mm Hg, HR >120 beats/min, cool, clammy skin
Aspiration pneumonia	↑ Temperature, decreased breath sounds, ↓ Pao_2 and Sao_2
Myocardial, cerebral ischemia	ST-T wave changes, chest pain, decreased LOC
DIC	Abnormal clotting factors, uncontrolled bleeding from all orifices
Peptic ulcer disease	
Perforation of stomach or intestine	Profound shock, sudden change in the character of the pain to include back pain and boardlike abdominal pain, rebound tenderness, absent bowel sounds
Gastric outlet obstruction	Protracted vomiting, visual peristaltic waves
Peritonitis	Elevated temperature, abdominal pain, ↑ WBCs

GI

sponse to therapy. Calculate MAP, an indicator of tissue
perfusion. MAP <60 mm Hg adversely affects cerebral
and renal perfusion. Orthostatic vital signs indicate a
loss of 10% to 15% of circulating blood volume.

2. Monitor fluid volume status: measure urine output
   hourly to evaluate renal perfusion; measure blood loss if
   possible; determine fluid balance q8h. Compare serial
   weights to evaluate rapid (0.5-1.0 kg/day) changes suggesting
   fluid volume imbalance.

3. Continuously monitor ECG for dysrhythmias and myocardial
   ischemia (ST, T wave changes) associated with
   reduced oxygen-carrying capacity associated with blood
   loss.

PHYSICAL ASSESSMENT

1. Assess patient for increased restlessness, apprehension,
   or altered consciousness, which may indicate decreased
   cerebral perfusion.

2. Assess hydration status: note skin turgor on inner thigh

or forehead, condition of buccal membranes, development of edema or crackles.
3. Be alert for recurrence of bleeding.
4. Assess the patient for development of clinical sequelae (see Table 5-31).

DIAGNOSTICS ASSESSMENT
1. Review Hgb and Hct levels to determine the effectiveness of treatment or worsening of the patient's condition. The Hct should rise 2-3 points for every 500 ml of PRBCs given.
2. Review clotting factors and serum calcium levels if multiple transfusions have been given.
3. Review serial BUN levels; elevated BUN (with a normal creatinine) can provide information about the degree of blood loss.
4. Review serial ABGs to evaluate oxygenation and acid-base status. Hypoxia can lead to lactic acidosis.
5. Review the results of endoscopic evaluation or arteriogram if available.

PATIENT MANAGEMENT
1. Maintain a patent airway; administer supplemental oxygen as ordered; intubation and mechanical ventilation may be required.
2. Administer NS or LR or colloids as ordered to restore intravascular volume. Intravenous fluids should contain thiamine with dextrose in patients with alcohol abuse. Carefully monitor patient response: note CVP, PA pressures, and BP.
3. Type and cross-match for at least 6 units of PRBCs. Transfuse the patient with blood or blood products to improve tissue oxygenation and correct coagulation deficiencies. Observe for transfusion reaction. (See Blood administration in Chapter 6, Therapeutic Modalities.)
4. Evacuate the stomach contents and initiate lavages to clear blood clots from the stomach. Keep HOB elevated to reduce the risk of aspiration.
5. Continue to monitor the patient closely once stabilized; rebleeding can occur even up to 1 week after the initial bleeding. Test all gastric secretions and stools for occult blood.
6. Vitamin K and/or fresh-frozen plasma may be ordered to correct coagulation deficiencies.
7. Administer H_2 receptor antagonists (ranitidine, cimeti-

dine) as ordered to decrease gastric acid secretion and neutralize gastric pH; cytoprotection may be provided with sucralfate to prevent mucosal lesion development; antacids may be used to reduce luminal acid. Gastric pH should be kept >3.5 or the value established by physician.

8. Explain all procedures and tests to the patient to help alleviate anxiety and decrease tissue oxygen demands.

9. Anticipate GI surgery (e.g., pyloroplasty, vagotomy, gastrectomy).

MANAGEMENT OF ESOPHAGEAL VARICES

1. Administer fluids conservatively and monitor CVP (keep <8 mm Hg), since rapid volume expansion can increase portal and variceal pressures, causing further rupture and bleeding.

2. Administer vasopressin as ordered to control esophageal bleeding. Intraarterial or intravenous vasopressin is thought to constrict hepatic artery and splanchnic arterioles, thus decreasing portal venous pressure. Generally, vasopressin is administered as a bolus 20 U over 20 min, followed by an infusion of 40 U/250 ml D_5W at a rate of 2-6 U/min. Subcutaneous infiltration can cause necrosis; therefore avoid peripheral veins if at all possible. Vasopressin can be given up to 24 hours after the bleeding has stopped. Observe for hypertension and myocardial and/or bowel ischemia. NTG may be given along with vasopressin to reduce the ischemic effects. Titrate the dose to desired effect; keep BP >90 mm Hg.

3. Anticipate balloon tamponade to temporarily control esophageal bleeding. (See Sengstaken-Blakemore tube, p. 521.)

4. Anticipate endoscopic sclerotherapy to obliterate the varices. (See Endoscopy, p. 58.)

5. Anticipate portosystemic shunting (see Chapter 6).

High risk for aspiration related to vomiting, esophageal tamponade, ileus, increased intragastric pressure, and altered mentation

PATIENT OUTCOMES
- Lungs clear to auscultation
- Pao_2 80-100 mm Hg
- O_2 sat >95%
- Afebrile
- Absence of vomiting

GI

Patient Monitoring

1. Monitor temperature q4h; elevation may indicate aspiration pneumonia.
2. Continuously monitor oxygen saturation with pulse oximetry (Spo_2). Monitor interventions and patient activities that may adversely affect oxygen saturation.

Physical Assessment

1. Assess LOC; patient may not be able to protect the airway if mentation is altered.
2. Assess respiratory status: auscutate lungs for excessive secretions or absence of breath sounds that may indicate pneumonia.
3. Assess abdomen: ausculate bowel sounds; absence of intestinal peristalsis can cause increased intragastric pressure and vomiting.
4. Assess placement of nasoenteric tube.

Diagnostics Assessment

1. Review serial chest radiographs to evaluate placement of nasoenteric tubes and assess lung fields.
2. Review serial ABGs, since aspiration can decrease gas exchange.

Patient Management

1. Elevate HOB if the patient is hemodynamically stable; a right side−lying position may enhance gastric emptying if the patient can tolerate this position.
2. Maintain patency of the NG tube to promote adequate decompression of the stomach.
3. Secure all tubes to prevent dislodgement and excessive movement that can cause gastric irritation.
4. Restrain or sedate patient if necessary to prevent tubes from being inadvertently pulled out.
5. Maintain esophageal tamponade with Sengstaken-Blakemore type tubes. Patient should be intubated, and scissors should be available to deflate the balloon tamponade if the patient manifests signs of respiratory distress (see p. 521).

Endocrine Disorders

ADRENAL CRISIS
Clinical Brief
Adrenal crisis or acute adrenal insufficiency (AI) is the inability of the body to tolerate stress resulting from a deficiency of glucocorticoids and mineralocorticoids and consequently is a life-threatening condition. Adrenocortical insufficiency is classified as either primary (e.g., destruction of adrenal gland [Addison's disease]) or secondary (e.g., inadequate ACTH secretion as a result of an interruption in the hypothalamic-pituitary-adrenal axis).

Autoimmune destruction of the adrenal gland is the most common cause of adrenal insufficiency, but metastatic disease and fungal infections can also cause the disorder. Secondary adrenal insufficiency has increased because of steroid therapy. Abrupt withdrawal or insufficient amounts of the exogenous steroid during stress can precipitate an adrenal crisis.

Presenting signs and symptoms
GI symptoms will be manifested: anorexia, nausea, vomiting, and diarrhea. The patient may be anxious and complain of muscle weakness and fatigue or manifest the signs of shock.

Physical examination
BP low or orthostatic hypotension (primary AI)
HR tachycardia (primary AI)
RR increased
T hypothermic or hyperthermic
Skin: Pale
      Hyperpigmentation (primary AI)
      Dehydrated, decreased turgor
Neurological: Confusion, lassitude, progressing to unresponsiveness

Diagnostic findings
There should be a high index of suspicion if unexplained hypotension, hypothermia, hyperkalemia, and hyponatremia are present. A lack of a response to IV cosyntropin confirms AI. (A normal response is an increase in the cortisol level of

at least 7 μg/dl over the basal level and a serum cortisol level to at least 20 μg/dl).

Acute Care Patient Management

Goals of treatment

Replace glucocorticoids or mineralocorticoids
  Hydrocortisone
  Desoxycorticosterone
Restore fluid, glucose, and electrolyte balance
  Crystalloids
  Electrolyte therapy
Reduce stress
  Stress-free environment

Priority nursing diagnoses

Fluid volume deficit
Altered protection
Altered nutrition: less than body requirements (see p. 149)
High risk for altered family process (see p. 150)

▶ **Fluid volume deficit** related to increased sodium and water excretion secondary to insufficient adrenocorticoids

PATIENT OUTCOMES

- Patient will be alert and oriented
- CVP 2-6 mm Hg
- PAP $\frac{15\text{-}30}{5\text{-}15}$ mm Hg
- SBP 90-140 mm Hg
- MAP 70-105 mm Hg
- HR 60-100 beats/min
- Serum sodium 135-145 mEq/L
- u/o 30 ml/hr or 0.5-1 ml/kg/hr
- Intake approximates output
- Elastic skin turgor
- Moist mucous membranes

PATIENT MONITORING

1. Obtain CVP, PA pressures, and BP hourly or more frequently to evaluate hypovolemia and patient response to therapy. Calculate MAP; MAP <60 mm Hg adversely affects cerebral and renal perfusion.
2. Monitor temperature hourly, since hyperpyrexia often occurs in adrenal crisis.
3. Monitor fluid volume status: measure u/o hourly; determine fluid balance q8h; compare serial weights for a rapid decrease (0.5-1 kg/day), suggesting fluid loss.
4. Continuously monitor ECG for dysrhythmias secondary to electrolyte imbalance.

PHYSICAL ASSESSMENT
1. Assess hydration status: skin turgor on inner thigh or forehead, buccal membranes, pulse pressure, development of edema or crackles.
2. Assess indicators of tissue perfusion: note level of consciousness, skin color and temperature, peripheral pulses, and capillary refill. (See Hypovolemic shock, p. 406.)

DIAGNOSTICS ASSESSMENT
1. Review serial serum sodium and potassium levels to evaluate the patient's response to therapy.
2. Review serial serum glucose levels; symptoms usually appear when level is <50 mg/dl.

PATIENT MANAGEMENT
1. Administer D_5NS rapidly to restore volume and provide a glucose source, since the patient may be hypoglycemic. Carefully monitor CVP, PA pressures, and BP to determine fluid needs and signs of fluid volume overload.
2. Administer glucocorticoids (hydrocortisone) as ordered, usually 100 mg IV q6h initially, then tapering the dosage as patient condition allows to an oral maintenance dose of 20 mg AM and 10 mg PM. If a diagnosis is not established, dexamethasone 1-4 mg IV may be required while giving the cosyntropin stimulation test. Long-term replacement therapy may include glucocorticoid preparations such as prednisone, methylprednisolone, or hydrocortisone.
3. Colloids and a sympathomimetic agent (dopamine) may be required if fluids and steroid administration do not improve intravascular volume.
4. Fludrocortisone may be required in patients with primary AI to help maintain sodium and potassium balance and control postural hypotension.
5. If the patient is able to take oral fluids, encourage fluids high in sodium to combat excessive sodium excretion.

▶ **Altered protection** related to maladaptive stress response secondary to insufficient adrenocorticoids

PATIENT OUTCOMES
• T 36.5° C-38.5° C (97.7° F-101.3° F)
• Absence of aspiration
• Patient will not injure self

PATIENT MONITORING
1. Monitor temperature hourly, since hyperpyrexia is common. Note the patient's response to therapy.

ENDO

PHYSICAL ASSESSMENT

1. Assess level of consciousness since fluid and electrolyte imbalance can alter mentation, which increases the risk of patient injury.
2. Assess respiratory status, since a patient with altered mentation may be unable to protect the airway and is at risk for aspiration and respiratory distress. Note rate and depth of respirations; auscultate lungs for decreased or adventitious breath sounds.
3. Assess level of anxiety, since added stressors may further compromise patient condition.

DIAGNOSTICS ASSESSMENT

None specific

PATIENT MANAGEMENT

1. Protect the patient from stimuli or stressors, maintain a quiet, dimly lit room; control room temperature to avoid extremes; screen visitors to those who promote patient relaxation.
2. Explain all procedures and ICU routine so that the patient is not unnecessarily surprised.
3. Maintain bed rest and limit activities until the patient's condition stabilizes.
4. Maintain a patent airway and supply supplemental oxygen as ordered.
5. Keep the patient NPO until nausea and vomiting resolve and patient mentation improves.
6. Maintain sterile technique when performing invasive procedures to prevent infection.

DIABETIC KETOACIDOSIS (DKA)

Clinical Brief

Diabetic ketoacidosis is characterized by hyperglycemia, acidosis, and ketones as a result of a relative or absolute lack of insulin. Despite the hyperglycemia, cells are unable to use the glucose as their energy source. Thus fatty acids and protein are used for energy, and fatty acids are converted to ketone bodies. Osmotic diuresis leading to cellular dehydration, hypotension, and electrolyte loss, and severe metabolic acidosis ensue. In 50% of the DKA episodes, insufficient insulin, an increase in the ingestion or production of glucose, or infection are precipitating factors. Other risk factors include pharmacotherapy with some medications (e.g., steroids, phenytoin sodium [Dilantin], thiazide diuretics) and stressful events (e.g., surgery, myocardial infarction, illnesses).

Presenting signs and symptoms

Neurological response may range from alert to comatose. Respirations are deep and rapid (Kussmaul) with a "fruity" acetone breath. The patient may be dehydrated and complain of extreme thirst, polyuria, and weakness. Nausea, vomiting, severe abdominal pain, and bloating are often present and can be mistaken for manifestations of an acute condition of the abdomen. Headache, muscle twitching, or tremors may also be present.

Physical examination

BP orthostatic hypotension
HR tachycardia
RR tachypnea to Kussmaul breathing
T may be elevated (infection)
Skin: Dry, flushed
       Decreased turgor
       Dry buccal membranes
Pulmonary: Lungs clear
             Pleuritic pain, friction rubs (dehydration)
Abdominal: Tender, guarding
           Decreased bowel sounds
           Rigid, absent BS, rebound tenderness (severe DKA)
Musculoskeletal: Weakness
                Decreased deep tendon reflexes

Diagnostic findings

Serum glucose >300 mg/dl but not >800 mg/dl
Urine ketones strongly positive
Serum ketones >3 mOsm/L
Blood pH <7.30
Serum bicarbonate <15 mEq/L
Serum osmolality increased but usually < 330 mOsm/L

Acute Care Patient Management

Goals of treatment

Provide cellular nutrition
   Insulin therapy
Restore fluid and electrolyte balance
   Crystalloids
   Colloids
   Electrolyte therapy
Determine and treat the cause
   Appropriate treatment
Detect/prevent clinical sequelae
   See Table 5-32

ENDO

Priority nursing diagnoses
Fluid volume deficit
Altered nutrition: less than body requirements
Altered thought processes
High risk for altered protection (see p. 145)
High risk for altered family process (see p. 150)
▶ **Fluid volume deficit** related to osmotic diuresis secondary to hyperglycemia and lack of adequate oral intake

PATIENT OUTCOMES
- CVP 2-6 mm Hg
- PAP $\frac{15\text{-}30}{5\text{-}15}$ mm Hg
- SBP 90-140 mm Hg
- HR 60-100 beats/min
- RR 12-20/min
- Urine specific gravity 1.003-1.035
- u/o 30 ml/hr or 0.5-1.0 ml/kg/hr
- Serum glucose 150-250 mg/dl
- Serum osmolality 280-300 mOsm/kg
- Serum sodium 135-145 mEq/L
- Serum potassium 3.5-5.5 mEq/L
- Elastic skin turgor
- Moist buccal membranes

PATIENT MONITORING
1. Obtain PAP and CVP hourly or more frequently if the patient's condition is unstable or during fluid resuscitation. Both parameters reflect the capacity of the vascular system to accept volume and can be used to monitor

TABLE 5-32 Clinical Sequelae Associated with DKA

Complications	Signs and symptoms
Circulatory collapse	SBP <90 mm Hg, HR >120 beats/min, change in mental status, cool clammy skin, diminished pulses
Renal failure	Oliguria, increasing BUN and creatinine
Electrolyte imbalances	Life-threatening dysrhythmias, ileus
Cerebral edema	Lethargy, drowsiness, headache during successful therapy

fluid volume status. Increasing values suggest fluid overload; decreasing values suggest hypovolemia.

2. Continuously monitor ECG to detect life-threatening dysrhythmias that may be caused by hypokalemia.

3. Perform bedside glucose monitoring with finger-stick to evaluate the patient's response to therapy.

4. Accurately monitor fluid volume status: measure urine output hourly, determine fluid balance q8h, and compare serial weights. Average water deficit is 6 L.

PHYSICAL ASSESSMENT

1. Obtain VS: BP, HR, RR, and PP hourly or more frequently if the patient's condition is unstable or during fluid resuscitation to evaluate the patient's response to therapy. Kussmaul breathing is associated with a pH <7.2.

2. Assess hydration status: note skin turgor on inner thigh or forehead, condition of buccal membranes, development of edema or crackles.

3. Assess LOC carefully during fluid resuscitation, since brain edema may result from overly aggressive volume replacement.

4. Assess respiratory status to determine the rate and depth of respirations or adventitious breath sounds. Potassium imbalance can cause respiratory arrest; rapid fluid resuscitation may cause fluid overload.

5. Assess GI status: nausea, abdominal distention, and absence of bowel sounds may indicate ileus.

6. Assess the patient for development of clinical sequelae (see Table 5-32).

DIAGNOSTICS ASSESSMENT

1. Review serial serum glucose levels (in addition to bedside monitoring) to evaluate patient response to insulin therapy.

2. Review serum electrolytes, since imbalances are associated with osmotic diuresis. Seizures may be associated with hyponatremia; ileus and dysrhythmias may result with potassium imbalances.

3. Review indicators of renal function: creatinine and BUN.

4. Review ABGs to evaluate oxygenation status and resolution or worsening of metabolic acidosis.

5. Review serial urine specific gravity, sugar, and acetone.

6. Review culture reports to identify presence of infecting organism.

ENDO

PATIENT MANAGEMENT

1. Administer crystalloids as ordered to correct dehydration. NSS boluses of up to 1000 ml/hr may be required until urine output, VS, and clinical assessment reflect an adequate hydration state. Half-strength solutions may follow once the patient's condition is stabilized or manifestations of congestive heart failure develop.
2. Offer small, frequent sips of water or ice chips if the patient is permitted to take fluids by mouth.
3. Provide frequent oral hygiene, since dehydration causes drying of the mucous membranes.
4. Provide insulin therapy as ordered.

▶ **Altered nutrition:** less than body requirements related to impaired glucose utilization secondary to lack of insulin

▶ **Altered thought processes** related to impaired cerebral cellular glucose utilization secondary to lack of insulin

PATIENT OUTCOMES

- Patient will be alert and oriented
- Serum glucose 150-250 mg/dl
- Absence of serum/urine ketones
- pH 7.35-7.45
- Serum bicarbonate 22-26 mEq/L
- Patient will not injure self

PATIENT MONITORING

None

PHYSICAL ASSESSMENT

1. Assess LOC, which may range from confusion to frank coma. Too rapid a reduction in serum glucose (>100 mg/dl/hr) may also impair cerebral function. If patient experiences headache, lethargy, or drowsiness during successful therapy, suspect cerebral edema.
2. Assess the patient for development of clinical sequelae (see Table 5-32).

DIAGNOSTICS ASSESSMENT

1. Review serial serum glucose levels (in addition to bedside monitoring) to evaluate the patient's response to insulin therapy.
2. Review ABGs to evaluate oxygenation status and resolution or worsening of metabolic acidosis.

PATIENT MANAGEMENT

1. Administer regular insulin as ordered. Generally, 10 U is given initially as an IV bolus, followed with a continuous insulin infusion, 100 U/100 ml NS, infused at

5-10 U/hr (0.1 U/kg). Because insulin adheres to plastic and may affect the infusion dosage, it is recommended that the IV tubing be flushed with the insulin solution before patient use. Glucose should drop 40-80 mg/dl/hr. Too rapid a fall in serum glucose levels can cause cerebral edema. If the serum glucose level does not decrease in 2 hours, doubling the dose of insulin infusion may be necessary. If cerebral edema occurs, anticipate mannitol administration.

2. Dextrose (D_5W) may be infused at 5-20 g/hr when the patient is no longer in ketoacidosis (i.e., glucose level 250-300 mg/dl), urine ketones are absent, pH is >7.2, and the patient does not manifest signs of shock.

3. Subcutaneous administration of regular insulin can be started when serum glucose is <250 mg/dl, pH is >7.2, or CO_2 is 15-18 mEq/L, and the patient is able to take fluids orally. Generally, an insulin infusion will be discontinued 1-2 hours after the patient receives subcutaneous insulin.

4. Anticipate K^+ supplementation (KCl, KPO_4, K acetate) to replace potassium loss as a result of urinary excretion, correction of metabolic acidosis, or secondary to cellular uptake with insulin therapy. Validate urine output before administering potassium.

5. Na bicarbonate is considered only if the serum pH is <7.1.

6. NG intubation may be required to reduce the risk of vomiting and aspiration in the patient with altered mentation. Keep the patient NPO until the patient is alert, vomiting has ceased, and bowel sounds have returned.

7. Intubation and mechanical ventilation may be required if the patient is unable to protect the airway or adequately ventilate and oxygenate.

8. Cough and deep breathe the conscious patient to prevent pulmonary stasis and atelectasis. Reposition the unconscious patient every 1-2 hours and suction secretions as needed.

9. Provide meticulous skin care to prevent impaired skin integrity; inspect bony prominences. Maintain body alignment in the unconscious patient.

10. Frequently orient the patient to the surroundings. Keep the bed in low position and side rails up.

ENDO

HYPERGLYCEMIC HYPEROSMOLAR NONKETOTIC COMA (HHNC)
Clinical Brief
HHNC is a condition of extreme hyperglycemia, dehydration, and minimal or absence of ketosis or acidosis. It occurs most often in the older population, either as a first symptom in a patient with undiagnosed type II diabetes or from an acute illness or infection in a patient with previously mild type II diabetes. Enteral or parenteral nutrition or certain medications have also been linked to the development of HHNC. Corticosteroids are the leading precipitator followed by thiazide diuretics, furosemide, cimetidine, phenytoin sodium, diazoxide, and propranolol hydrochloride. Regardless of the cause, the body does not have sufficient insulin for glucose utilization, yet enough insulin is present to prevent lipolysis.

It is most clearly distinguished from diabetic ketoacidosis (DKA) by the lack of or mild ketoacidosis and higher serum glucose levels, which can reach 2000 mg/dl or more.

Presenting signs and symptoms
Signs and symptoms include severe dehydration with mild or no nausea and vomiting. HHNC will resemble DKA in many ways (with the exception of the profound dehydration): polyuria, polyphagia, weakness, and confusion. Focal neurological signs such as hemisensory deficits, hemiparesis, aphasia, and seizures may mimic a cerebrovascular accident.

Physical examination
HR tachycardia

BP low systolic, orthostatic hypotension

RR rapid and shallow (not Kussmaul), absence of fruity breath

T normothermic or hyperthermic, depending on underlying process

Neurological: Altered mental status
Focal neurological signs may be present
+4 reflexes

Skin: Pale, dry, with decreased turgor
Dry buccal membranes
Tongue dry, furrowed

Cardiovascular: Pulse weak and thready
Capillary refill >3 sec

Diagnostic findings
Serum glucose >800 mg/dl, averaging 1200 mg/dl

Serum sodium >147 mEq/L

Serum potassium 3.4-4.5 mEq/L decreasing to
    <3.4 mEq/L
pH normal to mild acidosis <7.3
Serum bicarbonate 22-26 mEq/L
Serum osmolality >350 mOsm/kg
Urine acetone negative or slight
Urine specific gravity >1.022

Acute Care Patient Management

Goals of treatment

Restore fluid and electrolyte balance
    Crystalloids
    Electrolyte therapy
Improve glucose/insulin ratio
    Insulin therapy
Determine and treat the cause
    Appropriate therapy
Detect/prevent clinical sequelae
    See Table 5-33

Priority nursing diagnoses

Fluid volume deficit
Altered nutrition: less than body requirements
Altered thought processes
High risk for altered protection (see p. 145)
High risk for altered family process (see p. 150)

▶ **Fluid volume deficit** related to osmotic diuresis, inability to
take oral fluids, and nausea and vomiting

PATIENT OUTCOMES
• CVP 2-6 mm Hg
• PAP $\frac{15\text{-}30}{5\text{-}15}$ mm Hg

ENDO

TABLE 5-33 Clinical Sequelae Associated with HHNC

Complications	Signs and symptoms
Neurological deficits	Focal, generalized seizures, hemiparesis, sensory deficits
Hypovolemic shock	SBP <90 mm Hg, HR >120 beats/min, weak thready pulse, progressive deterioration in LOC
Renal failure	Decreased urinary output, increasing BUN and Cr
Embolic phenomenon	Calf pain, SOB, neurological deficits

- SBP 90-140 mm Hg
- MAP 70-105 mm Hg
- Absence of nausea/vomiting
- Moist buccal membranes
- Elastic skin turgor
- Serum osmolality 280-300 mOsm/kg
- u/o 30 ml/hr or 0.5-1.0 ml/kg/hr

PATIENT MONITORING

1. Obtain CVP, PA, and BP readings q15min during fluid resuscitation and evaluate the patient's response to therapy. Calculate MAP; MAP <60 mm Hg adversely affects cerebral and renal perfusion.
2. Monitor fluid volume status: measure urine output hourly, determine fluid balance q8h, compare serial weights for rapid (0.5-1.0 kg/day) changes that suggest fluid imbalance.
3. Continuously monitor ECG, since dysrhythmias may be precipitated by electrolyte imbalance associated with diuresis.

PHYSICAL ASSESSMENT

1. Monitor HR, RR, and BP q15min during fluid resuscitation and note the patient's response to therapy.
2. Assess the patient's hydration status: note skin turgor on inner thigh or forehead, buccal membranes, development of edema or crackles.
3. Assess tissue perfusion: note level of consciousness, peripheral pulses, skin temperature and moisture. Hypovolemia may lead to shock.
4. Assess for gastric distention and absent bowel sounds, which would suggest ileus.
5. Assess the patient for development of clinical sequelae (see Table 5-33).

DIAGNOSTICS ASSESSMENT

1. Review serial ABGs to evaluate hypoxemia and acidosis, which may be present with shock.
2. Review serial electrolyte levels (e.g., Na^+ and K^+) to evaluate the need for replacement or patient response to therapy.
3. Review serial serum osmolality and evaluate patient's response to therapy.
4. Review serial Hgb and Hct levels; increased levels are associated with profound diuresis and increase blood viscosity.

5. Review urine specific gravity; as osmotic diuresis is corrected, specific gravity will normalize.

PATIENT MANAGEMENT

1. Fluid resuscitation with NSS at 1 L/hr may be required if the patient is hypotensive and tachycardic. Fluid requirements may exceed 9 L; 1/2 NSS may be used if hypernatremia is present or the patient manifests signs and symptoms of CHF. D_5W is administered when serum glucose reaches 250-300 mg/dl.
2. Administer insulin as ordered, usually 0.1 U/kg/hr.
3. Plasma expanders may be required if isotonic solutions do not improve intravascular volume.
4. Administer K^+ supplements as ordered to prevent adverse effects on the myocardium, gastrointestinal, and respiratory muscles; validate adequate urine output before potassium administration.
5. Keep the patient NPO while nauseated and vomiting; NG intubation may be required if ileus develops or the patient is at risk for aspiration.
6. Prophylactic low-dose heparin therapy may be ordered to prevent clotting associated with increased blood viscosity secondary to profound diuresis.
7. Antibiotic therapy will be ordered if the patient has an underlying infection.
8. See electrolyte imbalances, pp. 361-383.

▶ **Altered nutrition:** less than body requirements related to insulin insufficiency

▶ **Altered thought processes** related to cerebral edema or cellular dehydration

PATIENT OUTCOMES

- Patient will be alert and oriented to person, place, and time
- Patient will not injure self
- Absence of seizure activity
- Serum sodium 135-145 mEq/L
- Serum glucose <250 mg/dl
- Serum osmolality 280-300 mOsm/kg

PATIENT MONITORING

1. Monitor bedside serum glucose levels at least hourly.

PHYSICAL ASSESSMENT

1. Assess neurological status q15-30min during fluid resuscitation when risk of cerebral edema is especially high. LOC will improve as osmolality decreases.

ENDO

2. Assess the patient for development of clinical sequelae (see Table 5-33).

DIAGNOSTICS ASSESSMENT

1. Evaluate serum glucose and serum osmolality to determine effectiveness of therapy.
2. Carefully monitor hourly potassium levels; as hyperglycemia and fluid volume deficit are corrected, potassium will shift intracellularly, resulting in hypokalemia.

PATIENT MANAGEMENT

1. Administer insulin as ordered. Generally, a bolus of regular insulin 10-15 U is given IV, followed by an insulin infusion at 0.1 U/kg/hr until the serum glucose reaches 250 mg/dl. Lowering serum glucose too rapidly (>100 mg/dl/hr) may result in hypoglycemia.
2. Institute seizure precautions: pad side rails, reduce environmental stimuli, place bed in low position, have emergency equipment (oral airway, suction) available.
3. Keep HOB elevated, if BP has stabilized, and NG tube patent to decrease the risk of aspiration.

HYPOGLYCEMIA (HYPERINSULINISM, INSULIN SHOCK, INSULIN COMA)

Clinical Brief

Hypoglycemia is a condition characterized by a serum glucose level less than 50 mg/dl caused by an absolute or relative excess of insulin. Failure to eat, gastroparesis, or excessive exercise after insulin injection can also cause hypoglycemia in the diabetic patient. Alcohol or salicylate ingestion, use of β-adrenergic blocking agents, and tapering of steroids can be contributing factors. Onset is rapid and the symptoms are varied. Iatrogenically induced hypoglycemia can result if serum glucose is rapidly reduced in the treatment of DKA. Repeated or prolonged periods of hypoglycemia can lead to permanent neurological damage (especially in children) or death. Elderly patients who have other disease conditions that cause them to be debilitated and patients with "hypoglycemia unawareness" (low blood sugar episodes without early-stage symptoms) are at risk for developing severe hypoglycemia.

Presenting signs and symptoms

Mild hypoglycemia is associated with adrenergic symptoms: pallor, diaphoresis, tachycardia, palpitations, hunger, paresthesia, and shakiness. Patients who are taking β-adrenergic blocking agents may not exhibit these symptoms. Patients are totally alert during mild hypoglycemic episodes.

Moderate hypoglycemia is characterized by neuroglycopenic signs: inability to concentrate, confusion, irrational behavior, slurred speech, blurred vision, fatigue, or somnolence. Severe hypoglycemia includes neuroglycopenic signs or loss of consciousness and seizures.

Physical examination
HR tachycardia
BP hypertension initially, progressing to shock
RR shallow and rapid initially, progressing to bradypnea
T normal
Neurological: Visual disturbances
Dilated pupils
Numbness of tongue and lips
Change in level of consciousness
Seizures
Skin: Pallor, diaphoresis, cool to touch
Paresthesias or paralysis

Diagnostic findings
Serum glucose <50 mg/dl
Serum ketones negative

Acute Care Patient Management
Goals of treatment
Restore serum glucose level
10%-50% dextrose IV
IV therapy with 5%-10% glucose solution

Priority nursing diagnoses
Sensory-perceptual alteration
High risk for altered protection (see p. 145)
Altered nutrition: less than body requirements (see p. 149)
High risk for altered family process (see p. 150)
Sensory-perceptual alteration related to CNS dysfunction secondary to lack of glucose energy source

PATIENT OUTCOMES
- Patient will be alert and oriented to person, place, and time
- Absence of seizures
- Serum glucose between 80-120 mg/dl

PATIENT MONITORING
1. Bedside glucose monitoring with finger-stick for quick evaluation of glucose level. May be performed hourly during initial treatment. Glucose should be raised to 100 mg/dl.

ENDO

PHYSICAL ASSESSMENT

1. Observe for adrenergic symptoms: tachycardia, hypertension. Note onset of palpitations, shakiness, pallor, or diaphoresis. These symptoms may indicate recurrence of a hypoglycemic episode.
2. Assess for changes in LOC, speech, vision, and behavior, which may signal neuroglycopenia.

DIAGNOSTICS ASSESSMENT

1. Review daily serum glucose levels to monitor the patient's response to nutritional and glucose support.
2. If the patient remains unconscious with a serum glucose of 200 mg/dl, suspect neurological residual.

PATIENT MANAGEMENT

1. If the patient is symptomatic but conscious, administer 4 oz of orange juice or apple juice. At least 10 g of carbohydrate are required to raise the blood sugar. Repeat q5-10min until symptoms begin to subside. Recheck glucose level in 20-30 minutes. IV therapy of D_5W may be ordered for continued glucose support.
2. If the patient is unconscious, administer dextrose 10%-50% solution intravenously as ordered. IV therapy of D_5W may be ordered for continued glucose support.
3. If long-acting oral hypoglycemic agents (e.g., sulfonylureas) have been implicated as the cause of the hypoglycemic episode, the patient is at risk for recurrences.
4. Institute seizure precautions: pad side rails, place the bed in low position; have emergency equipment available, such as oral airway and suction.
5. Alcoholic patients may require thiamine, since it promotes carbohydrate metabolism to prevent Wernicke-Korsakoff syndrome.

DIABETES INSIPIDUS (DI)

Clinical Brief

Diabetes insipidus is a disorder characterized by increased total body sodium and free water deficiency. A deficiency in ADH secretion or an unresponsive end-organ (kidneys) is responsible for the inability of the distal renal tubules to reabsorb water; thus excessive water loss and hyperosmolality result. DI is classified as either central, nephrogenic, or psychogenic. DI may be transitory or permanent, depending on the cause; however, profound diuresis regardless of the cause will occur. Central DI may be idiopathic or result from pituitary surgery or conditions that disturb the hypothalamus (e.g., head trauma, infection, cancerous brain tumors, or anoxic brain death). Nephrogenic DI occurs if the renal receptors are insensitive to circulating ADH. Causes include diseased kidneys or drug therapies (lithium carbonate, demeclocycline). Psychogenic DI occurs with compulsive water consumption. Patients can excrete from 4-24 L/day. As long as patients are able to respond to the thirst mechanism, serum osmolality will remain normal and dehydration will be prevented.

Presenting signs and symptoms
The alert patient will complain of polydipsia, polyuria, and fatigue as a result of lack of sleep from nocturia. Unresponsive patients will have profound dehydration or hypovolemic shock.

Physical examination
BP postural hypotension
HR tachycardia
RR eupnea
T normothermic
Cardiovascular: Cool, clammy skin
　　　　　　　　　Capillary refill >3 sec
　　　　　　　　　Pulse weak, thready
Skin: Decreased turgor; dry, sticky mucous membranes

Diagnostic findings
Water deprivation test demonstrates the following:
Serum osmolality >300 mOsm/kg
Serum sodium >145 mEq/L
Urine osmolality <300 mOsm/L
In addition:
Decreased serum ADH (nl = 1-5 pg/ml)
Urine specific gravity <1.005

Acute Care Patient Management
Goals of treatment
Restore fluid balance
　Hypotonic fluid replacement
　Vasopressin
　Treatment of the cause
Detect/prevent clinical sequelae
　See Table 5-34

Priority nursing diagnoses
Fluid volume deficit
High risk for altered protection (see p. 145)
High risk for altered family process (see p. 150)
Altered nutrition: less than body requirements (see p. 149)

ENDO

TABLE 5-34 Clinical Sequelae Associated with DI

Complication	Signs and symptoms
Circulatory collapse	Tachycardia, decreasing trend in BP, decreasing trend in u/o, diminished pulse, decreased sensorium, cool clammy skin, restlessness

▶ **Fluid volume deficit** related to excessive diuresis of dilute urine secondary to inadequate ADH secretion/response
  PATIENT OUTCOMES
  • Patient will be alert and oriented to person, place, and time
  • Moist buccal membranes
  • Elastic skin turgor
  • CVP 2-6 mm Hg
  • PAP $\frac{15\text{-}30}{5\text{-}15}$ mm Hg
  • SBP 90-140 mm Hg
  • MAP 70-105 mm Hg
  • Intake approximates output
  • Urine osmolality 300-1400 mOsm/L
  • Serum osmolality 285-300 mOsm/L
  • Urine specific gravity 1.010-1.030
  • Serum sodium 135-145 mEq/L
  PATIENT MONITORING
  1. Monitor CVP and PAP hourly or more frequently to evaluate volume status. Hypovolemic shock can occur.
  2. Calculate MAP; MAP <60 mm Hg adversely affects cerebral and renal perfusion.
  3. Monitor urine output hourly and determine fluid balance each shift. Urine output can exceed 1 L/hr. Compare daily weights; dramatic weight loss can occur if fluid replacement is inadequate. Neurosurgical patients (neurohypophysis destruction) may develop polyuria immediately after surgery, which lasts for approximately 5 days, followed by oliguria for approximately 5 days before developing permanent polyuria and polydipsia.
  PHYSICAL ASSESSMENT
  1. Obtain VS hourly or more often if the patient's condition is unstable; hypovolemic shock can occur. Signs

and symptoms include restlessness, cool clammy skin, tachycardia, SBP <90 mm Hg.

2. Assess hydration status to evaluate the patient's response to therapy. Note skin turgor on inner thigh or forehead, buccal membranes, resolution of postural hypotension.

3. Assess LOC; changes in sensorium can be caused by decreased perfusion or dehydration.

4. Assess the patient for development of clinical sequelae (see Table 5-34).

DIAGNOSTICS ASSESSMENT

1. Monitor serum sodium, potassium, and osmolality as well as urine specific gravity and osmolality to evaluate water deficiency and the patient's response to therapy. Serum osmolality can be calculated:

$$2Na + K + BUN/3 + Glucose/18.$$

PATIENT MANAGEMENT

1. Administer hypotonic fluids as ordered to reduce serum hyperosmolality and prevent circulatory collapse. Monitor the patient for fluid volume overload. NS may be used if signs of circulatory collapse are present.

2. Recognize risk factors that may potentiate osmolality problems such as the administration of TPN or enteral feedings.

3. Aqueous vasopressin (Pitressin) will be required in patients who are unable to synthesize ADH; DDAVP 50-100 µg intranasally may be used. Observe for abdominal cramps, hypertension, and coronary insufficiency with vasopressin administration.

4. In patients with nephrogenic DI, thiazide diuretics may be used to deplete Na^+ and cause increased renal water reabsorption. Nephrogenic DI does not respond to hormonal replacement.

5. Carbamazepine, clofibrate, or chlorpropamide may be helpful to produce and release endogenous vasopressin in patients with insufficient amounts of circulating ADH.

6. Restrict salt and protein intake for patients with nephrogenic DI.

7. Encourage iced fluids when the patient is able to take oral fluids.

8. Provide oral hygiene and meticulous skin care to preserve skin integrity. Vasopressin therapy may cause diarrhea, a risk factor for skin breakdown.

9. For hypernatremia, see p. 366.

ENDO

SYNDROME OF INAPPROPRIATE ANTIDIURETIC HORMONE (SIADH)

Clinical Brief

SIADH is a condition that results from oversecretion of antidiuretic hormone (ADH), resulting in hyponatremia and hemodilution. The kidneys respond by reabsorbing water in the tubules and excreting sodium; thus the patient becomes severely water intoxicated. SIADH can be the result of CNS disorders, such as Guillain-Barré syndrome, meningitis, and brain tumors. Head trauma, stress, and pain often cause SIADH. Bronchogenic cancer and other pulmonary-related conditions, such as pneumonia, and positive-pressure ventilation can cause SIADH. Pharmacological agents, such as bronchodilators, chemotherapeutic agents, diuretics, and analgesics, are also associated with SIADH release.

Presenting signs and symptoms

Signs and symptoms depend on the degree of water intoxication. The patient may complain of a headache and lethargy or have seizures or coma. If alert, the patient usually complains of nausea, vomiting, and anorexia with related muscle loss. Weight gain may result from increased water retention, although the patient does not appear edematous.

Physical examination

BP ↑ or may be normal

HR tachycardia

T ↓ or may be normal

Neurological: Alert to unresponsiveness
　　　　　　　Seizures

Cardiovascular: Bounding pulses

Pulmonary: Crackles may be present

GI: Cramps
　　Decreased bowel sounds
　　Vomiting

Musculoskeletal: Weakness
　　　　　　　　Cramps
　　　　　　　　Absent deep tendon reflexes

DIAGNOSTIC FINDINGS

A water load test confirms the diagnosis:

Serum sodium <120 mEq/L, normalizes with water restriction

Serum osmolality <250 mOsm/kg

Serum potassium <3.8 mEq/L

Serum calcium <8.5 mg/dl

Serum aldosterone level <5 ng/dl
Serum ADH >5 pg/ml
Urine osmolality >1090 mM/kg, 50-150 mOsmol/L
Urine sodium >200 mEq/24 hr, 20 mEq/L

Acute Care Patient Management

Goals of treatment

Restore fluid and electrolyte balance
  Fluid restriction <1000 ml/day
  Diuretic therapy
  Potassium supplementation
Control ADH excretion
  Lithium
  Demeclocycline
  Phenytoin
  Surgery
Prevent seizures
  Hypertonic saline
  Phenytoin
Treat the cause
  Appropriate therapy

Priority nursing diagnoses

Fluid volume excess
High risk for injury
High risk for altered protection (see p. 145)
Altered nutrition: less than body requirements (see p. 149)
High risk for altered family process (see p. 150)

Fluid volume excess related to excessive amounts of ADH secretion

PATIENT OUTCOMES

• Intake approximates output
• Serum potassium 3.5-5.0 mEq/L
• Serum sodium 135-145 mEq/L
• Serum chloride 95-105 mEq/L
• Serum osmolality 280-300 mOsm/kg
• Urine specific gravity 1.003-1.035
• CVP 2-6 mm Hg
• PAWP 4-12 mm Hg

PATIENT MONITORING

1. Monitor PA pressures and CVP hourly (if available) or more frequently to evaluate the patient's response to treatment. Both parameters reflect the capacity of the vascular system to accept volume and can be used to monitor fluid volume status.

ENDO

2. Monitor urine output and determine fluid balance q8h. Compare serial weights and note rapid (0.5-1.0 kg/day) changes in weight suggesting fluid imbalance.
3. Continuously monitor ECG for dysrhythmias resulting from electrolyte imbalance.

PATIENT ASSESSMENT
1. Obtain VS q1h or more frequently until the patient's condition is stable.
2. Evaluate hydration status q4h. Note skin turgor on inner thigh or forehead, buccal membranes, development of edema or crackles.

DIAGNOSTICS ASSESSMENT
1. Review serum sodium and potassium, serum osmolality, urine specific gravity, and urine osmolality to evaluate the patient's response to therapy.

PATIENT MANAGEMENT
1. Restrict fluid as ordered, generally <500 ml/day in severe cases and 800-1000 ml/day in moderate cases.
2. Administer potassium supplements as ordered; assess renal function and ensure adequate urine output before administering potassium.
3. As adjuncts to water restriction, demeclocyline may be ordered to inhibit the renal response to ADH in patients with lung malignancies; lithium carbonate may be used to alter psychogenic behavior.
4. Avoid hypotonic enemas to treat constipation, since water intoxication can be potentiated.

▶ **High risk for injury** related to low serum sodium

PATIENT OUTCOMES
• Patient will be alert and oriented to person, place, and time
• Patient will be free of seizures
• Serum sodium 135-145 mEq/L

PATIENT MONITORING
1. Obtain PA pressures and CVP (if available) hourly or more frequently during hypertonic saline infusions to monitor for development of fluid overload.

PATIENT ASSESSMENT
1. Assess LOC hourly to evaluate effects of water intoxication. Patients may become symptomatic (e.g., confusion, seizures, coma) at sodium levels <125 mEq/L.

DIAGNOSTICS ASSESSMENT
1. Review serial serum sodium levels to evaluate the patient's response to therapy.

PATIENT MANAGEMENT

1. If the patient's sodium level <105 mEq/L, hypertonic saline (3% NaCl) may be used to slowly raise serum sodium to 125 mEq/L. Too rapid an increase in serum sodium may further impair neurological function. Closely monitor for fluid overload and pulmonary edema during hypertonic infusion: dyspnea, increased respiratory rate, crackles, moist cough, bounding pulses. Furosemide or other diuretic agents may be administered with hypertonic saline infusions to prevent pulmonary edema.
2. Maintain airway.
3. Institute seizure precautions.

THYROID STORM
Clinical Brief
A thyroid storm is a life-threatening condition in which patients with underlying thyroid dysfunction exhibit exaggerated signs and symptoms of hyperthyroidism. Thyroid storm is precipitated by stressors such as infection, trauma, DKA, surgery, heart failure, or stroke. The condition can result from discontinuation of thyroid medication or as a result of untreated or inadequate treatment of hyperthyroidism. The excess thyroid hormones increase metabolism and affect the sympathetic nervous system, thus increasing oxygen consumption and heat production and altering fluid and electrolyte levels.

Presenting signs and symptoms
Signs and symptoms include abrupt onset of fever and tachycardia. The patient may be restless, confused, or unresponsive. GI symptoms may be present: nausea, vomiting, and diarrhea.

Physical examination
BP systolic hypertension or hypotension (if shock)
HR tachycardia disproportionate to the degree of fever
RR >20/min
T >37.8° C (100° F), can be up to 40.7° C (105.3° F)
Neurological: Agitated, tremulous, delirious to coma
Cardiovascular: Bounding pulses, systolic murmur, widening pulse pressure; ↑ JVP, S_3, weak thready pulses (depending on the degree of CV compromise)
Pulmonary: Tachypnea, crackles may be present
GI: ↑ Bowel sounds

ENDO

Diagnostic findings

Diagnosis is based on a high index of suspicion (fever, tachycardia out of proportion to the fever, and central nervous system dysfunction), and treatment should not be withheld until laboratory results confirm hyperthyroidism. Studies indicating hyperthyroidism include the following:

↑ T_4
↑ T_3 resin uptake
↓ TSH

ECG may reveal atrial fibrillation, SVT

Acute Care Patient Management

Goals of treatment

Reduce oversecretion of thyroid hormone
    Antithyroid agents
    β-Adrenergic blocking agents
    Glucocorticoids
    Surgery
    Treatment of precipitating factor
Restore hemodynamic stability
    Supplemental oxygen
    Crystalloids
    Vasopressor agents
    Inotropic agents
    Diuretic agents
Restore normothermia
    Cooling methods
    Acetaminophen
Support nutrition
    Supplemental feedings
    TPN
Detect/prevent clinical sequelae
    See Table 5-35

Priority nursing diagnoses

Altered body temperature: hyperthermia
Decreased cardiac output
Ineffective breathing pattern
Altered nutrition: less than body requirements
Altered protection (see p. 145)
High risk for altered family process (see p. 150)

▶ **Altered body temperature:** hyperthermia related to increased metabolism

PATIENT OUTCOMES
- T 36.5° C-37.8° C (97.7° F-100° F)
- SBP 90-140 mm Hg

TABLE 5-35 Clinical Sequelae Associated with Thyroid Storm

Complications	Signs and symptoms
Shock	SBP <90 mm Hg, HR >120 beats/min, altered mental state, cool clammy skin, ↓ u/o
Respiratory Failure	Pao_2 <50 mm Hg, $Paco_2$ >50 mm Hg, paradoxical breathing, restlessness, RR >30/min
Cardiac failure/pulmonary edema	Tachycardia, S_3, hypotension, ↑ JVP, crackles, tachypnea, dyspnea, frothy sputum

PATIENT MONITORING
1. Continuously monitor core temperature (if possible) to evaluate the patient's response to therapy.
2. Continuously monitor BP, since fever increases peripheral vasodilation, which can lead to hypotension.

PHYSICAL ASSESSMENT
1. Assess the patient for diaphoresis and shivering; shivering increases metabolic demand.
2. Assess the patient for development of clinical sequelae.

DIAGNOSTICS ASSESSMENT
1. Review culture reports for possible infection.

PATIENT MANAGEMENT
1. Administer antithyroid pharmacological agents as prescribed:

   Propylthiouracil (PTU): Blocks thyroid hormone synthesis and inhibits conversion of T_4 to T_3; loading dose of 600 to 1000 mg, then 150 to 200 mg tid-qid.

   Iodide: Inhibits the release of thyroid hormone and should be given at least 1 hr after PTU has been administered; SSKI—10 gtt q12h or Lugol's solution—4 gtt q12h or sodium iodide—500-1000 mg q12h may be ordered.

   Methimazole: Inhibits thyroid hormone synthesis; loading dose of 60-100 mg, then 10-20 mg tid.

   Dexamethasone: May be used to suppress conversion of T_4 to T_3 and to replace rapidly metabolized cortisol; 2 mg q6h.

   Colestipol: May be used in extreme cases; 10 g q8h.

2. Institute cooling methods; a hypothermia blanket may be necessary to reduce body temperature (see p. 452).

3. Avoid aspirin administration, since salicylates increase circulating thyroid hormones.

4. Administer acetaminophen as ordered and evaluate the patient's response.

5. Provide comfort measures, checking the patient for diaphoresis and changing patient's gown and bed linens as necessary.

6. Peritoneal dialysis and plasmapheresis have been reported to reduce thyroid hormone levels in extreme cases.

▶ **Decreased cardiac output** related to increased cardiac work secondary to increased adrenergic activity and **Fluid volume deficit** secondary to increased metabolism and diaphoresis

PATIENT OUTCOMES

- Patient will be alert and oriented to person, place, and time
- Peripheral pulses palpable
- Lungs clear to auscultation
- u/o 30 ml/hr or 0.5-1.0 ml/kg/hr
- SBP 90-140 mm Hg
- MAP 70-105 mm Hg
- HR 60-100 beats/min
- Absence of life-threatening dysrhythmias
- PAP $\frac{15-30}{5-15}$ mm Hg
- PAWP 4-12 mm Hg
- CO 4-8 L/min
- CI 2.5 L/min/m^2

PATIENT MONITORING

1. Continuously monitor ECG for dysrhythmias or HR >140 beats/min that can adversely affect CO and monitor for ST segment changes indicative of myocardial ischemia.

2. Continuously monitor oxygen saturation with pulse oximetry (Spo_2). Be alert for patient activities or interventions that adversely affect oxygen saturation.

3. Continuously monitor PAP, CVP (if available), and BP. Obtain CO and PAWP to evaluate cardiac function and patient response to therapy. Calculate MAP; a MAP <60 mm Hg adversely affects cerebral and renal perfusion.

4. Monitor fluid volume status: measure urine output hourly, determine fluid balance q8h. Compare serial weights; a rapid (0.5-1.0 kg/day) change suggests fluid imbalance.

PHYSICAL ASSESSMENT

1. Assess cardiovascular status: note extra heart sounds (S_3 is a hallmark of congestive heart failure), ↑ JVP, crackles, and prolonged capillary refill suggesting heart failure, which can progress to pulmonary edema (increasing dyspnea, frothy sputum). Assess the patient for myocardial ischemic pain.
2. Assess hydration status (thirst, dry mucous membranes, poor skin turgor), since dehydration can further decrease circulating volume and compromise CO.
3. Assess the patient for development of clinical sequelae (see Table 5-35).

DIAGNOSTICS ASSESSMENT

1. Review thyroid studies as available.
2. Review serial serum electrolytes, serum glucose, and serum calcium levels to evaluate the patient's response to therapy.
3. Review serial ABGs for hypoxemia and acid-base imbalance, which can adversely affect cardiac function.
4. Review serial chest radiographs for cardiac enlargement and pulmonary congestion.

PATIENT MANAGEMENT

1. Administer dextrose-containing IV fluids as ordered to correct fluid and glucose deficits. Carefully assess the patient for heart failure or pulmonary edema. Dopamine may be used to support BP.
2. Provide supplemental oxygen as ordered to help meet increased metabolic demands. Once patient is hemodynamically stable, provide pulmonary hygiene to reduce pulmonary complications.
3. Administer β-adrenergic blocking agents such as propranolol to control tachycardia secondary to catecholamine effects on the heart; 1 mg IV q5″ to achieve a HR ~ 90-100 beats/min, and q6h. Monitor HR for bradycardia and PA pressures (if available) to evaluate left ventricular function. A short-acting β-adrenergic blocking agent such as esmolol may also be tried. (See Chapter 7, Pharmacology, for specific drug information.)

ENDO

4. If the patient is in heart failure, typical pharmacological agents include digitalis, furosemide, potassium supplements, and afterload-reduction agents. (See Congestive heart failure, p. 254.)

5. Reduce oxygen demands: decrease anxiety, reduce fever, decrease pain, and limit visitors if necessary. Schedule uninterrupted rest periods. Approach the patient in a calm manner, explain procedures or provide information to decrease misperceptions. Keep the room cool and dimly lit and reduce external stimuli as much as possible.

6. Anticipate aggressive treatment of precipitating factor.

▶ **Ineffective breathing pattern** related to intercostal muscle weakness

PATIENT OUTCOMES
- Patient will be alert and oriented
- RR 12-20/min, eupnea
- Pao_2 80-100 mm Hg
- $Paco_2$ 35-45 mm Hg
- pH 7.35-7.45
- O_2 sat >95%

PATIENT MONITORING
1. Continuously monitor oxygen saturation with pulse oximetry (Spo_2). Monitor patient activities and interventions that can adversely affect oxygen saturation.
2. Continuously monitor ECG for dysrhythmias that may be related to hypoxemia or acid-base imbalance.

PHYSICAL ASSESSMENT
1. Assess respiratory status: note respiratory rate, rhythm, depth, and use of accessory muscles. Observe for paradoxical breathing pattern and increased restlessness, increased complaints of dyspnea, and changes in level of consciousness. Cyanosis is a late sign of respiratory distress.
2. Assess patient for development of clinical sequelae (see Table 5-35).

DIAGNOSTICS ASSESSMENT
1. Review serial ABGs to evaluate oxygenation and acid-base balance.
2. Review serial chest radiographs for pulmonary congestion.

PATIENT MANAGEMENT
1. Administer supplemental oxygen as ordered. If the patient is intubated and the lungs are mechanically ventilated, see p. 463.

2. Reposition the patient to improve oxygenation and mobilize secretions. Evaluate the patient's response to position changes with ABGs to determine the best position for oxygenation.
3. As the patient's hemodynamics stabilize, provide pulmonary hygiene to prevent complications.
4. Decrease oxygen demands (i.e., reduce fever, alleviate anxiety, limit visitors if necessary, schedule uninterrupted rest periods).
5. Administer antithyroid medications as prescribed.

▶ **Altered nutrition:** less than body requirements related to increased metabolism

PATIENT OUTCOMES
• Stabilized weight

PATIENT MONITORING
1. Conduct calorie counts to provide information about the adequacy of intake required to meet metabolic needs.
2. Compare serial weights; rapid (0.5-1.0 kg/day) changes indicate fluid imbalance and not an imbalance between nutritional needs and intake.

PHYSICAL ASSESSMENT
1. Assess GI status: absent or hyperactive bowel sounds, vomiting, diarrhea, or abdominal pain may interfere with nutritional absorption.
2. Assess the patient for development of clinical sequelae (see Table 5-35).

DIAGNOSTICS ASSESSMENT
1. Review serial serum glucose levels for hyperglycemia, since excessive circulating thyroid hormones increase glycogenolysis and decrease insulin levels.

PATIENT MANAGEMENT
1. Consult with a nutritionist to maximize intake of calories and protein to reverse the negative nitrogen balance.
2. Assist the patient with small, frequent feedings. TPN may be required. (See Chapter 6, Therapeutic Modalities, for information on parenteral nutrition.)
3. Insulin therapy may be required to control hyperglycemia.
4. Avoid caffeine products, which may increase peristalsis.

MYXEDEMA COMA

Clinical Brief

Myxedema coma is a life-threatening condition in which patients with underlying thyroid dysfunction exhibit exagger-

ENDO

ated manifestations of hypothyroidism. Precipitating factors may include (but are not limited to) infection, trauma, surgery, congestive heart failure, stroke, or CNS depressants. Hypothyroidism depresses metabolic rate, thus seriously affecting all body systems.

Presenting signs and symptoms
The patient may be lethargic, progressing to comatose, and hypothermic. Signs and symptoms of cardiac or respiratory failure may also be present.

Physical examination
BP hypotension or hypertension
HR bradycardia
RR bradypnea
T hypothermic; <34.4° C (94° F)
Skin: Coarse and dry, possibly carotene color, edema
Neurological: Obtunded, coma or seizures
　　　　　　　　Delayed reflexes

Diagnostic findings
Diagnosis is based on a high index of suspicion, and treatment should not be withheld until laboratory results confirm the diagnosis. Thyroid studies indicating primary hypothyroidism include the following:
Low free thyroxine index and elevated TSH level
Other: Hyponatremia and hypoglycemia may be present;
　　　　ECG demonstrates low voltage, prolonged QT
　　　　interval, flattened or inverted T wave
Cortisol level is usually low

Acute Care Patient Management
Goals of treatment
Increase thyroid hormone levels
　Thyroid replacement
Improve ventilation/oxygenation
　Supplemental oxygen
　Intubation/mechanical ventilation
Restore normothermia
　Warming methods
Restore hemodynamic stability
　Crystalloids
　Vasopressor agents
　Corticosteroids

Priority nursing diagnoses
Altered body temperature: hypothermia
Impaired gas exchange

Decreased cardiac output

Fluid volume excess

Altered protection (see p. 145)

High risk for altered family process (see p. 150)

▶ **Altered body temperature:** hypothermia related to decreased metabolism secondary to hypothyroidism

PATIENT OUTCOME

• T 36.5° C-37.8° C (97.7° F-100° F)

PATIENT MONITORING

1. Continuously monitor core temperature (if possible) to evaluate the patient's response to therapy.

PHYSICAL ASSESSMENT

1. Assess neurological status: note LOC.

DIAGNOSTICS ASSESSMENT

None specific

PATIENT MANAGEMENT

1. Administer thyroid hormone as ordered and carefully monitor cardiac patients for myocardial ischemia, chest pain, and ECG changes:

   Thyroxine: A loading dose is 300-500 μg, followed by a daily dose of 75-100 μg.

   Combination therapy may be ordered: Thyroxine 200-300 μg + 25 μg triiodothyronine q12h initially, then reducing thyroxine dose to 100 μg on day 2, and 50 μg per day thereafter.

   Triodothyronine alone may be ordered: 12.5-25 μg q6h.

   Dexamethasone may also be administered.

2. Institute passive rewarming methods; a thermal blanket may be necessary to increase body temperature. Use cautiously; rewarming may cause vasodilation and hypotension. (See Chapter 6, Therapeutic Modalities, for information about thermal regulation.)

▶ **Impaired gas exchange** related to respiratory muscle weakness and blunted central respiratory response to hypoxemia and hypercapnia

PATIENT OUTCOMES

• Patient alert and oriented to person, place, and time

• RR 12-20/min, eupnea

• Pao_2 80-100 mm Hg

• $Paco_2$ 35-45 mm Hg

• pH 7.35-7.45

• O_2 sat >95%

ENDO

PATIENT MONITORING

1. Continuously monitor oxygen saturation with pulse oximetry (Spo_2). Monitor interventions that can adversely affect oxygen saturation.
2. Continuously monitor ECG for dysrhythmias that may be related to hypoxemia or acid-base imbalance.

PHYSICAL ASSESSMENT

1. Assess respiratory status: note respiratory rate, rhythm, and depth. Patients are generally intubated and their lungs are mechanically ventilated.

DIAGNOSTICS ASSESSMENT

1. Review serial ABGs to evaluate oxygenation and acid-base balance.

PATIENT MANAGEMENT

1. Administer supplemental oxygen as ordered. If the patient is intubated and the lungs are mechanically ventilated, see Chapter 6, Therapeutic Modalities.
2. Administer thyroid medication as prescribed.
3. Reposition the patient to improve oxygenation and mobilize secretions. Evaluate the patient's response to position changes with ABGs to determine the best position for oxygenation.
4. As the patient stabilizes hemodynamically, provide pulmonary hygiene to prevent complications.
5. Avoid administering CNS depressants, since they are slowly metabolized by the hypothyroid patient.

▶ **Decreased cardiac output** related to bradycardia and decreased stroke volume

PATIENT OUTCOMES

- Patient will be alert and oriented to person, place, and time
- SBP 90-140 mm Hg
- MAP 70-105 mm Hg
- HR 60-100 beats/min
- u/o 30 ml/hr or 0.5-1.0 ml/kg/hr
- Peripheral pulses palpable
- PAP $\frac{15\text{-}30}{5\text{-}15}$ mm Hg
- CO 4-8 L/min

PATIENT MONITORING

1. Continuously monitor ECG for dysrhythmias or profound bradycardia that can adversely affect CO. A prolonged QT interval is associated with torsade de pointes.

2. Continuously monitor PA pressures, CVP (if available), and BP. Obtain CO and PAWP to evaluate cardiac function and the patient's response to therapy. Calculate MAP; a MAP <60 mm Hg adversely affects cerebral and renal perfusion.
3. Monitor fluid volume status: measure urine output hourly, determine fluid balance q8h; compare serial weights; a rapid (0.5-1.0 kg/day) change suggests fluid imbalance.

PHYSICAL ASSESSMENT
1. Assess cardiovascular status: note quality of peripheral pulses and capillary refill. Observe for increase in JVP and pulsus paradoxus, which may indicate pericardial effusion. Auscultate heart sounds, heart rate, and breath sounds for development of heart failure. Observe for tachycardia and myocardial ischemia as thyroid hormone is being replaced.

DIAGNOSTICS ASSESSMENT
1. Review thyroid studies as available. TSH levels should decline within 24 hr of therapy and should normalize after 7 days of therapy.

PATIENT MANAGEMENT
1. Administer IV fluids as ordered to maintain SBP >90 mm Hg; carefully monitor for fluid overload and development of heart failure.
2. Vasopressor agents may be used if hypotension is refractory to volume administration and if thyroid replacement has not had time to act. Carefully monitor the patient for lethal dysrhythmias.

▶ **Fluid volume excess** related to impaired free water clearance

PATIENT OUTCOMES
• Intake approximates output
• Serum sodium 135-145 mEq/L
• Serum osmolality 285-295 mOsm/L
• Urine specific gravity 1.010-1.030

PATIENT MONITORING
1. Monitor fluid volume status: measure intake and output hourly, determine fluid balance q8h. Compare serial weights; a rapid (0.5-1.0 kg/day) change indicates fluid imbalance. Weight gain without edema may be observed.
2. Monitor LOC with Glasgow coma scale.

ENDO

PHYSICAL ASSESSMENT

1. Assess hydration status: note skin turgor on inner thigh or forehead, observe buccal membranes, and assess thirst (if the patient is awake).
2. Assess the patient's lungs for adventitious sounds; assess heart sounds for development of S_3 (a hallmark of heart failure).

DIAGNOSTICS ASSESSMENT

1. Review serum sodium, serum osmolality, and urine specific gravity. Hyponatremia may be contributing to the obtunded state.

PATIENT MANAGEMENT

1. If the sodium level is <120 mEq/L, isotonic saline may be administered and free water restricted. (See p. 366 for management of hyponatremia.)
2. Institute seizure precautions.
3. Hydrocortisone 100 mg IV q6-8h may be ordered until adrenal function normalizes.

Renal Disorders

ACUTE RENAL FAILURE
Clinical Brief
Acute renal failure is a clinical syndrome characterized by a sudden, rapid deterioration in kidney function, which results in fluid, electrolyte, and acid-base imbalances. Causes of acute renal failure can be divided into three categories.

Prerenal: Factors that decrease renal perfusion, e.g., shock, intravascular volume depletion, and occlusion or damage to the renal arteries

Intrarenal: Factors that damage the renal parenchyma, e.g., nephrotoxic agents (antibiotics, contrast media, pesticides, myoglobin), inflammation, trauma, and any prerenal process that results in renal ischemia; acute tubular necrosis (ATN) is a type of intrarenal failure

Postrenal: Factors that result from obstruction of urine flow from the kidneys to the external environment, e.g., prostatic hypertrophy, kidney stones, or bladder tumor

Presenting signs and symptoms
The acute onset of renal failure is often accompanied by oliguria (less than 400 ml of urine in 24 hours), but may be nonoliguric, and azotemia (accumulation of nitrogen waste products).

Physical examination
↑ or ↓ BP
↑ HR
↑ RR
Normal or ↑ T
Neurological: Irritability, restlessness, change in LOC
Cardiovascular: S_3, S_4, JVD may be present
Pulmonary: Deep and rapid respirations, crackles
GI: Nausea, vomiting, anorexia

Diagnostic findings
Diagnostic findings vary with category (see Table 5-36).
NOTE: Diuretic administration will affect urine analysis.

TABLE 5-36 Categories of Acute Renal Failure and Related Laboratory Values

	Prerenal	Intrarenal (ATN)	Postrenal
Urine			
Volume	Low	Low or high	Low or high
Sodium	< 20 mEq/L	> 20 mEq/L	> 40 mEq/L
Osmolality	> 350 mOsm	< 300 mOsm (fixed)	< 350 mOsm (varies)
Specific gravity	> 1.020	< 1.010	
Creatinine	~Normal	Low	Low
FEna	≤ 1%	> 1%	
Plasma			
Urea (BUN)	High	High	High
Creatinine	~Normal	High	High
BUN:creatinine	20:1 or more	10:1 to 15:1	10:1

Acute Care Patient Management
Goals of treatment
Optimize renal perfusion and urine output
    Correction of suspected cause
    Fluid challenge
    Low-dose dopamine
    Diuretic agents
    Antihypertensive agents
    Vasodilator agents
    Avoidance of nephrotoxic agents
Normalize fluid status
    Fluid challenge in prerenal patients
    Fluid restriction in oliguric patients
    Diuretic agents
    Dialysis
Remove nitrogen waste products
    Restriction of protein intake
    Increase in caloric intake
    Dialysis
Maintain electrolyte balance
    Restriction of sodium
    Restriction of potassium
    Phosphate-binding antacids

TABLE 5-37 Clinical Sequelae Associated
with Acute Renal Failure

Complications	Signs and symptoms
Hyperkalemia	Peaked T waves, prolonged PR interval, prolonged QRS duration, dysrhythmias; twitching, cramps, hyperactive reflexes
Pericarditis	Chest discomfort aggravated by supine position or deep inspiration, intermittent friction rub and/or fever may be present
Metabolic acidosis	pH < 7.35 with $\downarrow$ HCO_3 and normal or $\downarrow$ $Paco_2$; Kussmaul respirations (hyperventilation); headache, fatigue, altered mental status
Anemia	Decreasing hematocrit, active bleeding; pale, weak, tired; SOB
GI bleed	Occult or visible blood in stools or gastric contents, decreasing hematocrit
Infection	Elevated temperature (may be subtle); pneumonia, UTI, or wound sepsis may be sources
Uremia	Lethargy progressing to coma, seizures, asterixis, heart failure, volume disturbances, pericarditis, N/V, anorexia, diarrhea, GI bleeding

For hyperkalemia: Kayexalate (with sorbitol)
                  Glucose with insulin
                  Sodium bicarbonate
Treat hypercatabolism
    Dialysis
    Nutrition: high calorie, low protein, high essential
               amino acids
Detect/prevent clinical sequelae
See Table 5-37
Priority nursing diagnoses
Fluid volume excess
Fluid volume deficit
Altered nutrition: less than body requirements
High risk for injury: electrolyte and acid-base imbalance
Altered protection (see p. 145)
High risk for altered family process (see p. 150)

KENAL

▶ **Fluid volume excess** related to decreased renal excretion (oliguria)

PATIENT OUTCOMES
- Patient at target body weight
- Intake approximates output
- MAP 70-105 mm Hg
- SBP 90-140 mm Hg
- Absence of edema
- Clear breath sounds
- Patient alert and oriented
- Absence of heart failure
- CVP 2-6 mm Hg
- Electrolytes WNL
- Cr 0.6-1.2 mg/dl
- Urine specific gravity 1.003-1.030

PATIENT MONITORING
1. Monitor fluid volume status: measure urine output hourly, determine fluid balance q8h and include other bodily drainage. Compare serial weights for rapid changes; an increase of 1 to 2 pounds/day indicates fluid retention. The oliguric phase (u/o < 400 ml/day) in ATN usually lasts 10 to 16 days, followed by a diuretic phase.
2. Obtain CVP, PAP (if available), and BP hourly or more frequently to evaluate the extent of fluid volume excess and the patient's response to therapy. Calculate MAP, an indicator of tissue perfusion; a decrease in MAP further insults the kidney.
3. Continuously monitor ECG for dysrhythmias secondary to electrolyte imbalance.

PHYSICAL ASSESSMENT
1. Assess fluid volume status; note any onset of S_3 and crackles, presence of edema, cough, or frothy sputum, increased work of breathing, decreased peripheral perfusion, and increased JVP to determine development of heart failure or pulmonary edema.
2. Assess the patient for development of clinical sequelae (see Table 5-37).

DIAGNOSTICS ASSESSMENT
1. Review BUN, creatinine, and BUN/creatinine ratio. Serum creatinine reflects GFR. Estimating GFR is not accurate in acute renal failure and is assumed to be < 10. Uremic symptoms may manifest if BUN is > 70-100

mg/dl or GFR is < 10-15 ml/min. A rise in BUN without a corresponding rise in creatinine may indicate bleeding.
2. Review urine sodium, urine osmolality, and urine specific gravity to evaluate renal function.
3. Review serial chest radiographs to evaluate pulmonary congestion.
4. Review serial ABGs to evaluate extent of acid-base imbalances.
5. Review serial electrolytes: hyperkalemia, hyponatremia, hypocalcemia, hyperphosphatemia, and hypermagnesemia are common in acute renal failure.

PATIENT MANAGEMENT

1. Restrict fluids to ~600 ml/day plus insensible losses in oliguric patients and restrict sodium intake to reduce fluid volume. Restrict protein intake to limit nitrogen accumulation. Increase caloric intake to minimize protein catabolism.
2. Concentrate medications when possible to minimize fluid intake.
3. Administer diuretics (furosemide, bumetanide) as ordered to produce diuresis. Closely monitor for signs of peripheral vascular collapse, hypovolemia, hypokalemia, and hyponatremia during rapid diuresis. If possible, obtain a urine specimen for laboratory analysis before administering diuretics.
4. Administer dopamine in low doses (1-5 μg/kg/min) to increase renal perfusion by vasodilating renal vasculature. Monitor urine output. (See Chapter 7, Pharmacology, for specific drug information.)
5. If the patient is hypertensive, administer vasodilators or antihypertensive agents as ordered. Carefully monitor BP before administration; generally SBP should be > 90 mm Hg. (See Chapter 7, Pharmacology, for specific drug information.)
6. Raise HOB if the patient is SOB without being hypotensive.
7. Provide meticulous skin care to prevent skin breakdown and infection.
8. Anticipate dialysis to remove excessive fluid, especially in conditions of congestive heart failure, myocardial damage, pulmonary edema, uremic pericarditis, hyperkalemia, or BUN > 100 mg/dl. PD or CAVH may be re-

RENAL

quired if the patient is hemodynamically unstable. (See Chapter 6, Therapeutic Modalities.)

9. Avoid administration of nephrotoxic agents or administer at reduced dosage or frequency to prevent additional renal damage.

▶ **Fluid volume deficit** related to volume depletion (diuretic phase)

PATIENT OUTCOMES
- MAP 70-105 mm Hg
- u/o 30 ml/hr or 0.5-1.0 ml/kg/hr
- Intake approximates output
- Elastic skin turgor
- Moist mucous membranes
- HR 60-100 beats/min
- Electrolytes WNL

PATIENT MONITORING
1. Monitor I & O hourly to assess the fluid balance trend, reflective of renal function. Diuretic phase (> 400 ml/day) of ATN may last 2 to 3 days or up to 12 days.
2. Compare daily weights to assess fluid volume loss.
3. Obtain CVP, PAP (if available), HR, and BP hourly or more frequently as patient condition dictates. Calculate MAP, an indicator of tissue perfusion; a MAP < 70 mm Hg further insults the kidney. Be alert for tachycardia and postural hypotension, which may indicate volume depletion.

PHYSICAL ASSESSMENT
1. Assess hydration state: note skin turgor on inner thigh or forehead, condition of buccal membranes, flat neck veins, complaints of thirst, decreased sensorium, which may signal volume depletion.
2. Assess the patient for development of clinical sequelae.

DIAGNOSTICS ASSESSMENT
1. Review urine sodium, osmolality, and specific gravity to assess volume status.
2. Review serial electrolytes, since severe imbalances can occur.

PATIENT MANAGEMENT
1. Administer aggressive fluid and electrolyte replacements as ordered to increase volume and maintain normal electrolyte and acid-base balance. Carefully monitor for increase in urine output and early signs of fluid volume excess when administering fluid challenges.
2. Avoid administration of nephrotoxic agents or adminis-

ter at reduced dosage or frequency to prevent additional renal damage.

3. Avoid rapidly placing the patient in an upright position, because postural hypotension may result.

4. Provide meticulous skin care to avoid skin breakdown and oral care to soothe dry mucous membranes.

5. Check for occult blood in stools and NG aspirate, since GI bleeding can occur in patients with renal failure, contributing to signs and symptoms of volume deficit.

6. Restrict protein intake to reduce nitrogen waste product accumulation. Increase caloric intake to minimize protein catabolism.

ELECTROLYTE IMBALANCE: POTASSIUM

Clinical Brief

Potassium imbalances occur as a result of changes in the concentration of potassium ions in the extracellular fluid. Hypokalemia is most frequently caused by losses of GI secretions, diuretic usage, decreased potassium intake, alkalemia, and aldosterone excess. Hyperkalemia occurs with decreased urine output, increased catabolism, increased potassium intake, acidemia, and hypoaldosteronism.

Presenting signs and symptoms

Signs and symptoms depend on the severity of the imbalance (see Physical examination).

Physical examination

Appearance: Weak, tired

Hypokalemia	Hyperkalemia
Cardiovascular:	
ECG: Flat T waves; U waves; peaked P waves, ST depression, dysrhythmias	ECG: Tall, peaked T waves, prolonged PR interval, flat or absent P waves, prolonged QRS duration, dysrhythmias
Pulmonary: SOB may progress to respiratory arrest	SOB may progress to respiratory arrest
Neuromuscular: Hypoactive reflexes, numbness, cramps, weakness, paralysis	Hyperactive reflexes, numbness, tingling, paralysis
GI: GI irritability, distention, ileus	Nausea, cramps, diarrhea

RENAL

Diagnostic findings

Hypokalemia is defined as a serum potassium < 3.5 mEq/L; hyperkalemia is a serum potassium > 5.5 mEq/L.

Acute Care Patient Management
Goals of treatment

	Hypokalemia	Hyperkalemia
Normalize serum potassium level	Treat underlying cause High-potassium diet Correct alkalosis Oral potassium supplements Intravenous potassium	Treat underlying cause Low-potassium diet Kayexalate with sorbitol Hypertonic glucose and insulin Sodium bicarbonate (if not fluid overloaded) Calcium gluconate Correct hypomagnesemia

Priority nursing diagnoses: Hypokalemia

▶ **High risk for injury** related to hypokalemia

PATIENT OUTCOMES

- Serum potassium level 3.5-5.5 mEq/L
- Rounded P and T waves
- PR interval 0.12 to 0.20 seconds
- QRS duration 0.04 to 0.10 seconds
- Absence of dysrhythmias
- MAP 70-105 mm Hg
- RR 12-20/min
- Nonlabored respirations
- Deep, symmetrical chest expansion
- Normal reflex activity
- Normal peripheral sensation and movement
- Active bowel sounds
- Absence of injury

PATIENT MONITORING

1. Monitor ECG for changes in complex configuration, waveform duration; ST segment depression, broad T waves, and U waves may be present. Dysrhythmias such as PVCs, heart blocks, VT, and VF may occur.
2. Monitor changes in intake or output that might affect

potassium balance. Hypokalemia may occur with osmotic diuresis, renal insufficiency, and GI losses.

PHYSICAL ASSESSMENT

1. Observe for signs of alkalosis (pH > 7.45, decreased respiratory rate, tingling, dizziness), since alkalosis shifts potassium into the cells, resulting in hypokalemia.
2. Assess patients on digitalis for signs of digitalis toxicity, since hypokalemia increases sensitivity to digitalis.
3. Assess muscle strength and monitor deep tendon reflex activity, since hypokalemia is associated with muscle weakness and hyporeflexia that may progress to tetany and respiratory arrest.
4. Assess abdomen size, shape, and bowel sounds q4h, since hypokalemia is associated with paralytic ileus.

DIAGNOSTICS ASSESSMENT

1. Review serial potassium levels to evaluate response to therapy and prior to administering diuretics. NOTE: Furosemide, dopamine, catecholamines, and antibiotics such as carbenicillin and gentamicin can cause hypokalemia.
2. Review magnesium levels, since abnormalities in magnesium are often mistaken for potassium imbalances.

PATIENT MANAGEMENT

1. Ensure adequate u/o before administering potassium.
2. When administering oral potassium supplements, dilute in fluid and administer with food or immediately after meals to minimize GI irritation and diarrhea.
3. Ensure patency of the intravenous line before and during potassium administration, since potassium is irritating and potentially damaging to tissues. Dilute intravenous potassium to minimize irritation to the veins. A central line is preferable for potassium infusions. Administer intravenous potassium at a rate not to exceed 20 mEq/100 ml/hr; continuous cardiac monitoring should be employed. Rapid potassium infusions can result in cardiac arrest; potassium should never be given as a bolus. Check the potassium level and be alert for overcorrection of hypokalemia.
4. Withhold oral intake and notify the physician if bowel sounds are severely diminished or absent. Otherwise, encourage foods rich in potassium, such as apricots, bananas, cantaloupes, dates, raisins, avocados, beans, meats, potatoes, and orange juice.

RENAL

5. If cardiac dysrhythmias or respiratory distress occurs, institute immediate treatment for hypokalemia while supporting cardiac and respiratory functioning.

Priority nursing diagnoses: hyperkalemia

▶ **High risk for injury** related to hyperkalemia

PATIENT OUTCOMES

- Serum potassium level 3.5-5.5 mEq/L
- Rounded P and T waves
- PR interval 0.12-0.20 seconds
- QRS duration 0.04-0.10 seconds
- Absence of dysrhythmias
- MAP 70-105 mm Hg
- RR 12-20/min
- Nonlabored respirations
- Deep, symmetrical chest expansion
- Normal reflex activity
- Normal peripheral sensation and movement
- Active bowel sounds
- Absence of injury

PATIENT MONITORING

1. Monitor ECG for changes in complex configuration, waveform, and duration; tall peaked T waves and a shortened QT interval occur with $K^+ > 6.5$ mEq/L; the PR interval increases and QRS widens with $K^+ > 8.0$ mEq/L. Cardiac and renal patients are especially at risk for lethal effects of increased potassium on the electrical conduction system of the heart. Dysrhythmias such as bradycardia, heart blocks, extrasystoles, junctional rhythm, idioventricular rhythm, ventricular tachycardia or fibrillation, sine wave, and asystole can occur.

2. Note changes in I & O that might affect potassium balance. A decrease in renal function, as with acute renal failure, is a risk factor for hyperkalemia.

PHYSICAL ASSESSMENT

1. Observe for signs of acidosis (pH < 7.35, increased respiratory rate and depth, confusion, drowsiness, headache), since acidosis shifts potassium out of the cells, resulting in hyperkalemia.

2. Assess muscle strength and monitor deep tendon reflex activity, since hyperkalemia is associated with muscle weakness and hyperreflexia. Numbness, tingling, muscle flaccidity, or paralysis may develop. Respiratory arrest may also occur.

DIAGNOSTICS ASSESSMENT

1. Review serial potassium levels and note the patient's response to therapy. Potassium-sparing diuretics (spironolactone, triamterene and amiloride), penicillin G, succinylcholine, angiotensin-converting enzyme inhibitors, β-adrenergic blocking agents, or salt substitutes can cause hyperkalemia, as well as hemolyzed blood samples.
2. Review magnesium levels, since abnormalities in magnesium are often mistaken for potassium imbalances.
3. Review serial ABGs, since metabolic acidosis is associated with hyperkalemia.

PATIENT MANAGEMENT

1. Administer kayexalate with sorbitol orally (15 g 1-4×/day) or rectally (30-50 g) as ordered to treat mild hyperkalemia (K^+ of 5.5 to 6.5 mEq/L). If administered rectally, encourage retention for 30 to 60 minutes for maximum effect. Kayexalate increases potassium excretion in the GI tract and each gram will remove 1 mEq of potassium. If kayexalate is used for several days, monitor for hypocalcemia, hypomagnesemia, and fluid overload (as a result of hypernatremia).
2. Anticipate furosemide and NS infusion to rid the body of excess potassium.
3. Administer hypertonic glucose (25 g of 50% dextrose) and insulin (10 U regular) for K^+ of 6.5-7.5 mEq/L to temporarily shift potassium into the cells.
4. A bolus of sodium bicarbonate (44 mEq) followed by an infusion (88-132 mEq $NaHCO_3$/L D_5NS) may be ordered to temporarily shift potassium into the cells. Carefully assess for signs of hypernatremia and fluid volume overload.
5. To antagonize the cardiac suppression associated with hyperkalemia, calcium gluconate may be ordered for severe hyperkalemia (K^+ of > 7.5 mEq/L). Administer calcium gluconate slowly over 2 to 3 minutes while observing for ECG changes. Stop the infusion if bradycardia occurs.
6. While administering medications to treat hyperkalemia, monitor for correction of hyperkalemia and signs of hypokalemia that might result from overcorrection. Observe closely for returning signs of hyperkalemia 30 minutes after calcium administration and 2 to 3 hours after sodium bicarbonate or insulin with glucose treatment.

RENAL

7. After emergency treatment of hyperkalemia, consult with the physician regarding follow-up treatment to permanently remove potassium.
8. Restrict foods rich in potassium such as apricots, bananas, coffee, cocoa, tea, dried fruits, cantaloupes, avocados, beans, meats, potatoes, and orange juice.

ELECTROLYTE IMBALANCE: SODIUM
Clinical Brief
Sodium imbalances occur as a result of changes in sodium ion concentrations in extracellular fluid. Hyponatremia is a deficiency of sodium relative to water and can occur from (1) excess water, as with excessive water intake or syndrome of inappropriate antidiuretic hormone release (SIADH); (2) sodium depletion, as with GI losses, diaphoresis, diuretics, renal excretion of sodium, and adrenal insufficiency; and (3) combined water and sodium retention, as with congestive heart failure, cirrhosis, or nephrotic syndrome. Hypernatremia is an excess of sodium relative to water and can occur from water depletion, as with diuretics, decreased intake, GI losses, hyperglycemia, diabetes insipidus; and sodium excess, as with large sodium intake (rare).

Sodium concentration is largely responsible for determining plasma osmolality. Symptoms associated with sodium imbalances are largely determined by the patient's volume status.

Presenting signs and symptoms
Signs and symptoms include complaints associated with dehydration or fluid retention. Patients with hyponatremia can have dehydration (circulatory insufficiency) or overhydration (fluid overload, pulmonary edema). Patients with hypernatremia usually have an ECF volume deficit (dehydration).

Physical examination
Dehydration (hyponatremia or hypernatremia)
Appearance: Fatigued, lethargic, loss of skin turgor, dry mucous membranes; with hypernatremia, flushed skin
VS: HR ↑
  BP ↓ or orthostatic BP
  T ↑
Cardiovascular: Weak peripheral pulses, flat neck veins
Neurological: Confused, decreased mentation; irritability, twitching, and seizures (associated with sodium imbalances)

GU: Decreased u/o
GI: Abdominal cramps and nausea (hyponatremia)
Overhydration (hyponatremia or hypernatremia)
Appearance: Malaise, edema, flushed skin (hypernatremia)
VS: ↑ BP
Cardiovascular: ↑ CO—bounding pulses, hypertension *or*
　　　　　　　　↓ CO—weak pulses, S_3, JVD
Pulmonary: Crackles, dyspnea
Neurological: Headache, confusion; irritability, twitching,
　　　　　　　and seizures (associated with sodium im-
　　　　　　　balances)
GI: Abdominal cramps and nausea (hyponatremia)

Diagnostic findings
Hyponatremia is defined as a serum sodium of < 135 mEq/
L; hypernatremia is a serum sodium of > 145 mEq/L.

Acute Care Patient Management
Goals of treatment

	Hyponatremia	**Hypernatremia**
Maintain normal serum sodium and osmolality level	Correct underlying problem	Correct underlying problem
	High sodium intake 3% saline 0.45 NS or 0.9 NS	Low sodium intake
Normalize fluid status and serum osmolality	Correct underlying problem	Correct underlying problem
	If volume deficit: Fluids	If volume deficit: Fluids without salt
	If volume excess: Restrict fluids Diuretics	If volume excess: Restrict fluids Diuretics

Priority nursing diagnoses
Fluid volume deficit
Fluid volume excess
High risk for injury: neurological dysfunction
Fluid volume deficit related to hypernatremia (hypertonic
dehydration) or hyponatremia (hypotonic dehydration) as-
sociated with decreased fluid intake, GI losses, diaphoresis,
diuretics, diabetes insipidus, increased renal excretion of so-
dium, or adrenal insufficiency
PATIENT OUTCOMES
• Patient will be alert and oriented
• Serum sodium 135-145 mEq/L

RENAL

- Serum osmolality 280-295 mOsm/L
- MAP 70-105 mm Hg
- SBP 90-105 mm Hg
- u/o 30 ml/hr or 0.5-1.0 ml/kg/hr
- CVP 2-6 mm Hg

PATIENT MONITORING

1. Monitor fluid volume status: obtain hourly I & O; include gastric and diarrheal fluid and diaphoresis in output when calculating fluid balance. Compare serial weights; a rapid decrease in weight (0.5-1 kg/day) suggests fluid volume loss.
2. Monitor BP, HR, and hemodynamic parameters (if available) to evaluate fluid volume status. An orthostatic BP suggests hypovolemia. Calculate MAP; a MAP < 70 mm Hg adversely affects renal and cerebral perfusion.

PHYSICAL ASSESSMENT

1. Assess hydration state: note poor skin turgor on inner thigh or forehead, dry buccal membranes, flat neck veins, complaints of thirst, and decreased sensorium, which may signal volume depletion.
2. Assess for the development of hypovolemic shock: decreased weight, O > I, decreased mentation, SBP < 90 mm Hg, u/o < 0.5 ml/kg/hr, weak pulses, cool and clammy skin.

DIAGNOSTICS ASSESSMENT

1. Review serial serum sodium, serum osmolality, urine osmolality, and specific gravity to assess fluid volume status. Na^+ < 135 mEq/L, specific gravity < 1.010, and serum osmolality < 285 suggest overhydration; Na^+ > 145 mEq/L, specific gravity > 1.015, and serum osmolality > 295 suggest dehydration.

PATIENT MANAGEMENT

1. Adjust oral intake of sodium as indicated by the serum sodium level. For a patient with *hyponatremia,* encourage fluids high in sodium, such as chicken or beef broths and canned tomato juice. For a patient with *hypernatremia,* encourage fluids low in sodium, such as distilled water, coffee, tea, and orange juice. Assist the patient with hypernatremia to avoid foods high in sodium.
2. Administer fluids and electrolytes as ordered. LR or 0.9 NS may be ordered for patients with hypovolemic hyponatremia. Patients should be carefully monitored for possible fluid overload as ECF volume is replaced.
3. Keep the patient supine until volume has been replaced.

Assist the patient with position changes or ambulation, since orthostatic changes may occur while the patient is volume depleted.

▶ **Fluid volume excess** related to hypernatremia or hyponatremia (excess fluid intake, CHF, cirrhosis, or nephrotic syndrome)

PATIENT OUTCOMES
- Patient will be alert and oriented
- Serum sodium 135-145 mEq/L
- Serum osmolality 280-295 mOsm/L
- MAP 70-105 mm Hg
- SBP 90-140 mm Hg
- Clear breath sounds
- CVP 2-6 mm Hg
- Intake approximates output

PATIENT MONITORING
1. Monitor fluid volume status: obtain hourly I & O; calculate fluid balance q8h. Compare serial weights; a rapid increase in weight (0.5-1 kg/day) suggests fluid volume retention.
2. Monitor BP, HR, and hemodynamic parameters (if available) to evaluate fluid volume status.

PHYSICAL ASSESSMENT
1. Assess fluid volume status; note the onset of S_3 and crackles, presence of edema, cough, or frothy sputum, increased work of breathing, decreased peripheral perfusion, and increased JVP to determine development of heart failure or pulmonary edema.
2. Assess for headache, blurred vision, and altered mentation and note pupil size and reaction, speech, motor strength, and tremors to determine development of cerebral edema. Neurological dysfunction is a major concern with hypernatremia.

DIAGNOSTICS ASSESSMENT
1. Review serial serum sodium, serum osmolality, urine osmolality, and specific gravity to assess fluid volume status. $Na^+ < 135$ mEq/L, specific gravity < 1.010, and serum osmolality < 285 suggest overhydration; $Na^+ > 145$ mEq/L, specific gravity > 1.015, and serum osmolality > 295 suggest dehydration.

PATIENT MANAGEMENT
1. Restrict salt and fluid intake in patients with hypervolemic hyponatremia. Concentrate medications when possible to minimize fluid intake.

RENAL

2. Hypotonic fluids may be administered to patients with hypervolemic hypernatremia.
3. Administer diuretics as ordered to rid the body of excess fluid. Be alert for rapid diuresis and signs of volume depletion; check VS and potassium level.

▶ **High risk for injury:** neurological dysfunction related to hypernatremia or hyponatremia

PATIENT OUTCOMES
• Patient will be alert and oriented to person, place, and time
• Absence of neurological deficits
• Serum sodium 135-145 mEq/L

PATIENT MONITORING
None specific

PHYSICAL ASSESSMENT
1. Assess neurological status: note any change in mental status, presence of neuromuscular irritability, focal neurological deficits, or seizure activity.

DIAGNOSTICS ASSESSMENT
1. Review serial serum sodium levels. Neurological signs generally manifest at sodium levels < 125 mEq/L and become more severe at levels < 115 mEq/L.

PATIENT MANAGEMENT
1. Primary problems (e.g., DI, SIADH, or AI) should be treated.
2. If the patient is hyponatremic, restrict fluids. If the Na^+ level is < 120 mEq/L, or the patient is symptomatic, NS may be administered to replace sodium. If Na^+ levels < 105 mEq/L, hypertonic saline (3% NaCL) in conjunction with diuretics may be administered. Generally, Na^+ levels should be corrected no faster than 1 mEq/L/hr to 120 mEq/L or until symptoms subside.
3. If patient is hypernatremic, hypotonic solutions may be used to gradually lower serum sodium. Rapid lowering of sodium can result in cerebral edema; carefully monitor neurological status.

ELECTROLYTE IMBALANCE: CALCIUM

Clinical Brief

Calcium imbalances occur as a result of changes in calcium ion concentrations in extracellular fluid. Because approximately half of the calcium is bound to albumin, evaluation of calcium levels must be done in conjunction with albumin levels. A falsely low calcium level is seen in the presence of low albumin levels. Changes in pH alter the amount of calcium bound to albumin, requiring that assessment of serum calcium levels ideally be done when the pH is normal.

Hypocalcemia frequently results from respiratory alkalosis associated with hyperventilation, receiving large amounts of stored blood, acute pancreatitis, decreased intake, or decreased absorption (from vitamin D deficiency, decreased parathyroid hormone release, hyperphosphatemia, chronic renal failure, or malabsorption). Hypercalcemia commonly occurs with hypermetastatic bone disease and hyperparathyroidism. However, immobility and resumption of kidney function following renal transplantation can also cause hypercalcemia.

Presenting signs and symptoms
Signs and symptoms depend on the severity of the imbalance. (See Physical examination.)

Physical examination

	Hypocalcemia	**Hypercalcemia**
Appearance:	Tired	Tired, lethargic, bone pain
Cardiovascular:	ECG: Prolonged QT interval Palpitations Decreased CO Dysrhythmias	ECG: Shortened QT interval Dysrhythmias, especially heart block; cardiac arrest
Pulmonary:	Stridor, bronchospasm, laryngospasm	
Neurological:	Cramping of hands, feet, circumoral paresthesia, hyperreflexia, tetany, carpal and pedal spasm, numbness, tingling, twitching, seizures, altered mental status	Hyporeflexia, altered mental status, headache
GI:	Abdominal cramps	Anorexia, thirst, nausea, vomiting, constipation

RENAL

Diagnostic findings
Hypocalcemia is defined as an ionized serum calcium level of less than 4.5 mg/dl (total calcium of less than 9.0 mg/dl); hypercalcemia is an ionized calcium of greater than 5.5 mg/dl (total greater than 11.0 mg/dl).

Acute Care Patient Management
Goals of treatment

	Hypocalcemia	Hypercalcemia
Maintain normal serum calcium level	Correct underlying problem	Correct underlying problem
	High-calcium diet Vitamin D Oral calcium supplements 10% calcium gluconate Phosphate-binding antacids	Low-calcium diet Normal saline and diuretics Corticosteroids Calcitonin Mithramycin Etidronate Phosphates

Priority nursing diagnoses: hypocalcemia
▶ High risk for injury related to calcium imbalance: hypocalcemia

PATIENT OUTCOMES
- Serum calcium 4.5-5.5 mg/dl (total 9-11 mg/dl)
- Normal reflex activity
- Normal peripheral sensation and movement
- Patient alert and oriented
- HR 60-100 beats/min
- PR interval 0.12-0.20
- QT interval $< \frac{1}{2}$ of R-R interval
- Absence of life-threatening dysrhythmias
- MAP 70-105 mm Hg
- Absence of injury
- Absence of seizure activity
- RR 12-20/min
- Nonlabored respirations
- Absence of laryngeal stridor
- Absence of Trousseau's sign
- Absence of Chvostek's sign

PATIENT MONITORING
1. Continuously monitor ECG for dysrhythmias. Measure serial QT intervals; torsade de pointe is associated with prolonged QT intervals.
2. Monitor BP, since decreased myocardial contractility and hypotension are cardiovascular manifestations associated with hypocalcemia.

PHYSICAL ASSESSMENT
1. Assess for presence of cramps in hands, feet, and legs, and assess for circumoral paresthesia.

2. Assess respiratory rate and depth, work of breathing, and breath sounds at least q4h. Airway obstruction and respiratory arrest can occur. Monitor for stridor, bronchospasm, and laryngospasm.
3. Assess for signs of tetany; numbness and tingling in the fingers, around the mouth, and over the face, which may be followed by spasms of the face and extremities.
4. Assess for Trousseau's sign by inflating a blood pressure cuff above SBP for 2 to 5 minutes and assessing for carpopedal spasm of the hand. A positive test, which results when carpopedal spasm is present, is associated with hypocalcemia.
5. Assess for Chvostek's sign by tapping the facial nerve anterior to the ear and observing for lip and cheek spasms. Spasms indicate a positive test result and are associated with hypocalcemia.
6. Be alert for seizures, since hypocalcemia causes CNS irritability.
7. Assess patients taking digitalis for signs of digitalis toxicity; increasing calcium may cause digitalis toxicity.

DIAGNOSTICS ASSESSMENT

1. Review albumin levels, since hypoalbuminemia is the most common cause of hypocalcemia.
2. Review serial serum calcium levels in conjunction with pH and albumin levels, since alkalosis and hypoalbuminemia decrease calcium ionization. To correct for calcium in the presence of hypoalbuminemia, the following formula can be used: Corrected Ca = Total calcium + 0.8 (4.0 − albumin). In addition, drugs can cause hypocalcemia: aminoglycosides, aluminum-containing antacids, corticosteroids, and loop diuretics.

PATIENT MANAGEMENT

1. Initiate seizure precautions by padding side rails, minimizing stimulation, assisting the patient with all activities, and keeping airway management equipment available. If seizures do occur, protect the patient and be prepared to correct hypocalcemia and administer antiseizure medications if ordered.
2. Have a tracheostomy tray available; be prepared to administer humidified air or oxygen, administer bronchodilators and/or assist with a tracheostomy if bronchospasm and laryngospasm occur.
3. If respiratory arrest occurs, institute emergency respiratory and cardiac support.

RENAL

4. For symptomatic hypocalcemia, 10% calcium gluconate will be required. Administer undiluted at 1 ml/min for emergency replacement of calcium. Too rapid IV administration of calcium can lead to cardiac arrest.
5. Phosphate-binding antacids may be used to reduce phosphate absorption and cause an inverse increase in calcium. Administer antacids before meals.
6. Administer vitamin D and oral calcium supplements 1 hour after meals and at bedtime to maximize calcium absorption and utilization.
7. Encourage foods high in calcium, e.g., milk products, meats, and leafy green vegetables.
8. Assist with self-care activities, since the patient may develop poor coordination.

Priority nursing diagnoses: hypercalcemia

▶ **High risk for injury** related to calcium imbalance: hypercalcemia

PATIENT OUTCOMES
• Serum calcium 4.5-5.5 mg/dl (total 9.0-11 mg/dl)
• Normal reflex activity
• Normal peripheral sensation and movement
• Patient alert and oriented
• HR 60-100 beats/min
• PR interval 0.12-0.20
• QT interval < ½ of R-R interval
• Absence of life-threatening dysrhythmias
• MAP 70-105 mm Hg
• Absence of injury

PATIENT MONITORING
1. Continuously monitor ECG for dysrhythmias. Measure the QT interval.
2. Monitor fluid volume status: measure I & O hourly; hypercalcemia impairs the kidneys to concentrate urine and diuretic therapy will cause u/o to increase. Patients may receive an intake of up to 10 L of fluid a day.

PHYSICAL ASSESSMENT
1. Assess mentation and observe for behavior changes. Patients may be confused or develop psychotic behavior.
2. Assess patients receiving digitalis for signs of digitalis toxicity, since the inotropic effect of digitalis is enhanced by calcium. Digitalis dosage may need to be reduced.
3. Assess GI function: note abdominal distention and absent bowel sounds, anorexia, or N/V, which may suggest paralytic ileus.

Diagnostics Assessment

1. Review serial calcium levels to evaluate patient response to therapy.

Patient Management

1. Anticipate the administration of normal saline to expand ECF volume along with diuretics to increase urinary excretion of calcium. Monitor for signs of fluid volume imbalances. Thiazide diuretics are avoided because they inhibit calcium excretion.

2. Etidronate may be administered intravenously for hypercalcemia associated with malignancy. Generally, 7.5 mg/kg is given qd for 3 days.

3. Calcitonin may be required if serum calcium is > 15 mg/dl or in patients who cannot tolerate sodium. Administer 3-4 U/kg subcutaneously q12-24h.

4. Corticosteroids may be initiated if hypercalcemia is associated with some types of granulomatous disorders.

5. Mithramycin may be given in hypercalcemia associated with malignancy. Administer over 4 hours to reduce nausea. Dilute medication to minimize irritation to the veins. Be alert for thrombocytopenia, hepatotoxicity, and nephrotoxicity.

6. Phosphates administered intravenously may be given as a last resort to lower calcium; fatal hypotension and widespread metastatic calcification may occur.

7. If the patient develops heart block, check BP, HR, pulse pressure; be prepared to administer atropine, calcium, and to assist with pacemaker insertion. Be prepared to initiate immediate emergency measures for cardiac arrest.

8. Encourage a diet low in calcium and protein.

9. Encourage mobility as soon as possible, since immobility results in the release of bone calcium; assist with ambulation, since muscle weakness may be present.

10. To prevent the formation of kidney stones, encourage a high fluid intake (avoiding milk products, which are high in calcium), distributed throughout the entire 24-hour period, to a level that maintains u/o of 2500 ml/day. Encourage prune or cranberry juice to maintain acidic urine, since calcium solubility is increased in acidic urine.

11. If the patient develops bone pain or pain from a kidney stone, initiate comfort measures (e.g., positioning, darkened room). Administer pain medications.

RENAL

ELECTROLYTE IMBALANCE: PHOSPHORUS
Clinical Brief
Phosphorus imbalances occur as a result of changes in phosphorus ion concentrations in extracellular fluid. Phosphorus concentration in the extracellular fluid is in an inverse relationship with calcium concentration. Hypophosphatemia is associated with hyperparathyroidism, excessive diuresis, chronic alcohol abuse, carbohydrate load, hyperalimentation without phosphorus supplementation, respiratory alkalosis secondary to mechanical ventilation, malabsorption syndromes, and chronic use of antacids. Hyperphosphatemia occurs with hypoparathyroidism, acute and chronic renal failure, rhabdomyolysis, cytotoxic agents, metabolic acidosis, and excessive phosphate intake.

Presenting signs and symptoms
See Physical examination

Physical examination

	Hypophosphatemia	Hyperphosphatemia
Neuromuscular:	Malaise, muscle pain, muscle weakness, paresthesia, neuroirritability, confusion, tremors, seizures, coma	Fatigue, S/S of tetany
GI:	Anorexia	

Diagnostic findings
Hypophosphatemia is defined as a serum phosphorus level less than 3.0 mg/dl or 1.8 mEq/L. Hyperphosphatemia is a serum phosphorus level greater than 4.5 mg/dl or 2.6 mEq/L.

Acute Care Patient Management
Goals of treatment

	Hypophosphatemia	Hyperphosphatemia
Maintain normal serum phosphorus level	High-phosphorus diet Low-calcium diet Correct hypercalcemia Phosphorus	Low-phosphorus diet High-calcium diet Correct hypocalcemia Phosphate-binding antacids (aluminum hydroxide, aluminum carbonate)

Priority nursing diagnoses: hypophosphatemia
▶ High risk for injury related to phosphorus imbalance: hypophosphatemia

PATIENT OUTCOMES
- Serum phosphorus 3.0-4.5 mg/dl (1.8-2.6 mEq/L)
- Serum calcium 4.5-5.5 mg/dl (total 9-11 mg/dl)
- Normal peripheral sensation and movement
- Absence of injury
- Hg 12.0-16.0 g/dl
- Hct 40%-48%

PATIENT MONITORING
None specific

PHYSICAL ASSESSMENT
1. Assess peripheral sensation and strength. Muscle weakness, muscle pain, numbness, and tingling often occur in patients with hypophosphatemia.
2. Assess neurological status for changes in mentation, confusion, or decreased LOC.
3. Be alert for development of hemolytic anemia: pallor, dyspnea, weakness, tachycardia, dysrhythmias.

DIAGNOSTICS ASSESSMENT
1. Review serum phosphorus levels in conjunction with calcium levels, since hypophosphatemia is usually associated with hypercalcemia.

PATIENT MANAGEMENT
1. Because patients with hypophosphatemia often experience muscle weakness, teach the patient methods for conserving energy and provide for rest periods.
2. Assist with self-care activities and ambulation.
3. Encourage a diet high in phosphorus by encouraging intake of hard cheeses, meats, fish, nuts, eggs, dried fruits and vegetables, and legumes.
4. When administering oral phosphorus supplements, mix them with ice water to increase palatability. Monitor for diarrhea.
5. Administer intravenous phosphate slowly, infusing no more that 20 mM over 8 hours, to avoid rapidly decreasing calcium levels. Observe for signs and symptoms of hypocalcemia, including tetany, fatigue, palpitations, hypotension, numbness and tingling, positive Trousseau's sign, and positive Chvostek's sign.
6. If hemolytic anemia occurs, be prepared to administer oxygen, fluids, and blood products.

Priority nursing diagnoses: hyperphosphatemia
High risk for injury related to phosphorus imbalance: hyperphosphatemia

RENAL

PATIENT OUTCOMES
- Serum phosphorus 3.0-4.5 mg/dl (1.8-2.6 mEq/L)
- Serum calcium 4.5-5.5 mg/dl (total 9-11 mg/dl)
- Normal peripheral sensation and movement
- Absence of injury
- Absence of seizure activity

PATIENT MONITORING
None specific

PHYSICAL ASSESSMENT
1. Assess BP to detect hypotension resulting from the hypocalcemia that often accompanies hyperphosphatemia.
2. Observe for signs and symptoms of hypocalcemia, including tetany, fatigue, palpitations, hypotension, numbness and tingling, positive Trousseau's sign, and positive Chvostek's sign, since hypocalcemia often accompanies hyperphosphatemia.
3. Be alert for the development of tremors and seizures.

DIAGNOSTICS ASSESSMENT
1. Review serial serum phosphorus levels in conjunction with calcium levels, since hyperphosphatemia is usually associated with hypocalcemia.

PATIENT MANAGEMENT
1. Restrict food high in phosphorus such as hard cheeses, meats, fish, nuts, eggs, dried fruits and vegetables, and legumes.
2. Because seizures may result from hyperphosphatemia, initiate seizure precautions by padding side rails, minimizing stimulation, assisting the patient with all activities, and keeping airway management equipment available. If seizures do occur, protect the patient and be prepared to correct hyperphosphatemia and hypocalcemia and administer antiseizure medications if ordered.
3. If ordered, administer phosphate-binding antacids (aluminum hydroxide, aluminum carbonate) before meals to reduce absorption of phosphorus.
4. In extreme situations, calcium administration may be required.

ELECTROLYTE IMBALANCE: MAGNESIUM

Clinical Brief

Magnesium imbalances occur as a result of changes in magnesium ion concentrations in extracellular fluid. Hypomagnesemia occurs as a result of malabsorption, starvation, hyperalimentation without magnesium, alcoholism, excessive

diuretics, GI losses, pancreatitis, pregnancy toxemia, hypocalcemia, and hyperaldosteronism. Hypermagnesemia is associated with chronic renal failure, acidosis, adrenal insufficiency, hyperparathyroidism, and increased magnesium
intake. Abnormalities in magnesium are often mistaken for
potassium imbalances.

Presenting signs and symptoms
See Physical examination

Physical examination

	Hypomagnesemia	Hypermagnesemia
Appearance:	Weak, dizzy, cramping	Lethargic, flushed
VS:	↑ HR, ↑ BP	↓ RR, ↓ HR, ↓ BP
Cardiovascular:	ECG: Flat or inverted T waves, prolonged PR or QT interval, dysrhythmias	ECG: Peaked T waves, wide QRS; prolonged QT interval, bradycardia, cardiac arrest
Pulmonary:	Stridor, bronchospasm, laryngospasm	Shallow respirations, apnea
Neurological:	Confusion, altered mental status, tremors, tetany, hyperreflexia, seizures	Altered mental status, hyporeflexia, seizures, muscle paralysis, coma
GI:	Anorexia, nausea	

Diagnostic findings
Hypomagnesemia is defined as a serum magnesium level less
than 1.5 mEq/L. Hypermagnesemia is a serum magnesium
level greater than 2.5 mEq/L.

Acute Care Patient Management
Goals of treatment

	Hypomagnesemia	Hypermagnesemia
Normalize serum magnesium levels	High-magnesium diet Magnesium sulfate	Low-magnesium diet Diuretics Calcium gluconate

Priority nursing diagnoses: hypomagnesemia
High risk for injury related to magnesium imbalance: hypomagnesemia

RENAL

PATIENT OUTCOMES

- Serum magnesium 1.5-2.5 mEq/L
- Normal reflex activity
- Normal peripheral sensation and movement
- HR 60-100 beats/min
- PR interval 0.12-0.20
- QT interval $<$ ½ of R-R interval
- T wave rounded
- Absence of life-threatening dysrhythmias
- MAP 70-105 mm Hg
- RR 12-20/min
- Nonlabored respirations
- Absence of laryngeal stridor
- Absence of injury
- Absence of seizure activity

PATIENT MONITORING

1. Continuously monitor ECG for changes in rate and rhythm. Measure PR and QT intervals. Torsade de pointes is associated with prolonged QT intervals. Dysrhythmias may occur: premature ventricular contractions, ventricular tachycardia, and ventricular fibrillation.

PHYSICAL ASSESSMENT

1. Assess mentation, changes in behavior, and ability to swallow.
2. Assess respiratory rate and depth, work of breathing, and breath sounds at least q4h. Monitor for stridor, bronchospasm, and laryngospasm, which can occur during acute hypomagnesemia.
3. Assess for signs of hypocalcemia, which often accompanies hypomagnesemia: muscle weakness, muscle pain, numbness and tingling, positive Trousseau's sign, and positive Chvostek's sign.
4. Assess patients taking digitalis for signs of digitalis toxicity, since hypomagnesemia predisposes the patient to toxicity. Digitalis dosage may need to be adjusted.
5. Be alert for seizures.

DIAGNOSTICS ASSESSMENT

1. Review magnesium levels when available, although serum levels do not reflect total body magnesium stores and thus are a poor indicator of magnesium deficiency.
2. Review potassium levels, since magnesium imbalances are often mistaken for potassium imbalances.
3. Review calcium levels, since hypocalcemia often accompanies hypomagnesemia.

Patient Management

1. Encourage foods high in magnesium, such as seafood, green vegetables, bananas, grapefruits, oranges, nuts and legumes. Diet can correct mild hypomagnesemia.
2. For symptomatic hypomagnesemia, administer intravenous magnesium as ordered. A rapid infusion may result in cardiac or respiratory arrest; 10% magnesium sulfate should be administered no faster than 1.5 ml/min.
   a. Assess renal function before administering magnesium, since magnesium is removed from the body through the kidneys.
   b. Obtain BP, HR, and respirations every 15 minutes during infusion of large doses of magnesium, since vasodilation and respiratory depression may occur.
   c. Before and during the administration of magnesium, monitor for hypermagnesemia by assessing the patellar (knee-jerk) reflex. If the reflex is absent, stop the magnesium infusion and notify the physician. Hyporeflexia will precede respiratory depression.
   d. If hypotension or respiratory depression occurs during magnesium infusion, stop the magnesium infusion, notify the physician, and be prepared to administer calcium and to support cardiac and respiratory functioning.
3. Seizures may result from hypomagnesemia. Initiate seizure precautions by padding side rails, minimizing stimulation, assisting the patient with all activities, and keeping airway management equipment available. If seizures do occur, protect the patient and be prepared to correct hypomagnesemia and administer antiseizure medications if ordered.
4. Have a tracheostomy tray available. Be prepared to administer humidified air or oxygen, administer bronchodilators, and/or assist with a tracheostomy if bronchospasm and laryngospasm occur.
5. If dysrhythmia occurs, be prepared to begin treatment to increase the serum magnesium level. Be aware that antidysrhythmic agents and defibrillation are often ineffective in the presence of hypomagnesemia.
6. If respiratory arrest occurs, institute emergency respiratory and cardiac support.
7. Correct the magnesium level before correcting the potassium level, since hypokalemia is difficult to treat in the presence of hypomagnesemia.

RENAL

8. Because patients with hypomagnesemia often experience muscle weakness, teach the patient methods for conserving energy; provide for rest periods and assist with self-care activities and ambulation.

Priority nursing diagnoses: hypermagnesemia

▶ **High risk for injury** related to magnesium imbalance: hypermagnesemia

PATIENT OUTCOMES

- Serum magnesium 1.5-2.5 mEq/L
- Normal reflex activity
- Normal peripheral sensation and movement
- HR 60-100 beats/min
- PR interval 0.12-0.20
- QT interval $<\frac{1}{2}$ of R-R interval
- T wave rounded
- Absence of life-threatening dysrhythmias
- MAP 70-105 mm Hg
- RR 12-20/min
- Nonlabored respirations
- Absence of laryngeal stridor
- Absence of injury

PATIENT MONITORING

1. Continuously monitor the ECG for bradycardia and heart block. Measure PR and QT intervals.
2. Monitor BP for hypotension.

PHYSICAL ASSESSMENT

1. Assess LOC and note lethargy or drowsiness.
2. Assess the respiratory rate and pattern; note shallow respirations or periods of apnea.
3. Monitor patellar (knee-jerk) reflex, since absence of the reflex indicates severe hypermagnesemia that may proceed to respiratory or cardiac arrest.

DIAGNOSTICS ASSESSMENT

1. Review magnesium levels when available.
2. Review potassium levels, since magnesium imbalances are often mistaken for potassium imbalances.
3. Review calcium levels, since hypercalcemia often accompanies hypermagnesemia.

PATIENT MANAGEMENT

1. Restrict food high in magnesium, including seafood, green vegetables, bananas, grapefruits, oranges, nuts, and legumes.

2. Administer normal saline and diuretics as ordered to increase renal excretion of magnesium (if patient has urine output). If the patient is anuric, dialysis may be used.

3. If the patient is symptomatic (e.g., hypotension, shallow respirations, and/or decreased LOC), administer calcium gluconate (5-10 ml of 10% solution) as ordered.

4. If dysrhythmia occurs, be prepared to begin treatment to decrease the serum magnesium level and to administer antidysrhythmic agents as ordered.

5. If respiratory or cardiac arrest occurs, institute emergency respiratory and cardiac support.

Multisystem Disorders

ACQUIRED IMMUNODEFICIENCY SYNDROME (AIDS)

Clinical Brief

HIV disease is grouped according to clinical findings. Mononucleosis-like symptoms characterize the early stage of the infection. The second stage of this disease includes an asymptomatic period, which may last for years, depending on the patient's age, the route of infection, or immunocompetence of the patient. Generalized lymphadenopathy without any obvious reason characterizes the third stage of this disease. The final stage of the infectious process is characterized by the presence of certain opportunistic infections or malignancies and does not require serologic evidence for the diagnosis of AIDS.

AIDS is caused by a retrovirus, human immunovirus (HIV), which infects and destroys T-helper lymphocytes and impairs the immune system. AIDS is transmitted via entry of infected body fluids, such as blood and semen, into the bloodstream. The virus can also be spread from an infected mother to her fetus. High-risk groups include homosexual and bisexual males, intravenous drug users, hemophiliacs, and recipients of blood transfusions.

Presenting signs and symptoms

Signs and symptoms vary, depending on the stage of illness and the presence of an opportunistic infection. Fatigue, night sweats, fever, and diarrhea are common; respiratory distress and coma may occur.

Physical examination

Skin: Purplish lesions (Kaposi's sarcoma)

Neurological: Irritability, depression, personality changes to coma; weakness to paralysis; seizures (CNS involvement)

Pulmonary: Dyspnea, dry, nonproductive cough *(Pneumocystis carinii)*

GI: Watery diarrhea

Diagnostic findings

Positive result to Western blot test

Polymerase chain reaction (PCR)

Acute Care Patient Management

Goals of treatment

Minimize further immune system damage
  Antiviral agents: zidovudine
Treat opportunistic infections
  Pneumocystis carinii
    Antiprotozoal agents:
    Trimethoprim/sulfamethoxazole
    Pentamidine isethionate
    Dapsone and trimethoprim
    Steroids
    Intubation/mechanical ventilation
  Kaposi's sarcoma
    Interferon alfa-2A
    Vinblastine, vincristine
  Toxoplasmosis
    Pyrimethamine + sulfadiazine
    Clindamycin
  Herpes
    Acyclovir
  Cytomegalovirus
    Ganciclovir
    Foscarnet sodium
    Acyclovir
  Cryptococcus
    Amphotericin B
    Flucytosine
    Ketoconazole
  Candida
    Nystatin
    Amphotericin B
    Ketoconazole
  Mycobacterium tuberculosis
    Isoniazid, ethambutol, rifampin
Detect/prevent clinical sequelae
  See Table 5-38

Priority nursing diagnoses

Impaired gas exchange
Altered protection
Fluid volume deficit
Altered nutrition: less than body requirements (see p. 149)
High risk for altered family process (see p. 150)

TABLE 5-38 Clinical Sequelae Associated with HIV

Complications	Signs and symptoms
Respiratory failure	Restlessness, tachypneic, $Pao_2 < 50$ mm Hg, $Paco_2 > 50$ mm Hg, pH < 7.35
Septic shock	SBP < 90 mm Hg, altered mental status, hypoxia, plasma lactate > 2 mmol/L, u/o < 0.5ml/kg/hr, HR > 90 beats/min, RR > 20/min
DIC	Bleeding from any orifice and mucous membranes; cool, clammy skin; abnormal clotting studies
AIDS dementia complex	Forgetfulness, personality changes, clumsiness, ataxia, weak or paralyzed extremities, aphasia
Meningitis	Nuchal rigidity, headache, fever, lethargy, confusion, seizures
Lymphoma (CNS)	Symptoms depend on tumor site, paresthesia, visual loss, ataxia, paresis, seizures
CMV retinitis	Progressive visual loss
Peripheral nervous system disease	Ascending paralysis, burning pain in feet, absent achilles tendon reflex, hypersensitivity, decreased sensation, muscle weakness

Impaired gas exchange related to infectious processes (pneumocystis carinii) impairing oxygen diffusion and decreasing lung compliance

PATIENT OUTCOMES

- Patient will be alert and oriented to person, place, and time
- Pao_2 60-100 mm Hg
- pH 7.35-7.45
- $Paco_2$ 35-45 mm Hg
- O_2 sat > 90%
- RR 12-20, eupnea
- Lungs clear
- Minute ventilation <10 L/min

MULTI

- Vital capacity 15 ml/kg
- Lung compliance 60-100 ml/cm H_2O

PATIENT MONITORING

1. Continuously monitor oxygenation status with pulse oximetry (Spo_2). Be alert for effects of interventions and patient activities, which may adversely affect oxygen saturation.
2. Monitor serial lung compliance values to assess progression of lung stiffness.
3. Monitor pulmonary function by assessing minute ventilation and vital capacity measurements. A vital capacity of > 15ml/kg is generally needed for spontaneous breathing.

PHYSICAL ASSESSMENT

1. Assess respiratory status: RR >30/min suggests impending respiratory dysfunction. Note the use of accessory muscles and the respiratory pattern. Note the presence of breath sounds and adventitious sounds suggesting worsening pulmonary congestion.
2. Assess for signs and symptoms of hypoxia: increased restlessness, increased complaints of dyspnea, changes in LOC. Cyanosis is a late sign.
3. Assess the patient for development of clinical sequelae (see Table 5-38).

DIAGNOSTICS ASSESSMENT

1. Review ABGs for decreasing trends in Pao_2 (hypoxemia) or pH (acidosis), which would reflect respiratory distress. O_2 sat should be $> 90\%$.
2. Review serial chest radiographs to evaluate patient progress or worsening lung condition.
3. Review culture reports for identification of the infecting organism.

PATIENT MANAGEMENT

1. Provide supplemental oxygen as ordered. If the patient develops respiratory distress, be prepared for intubation and mechanical ventilation. (See Chapter 6, Therapeutic Modalities.)
2. Promote pulmonary hygiene with chest physiotherapy and postural drainage if necessary. C & DB the patient and reposition the patient at least q2h. Encourage incentive spirometry to decrease risk of atelectasis. Suction secretions prn and note the color and consistency of sputum. Position the patient for maximum chest excursion.

3. Minimize oxygen demand by decreasing anxiety, fever, and pain.
4. Administer chemotherapeutic agents as ordered. Be alert for further decreases in WBC, RBC, platelets, and fluid and electrolyte imbalance. Orthostatic hypotension can occur with parenteral pentamidine administration.
5. Steroids may be administered to decrease the interstitial inflammatory response.

▶ **Altered protection** related to immune dysfunction, chemotherapeutic agents, and central nervous system involvement

PATIENT OUTCOMES
- Absence of injury
- Absence of aspiration
- Absence of additional infections
- T 36.5° C (97.7° F)–38.5° C (101.3° F)
- u/o 30 ml/hr or 0.5-1.0 ml/kg/hr
- BUN 10-20 mg/dl
- Creatinine 0.6-1.2 mg/dl
- WBCs 5-10 × 10^3/μl
- RBCs 4.2-6.2 × 10^6/μl
- Platelets > 150 × 10^3/μl

PATIENT MONITORING
1. Monitor urine output hourly and note a decreasing trend, which may suggest renal insufficiency.

PHYSICAL ASSESSMENT
1. Assess for fever, chills, and night sweats. Hypotension may signal sepsis.
2. Assess neurological status: changes in LOC, cognition, personality; the onset of numbness/tingling, weakness of extremities, uncoordination, or paralysis; or visual loss may indicate CNS infection or side effects of chemotherapeutic agents. Assess for nuchal rigidity, which may indicate meningitis.
3. Assess for signs and symptoms of infection: redness, tenderness, drainage at IV sites; cloudy urine; purulent sputum; white patches on oral mucosa.
4. Assess for bleeding: test urine and stool; note gingival bleeding or oozing of blood from IV sites; note any petechiae.
5. Inspect skin for new lesions, rashes, or breaks in skin.
6. Assess the patient for clinical sequelae (see Table 5-38).

DIAGNOSTICS ASSESSMENT
1. Review serial WBC with differential and cultures to evaluate course of infection.

MULTI

2. Review serial Hgb, Hct, and platelets to evaluate anemia and extent of thrombocytopenia.
3. Review serial BUN and creatinine levels to evaluate renal function.

PATIENT MANAGEMENT
1. Provide oral hygiene before and after meals to treat stomatitis associated with chemotherapy. Apply lip balm to prevent cracks and crustations.
2. Provide meticulous body hygiene, especially after diarrheal episodes to prevent spread of organisms from stool. Use of A & D ointment or zinc oxide may prevent skin excoriation around the anorectal area.
3. Turn and reposition the patient at least q2h and provide ROM and skin care to improve circulation and prevent skin breakdown. A therapeutic bed may be required.
4. Encourage fluids to maintain hydration and minimize nephrotoxic effects of drugs.
5. Keep HOB elevated or the patient in a side-lying position to prevent aspiration if the level of consciousness is decreased and/or the patient is receiving enteral feedings. Keep suction equipment available.
6. Ensure a safe environment: bed in low position, call bell in reach, soft restraints if indicated.
7. Institute seizure precautions as necessary.
8. Institute bleeding precautions if the patient is thrombocytopenic.
9. Assist the patient with activities to prevent falls.
10. Hematest body fluids for occult blood. Spontaneous bleeding (e.g., hemoptysis, hematuria) may indicate DIC.
11. Orient the patient as needed.

▶ **Fluid volume deficit** related to severe diarrhea, vomiting, poor oral intake, and intestinal malabsorption

PATIENT OUTCOMES
• Moist mucous membranes
• Elastic skin turgor
• Intake approximates output
• Urine specific gravity 1.001-1.035
• Serum osmolality 275-295 mOsm/kg
• SBP 90-140 mm Hg

PATIENT MONITORING
1. Continuously monitor CVP and PAP (if available) to evaluate trends. Decreasing trends suggest hypovolemia.

2. Monitor fluid status: hourly I & O to determine fluid balance. Compare daily weights; a loss of 0.25-0.5 kg/day reflects excess fluid loss. Include an accurate stool count, since patients may exceed 10 L of fluid per day with watery diarrhea.
3. Measure urine specific gravity to evaluate hydration status. Increased values reflect dehydration or hypovolemia.
4. Calculate MAP; a value < 60 mm Hg adversely affects renal and cerebral perfusion.

PHYSICAL ASSESSMENT

1. Obtain BP and HR q1h to evaluate the patient's fluid volume status: HR > 120 and SBP < 90 mm Hg suggest hypovolemia; orthostatic hypotension reflects hypovolemia.
2. Evaluate mucous membranes by checking the area where the cheek and gum meet; dry, sticky membranes are associated with hypovolemia. Test skin turgor on the sternum or the inner aspects of thighs for best assessment.
3. Assess the patient for clinical sequelae (see Table 5-38 on p. 387).

DIAGNOSTICS ASSESSMENT

1. Review stool cultures for identification of any infectious agent.
2. Review serial electrolytes, since diarrhea and vomiting can result in a severe electrolyte imbalance.
3. Review serial serum osmolality to evaluate hydration status; increased values are associated with dehydration/hypovolemia.

PATIENT MANAGEMENT

1. Administer fluids as ordered, carefully monitoring CVP and PAP for increasing trends that suggest fluid overload.
2. Administer antidiarrheal agents as ordered to help control diarrhea.
3. Administer antiemetic agents as ordered to help control vomiting and increase the patient's ability to take oral food and fluids. Anticipate administration of nutritional supplementation either parenterally or enterally. Consult with a nutritionist to assess the patient's needs.
4. Provide small portions of food more frequently. Include high-caloric, high-protein snacks. Avoid spicy or greasy foods. Cold entrees may be more palatable.
5. Low-fiber, lactulose-free, or pectin-containing formulas may help reduce diarrheal episodes.

MULTI

BURNS
Clinical Brief
Thermal, electrical, or chemical media are common causes of burns. The severity of the burn is determined by the percentage or extent of the burn wound size and the degrees or depth of the burn wound. In addition to burn depth and percentage, the patient's age, medical history, and cause and location of the burn are investigated. According to the American Burn Association, burn injuries requiring care in burn centers include the following:

Full-thickness burn > 10% BSA

Partial-thickness burn > 20% BSA and full-thickness burn > 10% BSA in adults

Burn injuries involving the face, hands, feet, perineum, genitalia, or major joints

Circumferential burns of an extremity or chest wall

Chemical, electrical, or inhalation burns

Burns associated with other major injuries

Presenting signs and symptoms
Superficial partial-thickness (first degree): Skin is red, blanches, and is painful (e.g., sunburn).

Deep partial-thickness (second degree): Involves entire epidermal layer and part of the dermis; epidermis is blistered; wound is red, shiny and wet if vesicles are broken. The wound is very painful.

Full-thickness (third degree): Involves all layers of the skin and subcutaneous tissue; the wound varies from waxy white or charred, red or brown and leathery; the area is edematous and insensitive to pain. Injury may involve muscles, tendons, or bones.

Inhalation injury: Chest tightness, hoarseness, dyspnea, tachypnea.

Physical examination
Skin: Area of body burned (Figure 5-2), depth of burn

Burns of head/neck/face/chest/mouth/nose/pharynx correlate with inhalation injury

Hallmark of smoke inhalation: hypercapnea, hypoxemia, widened alveolar-arterial oxygen gradient, and increased carboxyhemoglobin levels. Stridor, crackles, and carbonaceous sputum may be present.

Diagnostic findings
Other findings may include the following:

SBP < 90 mm Hg and HR > 120 beats/min if shock is present

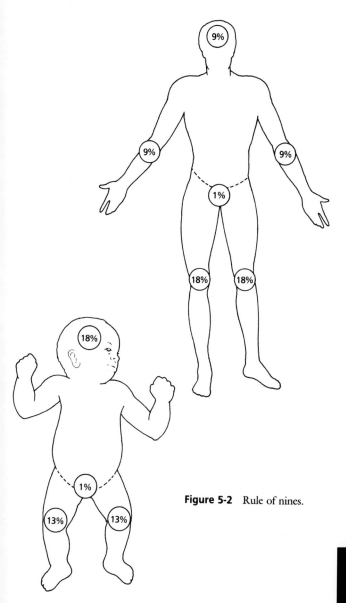

Figure 5-2   Rule of nines.

Burns can be classified as the following:

Minor: < 15% BSA
   < 2% BSA full-thickness injury
   No preexisting disease

Moderate: 15-25% BSA
   < 10% BSA full-thickness injury
   No concurrent injury
   No preexisting disease

Major: > 25% BSA
   > 10% BSA full-thickness injury
   Face, eyes, ears, hands, feet, perineum involvement
   Presence of existing disease

Acute Care Patient Management

Goals of treatment

Maintain airway and oxygenation
   Supplemental oxygen
   Intubation/mechanical ventilation
Restore intravascular volume
   Crystalloids, colloids
Control pain
   Morphine sulfate, midazolam
Maximize wound closure
   Topical antimicrobials, wound management
Detect/prevent clinical sequelae
   See Table 5-39

Priority nursing diagnoses

Impaired gas exchange
Fluid volume deficit
Altered tissue perfusion
Pain
Impaired skin integrity
Altered nutrition: less than body requirements (see p. 149)
Altered protection (see p. 145)
High risk for altered family process (see p. 150)

▶ **Impaired gas exchange** related to inhalation injury: carbon monoxide poisoning, chemical pneumonitis, and upper airway obstruction

PATIENT OUTCOMES

- Patient will be alert and oriented to person, place, and time
- Pao_2 60-100 mm Hg
- $Paco_2$ 35-45 mm Hg
- pH 7.35-7.45

TABLE 5-39 Clinical Sequelae Associated with Burns

Complications	Signs and symptoms
Burn shock (hypovolemic)	SBP < 90 mm Hg, HR > 100 beats/min, u/o < 0.5 ml/kg/hr, cool, clammy skin
Renal failure	u/o < 0.5 ml/kg/hr, steady rise in BUN, creatinine
Respiratory distress	Carbon flecks in sputum, carbon monoxide levels > 15%, RR >30/min, Pao_2 < 60 mm Hg, stridor, noisy respirations, restlessness, change in LOC
Loss of limb	Pulselessness, pain, paresthesia, paralysis
Burn wound sepsis	Purulent exudate; focal black, grey, or dark brown discoloration; hemorrhagic discoloration and vascular thrombosis of underlying fat; erythema or edema of unburned skin at the wound margins; unexpected rapid eschar separation; greater than 100,000 organism-per-gram tissue
Curling's ulcer	Blood in emesis, N/G aspirate, or stool; decreasing trend in Hgb and Hct
Septic shock	SBP < 90 mm Hg, HR >90 beats/min, RR >20/min, decreased sensorium, u/o < 30 ml/hr or < 0.5 ml/kg/hr, hypoxemia, serum lactate > 2.2 mmol/L

- O_2 sat > 90%
- Lungs clear
- RR 12-20/min, eupnea

PATIENT MONITORING

1. Continuously monitor oxygenation status with pulse oximetry (Spo_2). Be alert for effects of interventions and patient activities that may adversely affect oxygen saturation.

2. Calculate $P(a/A)o_2$ ratio to estimate intrapulmonary shunting and evaluate degree of lung dysfunction. The higher the ratio, the better the lung function.

PHYSICAL ASSESSMENT

1. Obtain BP, HR, RR q15min during the acute phase. Patients with carbon monoxide poisoning are tachycardic and tachypneic.
2. Assess for headache, confusion, n/v, and dyspnea. Note skin and mucous membranes—cherry red color reflects carbon monoxide poisoning. As the carbon monoxide level increases, the patient will become less responsive.
3. Assess the rate and depth of respirations; note stridor or noisy respirations that may indicate respiratory distress. Laryngeal edema can develop over 72 hours after the burn event. In patients with burns of the chest, carefully assess chest excursion, since burns to this area may result in hypoventilation and decreased compliance.
4. Note the presence of carbonaceous sputum, an indicator of inhalation injury.
5. Assess for signs and symptoms of hypoxia: increased restlessness, increased complaints of dyspnea, changes in LOC.
6. Assess the patient for development of clinical sequelae (see Table 5-39).

DIAGNOSTICS ASSESSMENT

1. Review carboxyhemoglobin levels for carbon monoxide reflecting smoke inhalation (normal is $< 5\%$ saturation of Hgb in nonsmokers; $< 10\%$ in smokers).
2. Review ABGs for decreasing trends in Pao_2 (hypoxemia) or pH (acidosis). O_2 sat should be $> 90\%$.
3. Review serial chest radiographs to evaluate the patient's progress or a worsening lung condition.
4. Review Hgb and Hct levels and note trends. Decreased RBCs can adversely affect oxygen-carrying capacity.

PATIENT MANAGEMENT

1. Maintain oral airway and administer supplemental oxygen as ordered. Fio_2 100% is used to treat carbon monoxide poisoning. Anticipate intubation and mechanical ventilation with PEEP for respiratory failure. (See Chapter 6, Therapeutic Modalities, for a discussion of mechanical ventilation.)
2. Anticipate escharotomies to a burned chest to improve compliance and ventilation.
3. Promote pulmonary hygiene: position the patient for

maximum chest excursion, cough and deep breathe to mobilize secretions, and encourage incentive spirometry to prevent atelectasis; chest physiotherapy and suction may be required.

4. Bronchodilators may be used to treat bronchospasm.

▶ **Fluid volume deficit** related to plasma loss, increased capillary permeability with interstitial fluid accumulation, and increased insensible water loss

PATIENT OUTCOMES
- Clear sensorium
- HR 60-100 beats/min
- SBP 90-140 mm Hg
- u/o 30-50 ml/hr or 0.5-1.0 ml/kg/hr
- Lungs clear
- Serum sodium 135-145 mEq/L
- Serum potassium 3.5-5.5 mEq/L

PATIENT MONITORING
1. Monitor fluid volume status: massive fluid shifts can occur within the first 72 hours of a burn event. Measure hourly I & O to determine fluid balance. Compare daily weights (1 kg ~ 1000 ml of fluid); a 15% to 20% weight gain within the first 72 hours can be anticipated. The diuresis phase begins approximately 48 to 72 hours after the burn event.

2. If a pulmonary artery catheter has been inserted, monitor PAWP to evaluate fluid status and detect development of pulmonary edema (PAWP > 18 mm Hg).

3. If a CVP line is indicated, frequently monitor pressure during fluid resuscitation to evaluate the patient's response to therapy and detect fluid volume overload.

4. Continuously monitor the ECG for dysrhythmias.

PHYSICAL ASSESSMENT
1. Obtain VS q15min during the acute phase to detect cardiopulmonary deterioration.

2. Assess fluid volume status: Dry mucous membranes, decreased pulse pressure, tachycardia, furrowed tongue, absent JVD, and complaints of thirst suggest hypovolemia. Bounding pulses, cough, dyspnea, and crackles suggest volume overload.

3. Assess the patient for development of clinical sequelae (see Table 5-39).

DIAGNOSTICS ASSESSMENT
1. Review serum K^+ and Na^+ levels closely during the fluid resuscitation period; either hyperkalemia or hy-

pokalemia can occur; hyponatremia is not uncommon. Electrolyte imbalances can occur as a result of loss of fluids via burns, shifts into interstitial spaces, drainage, or fluid resuscitation.

2. Review serial Hgb, Hct, osmolality, and urine specific gravity and note trends. An increase in values may indicate hypovolemia.

PATIENT MANAGEMENT

1. Fluid administration is usually instituted for burns > 20%. Administer LR as ordered. The American Burn Association (ABA) recommends 2-4 ml/kg/%BSA burned. Give the first half during the first 8 hours from the time of the burn injury and the second half during the next 16 hours. Colloids may be administered during the second 24 hours to maintain intravascular volume. As diuresis occurs, infusion rates may be decreased. Dextrose in water solutions may be used to maintain serum sodium within normal limits in the second 24 hours.

2. Blood or blood products may be administered as needed.

3. Administer potassium as ordered to replace potassium lost through the urine.

▶ **Altered tissue perfusion** related to hypovolemia, circumferential burns of extremities, and presence of myoglobin

PATIENT OUTCOMES

- Patient will be alert and oriented
- Peripheral pulses strong
- Bowel sounds present
- Absence of GI bleeding
- Gastric pH 5-7
- u/o 30-50 ml/hr or 0.5-1.0 ml/kg/hr
- SBP 90-140 mm Hg

PATIENT MONITORING

1. Measure hourly I & O and urine specific gravity to evaluate adequacy of hydration; if u/o falls below 30 ml/hr, suspect renal ischemia secondary to hypovolemia or damage to tubules by myoglobin.

2. Monitor the color of the urine; if it is a port-wine color, suspect myoglobinuria.

3. If a CVP line is indicated, continuously monitor pressure as an index of fluid volume status.

PHYSICAL ASSESSMENT

1. Assess for systemic hypoperfusion: absent/decreased peripheral pulses, cool pale skin, capillary refill < 3 sec.

2. Assess neurovascular status q15-30min the first 24 to 48 hours: pulselessness, pallor, pain, paresthesia, and paralysis can signal nerve ischemia. Damaged sensory nerve fibers may be misinterpreted as improvement in neurovascular status, when in fact a loss of a limb may be the outcome.

3. Assess GI status: test gastric pH, auscultate bowel sounds, and test stool for occult blood. Decreased perfusion to the GI system contributes to Curling's ulcer.

4. Assess the patient for development of clinical sequelae (see Table 5-39).

DIAGNOSTICS ASSESSMENT

1. Check the urinalysis for myoglobin level (myoglobin can cause tubular destruction and ATN).

2. Review serial BUN, creatinine, and potassium results for a steady rise in values, which may indicate renal failure.

3. Review Hgb and Hct levels for decreasing trends, which may suggest blood loss secondary to Curling's ulcer.

PATIENT MANAGEMENT

1. Administer fluids as ordered to optimize oxygen delivery and tissue perfusion.

2. Anticipate administration of mannitol, an osmotic diuretic, to flush kidneys if the patient has myoglobinuria.

3. Anticipate N/G intubation for abdominal distension secondary to reflex paralytic ileus, and/or antacid administration.

4. Maintain gastric pH at 5-7 with antacids and H_2 antagonists as ordered to help prevent Curling's ulcer.

5. Elevate edematous extremities to increase venous return and to decrease edema, which may adversely affect tissue perfusion. Be prepared for an escharotomy or fasciotomy to improve circulation.

6. Maintain a warmer than normal room temperature and keep wounds covered to prevent hypothermia and vasoconstriction.

Pain related to burned tissues and wound debridement

PATIENT OUTCOMES

• Pain relief

PATIENT MONITORING

None specific

PHYSICAL ASSESSMENT

1. Use a visual analogue scale (Figure 1-1) to evaluate pain and the patient's response to therapy. An increase in intensity of pain may indicate ischemia. A decrease in pain

MULTI

may be misinterpreted as an improvement, when in fact sensory nerve fibers may be damaged.

DIAGNOSTICS ASSESSMENT

None specific

PATIENT MANAGEMENT

1. Administer an analgesic as ordered (usually morphine sulfate) before debridement and at frequent intervals for controlled pain management. Pain increases catechol-amine release and the metabolic rate, which puts an added burden on an already hypermetabolic state.
2. Plan diversional activities appropriate for the patient's developmental level and the severity of burn incurred (e.g., music, television).
3. Promote relaxation through controlled breathing and guided imagery.
4. Reposition the patient frequently to promote comfort.
5. Keep partial-thickness burn wounds covered, since any stimulus to these wounds can cause pain.
6. If the open method of wound treatment is used, keeping the room warm (85° F, 29° C) and preventing drafts may help to decrease pain.

▶ **Impaired skin integrity** related to severe burns

PATIENT OUTCOMES

- T 36.5° C (97.7° F) to 38° C (100.4° F)
- Negative wound biopsy
- Healing by secondary intention or skin grafting without purulent drainage

PATIENT MONITORING

None specific

PHYSICAL ASSESSMENT

1. Obtain T q4h to monitor inflammatory response.
2. Assess the wound daily and note color, drainage, odor, and the presence of epithelial buds. Rapid eschar separa-tion, disappearance of well-defined burn margins, discol-oration, and purulent exudates are indicative of infec-tion. In skin grafts, bright red blood drainage and pool-ing of fluid will inhibit successful grafting. Check the donor site for infection development.
3. Assess the patient for development of clinical sequelae.

DIAGNOSTICS ASSESSMENT

1. Review wound biopsy reports for identification of the infecting organism (>100,000 organisms per gram tis-sue = burn wound sepsis).

2. Review serial WBC counts; silver sulfadiazine may decrease WBCs; an increase may be associated with sepsis, although the leukocytosis may be caused by the inflammatory process.

PATIENT MANAGEMENT

1. Avoid placing IV lines through burned skin. Avoid invasive lines if at all possible, or remove them as early as possible.
2. Verify tetanus prophylaxis.
3. Regulate environmental temperature to 85° F to 90° F (29° C-32° C) to avoid excess heat loss when wounds are open.
4. Wound management depends on institutional protocol:
   - Generally, wound cleansing and debridement are performed daily.
   - Strict aseptic technique is used. Hair may need to be clipped around burn wounds to prevent infection.
   - Open treatment involves exposure of the wounds; isolation technique is required.
   - Closed treatment involves covering wounds with dressings; treatment includes washing of the wound and applying dressings with a topical agent per protocol. Observe for impaired circulation caused by the dressings.
5. Anticipate a wound excision and skin grafting to speed healing, prevent contractures, and shorten convalescence.
6. Administer antibiotics as ordered when an invasive burn wound infection has been identified.
7. Anticipate nutritional support that supplies adequate protein, carbohydrate, and fat calories, zinc, vitamins, and minerals to promote tissue healing. Energy requirements may be as high as 5000 kcal/day. High-nitrogen diets by the enteral route may offer immunological benefits. The parenteral route may be required.

DISSEMINATED INTRAVASCULAR COAGULATION (DIC)

Clinical Brief

DIC is a coagulation disorder characterized by concurrent thrombus formation and hemorrhage secondary to overstimulation of the clotting cascade. It is a secondary complication of many underlying conditions (e.g., shock, sepsis, crush injuries, obstetrical complications, burns, and ARDS).

MULTI

Presenting signs and symptoms

Signs and symptoms include abdominal, back, or joint pain; bleeding from multiple orifices and mucous membranes; and a feeling of impending doom.

Physical examination

Depends on the underlying condition:

Appearance: Anxious, altered LOC

VS: HR >100 beats/min

BP < 90 mm Hg

RR > 20/min

Neurological: Restless, seizures, unresponsive

Skin: Mottled, cold fingers and toes; ecchymoses, petechiae, gingival bleeding

Cardiovascular: Tachycardia, murmurs may be noted

Pulmonary: Dyspnea, tachypnea, hemoptysis

GI: Hematemesis, melena, abdominal tenderness

Renal: u/o < 0.5 ml/kg/hr, hematuria

Other: Bleeding from any orifice

Diagnostic findings

Clinical manifestations are the basis for diagnosis. Usually sudden onset of bleeding with organ failure and unresponsive shock are suggestive of DIC. Other findings include the following:

Platelets < $150 \times 10^3/\mu l$

PT > 15 sec

PTT > 40 sec

Fibrinogen < 160 mg/dl

Fibrin split products > 8 $\mu g/ml$

Antithrombin III decreased

Blood smear shows schistocytes and burr cells

Positive protamine sulfate test results

Acute Care Patient Management

Goals of treatment

Treat primary problem

Surgery, antibiotics

Optimize oxygen delivery

Crystalloids

Supplemental oxygen/mechanical ventilation

RBCs

Positive inotropes: dopamine, dobutamine

Reverse clotting mechanism

Heparin (controversial)

Replace coagulation components

Platelets, FFP, cryoprecipitate

Correct hemostatic deficiency
   Folic acid, vitamin K
Detect/prevent clinical sequelae
   See Table 5-40
Priority nursing diagnoses
Altered tissue perfusion
Altered protection (see p. 145)
Altered nutrition: less than body requirements (see p. 149)
High risk for altered family process (see p. 150)
▶ **Altered tissue perfusion (peripheral, renal, cerebral, GI, and pulmonary)** related to concurrent thrombus formation and bleeding
PATIENT OUTCOMES
- Patient will be alert and oriented to person, place, and time
- Absence of neurological deficits
- Skin w/d
- Peripheral pulses strong
- Absence of acral cyanosis (mottled, cool toes and fingers)
- Absence of chest pain
- Absence of hemoptysis
- RR 12-20/min, eupnea
- Absence of hematemesis, melena
- Active bowel sounds
- u/o 30 ml/hr or 0.5-1.0 ml/kg/hr
- Absence of hematuria

TABLE 5-40 Clinical Sequelae Associated with DIC

Complications	Signs and symptoms
ARDS	Dyspnea, hypoxemia refractory to increases in Fio_2, cyanosis
Intracerebral bleeding	Change in sensorium, headache, seizures, extremity weakness/paralysis
GI dysfunction	Absent bowel sounds, abdominal pain, diarrhea, upper and lower GI bleeding
Renal failure	u/o < 0.5 ml/kg/hr, steady rise in creatinine
Shock	SBP <90 mm Hg, HR > 100 beats/min, patient anxious to unresponsive, cold clammy skin, u/o < 0.5 ml/kg/hr

MULTI

- Absence of pain, tenderness, redness, and venous distention in calves
- SBP 90-140 mm Hg
- MAP 70-105 mm Hg
- CI 2.5-4.0 L/min/m^2
- O_2 sat > 95%
- Svo_2 60%-80%
- Hct ~30%

PATIENT MONITORING

1. Monitor BP continuously via arterial cannulation, since cuff pressures can cause further injury and bleeding. Calculate MAP, an indicator that accurately reflects tissue perfusion. MAP < 60 mm Hg adversely affects cerebral and renal perfusion.
2. Obtain CO and calculate CI at least q8h or more frequently to evaluate the patient's progress or deterioration.
3. Calculate $\dot{D}O_2$ and $\dot{V}O_2$ to evaluate oxygen transport; inadequate oxygen delivery and consumption produce tissue hypoxia.
4. Monitor PAP and CVP hourly or more frequently to evaluate patient response to treatment. Both parameters reflect the capacity of the vascular system to accept volume and can be used to monitor for fluid overload and pulmonary edema.
5. Continuously monitor Svo_2. A decreasing trend may indicate decreased CO and increased tissue oxygen extraction.
6. Continuously monitor oxygen status with pulse oximetry. Be alert for effects of interventions and patient activities, which may adversely affect oxygen saturation.
7. Continuously monitor ECG to detect life-threatening dysrhythmias and ST-T wave changes.
8. Monitor fluid balance: record hourly I & O; include blood loss in determining fluid balance.

PHYSICAL ASSESSMENT

1. Obtain HR, RR, BP q15min to evaluate the patient's response to therapies and detect cardiopulmonary deterioration.
2. Assess peripheral pulses, capillary refill, and the color and temperature of extremities to evaluate thrombotic-ischemic changes.
3. Assess skin, mucous membranes, and all orifices for

bleeding. Test emesis, urine, stool, NG aspirate, and drainage from tubes, drains, and so on for blood. Assess invasive line sites for oozing of blood.

4. Assess for the presence of headache or any change in LOC that might suggest impaired cerebral perfusion or intracranial bleeding; check extremities for strength and movement to identify neurological involvement.

5. Assess the patient for development of clinical sequelae (see Table 5-40).

DIAGNOSTICS ASSESSMENT

1. Review coagulation studies: PT, PTT, TT, fibrinogen level, platelet count, fibrin degredation products, and factors II, V, VII, and VIII to evaluate resolution or worsening of DIC.

2. Review Hgb and Hct levels and note trends. Decreased RBCs can adversely affect oxygen-carrying capacity.

3. Review ABGs for hypoxemia and acidosis, which can signal pulmonary involvement and impaired gas exchange.

PATIENT MANAGEMENT

1. Administer blood and blood products as ordered to replace coagulation components. (See Chapter 6, Therapeutic Modalities.)

2. Administer crystalloids (LR or NS) as ordered to optimize oxygen delivery. Monitor CVP and PAWP to evaluate response to fluid resuscitation. A PAWP > 18 mmHg is associated with pulmonary edema.

3. Avoid dextran infusions for hypovolemia secondary to hemorrhage, since coagulation problems can occur and enhance the bleeding problem.

4. Heparin may be ordered in select cases. Observe the patient for increased bleeding.

5. Dopamine or dobutamine may be used to enhance contractility; dopamine may be used to improve renal and splanchic blood flow. (See Chapter 7, Pharmacology.)

6. Provide oxygen therapy as ordered.

7. Do not disturb established clots; use cold compresses or pressure to stop bleeding. Use an arterial line to minimize the number of peripheral sticks, thus minimizing thrombosis.

8. Avoid trauma and excessive manipulation of the patient to prevent further bleeding. Use gentle oral care, keep

the patient's lips moist, avoid tape on the skin, use an
electric razor, and use suction at the lowest pressure
possible.

9. Avoid aspirin products, which could potentiate bleeding.

10. Administer pharmacological agents such as folic acid
    and vitamin K as ordered to correct hemostatic deficiency.

SHOCK
Clinical Brief
Shock is a syndrome that reflects inadequate oxygen delivery
and oxygen consumption. The causes vary, as do the pathophysiological mechanisms. However, shock is a cyclic self-perpetuating condition that results in inadequate tissue perfusion, anaerobic metabolism, and the release of mediators
that damage tissues. Three major classifications of shock are
(1) hypovolemic, (2) cardiogenic, and (3) distributive (septic, anaphylactic, neurogenic).

HYPOVOLEMIC SHOCK
Clinical Brief
Hemorrhage is a major cause of hypovolemic shock. However, plasma loss and interstitial fluid accumulation (third
spacing) can also adversely reduce circulating volume and
consequently decrease oxygen availability to cells. The primary defect is decreased preload.

Presenting signs and symptoms
Appearance: Anxiety progressing to coma
BP normal to unobtainable
Palpable radial pulse reflects SBP of 80 mm Hg
Palpable femoral pulse reflects SBP of 70 mm Hg
Palpable carotid pulse reflects SBP of 60 mm Hg
HR normal to >140 beats/min
RR normal to > 35/min

Physical examination
Cardiovascular: Weak, thready pulse
Pulmonary: Deep or shallow rapid respirations, lungs usually clear
Skin: Cool, clammy skin, color pale
    Delayed/absent capillary refill
    Lips cyanotic (late sign)

Diagnostic findings
Clinical findings are the basis for diagnosis. Other findings include the following:

CI < 2 L/min/m^2

Lactate > 2 mmol/L

Svo_2 < 60%

MAP < 80 mm Hg

PAP declining trend

CVP declining trend

PAWP declining trend

Acute Care Patient Management

Goals of treatment
Reestablish intravascular volume
  Blood, blood products
  Autotransfusion
  Colloids, crystalloids
Optimize oxygen delivery
  Oxygen therapy, intubation, and mechanical ventilation
  Inotropes, vasodilators, vasopressors
Treat underlying problem
  Surgery
Detect/prevent clinical sequelae
  See Table 5-41

Priority nursing diagnoses

Altered tissue perfusion

Altered protection (see p. 145)

Altered nutrition: less than body requirements (see p. 149)

High risk for altered family process (see p. 150)

Altered tissue perfusion related to blood loss and hypotension

PATIENT OUTCOMES

- Patient will be alert and oriented to person, place, and time
- Skin w/d
- Peripheral pulses strong
- u/o 30 ml/hr or 0.5-1.0 ml/kg/hr
- Hct ~ 32%
- SBP 110-140 mm Hg
- MAP 80-105 mm Hg
- CI > 4.5 L/min/m^2
- O_2 sat > 95%
- Svo_2 60%-80%

MULTI

TABLE 5-41 Clinical Sequelae Associated with Hypovolemic Shock

Complications	Signs and symptoms
Cardiopulmonary arrest	Nonpalpable pulse, absent respirations
ARDS	Hypoxemia refractory to increases in Fio_2, decreased compliance
Acute tubular necrosis/renal failure	u/o < 0.5ml/kg/hr, steady rise in creatinine
GI dysfunction/bleeding	Blood in NG aspirate, emesis, stool; absent bowel sounds, abdominal pain, N/V, jaundice
DIC	Bleeding from puncture sites, mucous membranes; hematuria, ecchymoses; prolonged PT and PTT; decreased fibrinogen, platelets, factors V, VIII, XIII, II; increased FSP

- $\dot{D}O_2I > 600$ ml/min/m^2
- $\dot{V}O_2I > 170$ ml/min/m^2
- O_2ER 22%-30%

PATIENT MONITORING

1. Monitor BP continuously via arterial cannulation since cuff pressures are less accurate in shock states. Calculate MAP, an indicator that accurately reflects tissue perfusion. MAP < 60 adversely affects cerebral and renal perfusion.
2. Obtain CO and calculate CI at least q4h or more frequently to evaluate patient response to changes in therapies.
3. Calculate $\dot{D}O_2I$ and $\dot{V}O_2I$ to evaluate effectiveness of therapies. Inadequate oxygen delivery or consumption produces tissue hypoxia. Calculate O_2ER; a value > 35% suggests increased oxygen consumption, decreased oxygen delivery, or both.
4. Monitor PAP and CVP hourly or more frequently to evaluate patient response to treatment. Both parameters reflect the capacity of the vascular system to accept volume and can be used to monitor for fluid overload and pulmonary edema.

5. Continuously monitor Svo_2. A decreasing trend may indicate decreased CO and increased tissue oxygen extraction.
6. Continuously monitor ECG to detect life-threatening dysrhythmias or HR > 140 beats/min, which can adversely affect stroke volume.
7. Monitor hourly urine output to evaluate renal perfusion.
8. Measure blood loss (if possible) to quantify the loss and evaluate progression or improvement of the problem.

PHYSICAL ASSESSMENT
1. Obtain HR, RR, BP q15min to evaluate patient response to therapies and detect cardiopulmonary deterioration.
2. Assess mentation, skin temperature, and peripheral pulses to evaluate CO and state of vasoconstriction. Measure great toe temperature, an index of perfusion, and note trends. Normal is 28° C (82.4° F); < 22° C (77.6° F) is associated with low CO.
3. Assess the patient for development of clinical sequelae (see Table 5-41).

DIAGNOSTICS ASSESSMENT
1. Review Hgb and Hct levels and note trends. Decreased RBCs can adversely affect oxygen-carrying capacity.
2. Review lactate levels, an indicator of anaerobic metabolism. Increased levels may signal decreasing oxygen delivery or utilization.
3. Review ABGs for hypoxemia and acidosis, since these conditions can precipitate dysrhythmias and affect myocardial contractility. O_2 sat should be > 95%.
4. Review BUN, Cr, and electrolytes and note trends to evaluate renal function.

PATIENT MANAGEMENT
1. Use a large-bore (16- to 18-gauge) cannula for IVs to replace volume rapidly.
2. Administer blood and blood products as ordered to reestablish intravascular volume and improve oxygen-carrying capacity. (See Chapter 6, Therapeutic Modalities, for information on blood administration.)
3. Colloids (albumin) and crystalloids (LR or NS) can be administered in addition to blood. Monitor CVP and PAWP to evaluate response to fluid resuscitation. A PAWP > 18 mm Hg is associated with pulmonary edema.

MULTI

4. Avoid dextran infusions for hypovolemia secondary to hemorrhage, since coagulation problems can occur and enhance the bleeding problem.

5. Pharmacological agents may be used if intravasular volume is replaced, but CI, $\dot{D}O_2I$, and $\dot{V}O_2I$ are not improved. Correct acidotic state, since acidosis blocks or diminishes responsiveness to drug therapy. Inotropes (dopamine or dobutamine) may be used if HR < 130 beats/min. Vasodilators (nitroprusside or nitroglycerin) may be used to optimize CO unless MAP is < 80 mm Hg and SBP < 110 mm Hg. Vasopressors (dopamine or norepinephrine) may be used to maintain a MAP adequate for cerebral and coronary perfusion. (See Chapter 7 for emergency drug administration.)

6. Provide oxygen therapy as ordered. Anticipate intubation and mechanical ventilation if oxygenation status deteriorates or cardiopulmonary arrest ensues.

7. If the site of bleeding is known, e.g., GI bleeding, treat accordingly.

8. A pneumatic antishock garment or military antishock trousers may be used in addition to other therapies, although controversy in their use still exists.

9. Prepare the patient for surgical intervention if required.

CARDIOGENIC SHOCK
Clinical Brief
Left ventricular dysfunction resulting from myocardial infarction is the most common cause of cardiogenic shock. The loss of viable myocardium and consequently impaired contractility adversely affects stroke volume. Other causes include ventricular septal defect, papillary muscle rupture, pulmonary embolism, endstage cardiomyopathies, and valvular disorders. The primary defect in this acute circulatory failure is severe left ventricular dysfunction.

Presenting signs and symptoms
Restlessness progressing to unresponsiveness

VITAL SIGNS

HR > 100 beats/min

SBP < 80 mm Hg

RR > 20/min

Physical examination
Neurological: Agitation, restlessness progressing to unresponsiveness

Cardiovascular: Weak, thready pulses; rhythm may be irregular; S_3, S_4

Pulmonary: Crackles, rapid respirations

Skin: Cool, clammy skin, color pale, delayed capillary refill

Diagnostic findings

Clinical manifestations and hemodynamic findings are the basis for diagnosis.

CI < 1.8 L/min/m^2

PAWP >18 mm Hg

SVR > 1200 dynes/sec/cm^{-5}

PP narrowed

SI decreasing trend

LVSW decreasing trend

u/o < 0.5 ml/kg/hr

Acute Care Patient Management

Goals of treatment

Optimize oxygen delivery
  Supplemental oxygen
  Intubation and mechanical ventilation
  Morphine sulfate
  Inotropes: dopamine, dobutamine, amrinone
  Vasopressors: norepinephrine, epinephrine, phenylephrine, methoxamine hydrochloride
  Mechanical support: IABP, VAD
  ECMO
  PTCA, CABG

Reduce oxygen demand
  Morphine sulfate
  Diuretics: furosemide, bumetanide
  Vasodilators: nitroglycerin
  Mechanical support: IABP, VAD

Detect/prevent clinical sequelae
  See Table 5-42

Priority nursing diagnoses

Altered tissue perfusion

Impaired gas exchange

Altered protection (see p. 145)

High risk for altered family process (see p. 150)

Altered nutrition: less than body requirements (see p. 149)

Altered tissue perfusion related to **Decreased cardiac output** secondary to decreased contractility

PATIENT OUTCOMES

• Patient will be alert and oriented

TABLE 5-42 Clinical Sequelae Associated with Cardiogenic Shock

Complications	Signs and symptoms
Cardiopulmonary arrest	Nonpalpable pulse, absent respirations
Extension of MI	Cardiac pain, ST-T changes involving more leads
Pulmonary edema	Dyspnea, cough, frothy sputum, cyanosis
Renal failure	u/o < 0.5 ml/kg/hr, steady rise in creatinine
GI dysfunction/bleed	Blood in NG aspirate, emesis, stool; absent bowel sounds, distension

- Skin w/d
- Peripheral pulses strong
- HR 60-100 beats/min
- Absence of life-threatening dysrhythmias
- Coronary perfusion pressure 60-80 mm Hg
- u/o 30 ml/hr or 0.5-1.0 ml/kg/hr
- SBP 90-140 mm Hg
- MAP 70-105 mm Hg
- CI 2.5-4.0 L/min/m^2
- SVR < 1400 dynes/sec/cm^{-5}
- PVR < 250 dynes/sec/cm^{-5}
- O_2 sat > 95%
- Svo_2 60%-80%
- DO_2I 500-650 ml/min/m^2
- VO_2I 115-165 ml/min/m^2

PATIENT MONITORING

1. Monitor BP continuously via arterial cannulation since cuff pressures are less accurate in shock states. Calculate MAP, an indicator that accurately reflects tissue perfusion. MAP < 60 mm Hg adversely affects cerebral and renal perfusion.

2. Continuously monitor ECG to detect life-threatening dysrhythmias or HR > 140 beats/min, which can adversely affect stroke volume. Monitor for ischemia (ST-T changes) associated with decreased coronary perfusion.

Presenting signs and symptoms
SEPSIS SYNDROME
Appearance: Anxious; skin flushed, warm
VS: HR > 90 beats/min
    RR > 20/min
    BP normal
    T > 38.3° C (101° F) or < 35.5° C (96° F)
Other: Clinical evidence of an infection site
        Evidence of one organ underperfused, e.g., decreased sensorium, oliguria, hypoxemia, elevated serum lactate

Physical examination
Neurological: Anxiety or decreased level of consciousness
Cardiovascular: Full, bounding pulses
               HR > 90 beats/min
Pulmonary: Crackles may or may not be present
          Shallow, rapid respirations
Skin: Warm
     Color rubor

SEPTIC SHOCK
Signs and symptoms of sepsis syndrome, plus the following:
VS: SBP < 90 mm Hg
Other: Multiple organ involvement

Physical examination
Neurological: Unresponsive, difficult to arouse
Cardiovascular: Weak, thready pulses
Pulmonary: Crackles, wheezes, respiratory distress
Skin: Cool, clammy skin
    Color pale
Other: Evidence of multiple organ failure

Diagnostic findings
Clinical manifestations are the basis for diagnosis. Other findings include the following:

Sepsis syndrome: (hyperdynamic)	Normal or increased CO/CI SVR < 800 dynes/sec/cm^{-5} PAP decreasing trend PP widened
Septic shock: (hypodynamic)	CI < 2.2 L/min/m^2 SVR > 1300 dynes/sec/cm^{-5} PAWP > 18 mm Hg PP narrowed

MULTI

Acute Care Patient Management
Goals of treatment
Optimize oxygen delivery
  Colloids, crystalloids
  Inotropes: dobutamine
  Vasopressors: dopamine, norepinephrine, phenylephrine
  Vasodilators: nitroprusside, nitroglycerin, labetalol, pros-
    taglandin E
  Low-dose dopamine
  Intubation/mechanical ventilation
Treat underlying problem
  Antibiotics
  Surgery
Detect/prevent clinical sequelae
  See Table 5-43
Priority nursing diagnoses
Altered tissue perfusion
Impaired gas exchange
Ineffective thermoregulation
Altered protection (see p. 145)

TABLE 5-43 Clinical Sequelae Associated
with Septic Shock

Complications	Signs and symptoms
Cardiopulmonary arrest	Nonpalpable pulse, absent respirations
Multiple organ failure (MOF)	
ARDS	Hypoxemia refractory to increases in Fio_2, decreased compliance
Renal failure	u/o < 0.5 ml/kg/hr, steady rise in creatinine
GI bleed/dysfunction	Blood in NG aspirate, emesis, stool; absent bowel sounds, distention
Hepatic dysfunction	Jaundice, bilirubin > 3 mg %, rise in LFTs, decreased albumin
DIC	Bleeding from puncture sites and mucous membranes, hematuria, ecchymoses, prolonged PT and PTT; decreased fibrinogen, platelets, factors V, VIII, XIII, II; increased FSP

Altered nutrition: less than body requirements (see p. 149)
High risk for altered family process (see p. 150)

▶ **Altered tissue perfusion** related to maldistribution of blood flow and depressed myocardial function

PATIENT OUTCOMES
- Patient will be alert and oriented
- Skin w/d
- Peripheral pulses strong
- u/o 30 ml/hr or 0.5-1.0 ml/kg/hr
- SBP 90-140 mm Hg
- MAP 70-105 mm Hg
- CI ~ 4.5 L/min/m^2
- O$_2$ sat > 95%
- Svo$_2$ 60%-80%
- DO$_2$I > 600 ml/min/m^2
- VO$_2$I > 170 ml/min/m^2
- O$_2$ER 22%-30%

PATIENT MONITORING
1. Monitor BP continuously via arterial cannulation, since cuff pressures are less accurate in shock states. Calculate MAP, an indicator that accurately reflects tissue perfusion. MAP < 60 mm Hg adversely affects cerebral and renal perfusion.
2. Obtain CO and calculate CI at least q4h or more frequently to evaluate the patient's response to changes in therapies.
3. Calculate SVR and note trends; increasing values reflect a decompensating state (hypodynamic state).
4. Calculate DO$_2$I and VO$_2$I to evaluate effectiveness of therapies. Inadequate oxygen delivery or consumption produces tissue hypoxia. Calculate O$_2$ER; a value > 35% suggests increased oxygen consumption, decreased oxygen delivery, or both.
5. Monitor PAP and CVP hourly or more frequently to evaluate the patient's response to treatment. Both parameters reflect the capacity of the vascular system to accept volume and can be used to monitor for fluid overload and pulmonary edema.
6. Continuously monitor Svo$_2$. A decreasing trend may indicate decreased CO and increased tissue oxygen extraction (inadequate perfusion). Calculating Ca-vo$_2$ (arteriovenous oxygen content difference) also provides information regarding oxygen uptake at the tissue level.
7. Monitor hourly urine output to evaluate renal perfusion.

MULTI

PHYSICAL ASSESSMENT

1. Obtain HR, RR, BP q15min to evaluate patient response to therapy and detect cardiopulmonary deterioration.

2. Assess mentation, skin temperature, and peripheral pulses and the presence of cardiac or abdominal pain to evaluate CO and the state of vasoconstriction. Measure great toe temperature, an index of perfusion, and note trends. Normal is 28° C (82.4° F); < 22° C (77.6° F) is associated with low CO.

3. Assess the patient for development of clinical sequelae (see Table 5-43).

DIAGNOSTICS ASSESSMENT

1. Review ABGs for hypoxemia and acidosis, since these conditions can precipitate dysrhythmias or affect myocardial contractility. Hypoxemia refractory to increasing Fio_2 and PEEP may signal ARDS.

2. Review WBC counts for leukocytosis as the body attempts to fight infection or leukopenia as the bone marrow becomes exhausted.

3. Review culture reports for identification of the infecting pathogen.

4. Review Hgb and Hct levels and note trends. Decreased RBCs can adversely affect oxygen-carrying capacity.

5. Review lactate levels, an indicator of anaerobic metabolism. Increased levels may signal decreasing oxygen delivery.

6. Review BUN, Cr, and electrolytes and note trends to evaluate renal function.

PATIENT MANAGEMENT

1. Administer colloids (albumin) and crystalloids (LR or NS) to increase preload as ordered. Monitor CVP and PAWP to evaluate the patient's response to fluid resuscitation. A PAWP > 18 mm Hg is associated with pulmonary edema.

2. To increase oxygen transport, inotropes such as dobutamine may be required to increase myocardial contractility, stroke volume, cardiac output, and blood pressure.

3. Administer vasopressors such as dopamine, norepinephrine, or phenylephrine as ordered to oppose vasodilation. (See Chapter 7, Pharmacology, for specific drug information.)

4. Administer vasodilators, such as nitroprusside or nitroglycerin, as ordered to reduce afterload. As shock

progresses, SVR increases, and these agents can increase stroke volume and decrease myocardial oxygen consumption secondary to afterload reduction.

5. Correct an acidotic state since acidosis blocks or diminishes responsiveness to drug therapy.

6. Provide oxygen therapy as ordered. Anticipate intubation and mechanical ventilation if the oxygenation status deteriorates or cardiopulmonary arrest ensues.

7. Administer antibiotics as ordered. Antibiotic therapy may not be effective in the first 48 to 72 hours; thus interventions to support BP and oxygenation are required.

8. Treat dysrhythmias according to ACLS.

9. Prepare the patient for surgical intervention if required (e.g., abscess drainage).

▶ **Impaired gas exchange** related to increased pulmonary vascular resistance, pulmonary interstitial edema, and pulmonary microthrombi

PATIENT OUTCOMES
• Patient will be alert and oriented to person, place, and time
• pH 7.35-7.45
• Pao_2 60-100 mm Hg
• $Paco_2$ 35-45 mm Hg
• O_2 sat > 90%
• RR 12-20/min, eupnea
• Lungs clear

PATIENT MONITORING
1. Continuously monitor oxygenation status with pulse oximetry (Spo_2). Be alert for effects of interventions and patient activities, which may adversely affect oxygen saturation.

2. Continuously monitor PA systolic pressure, since hypoxia can increase sympathetic tone and increase pulmonary vasoconstriction.

PHYSICAL ASSESSMENT
1. Obtain HR, RR, BP q15min to evaluate patient response to therapy and detect cardiopulmonary deterioration.

2. Assess respiratory status: RR > 30 beats/min suggests impending respiratory dysfunction. Note the use of accessory muscles and respiratory pattern. Note the presence of breath sounds and adventitious sounds, suggesting worsening pulmonary congestion.

MULTI

3. Assess for signs and symptoms of hypoxia: increased restlessness, increased complaints of dyspnea, changes in LOC. Cyanosis is a late sign.
4. Assess the patient for development of clinical sequelae.

DIAGNOSTICS ASSESSMENT

1. Review ABGs for Pao_2 refractory to increases in Fio_2 that may suggest ARDS. O_2 sat should be > 90%.
2. Review serial chest radiographs to evaluate patient progress or worsening lung condition.
3. Review Hgb and Hct levels and note trends. Decreased RBCs can adversely affect oxygen-carrying capacity.

PATIENT MANAGEMENT

1. Provide supplemental oxygen as ordered. If the patient develops respiratory distress, be prepared for intubation and mechanical ventilation (see Chapter 6).
2. When hemodynamically stable, promote pulmonary hygiene: C & DB and reposition the patient q2h to mobilize secretions and prevent atelectasis.
3. Minimize oxygen demand by decreasing anxiety, fever, shivering, and pain.
4. Position patient for maximum chest excursion and comfort.

▶ **Ineffective thermoregulation** related to infecting pathogen

PATIENT OUTCOMES

• T 36.5° C (97.7° F) to 38° C (100.4° F)
• Absence of shivering

PATIENT MONITORING

1. Continuously monitor core temperature for any changes. T > 38.3° C (101° F) is common in sepsis syndrome; hypothermia, 35.6° C (96° F), may develop as shock progresses.

PHYSICAL ASSESSMENT

1. Obtain HR and BP during temperature spikes; obtain T after administering antipyretics to evaluate effectiveness.
2. Assess skin temperature and presence of diaphoresis. Note any chills or shivering, which increases oxygen demand.
3. Assess the patient for the development of clinical sequelae (see Table 5-43).

DIAGNOSTICS ASSESSMENT

1. Review culture reports for identification of infecting pathogen.
2. Review WBC counts; an increase suggests the body's

attempt to fight the infection; a decrease suggests bone marrow exhaustion, common in hypodynamic state.

PATIENT MANAGEMENT

1. Regulate environmental temperature to help maintain patient temperature between 36.5° C (97.7° F) to 38° C (100.4° F). (See Thermal regulation in Chapter 6.)
2. Apply extra bed linens or blankets during hypothermia and shivering episodes.
3. Remove extra linens during hyperthermia episodes.
4. Tepid sponge baths or a cooling blanket may be needed during hyperthermia episodes.
5. Administer antipyretics as ordered to reduce fever.
6. Administer antibiotics as ordered to eradicate infection.

NEUROGENIC SHOCK

Clinical Brief

Spinal cord injury and anesthesia can cause neurogenic shock. However, emotional experiences such as fright or stress, severe pain, or hyperinsulinism (although rare) may cause neurogenic shock. The primary defect in neurogenic shock is loss of sympathetic control of vasomotor tone and consequently maldistribution of blood flow. Venous and arterial dilation occur, resulting in a relative reduction in circulatory volume and blood flow to the brain, which causes the patient to faint. Neurogenic shock is usually of short duration and spontaneously resolves itself, unless it is associated with a spinal cord injury. (See Spinal cord injury, p. 155.)

Presenting signs and symptoms

HR < 50 beats/min
SBP < 90 mm Hg
Skin w/d

Physical examination

Neurological: May be restless to unresponsive
With spinal shock, loss of motor/sensory activity below lesion
Cardiovascular: Bradycardia
Hypotension
Skin: Warm, dry

Diagnostic findings

Clinical manifestations are the basis for diagnosis.

Acute Care Patient Management

See Spinal cord injury, p. 155
Correct the underlying cause
  e.g., stop anesthesia

MULTI

Optimize oxygen delivery
  Lower patient's head
  Crystalloids
Priority nursing diagnoses
Altered tissue perfusion: cerebral
Altered protection (see p. 145)
▶ **Altered tissue perfusion: cerebral** related to relative hypovolemia secondary to massive vasodilation and venous pooling

PATIENT OUTCOMES
- Patient will be alert and oriented to person, place, and time
- SBP 90-140 mm Hg
- HR 60-100 beats/min

PATIENT MONITORING
1. Continuously monitor ECG to identify changes in HR and the development of dysrhythmias.
2. Continuously monitor arterial BP (if available). Calculate MAP; a MAP < 60 mm Hg adversely affects cerebral and renal perfusion.
3. Monitor hourly urine output to evaluate end-organ perfusion.
4. Continuously monitor oxygenation status with pulse oximetry (if available).

PHYSICAL ASSESSMENT
1. Obtain VS q15min during acute phase to evaluate resolution of condition or patient response to therapy.
2. Assess mentation to evaluate cerebral perfusion.

DIAGNOSTICS ASSESSMENT
1. Review ABGs for hypoxemia and acidosis.

PATIENT MANAGEMENT
1. Placing the patient in a horizontal position usually promotes adequate venous return and sufficient CO to prevent progressive shock.
2. IV fluids may be ordered to increase intravascular volume and improve oxygen delivery.
3. Vasopressors are rarely used. Cardiopulmonary support should be continued until vasomotor tone has returned.

ANAPHYLACTIC SHOCK

Clinical Brief

Drugs, blood, and blood products can cause anaphylactic reactions. In addition, insect bites and vaccines can also produce this respiratory and circulatory emergency. A stimulus triggers a release of biochemical mediators, which causes a change in vascular permeability, leading to fluid accumulation in the interstitial spaces and a decreased circulating volume. Increased bronchial reactivity produces bronchial edema and bronchoconstriction, causing alveolar hypoventilation and respiratory distress.

Presenting signs and symptoms

Signs and symptoms include chest tightness, a feeling of impending doom, and itching.

Appearance: Anxiety, restlessness

VS: BP normal to hypotensive

    HR >100 beats/min

    RR rapid

Physical examination

Neurological: Anxiety progressing to unresponsiveness

Cardiovascular: Tachycardia with ectopic beats

Pulmonary: Stridor, wheezes, crackles

Skin: Erythema, urticaria, flushing, angioedema

Diagnostic findings

Clinical manifestations are the basis for diagnosis.

Acute Care Patient Management

Goals of treatment

Maintain airway

    Oxygen, intubation/mechanical ventilation

    Aminophylline

    Epinephrine

Optimize oxygen delivery

    Colloids (albumin)

    Epinephrine

    Vasopressors: dopamine, norepinephrine

Priority nursing diagnoses

Impaired gas exchange

Altered tissue perfusion

Altered protection (see p. 145)

High risk for altered family process (see p. 150)

▶ **Impaired gas exchange** related to bronchoconstriction, pulmonary edema, or obstructed airway

PATIENT OUTCOMES

- Patient will be alert and oriented to person, place, and time
- Pao_2 80-100 mm Hg
- pH 7.35-7.45
- $Paco_2$ 35-45 mm Hg
- O_2 sat >95%

MULTI

- Lungs clear
- RR 12-20/min, eupnea

PATIENT MONITORING

1. Continuously monitor oxygenation status via pulse oximetry (Spo_2).

PHYSICAL ASSESSMENT

1. Obtain Vs q15min during the acute phase.
2. Assess lung sounds and respiratory rate and depth to evaluate the degree of respiratory distress. Decreased air movement indicates severe respiratory distress.
3. Assess for signs and symptoms of hypoxia: increased restlessness, increased complaints of dyspnea, changes in LOC. Cyanosis is a late sign.

DIAGNOSTICS ASSESSMENT

1. Review ABGs to evaluate hypoxemia and acid-base status. Hypoxemia and acidosis are risk factors for dysrhythmias. O_2 sat should be $> 95\%$.

PATIENT MANAGEMENT

1. Establish/maintain an airway and provide supplemental oxygen. Endotracheal intubation or tracheostomy may be required.
2. Administer epinephrine 3-5 ml of 1:10,000 solution (0.3-0.5 mg) to reverse bronchoconstriction and hypotension. May be administered via ET tube if unable to establish IV access.
3. Administer aminophylline as ordered to relieve bronchoconstriction. Assess lungs for air movement and resolution of wheezes.
4. Position the patient for maximum chest excursion.
5. Administer CPR and follow the ACLS protocol should cardiopulmonary arrest occur.
6. Diphenhydramine and corticosteroids may be administered to decrease or control edema.

▶ **Altered tissue perfusion** related to decreased circulating volume associated with permeability changes and loss of vasomotor tone

PATIENT OUTCOMES

- Patient will be alert and oriented to person, place, and time
- Skin w/d
- Peripheral pulses strong
- u/o 30 ml/hr or 0.5-1.0 ml/kg/hr
- Absence of edema

- SBP 90-140 mm Hg
- MAP 70-105 mm Hg
- O_2 sat >95%

PATIENT MONITORING

1. Monitor BP continuously via arterial cannulation, since cuff pressures are less accurate in shock states. Calculate MAP, an indicator that accurately reflects tissue perfusion. MAP < 60 mm Hg adversely affects cerebral and renal perfusion.
2. Continuously monitor ECG to detect life-threatening dysrhythmias or HR > 140 beats/min, which can adversely affect stroke volume.
3. Continuously monitor oxygenation status via pulse oximetry (Spo_2).
4. Monitor hourly urine output to evaluate renal perfusion.
5. Monitor PAP and CVP (if available) hourly or more frequently to evaluate the patient's response to treatment. Both parameters reflect the capacity of the vascular system to accept volume and can be used to monitor for fluid overload and pulmonary edema.
6. Calculate SVR q8h or more frequently to evaluate afterload. SVR should increase with epinephrine administration.
7. Obtain CO and calculate CI at least q8h or more frequently to evaluate the patient's response to changes in therapies.

PHYSICAL ASSESSMENT

1. Obtain HR, RR, BP q15min to evaluate patient response to therapies and detect cardiopulmonary deterioration.
2. Assess mentation, skin temperature, and peripheral pulses to evaluate CO and state of vasoconstriction.
3. Assess periorbital area, lips, hands, feet, and genitalia to evaluate interstitial fluid accumulation.

DIAGNOSTICS ASSESSMENT

1. Review lactate levels, an indicator of anaerobic metabolism. Increased levels may signal decreasing oxygen delivery.
2. Review ABGs for hypoxemia and acidosis, since these conditions can precipitate dysrhythmias and affect myocardial contractility.
3. Review BUN, Cr, and electrolytes and note trends to evaluate renal function.

MULTI

PATIENT MANAGEMENT

1. Administer colloids (albumin) or crystalloids (LR) as ordered to restore intravascular volume. Monitor CVP and PAWP to evaluate response to fluid resuscitation. A PAWP > 18 mm Hg is associated with pulmonary edema.
2. Pharmacological agents such as dopamine or dobutamine may be used to improve cardiac contractility when intravascular volume is replaced. Correct an acidotic state, since acidosis blocks or diminishes responsiveness to drug therapy.
3. Vasoconstrictors such as norepinephrine or methoxamine hydrochloride may be used to oppose vasodilation.
4. Provide oxygen therapy as ordered. Anticipate intubation and mechanical ventilation if the oxygenation status deteriorates or cardiopulmonary arrest ensues.

BIBLIOGRAPHY

1. Allaire M: Implications of administering drugs in renal insufficiency, Focus 13(1):46, 1986.
2. Alspach JG and Williams SM: Core curriculum for critical care nursing, ed 3, Philadelphia, 1985, WB Saunders Co.
3. American Association of Neuroscience Nurses: Core curriculum for neuroscience nursing, vol I and II, Chicago, 1984, The Association.
4. American College of Surgeons: Thoracic trauma. In advanced trauma life support course for physicians manual, Chicago, 1989, The College.
5. American Heart Association: Adjuncts for airway control, ventilation, and supplemental oxygen, Dallas, 1987, The Association.
6. American Nurses Association and Association of Neuroscience Nurses: Neuroscience nursing practice: process and outcome criteria for selected diagnoses, Kansas City, 1986, The Association.
7. Ardrogue H, Barrero J, Ryan J and Dolson G: Diabetic ketoacidosis: a practical approach, Hosp Pract 24(2):83-112, 1989.
8. Atkins JM: New option: automated defibrillation for sudden cardiac death, Contemp Intern Med Jan 1990, 11-22.
9. Balk RA and Bone RC: Mechanical ventilation. In Bone RC, George RB and Hudson LD, editors: Acute respiratory failure, New York, 1987, Churchill Livingston, Inc.
10. Barone JE and Snyder AB: Treatment strategies in shock: use of oxygen transport measurements, Heart Lung 20(1):81-85, 1991.

11. Bayley E: Wound healing in the patient with burns, Nurs Clin North Am 25(1):205-222, 1990.
12. Beare PG, Rahr VA and Ronshausen CA: Nursing implications of diagnostic tests, ed 2, Philadelphia, 1985, JB Lippincott Co.
13. Bevan N: Nursing care of the patient with unilateral lung injury, Crit Care Nurse 10(7):85-88, 1990.
14. Blake, P: Precision moves that counter cardiogenic shock, RN May, 52-58, 1989.
15. Bracken MB and others: A randomized, controlled trial of methylprednisolone or naloxone in the treatment of acute spinal-cord injury: results of the second national acute spinal cord injury study, N Engl J Med 1405(2):322, 1990.
16. Bradley R: Adult respiratory distress syndrome, Focus Crit Care 14(5):48, 1987.
17. Braunwald E: Pericardial disease. In Braunwald E and others, editors: Harrison's principles of internal medicine, New York, 1987, McGraw-Hill Book Co.
18. Bridker NS and Kirschenbaum MA, editors: The kidney: diagnosis and management, New York, 1984, John Wiley & Sons.
19. Brundage DJ: Nursing management of renal problems, ed 2, St Louis, 1980, The CV Mosby Co.
20. Bryan CL: Classification of respiratory failure. In Kirby RR and Taylor RW, editors: Respiratory failure, Chicago, 1986, Year Book Medical Publishers, Inc.
21. Caine R: Families in crisis: making the critical difference. Focus Crit Care, 16(3):184-189, 1989.
22. Carroll-Johnson RM, editor: Classification of nursing diagnoses: proceedings of the eighth conference, Philadelphia, 1989, JB Lippincott Co.
23. Caspar W, Barbier DD and Klara PM: Anterior cervical fusion and caspar plate stabilization for cervical trauma, Neurosurgery 491(4):25, 1989.
24. Clinical Practice Committee: Outcome criteria and nursing diagnosis in ESRD patient care planning. I. Conservative management, ANNA J 14:36, 1987.
25. Cooper PR: Head trauma, Neurosurg Consult 1(6):1, 1990.
26. Currie RB: Pulmonary embolism. In Kirby RR and Taylor RW, editors: Respiratory failure, Chicago, 1986, Year Book Medical Publishers, Inc.
27. Dallen JE: Diseases of the aorta. In Braunwald E and others, editors: Harrison's principles of internal medicine, New York, 1987, McGraw-Hill Book Co.
28. Delaney MD, Spagnolo SV and Medinger A: Life-threatening pneumonia. In Spagnolo SV and Medinger A, editors: Handbook of pulmonary emergencies, New York, 1986, Plenum Medical Book Co.

29. Demling R: Management of the burn patient. In Shoemaker W. and others, editors: Textbook of critical care, ed 2, Philadelphia 1989, WB Saunders Co.

30. Devault G: Hypertensive emergencies: pathogenesis, diagnosis, therapy, J Crit Illness 5(8):802-814, 1990.

31. Devault G: Therapy in hypertensive emergencies. I. Vasodilators and sympatholytics, J Crit Illness 5(9):973-988, 1990.

32. Devita M and Greenbaum D: The critically ill patient with the acquired immunodeficiency syndrome. In Shoemaker W and others, editors: Textbook of critical care, ed 2, Philadelphia, 1989, WB Saunders Co.

33. Ditchek T and Steiner RM: Radiologic diagnosis of acute cardiopulmonary disorders in the critical care unit. In Applefeld JJ and Linberg SE, editors: Acute respiratory care, Boston, 1988, Blackwell Scientific Publications.

34. Dix-Sheldon DK: Pharmocologic management of myocardial ischemia, J Cardiovasc Nurs 3(4):17-30, 1989.

35. Doyle JE: The person with lower extremity arterial occlusive disease. In Guzetta CE and Dossey BM, editors: Cardiovascular nursing: bodymind tapestry, St Louis, 1984, The CV Mosby Co.

36. Doyle JE: Treatment modalities in peripheral vascular disease, Nurs Clin North Am 21:241, 1986.

37. Drummond BL: Preventing increased intracranial pressure: nursing care can make the difference, Focus Crit Care 116(2):17, 1990.

38. Edwards JD: Practical application of oxygen transport principles, Crit Care Med 18(1):S45-S48, 1990.

39. Ehrmann D and Sarne D: Early identification of thyroid storm and myxedema, J Crit Illness 3(3):111-118, 1988.

40. Emde KL and Searle LD: Current practices with thrombolytic therapy, J Cardiovasc Nurs 4(1):11-21, 1989.

41. Emergency Nurse's Association: Chest trauma. In Rea R, editor: Trauma nursing core course provider manual, Chicago, 1986, Award Printing Corp.

42. Enger E and Schwertz DW: Mechanisms of myocardial ischemia, J Cardiovasc Nurs 3(4):1-15, 1989.

43. Esparaz B and Green D: Disseminated intravascular coagulation, Crit Care Nurs Q 13(2):7-13, 1990.

44. Fain JA and Amato-Vealy E: Acute pancreatitis: a gastrointestinal emergency, Crit Care Nurse 8(5):47-60, 1989.

45. Gabrilove JL: Adrenocortical insufficiency, Hosp Med (supplement) 25(4), 1988.

46. Galambos MR and Galambos JT: How to cope with bleeding esophageal varices, J Crit Med 5(6):603, 1990.

47. Gordon D and Tedesco F: Systemic manifestations of acute pancreatitis, J Crit Illness 2(3):77-80, 1987.

48. Gouge T: Emergency: peritonitis, Hosp Med (supplement), April, 1988, 35-53.

49. Griffin K and Bidani A: How to manage disorders of sodium and water balance, J Crit Illness 5(10):1054-1084, 1990.

50. Gross D, Parris A and Safai B: Update on AIDS, Hosp Med 25(5):19-47, 1989.

51. Halloran T: Nursing responsibilities in endocrine emergencies. Crit Care Nurs Q 13(3):81, 1990.

52. Hansbrough J: Burn wound sepsis, J Intensive Care Med 2(6):313-327, 1987.

53. Hickey, JV: The clinical practice of neurological and neurosurgical nursing, ed 2, Philadelphia, 1987, JB Lippincott Co.

54. Hickey M: What are the needs of families of critically ill patients? Heart Lung 19(4):401-415, 1990.

55. Holloway NM: Nursing the critically ill adult, ed 3, Menlo Park, Calif, 1988, Addison-Wesley Publishing Co.

56. Holloway NM: Critical care care plans, Springhouse, Pa, 1989, Springhouse Publishers.

57. Houston M: Pathophysiology of shock, Crit Care Nurs Clin North Am 2(2):143-150, 1990.

58. Hoyt N: Preventing septic shock: infection control in the intensive care unit, Crit Care Nurs Clin North Am 2(2):287-297, 1990.

59. Hudak CM, Gallo BM and Benz JJ: Critical care nursing: a holistic approach, ed 5, Philadelphia, 1990, JB Lippincott Co.

60. Hunt WE and Hess RM: Surgical risk as related to time of intervention in the repair of intracranial aneurysms, J Neurosurg 14:28, 1968.

61. Hurn PD: Thoracic injuries. In Cardona VD and others, editors: Trauma nursing from resuscitation through rehabilitation, Philadelphia, 1988, WB Saunders Co.

62. Ingbar S and Braverman L: The thyroid, ed 5, Philadelphia, 1986, JB Lippincott Co.

63. Isley W: Thyroid disorders, Crit Care Nurs Q 13(3):39-49, 1990.

64. Isley W: Serum sodium concentration abnormalities, Crit Care Nurs Q Vol 13(3):82-88, 1990.

65. Jacoby AG and Wiegman MV: Cardiovascular complications of intravenous vasopressin therapy, Focus Crit Care 17(1):63, 1990.

66. Johanson BC, Wells SJ, Hoffmeister D and Dungca CU: Standards for critical care, ed 3, St Louis, 1988, The CV Mosby Co.

67. Kandel G: Management of nonvariceal upper GI hemmorrhage, Hosp Pract 25(1):167-184, 1990.

68. Karb VB: Electrolyte abnormalities and drugs which commonly cause them, J Neurosc Nurs 21:125, 1989.

69. Keck S, Anderson C and Rieth J: Cardiac tamponade: an initial study of a predictive tool, Heart Lung 12:505-509, 1983.

70. Kenner CV, Guzzetta CE and Dossey BM: Critical care nursing: body-mind-spirit, Boston, 1981, Little, Brown & Co.

71. Kenner CV, Guzzetta CE and Dossey BM: Critical care nursing: body-mind-spirit, ed 2, Boston, 1985, Little, Brown & Co.

72. Kinney MR, Packa DR and Dunbar SB: AACN'S clinical reference for critical-care nursing, ed 2, New York, 1988, McGraw-Hill Book Co.

73. Kirby R, Taylor R and Civetta J: Pocket companion of critical care: immediate concerns, Philadelphia, 1990, JB Lippincott Co.

74. Kitabchi A and Rumbak M. The management of diabetic emergencies, Hosp Pract 24(6):129-160,

75. Kocan MJ: Pulmonary considerations in the critical care phase. In Sullivan J, editor: Spinal cord injury, Crit Care Nurs Clin North Am 369(3):2, 1990.

76. Kohler RB: Selecting antibiotics in eight special pneumonia settings, J Resp Dis 11(10):918, 1990.

77. Kopitsky RG and Genton RE: Myocardial and valvular heart diseases. In Dunagin WC and Ridner ML, editors: Manual of medical therapeutics, Boston, 1989, Little, Brown & Co.

78. Lancaster LE: The patient with end stage renal disease, ed 2, New York, 1984, John Wiley & Sons.

79. Lee L and Bates E: Management of cardiogenic shock complicating acute myocardial infarction, Pract Cardiol 15(11):66-73, 1989.

80. Leste GW: Nondialytic treatment of established acute renal failure, Crit Care Q 1(2):11, 1978.

81. Levitzky MG, Cairo JM and Hall SM: Introduction to respiratory care, Philadelphia, 1990, WB Saunders Co.

82. Linton AL: Hypertensive crisis. In Sibbald WJ, editor: Synopsis of critical care, Baltimore, 1988, Williams & Wilkins Co.

83. Manifold SL: Aneurysmal SAH: cerebral vasospasm and early repair, Crit Care Nurse 62(8):10, 1990.

84. Markovchich VJ: Acute pericardial tamponade. In Rosen P and others, editors: Emergency medicine: concepts and clinical practice, St Louis, 1988, The CV Mosby Co.

85. Mars DR and Treloar D: Acute tubular necrosis—pathophysiology and treatment, Heart Lung 13:194, 1984.

86. Martin, L. Nursing implications of today's burn care techniques, RN 52(5):26-33, 1989.

87. McCormac M: Managing hemorrhagic shock, Am J Nurs 90(8):22-27, 1990.

88. McVan B: Respiratory care handbook, Springhouse, Pa, 1989, Springhouse Publishers.

89. Meijs C: Care of the family of the ICU patient, Crit Care Nurse 9(8):42-45, 1989.

90. Metheny NM and Snively WD: Nurses' handbook of fluid balance, ed 4, Philadelphia, 1983, JB Lippincott Co.

91. Meyer FB: Calcium antagonists and vasospasm. In Mayberg MR, editor: Neurosurg Clin North Am 367(2):1, 1990.

92. Micon L and others: Rupture of the distal thoracic esophagus following blunt trauma: case report, J Trauma 30(2):214, 1990.

93. Minamoto G and Armstrong D: Combating infections in patients with AIDS, J Crit Illness 1(9):37-48, 1986.

94. Moorhouse M, Geissler A and Doenges M: Critical care plans: guidelines for patient care, Philadelphia, 1987, FA Davis Co.

95. Mosley S: Inhalation injury: a review of the literature, Heart Lung 17(1):3-9, 1988.

96. Muizelaar JP: Perioperative management of subarachnoid hemorrhage, Contemp Neurosurg 1(17):12, 1990.

97. Munoz S and Maddrey W: Major complications of acute and chronic liver disease, Gastroenterol Clin North Am 17(2):265-281, 1988.

98. Newell DW and Winn R: Transcranial Doppler in cerebral vasospasm. In Mayberg MR, editor: Neurosurg Clin North Am 319(2):1, 1990.

99. Norris MKG: Acute tubular necrosis: preventing complications, DCCN 8(1):16, 1989.

100. Papadopoulos S and Sonntag V: Casper plate instrumentation, Perspectives Neurol Surg 87(1):1, 1990.

101. Parrillo JE: Cardiomyopathies: pathogenesis and treatment in a critical care environment. In Shoemaker and others, editors: Textbook of critical care, Philadelphia, 1989, WB Saunders Co.

102. Perdew S: Facts about AIDS: a guide for health care providers, Philadelphia, 1990, JB Lippincott Co.

103. Perez R and Francis PB: Acute respiratory failure in COPD: today's therapeutic approaches, J Crit Illness 3(7):12-28, 1988.

104. Petty TL: Adult respiratory distress syndrome. In Mitchell RS and Petty TL, editors: Synopsis of clinical pulmonary disease, ed 4, St Louis, 1989, The CV Mosby Co.

105. Petty TL and Nett LM: Rational respiratory therapy, New York, 1988, Thieme Medical Publishers, Inc.

106. Pierce J, Wilkerson E and Griffiths S: Acute esophageal bleeding and endoscopic injection sclerotherapy, Crit Care Nurse 13(9):67-72, 1990.

MULTI

107. Pierson DJ: Pneumonia. In Luce JM and Pierson DJ, editors: Critical care medicine, Philadelphia, 1988, WB Saunders Co.

108. Plum F and Posner J: The diagnosis of stupor and coma, ed 3, Philadelphia, 1980, FA Davis Co.

109. Pollak VE and others: Ancrod, a safe thrombolytic agent, causes rapid thrombolysis in acute stroke, Clin Res 37(2):549A, 1989.

110. Pontoppidan H, Geffin B and Lowenstein E: Acute respiratory failure in the adult, N Engl J Med 287:690, 1972.

111. Potts JR: Acute pancreatitis. In Sawyers JL and Williams LF, editors: Surg Clin North Am, The acute abdomen 68(2):281, April 1988 Philadelphia, WB Saunders Co.

112. Rakita L and Vrobel TR: Electrocardiography in critical care medicine. In Shoemaker WC and others, editors: Textbook of critical care, ed 2, Philadelphia, 1989, WB Saunders Co.

113. Ram CV and Hyman B: Hypertensive crises, J Intensive Care Med 2(3):151-162, 1987.

114. Randall E: Recognizing cardiac tamponade, J Cardiovasc Nurs 3(3):42-51, 1989.

115. Reasner C: Adrenal disorders, Crit Care Nurs Q 13(3):67-73, 1990.

116. Reedy J and others: Mechanical cardiopulmonary support for refractory cardiogenic shock, Part 1, Heart Lung 19(5):514-524, 1990.

117. Richard CJ: Comprehensive nephrology nursing, Boston, 1986, Little, Brown & Co.

118. Roberts S: Behavioral concepts and the critically ill patient, ed 2, Norwalk, Ct, 1986, Appleton-Century-Crofts.

119. Robichaud A: Alteration in gas exchange related to body position, Crit Care Nurse 10(1):56-58, 1990.

120. Rohatgi P: Catastrophic pleural disease. In Spagnolo SV and Medinger A, editors: Handbook of pulmonary emergencies, New York, 1986, Plenum Medical Book Co.

121. Rosamond TL and Fields LE: Hypertension. In Dunagin WC and Ridner ML, editors: Manual of medical therapeutics, Boston, 1989, Little, Brown & Co.

122. Ruppel G: Manual of pulmonary function tests, ed 4, St Louis, 1986, The CV Mosby Co.

123. Sabo CE and Michael SR: Diabetic ketoacidosis: pathophysiology, nursing diagnosis, and nursing intervention, Focus Crit Care 16(1):21, 1989.

124. Sahn SA: Pneumothorax and pneumomediastinum. In Mitchell RS and Petty TL, editors: Synopsis of clinical pulmonary disease, ed 4, St Louis, 1989, The CV Mosby Co.

125. Satler LF and Rackley CE: The medical emergency of cardiac tamponade: recognition and management. Cardiovasc Clin 16(3):181-189, 1986.

126. Schrier RW and Briner VA: The differential diagnosis of hyponatremia, Hosp Pract 25(9A):29-37, 1990.
127. Sheehy SB, Marvin JA and Jimmeson CL: Manual of clinical trauma care the first hour, St Louis, 1989, The CV Mosby Co.
128. Sheldon RL: Clinical application of the chest radiograph. In Wilkins RL, Sheldon RL and Krider SJ, editors: Clinical assessment in respiratory care, St Louis, 1990, The CV Mosby Co.
129. Sherman DW: Managing an acute head injury, Nurs 90, 46(4):20, 1990.
130. Shoemaker W: Therapy of shock based on pathophysiology, monitoring and outcome prediction, Crit Care Med (supplement) 18(1):S19-S25, 1990.
131. Shoemaker WC and others: Textbook of critical care, ed 2, Philadelphia, 1989, WB Saunders Co.
132. Sibbald WJ: Pulmonary edema. In Sibbald WJ, editor: Synopsis of critical care, Baltimore, 1988, Williams & Wilkins Co.
133. Sonntag VKH and Hadley MN: Management of nonodontoid upper cervical spine injuries. In Management of posttraumatic spinal instability, Park Ridge, Illinois, 1990, American Association of Neurological Surgeons.
134. Stanik J: Caring for the family of the critically ill surgical patient, Crit Care Nurse 10(1):43-47, 1990.
135. Stanley R: Drug therapy of heart failure, J Cardiovasc Nurs 4(3):17-34, 1989.
136. Stillwell S and Randall E: Pocket guide to cardiovascular care, St Louis, 1990, The CV Mosby Co.
137. Summers G: The clinical and hemodynamic presentation of the shock patient, Crit Care Nurs Clin North Am 2(2):161-166, 1990.
138. Szwed JJ: Pathophysiology of acute renal failure: rationale for signs and symptoms, Crit Care Q 1(2):1, 1978.
139. Taber J: Nutrition in HIV infection, Am J Nurs 89(11):1446-1451, 1989.
140. Talbot L and Meyers-Marquardt M: Pocket guide to critical care assessment, St Louis, 1989, The CV Mosby Co.
141. Taylor RW: The adult respiratory distress syndrome. In Kirby RR and Taylor RW, editors: Respiratory failure, Chicago, 1986, Year Book Medical Publishers, Inc.
142. Thelan LA, Davie JK and Urden LD: Textbook of critical care nursing, St Louis, 1990, The CV Mosby Co.
143. Thompson J and others, editors: Mosby's manual of clinical nursing, ed 2, 1989, The CV Mosby Co.
144. Timerding BL and others: Stroke patient evaluation in the emergency department before pharmacologic therapy, Am J Emergency Med 11(1):7, 1989.

MULTI

145. Tobin MJ: Essentials of critical care medicine, New York, 1989, Churchill Livingstone, Inc.

146. Turner DA, Tracy J and Haines SJ: Risk of late stroke and survival following carotid endarterectomy procedures for symptomatic patients, J Neurosurg 193(2):73, 1990.

147. Vasbinder-Dillon D: Understanding mechanical ventilation, Crit Care Nurse 8(7):42, 1988.

148. Vellman WP and Drake TR: Aortic aneurysms. In Rosen P and others, editors: Emergency medicine: concepts and clinical practice, St Louis, 1988, The CV Mosby Co.

149. Vesely D and Bone R: Coping with hyperalimentation-induced hyperosmolar nonketotic coma, J Crit Illness 2(6):38-48, 1987.

150. Vincent J-L and Van der Linden P: Septic shock: particular type of acute circulatory failure, Crit Care Med (supplement) 18(1):S70-S74, 1990.

151. Vukich D and Markovchich V: Pulmonary and chest wall injuries. In Rosen P and others, editors: Emergency medicine: concepts and clinical practice, St Louis, 1988, The CV Mosby Co.

152. Walleck CA: Neurological considerations in the critical care phase. In Sullivan J, editor: Spinal cord injury, Crit Care Nurs Clin North Am 357(3):2, 1990.

153. Williams SM: The pulmonary system. In Alspach JG and Williams SM, editors: Core curriculum for critical care nursing, Philadelphia, 1985, WB Saunders Co.

154. Winters B: Nursing implications of hyperosmolar coma, Heart Lung 12(4):439, 1983.

155. Winters C: Monitoring ventilator patients for complications, Nurs 88, 38, 1988.

156. Wright SM: Pathophysiology of congestive heart failure, J Cardiovasc Nurs 4(3):1-16, 1989.

157. Yeates S and Blaufuss J: Managing the patient in diabetic ketoacidosis, Focus Crit Care 17(3):240, 1990.

CHAPTER 6

Therapeutic Modalities

Miscellaneous Modalities

AUTOTRANSFUSION

Clinical Brief

A technique that allows for the collection, filtration, and transfusion of the patient's own blood. Autologous transfusions have several advantages: they are readily available, eliminate the risk of transfusion reactions, and eliminate the risk of blood-transmittable diseases.

Autotransfusion can be performed preoperatively and saved for future use, intraoperatively to replace blood loss, and postoperatively to replace blood shed, e.g., mediastinal chest drainage. It can also be used in the trauma patient with massive intrathoracic bleeding when banked blood is not readily available.

Contraindications include blood that is contaminated by bacteria, bile, urine, or feces; AIDS, cancer, or sickle cell anemia; or in patients with wound blood greater than 4 hours old.

Complications and Related Nursing Diagnoses

Coagulopathies	High risk for injury: excessive bleeding
Sepsis	High risk for infection
	Altered tissue perfusion
Emboli	Altered tissue perfusion

Patient Care Management Guidelines

Patient assessment

1. Obtain pretransfusion baseline hematology profile: CBC, platelet count, PT, PTT, hemoglobin, hematocrit; and electrolytes.
2. During the transfusion, obtain T, HR, RR, and BP q30min; measure u/o and hemodynamics (if available), PAP, PAWP, CVP hourly (more frequently if patient condition warrants).

3. Observe the patient for signs and symptoms of excessive bleeding: tachycardia, hypotension, decreased peripheral pulses, cool, clammy skin, decrease in CVP, PAP, PAWP, hematuria, hematemesis, increase in wound drainage, or chest tube drainage.
4. Observe the patient for signs and symptoms of emboli: SOB, change in LOC, absent or decreased pulses.

Patient management
1. Ensure optimal functioning of autotransfusion system.
2. Document the anticoagulant used on the salvaged blood and note any clot formation.
3. Accurately measure and record the amount of autotransfused blood. Anticipate administration of blood products (platelets, FFP) if more than 3 L of salvaged blood have been infused.
4. Note any foam forming in the blood, which suggests increased hemolysis.
5. Monitor CBC, platelet count, PT, PTT, Hgb, Hct, and electrolytes during and after the infusion.

Critical observations
Consult with the physician for the following:
1. Suspected blood hemolysis or clots in salvaged blood
2. Embolic phenomenon
3. Thrombocytopenia
4. Increasing temperature, unstable BP
5. Excessive bleeding
6. Electrolyte imbalance

BLOOD ADMINISTRATION

Clinical Brief
Multiple blood components are available for transfusion therapy in the critically ill patient. Despite advances to maximize the safety of blood, adverse reactions and the risk of transmitting infection still occur. Hepatitis can be transmitted by all forms of red cell products, plasma, cryoprecipitate, platelets, and coagulation concentrates. HIV can be transmitted by all forms of red cell transfusion, plasma, platelets, cryoprecipitate, and nonheated coagulation concentrates. CMV can be transmitted via blood products that contain white blood cells in which the virus is harbored.

Whole blood: Used to replace volume in acute massive hemorrhage.

Packed red blood cells (PRBCs): Used to increase the oxygen-carrying capacity with less risk of fluid overload.

Leukocyte-poor RBCs: Contains PRBCs with leukocytes and platelets removed. Used to transfuse patients who have had more than one febrile transfusion reaction, patients who are likely to require multiple transfusions (leukemia), and patients who are immunocompromised and at risk for organisms that can be transmitted via leukocytes.

Platelets: Used to restore platelets in patients who have a platelet defect and are bleeding; improve hemostasis in the thrombocytopenic patient who has received a massive transfusion, has undergone cardiac bypass surgery, or is in DIC. Prophylactic platelet transfusion is controversial.

Granulocytes: Used to treat patients with decreased WBC count secondary to radiation or chemotherapy. Febrile reactions are common.

Fresh frozen plasma (FFP): Used to treat patients with deficient coagulation factors (e.g., DIC, severe liver disease, massive transfusions).

Cryoprecipitate: Contains factor VIII, factor XIII, and fibrinogen. Used to treat von Willebrand's disease, hypofibrinogenemia, and to correct factor XIII deficiency.

Factor VIII concentrate: Contains factor VIII. Used to replace factor VIII in hemophilia A patients.

Factor IX concentrate: Contains factor IX. Used to supply factor IX in hemophilia B patients.

Albumin: Used to expand intravascular volume or replace colloids. Available in 5% solution, used to correct colloid loss. Available in 25% solution, used to correct profound hypoalbuminemia.

Plasma protein fraction (Plasmanate): Contains albumin and globulins. Used to expand intravascular volume or correct colloid loss.

Complications and Related Nursing Diagnoses

Hemolytic reaction	Altered tissue perfusion: shock Altered body temperature Impaired gas exchange
Febrile reaction	Altered body temperature Pain: lumbar/headache
Anaphylactic shock	Altered tissue perfusion: shock Impaired gas exchange
Circulatory overload	Fluid volume excess
Allergic reaction	Impaired skin integrity Ineffective breathing pattern

Patient Care Management Guidelines
Patient assessment
1. Obtain pretransfusion vital signs, and assess them again 15 minutes after initiating the transfusion. Obtain T, HR, RR, and BP q30min until the transfusion is completed. If transfusing granulocytes, measure VS q15min until the transfusion is complete.
2. Observe the patient for hemolytic reaction: high fever (39° C, 102.2° F); rigors; pain in the chest, loin, neck, or back; hematuria; oliguria; hypotension.
3. Observe the patient for an anaphylactic reaction: wheezing, edema of the tongue, larynx, and pharynx; stridor, hypotension, arrest.
4. Observe the patient for a febrile reaction: fever (38.3° C; 100.4° F), chills, headache or backache, hypotension, cough, dyspnea, nausea and vomiting.
5. Observe the patient for fluid overload: SOB, tachycardia, hypotension, increased CVP, cough, crackles, distended neck veins.
6. Observe the patient for an allergic reaction: pruritus, urticaria, headache, edema.
7. Assess the patient's response to therapy; check hemoglobin, hematocrit, prothrombin time, platelet count, sodium, potassium, and calcium levels.
8. Assess the patient for citrate toxicity if the patient is receiving a massive transfusion: tingling of extremities, hypotension, dysrhythmias, carpopedal spasm.

Patient management
1. Inspect the blood product for clots, bubbles, and discoloration.
2. Only NS can be used to prime or flush the blood administration set or to infuse simultaneously with the blood.
3. Do not administer medications through a blood infusion line.
4. Change blood filters if the infusion rate cannot be maintained, if the administration set has been in use for 4 hours, or after each 2 units of blood.
5. Use a blood warmer if large amounts of cold blood products are expected to be given over 4 hours or less, to postoperative hypothermic patients, and for patients with cold agglutinins. Warm blood to body tempera-

ture and monitor blood and body temperature throughout the infusion.

6. Verify the patient and blood product according to institution protocol. Generally, another nurse or health care professional is required to identify the patient and blood product. Information on the patient's ID bracelet, transfusion request, and blood product label should match. Do not administer the product if there is not a precise match. Be sure to check the expiration date.

7. Ensure patency of the IV. Most blood products can be infused through an 18-gauge catheter.

8. Administer the blood product at a rate of 2 ml/min during the first 15 minutes and stay with the patient. Signs of anaphylaxis or a hemolytic reaction usually occur after a small amount of blood has been infused.

9. If no reaction occurs, increase the infusion rate based on the patient's condition and the type of the blood product (Table 6-1). Monitor patients with cardiovascular, renal, or liver disease for fluid volume overload.

10. Discontinue the transfusion if the patient manifests any signs and symptoms of a reaction. Save the blood product and tubing for the blood bank, and follow institution protocol.

Critical observations
Consult the physician for the following:
1. Allergic reaction
2. Hemolytic reaction
3. Anaphylactic reaction
4. Febrile reaction
5. Volume overload

CENTRAL VENOUS CATHETERS
Clinical Brief
Used to administer various intravenous therapies (e.g., blood, chemotherapy, medications) and to obtain blood samples. These catheters can be partially implanted (Hickman, Broviac, Groshong) or totally implanted (Port-a-cath) beneath the skin and are available in single and multilumen capacities. Catheter selection is based on patient need; long-term catheters are usually indicated for therapies longer than 4 weeks. See Table 6-2 for types and characteristics of commonly used central venous catheters (CVCs).

TABLE 6-1 Blood Component Administration Guidelines

Blood component	Infusion rate	Filter	Volume	Comment
Whole blood	2-4 hr Max: 4 hr	Required	500 ml	Rapid infusion if need is urgent
Packed red blood cells	2-4 hr Max: 4 hr	Required	250 ml	Hgb rises 1 g/dl; Hct rises 3% after 1 unit
Leukocyte-poor red blood cells	2 hr	Required	Variable	
Fresh frozen plasma	1-2 hr, rapidly if bleeding	Use component filter	250 ml	Notify blood bank—takes 20 min to thaw
Platelets	Rapidly as patient tolerates	Use component filter	35-50 ml /unit	Usually 6-10 units are ordered. Request that blood bank pool all units
Albumin	1-2 ml/min in normovolemic patients	Special tubing	Varies	Comes in 5% and 25%; can increase intravascular volume quickly; infuse cautiously
Cryoprecipitate	30 min	Use component filter	10 ml/unit	Usually 6-10 units ordered
Granulocytes	2-4 hr	Use component filter	300-400 ml	Request that blood bank pool units VS q15min during infusion

TABLE 6-2 Characteristics of Central Venous Catheters

Catheter	Use	Volume	Heparinization*	Comment
Subclavian Multilumen	Short-term	0.5-0.6 ml/lumen	Required	Distal port can be used for CVP monitoring; distal port is 16 gauge; middle and proximal ports are 18 gauge; can be inserted at bedside
Implantable device Porta-cath Medi-port	Long-term	2 ml port 2 ml lumen	Required	OR insertion required; intraarterial, epidural, and intraperitoneal placements available

*For catheter lumens not used for continuous infusions.

Continued.

TABLE 6-2 Characteristics of Central Venous Catheters—cont'd

Catheter	Use	Volume	Heparinization*	Comment
Right atrial catheters				
Hickman	Long-term	1.8 ml/lumen	Required	OR insertion required; catheter is tunneled subcutaneously and contains a dacron mesh cuff to stabilize catheter
Broviac	Long-term	1.0 ml/lumen	Required	See Hickman
Groshong	Long-term	1.8 ml/lumen	Required	OR insertion required; catheter is tunneled subcutaneously; contains a three-position valve

*For catheter lumens not used for continuous infusions.

▶ Complications and Related Nursing Diagnoses

Air emboli	Ineffective breathing pattern Impaired gas exchange Pain: chest pain
Local or systemic infection	High risk for infection Impaired skin integrity
Loss of catheter function: • Catheter occlusion • Catheter dislodgment • Catheter migration • Catheter tear	High risk for injury

Patient Care Management Guidelines
Patient assessment

1. Review initial and serial chest radiographs to verify catheter placement.
2. Assess skin integrity at the insertion site or exit site of catheters each shift. Note any redness, tenderness, swelling, skin breakdown, fluid leakage, or purulent drainage at the site.
3. Monitor vital signs q4h, noting any trend in increase in temperature.
4. Assess for air embolus (increased risk occurs during tubing changes or with procedures requiring exposed catheter hub): chest pain, tachycardia, tachypnea, cyanosis, hypotension.
5. Monitor for any increased trend in WBC or blood glucose levels, which may signal infection.

Patient management: all CVCs
Prevent infection:

1. Use strict aseptic technique while manipulating catheters, e.g., dressing changes, accessing ports, changing injection caps. Povidone-iodine can be used as an antiseptic to cleanse the site and injection ports.

Prevent catheter dislodgment/disconnection:

1. Secure catheter and extension tubings to prevent catheter dislodgment or disconnection. Document catheter position, using markings on the catheter (except totally implanted ports). Have a clamp (without teeth) available. If an air embolus is suspected, clamp the catheter, turn the patient to the left side, and lower the HOB. Administer oxygen.

Catheter malfunction:

1. If unable to aspirate blood from the catheter, raise the patient's arm or have patient C & DB. Try flushing the catheter gently with NS. Catheter placement may need to be verified by a chest radiograph.

2. If unable to infuse IV fluid or medication, try flushing the catheter gently with NS—*do not use force*. Catheter placement may need to be verified by a chest radiograph. If catheter occlusion is suspected, urokinase may be ordered; follow institution protocol. Generally, 1 ml (5000 U/ml) is injected using a tuberculin syringe; wait 5-10 minutes and aspirate. The procedure can be repeated twice. If catheter patency has been achieved, withdraw 5 ml of fluid from the catheter and discard. Flush the catheter with NS and resume previous fluid administration.

Obtaining blood samples:

1. To obtain blood samples, turn off IV solution(s) for 1 minute; attach a syringe to the hub of the catheter; discard 3x the volume of the catheter lumen (see Table 6-2); and withdraw the amount of blood needed. Flush the lumen and resume IV fluids; if the lumen is not in use, flush and heparinize the lumen.

Catheter repair:

1. Inspect the catheter for cracks or tears—fluid and blood will leak from the damaged site.

2. For temporary repair, clamp the catheter between the site of insertion and the damaged section of the catheter. Cut the damaged section using sterile scissors. Insert a blunt-end needle of the appropriate gauge into the end of the catheter. Cap the needle and heparinize the catheter. An angiocath may be used; however, pull back on the stylet to avoid puncturing the CVC when inserting the angiocath into the catheter. A tongue blade can be used to splint or support the repaired area.

3. Permanent repair for long-term catheters should be done with the manufacturer's repair kit as soon as possible. Short-term multilumen catheters should be changed as soon as possible.

MULTILUMEN CVP

Patient management

1. Maintain a sterile occlusive dressing on the site; change the dressing q72h or more frequently if the dressing becomes soiled, wet, or loose.

MISC

2. Change injection caps q72h or more frequently if rubber coring occurs.
3. Tape piggybacked intermittent infusion lines securely to prevent inadvertent disconnection.
4. Flush the catheter lumen with heparinized saline q8-12h (or according to institution protocol) when not in use. Flush the catheter lumen with 2 ml NS before infusing intermittent medications. After the infusion is complete, flush with NS and heparinize the lumen.
5. To reduce the risk of introducing air into the catheter, draw up 3 ml of the normal saline or heparinized solution but inject only 2-2.5 ml. To prevent a backflow of blood into the catheter tip, withdraw the needle from the injection port while continuing to inject the solution (do not completely empty the syringe). Discard remaining NS or heparinized saline.

CATHETER REMOVAL

1. If catheter insertion is in a neck vein, place the patient in the Trendelenberg position (to prevent air embolus).
2. Using aseptic technique, remove sutures and steadily pull the catheter back. Apply pressure to the insertion site and apply a sterile occlusive dressing. Check to see if the catheter is intact.

BROVIAC OR HICKMAN
Patient management

1. Maintain a sterile occlusive dressing on the exit site.
2. Change dressing q72h or more frequently if the dressing becomes soiled, wet, or loose.
3. Change injection caps q72h or more frequently if rubber coring occurs.
4. Tape piggybacked intermittent infusion lines securely to prevent inadvertent disconnection.
5. Flush the catheter lumen with heparinized saline q8-12h (or according to institution protocol) when not in use. Flush the catheter lumen with 2 ml NS before infusing intermittent medications. After infusion is complete, flush with NS and heparinize the lumen.
6. To reduce the risk of introducing air into the catheter, draw up 3 ml of the normal saline or heparinized solution but inject only 2-2.5 ml. To prevent a backflow of blood into the catheter tip, withdraw the needle from the injection port while continuing to inject the solution (do not completely empty the syringe). Discard remaining normal saline or heparinized saline.

Groshong
Patient management
1. Maintain a sterile occlusive dressing to exit site.
2. Change dressing q72h or more frequently if the dressing becomes soiled, wet, or loose.
3. Change injection caps q72h or more frequently if rubber coring occurs.
4. Tape piggybacked intermittent infusion lines securely to prevent inadvertent disconnection.
5. Flush catheter vigorously with 5 ml normal saline after completion of intermittent infusions.
6. Flush the catheter lumen with 20 ml NS after blood infusions or obtaining blood samples.
7. A Groshong catheter requires no clamping because of its specially designed valve.

Implantable Devices
Patient management
1. Use aseptic technique when accessing the implanted port. Stabilize the port with thumb and index finger.
2. Cannulate the port using a Huber needle and extension tubing flushed with NS. A 90-degree-angled needle is recommended with continuous infusions for patient comfort and ease of dressing applications.
3. Push the Huber needle through the port until it touches the back of the port (to ensure that it is not in the rubber septum).
4. Aspirate for a blood return and flush the system with NS to confirm patency before initiating the infusion.
5. Flush the catheter with 5 ml NS after a bolus injection; follow with 5 ml heparinized saline.
6. Flush catheter with 20 ml NS after a blood sample has been withdrawn or blood has been administered.
7. Maintain a sterile dressing over the needle and port when in use; otherwise no dressing is required.
8. Change Huber needles q3-7days during continuous infusion.
9. Check the site for irritation or ulceration around the needle; rotate the insertion site prn; the skin area over the port is $\sim$ 1 inch $\times$ 1 inch.

Critical observations
Consult with the physician for the following:
1. Patient becomes febrile
2. Unable to inject fluid into or withdraw blood from catheter

3. Patient develops chest pain, dyspnea, cyanosis
4. Site is inflamed, tender, or is draining fluid or pus
5. Catheter tears/cracks

EPIDURAL ANALGESIA

Clinical Brief

Epidural analgesia is employed to provide continuous pain relief to postoperative patients without adversely affecting the patient's mentation and respiratory function, as is associated with intravenous or intramuscular administration of narcotics. Narcotics are administered via a catheter placed in the epidural space; they bind to spinal cord opioid receptors and thus interfere with pain transmission without causing blockade of sensory, motor, or sympathetic nerve fibers.

Narcotics commonly used are morphine (Duramorph) and fentanyl (Sublimaze). Fentanyl is 100 times more potent than morphine. It has an immediate onset with a duration of 12 hours, whereas the onset of morphine is within 1 hour and has a duration of 24 hours. Therefore patients must be monitored closely for adverse effects 6 hours (fentanyl) to 24 hours (morphine) after the epidural infusion has been discontinued.

Patients with a history of allergy to narcotics, increased ICP, coagulopathy or on anticoagulant therapy, bacteremia, infection at the puncture site, and prior laminectomy (if the dura was opened) are not candidates for epidural analgesia.

▶ Complications and Related Nursing Diagnoses

Migration of catheter	High risk for injury
Respiratory depression	Ineffective breathing pattern Impaired gas exchange
Side effects of narcotics:	
• Nausea/vomiting	Fluid volume deficit: potential
• Pruritis	Impaired skin integrity: potential
• Urinary retention	Altered urinary elimination
• Hypotension	Decreased cardiac output
Infection	Altered body temperature
Headache following dural puncture	Pain
Neurological sequelae: • Paresthesia • Motor deficit	Impaired physical mobility

Patient Care Management Guidelines
Patient assessment
1. If a bolus of narcotic is administered, monitor VS q15min × 4; q1h × 12; q2h × 12; then q4h.
2. Assess respiratory status q1h for 12-24 hours; q2h for 12 hours; then q4h during epidural infusion and 6 or 24 hours after it is discontinued. Count respirations for 1 full minute—note the rate and depth of respirations, skin color, and LOC.
3. Assess pain control q2-4h using a pain scale (see Figure 1-1).
4. Assess level of sedation (wide awake, drowsy, dozing intermittently, mostly sleeping, awakens only when aroused).
5. Check motor strength and sensation, since neurological changes can be caused by epidural hematoma or abscess.
6. Monitor temperature q4h; assess for signs and symptoms of meningitis.
7. Assess voiding; check for bladder distention or discomfort q4h.
8. Assess condition of dressing. Use a transparent dressing if at all possible for monitoring the epidural site.

Patient management
1. Isolate the infusion pump if possible and label the pump and IV tubing with "Epidural Precautions."
2. Tape all ports on the IV tubing to prevent accidental injection of substances.
3. Check patency of the catheter; examine the catheter for kinks or loose connections. If > 1 ml of clear fluid can be aspirated from the catheter, migration of the catheter to the subarachnoid space should be suspected. If blood is aspirated, the catheter may be in an epidural vein.
4. Maintain sterility when manipulating the catheter or dressing. Dressing changes can increase the risk for catheter dislodgement. Check the institution protocol for how often and who is responsible for dressing changes.
5. *Avoid* using alcohol or iodine to clean connections; these substances can be toxic to the nervous system.
6. Verify the solution with another nurse to ensure the correct concentration and correct *preservative-free* narcotic.
7. Check the infusion rate and verify correct dosage.

8. Ensure a patent emergency IV access during the infusion and 6 hours (fentanyl) or 24 hours (morphine) after it is discontinued.

9. Place the patient on a pulse oximeter or an apnea monitor during the infusion and 6 hours (fentanyl) or 24 hours (morphine) after it is discontinued.

10. Keep naloxone (Narcan) and a syringe at the bedside during the infusion and for 6 hours (fentanyl) or 24 hours (morphine) after it is discontinued.

11. If respiratory depression develops, follow institutional policy. Generally, if the rate is less than 8/min, Spo_2 less than 95%, or apnea greater than 10 sec, give naloxone 0.1-0.4 mg IVP. A naloxone infusion at 5 μg/kg/hr may be necessary.

12. If hypotension develops, place the patient flat and stop the epidural infusion; a fluid challenge may be needed.

13. An indwelling catheter may be necessary for the duration of the epidural analgesia. Low-dose (0.1 mg IV or IM) naloxone may be given for urinary retention.

14. Diphenhydramine (Benadryl) 25 mg IM may be given for pruritus. For severe pruritus, low-dose (0.1 mg) naloxone may be given.

15. Promethazine (Phenergan) 6.25-12.5 mg IV or IM may be given for nausea or vomiting. Metoclopramide (Reglan) 10 mg IV or droperidal (Inapsine) 0.25-0.625 mg IV may also be used to relieve nausea or vomiting.

CATHETER REMOVAL

1. Removal of the catheter is done by the anesthesiologist, nurse anesthetist, and in some institutions, the critical care nurse.

2. After slowly removing the catheter, check the tip of the catheter and note the presence of a colored mark. The colored mark denotes an intact catheter. Document this finding in the chart.

3. Check the site for infection. Do not clean the site with alcohol. Apply a sterile dressing to the site.

Critical observation

Consult with the physician for the following:

1. Respiratory rate < 8/min
2. Sustained Spo_2 < 95%
3. Inadequate analgesia
4. Oversedation
5. Persistent side effects

6. Signs of infection
7. Dislodged epidural catheter
8. Presence of paresthesia
9. Inability to remove epidural catheter
10. Absence of colored mark on catheter tip, or a broken or sheared catheter on removal

THERMAL REGULATION

Clinical Brief

Cooling and rewarming methods are used to control body temperature. Common thermoregulation disorders treated in the critical care units include hyperpyrexia (fever) and postoperative hypothermia, although heat stroke, malignant hyperthermia, and hypothermia resulting from burns or accidental exposure are also seen in the critical care setting.

External cooling methods can be used alone or in combination with antipyretic therapy. Rewarming methods are generally used in patients who have undergone elective hypothermia, e.g., cardiovascular, thoracic, and neurosurgical surgeries.

Cooling methods are used to treat hyperthermia. Hyperthermia refers to a body temperature greater than 37.2° C (99° F) and is classified as (1) *mild*—37.2° C to 38.8° C (99° F to 102° F); (2) *moderate*—38.8° C to 40° C (102° F to 104° F); (3) *critical*—≥40.5° C (≥ 105° F); and (4) *malignant*—0.5° C/15 min to 42.7° C (1° F/15 min to 109° F).

Rewarming methods are used to treat hypothermia. Hypothermia refers to a body temperature less than 37° C (98.6° F) and is classified as (1) *mild*—34° C to 36.5° C (93.2° F to 97° F); (2) *moderate*—28° C to 33.5° C (82° F to 92.3° F); (3) *severe*—17° C to 27.5° C (62.6° F to 81.5° F); and (4) *profound*—0 to 16.5° C (< 61.7° F).

▶ **Complications and Related Nursing Diagnoses**

External cooling methods

Vasoconstriction/decreased heat loss	Hyperthermia
Frostbite	Impaired skin integrity
Overshoot	Hypothermia

Rewarming methods

Shock	Altered tissue perfusion
Burns	Impaired skin integrity
Overshoot	Hyperthermia

Patient Care Management Guidelines
Cooling Methods
Patient assessment

1. Measure core temperature q15-30min during initial therapy. Anticipate an increase in HR, BP, and RR on initiation of therapy.
2. Assess LOC, presence of peripheral pulses, capillary refill, and skin temperature and condition.
3. Observe for shivering, which can cause an increase in metabolic rate and oxygen consumption. Tensing or clenching of the jaw muscles is an early sign of shivering. An ECG artifact associated with muscle tremor may also be observed.

Patient management

1. Maintain the environmental temperature at about 70° F (21° C); fans may be required to keep the room cool.
2. Use a wet sheet to cover the patient's torso; tepid baths may be given to lower the patient's temperature. Avoid cold baths, since shivering may occur.
3. A cooling blanket may be used:
   a. Precool the blanket if at all possible.
   b. Avoid layers of blankets; a single layer should be used to absorb perspiration.
   c. Turn the patient at least q2h and massage the skin. Keep the blanket in contact with patient during position changes.
   d. Monitor for drift (T change > 1° C in 15 min). Avoid overshoot (continual temperature reduction after device is turned off) by stopping the cooling blanket when the core temperature is 39° C (102.2° F).
4. For prolonged moderate hyperthermia (38.8° C to 40° C; 101.8° F to 104° F) or critical hyperthermia (≥40.5° C; 104.9° F):
   a. Ice packs can be applied to major artery sites or ice baths may be given.
   b. Gastric, bladder, and rectal irrigations with iced isotonic solution may be required.
5. Administer antipyretics as ordered; neuroleptic agents may be required to control shivering.

Patient Care Management Guidelines
Rewarming Methods
Patient assessment

1. Measure core temperature q15-30min during initial therapy. Anticipate increase in HR, BP, and RR on ini-

tiation of therapy. A drop in BP during rewarming may signal peripheral vasodilation, decreased venous return, and decreased CO (rewarming shock).

2. Continuously monitor ECG for dysrhythmias.
3. Assess LOC (hearing returns at ~ 34° C; 93.2° F); observe for signs of gastritis or ulceration, fluid volume excess, and thermal injury to skin.

Patient management

1. Minimize drafts and maintain room temperature; give warm fluids orally if the patient is alert and a gag reflex is present.
2. Apply a bath blanket and cover the head; peripheral vasodilation may occur with use of a hyperthermia blanket.
3. An external hyperthermia blanket may be used: turn the device off when core body temperature is within 1-2° of desired temperature. Monitor for drift (temperature drift may occur after the device is turned off).
4. In severe and profound hypothermia (< 27.5° C; 81.5° F) active rewarming methods may be used: gastric, peritoneal, rectal, or bladder irrigations with heated isotonic solutions, or extracorporeal circulation may be required.
5. If cardiopulmonary arrest occurs, raise the core temperature to 32° C to 33° C (92° F) to optimize conditions for defibrillation.
6. Monitor the patient for "bolus effect" of pharmacological agents given during a hypothermia episode, as vasodilation occurs with rewarming.
7. Maintain extremities below heart level until vasodilation and hemodynamic stability have been achieved. Cardiac dysrhythmias may result from venous return of acidemic peripheral blood when arms or legs are raised.
8. Do not exceed a rate of 2° C/hr to rewarm the patient.
9. If blood transfusions are required, use a blood warmer.

Critical observations

Consult with the physician for the following:

1. Hypothermia or hyperthermia unresponsive to therapeutic interventions
2. Excessive shivering
3. Hypotension
4. Dysrhythmias
5. Fluid and electrolyte disturbances
6. Hypoxemia and acid-base imbalance
7. Seizures
8. Cardiopulmonary arrest

Neurological Modalities

CRANIOTOMY

Clinical Brief

A craniotomy provides a "bone window" through which to evacuate hematomas, clip or ligate aneurysms or feeding vessels of an AVM, resect tumors, and biopsy the brain. Craniotomies are also used in the surgical treatment of epilepsy, i.e., intraoperative electroencephalography and resection of the cortex areas responsible for seizure activity. Pituitary tumors may be approached either transcranially through a craniotomy (especially when the tumor has a large suprasellar component) or by the transnasal transsphenoidal route.

Possible complications depend on the reason the surgery was performed, the location of the pathological condition, and underlying medical conditions.

Complications and Related Nursing Diagnoses

Cerebral hemorrhage, edema, ischemia	Altered tissue perfusion: cerebral
	High risk for injury: IICP
CSF leak	High risk for infection
Diabetes insipidus (DI)	Fluid volume deficit
Syndrome of inappropriate ADH (SIADH)	Fluid volume excess

Patient Care Management Guidelines

Patient assessment

1. Assess pupil size, reactivity, and visual fields, LOC, quality and comprehension of speech, and sensorimotor function. Test gag, swallow, and corneal reflexes.
2. Observe for signs and symptoms of meningitis: lethargy, severe headache, photophobia, nuchal rigidity, positive Kernig's sign.
3. Assess trends in ICP; initial readings may be required q15-30min. Calculate and record cerebral perfusion pressure readings (normal is 60-100 mm Hg) q1h. Note effects of patient and nursing activities on ICP and plan care accordingly.

4. Obtain BP and calculate MAP; CPP depends on adequate BP. Obtain CVP and PA pressures (if available) to determine imbalances in volume status that can adversely affect cerebral perfusion pressure.

5. Measure I & O hourly and determine fluid balance q8h. Measure specific gravity at least q8h and review serum electrolyte levels. DI and SIADH can develop in patients following a craniotomy.

6. Assess for CSF leaks. For transsphenoidal and transoral surgical approaches, question the patient about a feeling of a postnasal drip down the back of the throat. Apply moustache dressing to check for CSF leaks from either nostril (transsphenoidal approach). Assess patient's posterior pharynx for any signs of CSF leak (transoral approach).

7. Assess respiratory function. Monitor airway patency, oxygen saturation via pulse oximeter, and the patient's ability to handle secretions (i.e., gag/swallow reflex). Note rate, depth, and pattern of respirations and assess the lungs for adventitious sounds.

8. Examine the surgical dressing for bloody drainage or possible CSF drainage (CSF drainage will test positive for glucose).

Patient management

1. Administer analgesics as ordered and evaluate the effectiveness of medication. Maintain a quiet environment and provide uninterrupted rest periods.

2. Administer oxygen as ordered and monitor ABGs; hypoxia and hypercarbia are disturbances that can cause an increase in ICP. Promote pulmonary hygiene to prevent atelectasis and pneumonia.

3. Fluid management depends on the type of surgery and potential complications. Generally, hypotonic solutions are avoided, since they may cause an increase in ICP.

4. Keep HOB at 30-45 degrees or as ordered to promote cerebral venous drainage. Maintain the patient's head and neck in proper alignment; teach the patient to avoid the Valsalva maneuver; hyperoxygenate the patient's lungs before and after suctioning secretions, and limit suctioning to 15 seconds.

5. Pharmacological agents such as chlorpromazine may be needed to reduce shivering; pancuronium may be needed to prevent posturing; and anticonvulsants may be needed to control seizures.

6. Vasoactive agents may be required to control BP since CPP depends on an adequate BP. For hypotension, a dopamine or phenylephrine infusion may be titrated to the desired BP. For hypertension, labetalol or hydralazine HCl may be ordered (see Chapter 7).

7. If a ventriculostomy is being used, drain CSF according to established parameters (generally to maintain ICP < 20 mm Hg). Keep the CSF drainage system at the level ordered to prevent inadvertent collapse of the ventricles.

8. H_2 blocking agents may be ordered to decrease gastric acid secretion. If an NG tube is in place, sucralfate may be ordered to reduce the risk of ulcer formation.

9. Patients who have undergone transsphenoidal surgery may develop episodes of diabetes insipidus (DI) in the first 72 hours. Maintenance IVs plus replacement fluid and/or administration of aqueous pitressin may be ordered. Carefully measure urine output hourly; specific gravity measurements may be required q2h. Frequent serum Na^+, K^+, and serum osmolality levels should be monitored.

10. Patients who have undergone aneurysmal clipping and develop cerebral vasospasm may require calcium channel blockers, such as nimodipine, and/or hypervolemic hemodilution therapy to reduce the risk of cerebral ischemia. To increase intravascular volume and decrease hematocrit levels, crystalloid infusions may be used to maintain PAD pressure at 14-16 mm Hg or CVP at 12-15 cm H_2O. Hypertensive therapy may also be employed to treat suspected/documented vasospasm. A phenylephrine infusion may be titrated to raise SBP 25% to 40%.

Critical observations

Consult with the physician for the following:

1. Decreased LOC, pupillary inequality, hemiparesis or hemiplegia, visual changes, onset or worsening of aphasia, or any deterioration in neurological functioning
2. A loss of the gag or swallow reflexes
3. ICP > 20 mm Hg and unresponsive to ordered therapy
4. Suspected CSF leak
5. u/o >200 ml/hr for 2 hours (without diuretic) or u/o <30 ml/hr
6. Hypernatremia or hyponatremia
7. Sudden bloody drainage from ventriculostomy

CAROTID ENDARTERECTOMY
Clinical Brief
Carotid surgery can be performed to repair traumatic injuries to the artery or to improve cerebral circulation in patients with occlusive vascular disease.

Carotid endarterectomies are usually performed to remove atherosclerotic plaques that have significantly reduced the lumen of the artery or have become ulcerative and are the source of emboli. The symptoms in carotid disease are caused by a significant reduction in cerebral blood flow resulting from an area of tight stenosis or by transient ischemic attacks (TIAs) resulting from embolization of plaque fragments, platelet clumps, or small blood clots from the ulcer in the atheroma. The objective of endarterectomy is to remove the embolism source and improve cerebral circulation.

▶ Complications and Related Nursing Diagnoses

Embolic stroke	Altered tissue perfusion: cerebral
	Self-care deficit
Cranial nerve impairment (IX, X)	Ineffective airway clearance
	High risk for aspiration
	High risk for injury: dysrhythmia

Patient Care Management Guidelines
Patient assessment
1. Assess neurological status hourly and compare findings with the baseline. Note the integrity of the cough and gag reflexes, and visual fields and motor and sensory integrity. Monitor speech for comprehension and quality. Ask the patient to report signs and symptoms of TIAs.
2. Assess the patency of the carotid artery by palpating the superficial temporal artery and note the presence, quality, strength, and symmetry of pulses.
3. Assess vital signs hourly and carefully note BP; hypotension can occur secondary to carotid sinus manipulation during surgery.
4. Assess respiratory status: note rate and depth of respirations; observe respiratory pattern and note patient's ability to handle secretions (gag, cough, swallowing reflexes). Assess for hematoma or swelling at the operative site, which may adversely affect airway patency; note the presence of any tracheal deviation. Continuously monitor oxygen saturation via pulse oximetry (Spo_2).
5. Continuously monitor ECG for dysrhythmias secondary to intraoperative manipulation of carotid sinus.

6. Examine the surgical dressing for bloody drainage. Note any swelling or hematoma formation at the incision site.

Patient management

1. Keep HOB at 30 degrees unless hypotensive events occur, then lower HOB to enhance cerebral blood flow.
2. Maintain a dry, occlusive dressing at the incision site. Keep firm pressure over the dressing if bleeding occurs.
3. Administer analgesics as ordered and evaluate the effectiveness of medication.
4. Administer vasopressors and/or antihypertensive agents as necessary to maintain BP within set parameters.
5. Turn and position the patient to prevent airway obstruction and aspiration. Provide incentive spirometry and C & DB the patient. Keep the patient NPO until the gag and swallow reflexes return to normal.

Critical Observations

Consult with the physician for the following:
1. Symptoms reported by the patient that suggest TIAs
2. Hemiparesis/hemiplegia, pupillary irregularity, aphasia
3. Difficulty in breathing
4. Excessive bleeding at incision site
5. Dysrhythmias, hypotension, or hypertension

HYPERVENTILATION THERAPY

Clinical Brief

Cerebral edema resulting from head injury, brain tumors, or cerebrovascular accidents raises ICP. The use of hyperventilation therapy to lower Pa_{CO_2} has been shown to be a useful adjunct in the treatment of increased ICP.

Hypercarbia produces cerebral vasodilation and consequently increases intracranial pressure. Hypocarbia, induced by hyperventilation, produces vasoconstriction of the cerebral capillaries, which restricts venous blood pooling and decreases ICP. In the initial phase (24 to 48 hours) of therapy, ICP may be reduced as much as 25% to 30% with up to a 10 mm Hg drop in Pa_{CO_2}.

▶ Complications and Related Nursing Diagnoses

Respiratory alkalosis	Impaired tissue perfusion: systemic
Hypotension	Decreased cardiac output

Patient Care Management Guidelines

Patient assessment

1. Obtain ICP readings to assess the patient's response to hyperventilation therapy. Calculate CPP (normal is 60-

100 mm Hg). The inability to reduce ICP with hyperventilation is a poor prognostic indicator.

2. Monitor P_{ETCO_2} with capnometry to evaluate the patient's response to hyperventilation therapy. Generally, $Paco_2$ levels are maintained at 25 to 30 mm Hg. If $Paco_2$ drops below 20 mm Hg, cerebral hypoxia can occur as a result of severe vasoconstriction.

3. Review ABGs to assess oxygenation and acid-base balance. Respiratory alkalosis can occur as a result of hyperventilation therapy. Hypoxemia (Pao_2 <50 mm Hg) can lead to cerebral vasodilation.

4. Monitor body temperature. Hypothermia can shift the oxyhemoglobin dissociation curve to the left. This causes hemoglobin and oxygen to be more tightly bound and reduces oxygen availability to the tissues.

5. Continuously monitor arterial blood pressure and calculate MAP; monitor CVP and PA pressures (if available).

6. Monitor fluid volume status: measure intake and output hourly; determine fluid balance q8h.

Patient management

1. Sedatives may be used to reduce ICP caused by agitation. Monitor LOC carefully. (See Chapter 3 for information on ICP monitoring.)

2. Ensure airway patency; suction secretions only when necessary.

3. Inotropic or vasoactive agents may be ordered to maintain a MAP that results in a CPP of at least 60 mm Hg.

Critical observations

Consult with the physician for the following:

1. ICP unresponsive to maximum hyperventilation
2. CPP <60 mm Hg
3. O_2 sat <95%
4. Systolic blood pressure <90 mm Hg
5. pH consistently >7.45

BARBITURATE COMA

Clinical Brief

The use of barbiturates in treating cases of malignant ICP (sustained ICP >20 mm Hg) has remained controversial in its wide range of clinical applications. While barbiturates have been used for patients with severe head injury, there have been other opportunities for its use in the acute care setting. These include cases of intractable seizures, sagittal sinus thrombosis, Reye's syndrome, and ischemic stroke.

The mechanism of barbiturate action is not fully understood, but it is believed to play a role in the reduction of cerebral blood flow, oxygen demand, and cerebral metabolism, thereby reducing ICP. The use of barbiturates may also reduce swelling and promote resolution of cerebral edema.

In patients whose ICP has not responded well to CSF drainage, hyperventilation, or osmotic therapy and in whom there is no surgical lesion, barbiturate coma may be instituted. Since the clinical examination is not reliable during the drug-induced coma, a surgical lesion must be removed before barbiturate coma is instituted.

Serial EEG recordings guide induction of the coma and adjustments in dosage maintenance of barbiturate infusion.

Contraindications to barbiturate therapy include those patients whose ICP is normal or those patients who respond promptly to CSF drainage, hyperventilation, and/or osmotic therapy. Patients who suffer from cardiac disease, especially heart failure, are not candidates for barbiturate coma because of the myocardial depressive effects of barbiturates.

► **Complications and Related Nursing Diagnoses**

Hypotension	Decreased cardiac output
Hypostatic pneumonia	Impaired gas exchange
Aspiration	High risk for infection
	Impaired gas exchange
Hypothermia	Altered body temperature

Patient Care Management Guidelines
Patient assessment

1. Continuously monitor arterial BP; assess the patient for hypotension and tachycardia.
2. Obtain ICP readings and calculate cerebral perfusion pressure.
3. Continuously monitor oxygen saturation with pulse oximetry and P_{ETCO_2} with capnometry (if available). Review ABGs to evaluate oxygenation and acid-base status.
4. Obtain PA and wedge pressures as well as CO to evaluate the hemodynamic response to barbiturate coma.
5. Closely monitor body temperature; barbiturates reduce metabolism and can cause hypothermia.
6. Assess neurological status to evaluate degree of coma.

Patient management

1. Intubation and mechanical ventilation are required. Anticipate NG tube placement to maintain gastric decompression and prevent the risk of aspiration.

2. Portable EEG monitoring or compressed spectral analysis (CSA) will be necessary to monitor the patient's response to the loading dose and to adjust maintenance dosing. Obtaining hourly EEG printouts is recommended.

3. A loading dose of pentobarbital is 5-10 mg/kg IV at a rate no faster than 100 mg/min. Designate one IV line for pentobarbital infusion only. Have phenylephrine HCl 50 mg/250 ml D_5W available in case the patient becomes hypotensive; dopamine (ACLS concentration: Patient's wt in kg × 15 = Amount in 250 ml) may also be prepared and ready to infuse during the loading dose of pentobarbital. Maintain SBP > 90 mm Hg and cerebral perfusion > 60 mm Hg.

4. The maintenance dose is usually 3-5 mg/kg/hr and may be given hourly as a bolus or as a constant infusion. The dosage is adjusted according to electrical activity recorded on EEG or CSA.

5. During the first several hours of pentobarbital infusion, assess neurological function. The patient will become nonresponsive and flaccid; corneal, cough, gag, swallow, and/or pupillary reflexes will decrease or become absent; and spontaneous respirations will cease.

6. Osmotic therapy and CSF drainage may continue as needed for intermittent ICP control during barbiturate coma.

7. Once the ICP has been lowered and remains stable for greater than 48 hours, a slow taper of barbiturates may begin. Osmotic diuretics and CSF drainage may continue prn. If ICP does not respond to diuretics and CSF drainage (i.e., ICP >20 mm Hg), barbiturate therapy may be resumed.

Critical observations

Consult with the physician for the following:

1. ICP unresponsive to barbiturate administration
2. CPP < 60 mm Hg
3. Hypotension
4. O_2 sat <95%
5. Hypothermia
6. Suspected aspiration
7. Unilateral change in pupil size

Pulmonary Modalities

MECHANICAL VENTILATION
Clinical Brief

Various methods of mechanical ventilation can be used to improve alveolar ventilation in the critically ill patient who cannot effectively meet the body's metabolic needs. A variety of positive and negative pressure ventilators are available.

Negative pressure ventilators apply external subatmospheric pressure to the thorax, decreasing intrathoracic pressure and allowing air to enter the lungs. Examples include the iron lung, chest cuirass, and poncho wrap.

Positive pressure ventilators include time-cycled, pressure-cycled, or volume-cycled models; all of these apply positive pressure to the airways, causing air to enter the lungs.

The type of positive pressure ventilator is classified according to the physical parameter responsible for terminating inspiratory flow.

Time-cycled: Inspiratory flow ceases at a preset time regardless of the tidal volume delivered.

Pressure-cycled: Inspiratory flow is delivered until a preset airway pressure is reached.

Volume-cycled: Inspiratory flow is delivered until a preset tidal volume is reached, unless peak pressures are exceeded then the delivery of tidal volume is terminated to prevent possible barotrauma.

Ventilator settings: positive pressure ventilation

Fio_2: The Fio_2 is adjusted to maintain a Pao_2 of at least 60 mm Hg and a Sao_2 $\geq$90%.

PEEP: When patients require Fio_2 settings >0.60 to maintain an adequate Pao_2, PEEP can be added to decrease the Fio_2. It is desirable to decrease the Fio_2 to nontoxic levels (0.40) to prevent oxygen toxicity.

Tidal volume: Tidal volume is calculated to be 10-15 ml/kg.

Rate: The rate is adjusted to maintain a normal $Paco_2$. Initially, rates may be set at 10-15/min.

Inspiratory flow: The speed of air flow is usually set at 40-60 L.

Sigh: Sigh ventilations, if used, are set at 1.5 to 2.0 times the tidal volume. If PEEP or large tidal volumes are being used, sigh ventilations are unnecessary. Sigh is also undesirable in a patient with COPD or any patient with poor compliance because of the increased risk of barotrauma.

High-frequency ventilation is a special positive pressure ventilation used in some patient conditions. The various modes of high-frequency ventilation are listed in Table 6-3. Other modes of mechanical ventilation are discussed in Table 6-4.

Independent lung ventilation (ILV) is a technique that allows each lung to be ventilated separately. It is used predominantly in patients with unilateral lung disease. ILV requires intubation with a double lumen tube (Carlens, White, Bryce-Smith, Robertshaw, Broncho-cath) and one or two ventilators. The special endobronchial tube is generally placed in the mainstem bronchus of the affected lung. The unaffected lung is ventilated through a side port located on the opposite side of the tube.

Indications

Suggested parameters for ventilatory support are listed in the box on p. 466. In patients with acute respiratory failure, mechanical ventilation is required continuously. Nocturnal positive pressure ventilation may be indicated in patients with chronic disorders. The ventilator decreases the work of breathing and provides some rest for the respiratory system

TABLE 6-3 Modes of High-Frequency Ventilation

Type	Description
HF positive pressure ventilation (HFPPV)	Extremely short inspiratory times with V_T equivalent to deadspace at a rate of 60-100 cycles/min
HF jet ventilation (HFJV)	Small volumes, $\leq$ anatomical deadspace, are pulsed through a jet injector catheter at rates of 60-600 cycles/min
HF oscillation (HFO)	Small volume of gas is continually vibrated in the airways at rates of 900-3000 cycles/min

TABLE 6-4 Modes of Ventilatory Support

Type	Description
Assist-controlled mode ventilation (ACV)	Patient triggers a breath and the ventilator delivers a preset volume; the control mode takes over at a preset backup rate if patient becomes apneic
Bilevel CPAP (BiPAP)	Positive pressure applied during spontaneous breathing that allows the inspiratory positive airway pressure (IPAP) and expiratory positive airway pressure (EPAP) to be independently adjusted
Continuous positive airway pressure (CPAP)	Positive pressure applied during spontaneous breathing and maintained throughout the entire respiratory cycle; decreases intrapulmonary shunting
Controlled mandatory ventilation (CMV)	Ventilator delivers a preset tidal volume at a fixed rate regardless of the patient's efforts to breathe
Intermittent mandatory ventilation (IMV)	Patient may be able to breathe spontaneously but receives intermittent ventilator breaths at a preset rate and tidal volume; tidal volume stacking can occur
Inverse-ratio ventilation	Provides inspiratory time greater than expiratory time, thereby improving distribution of ventilation and preventing collapse of stiffer alveolar units
Positive end-expiratory pressure (PEEP)	Positive pressure applied during machine breathing and maintained at end-expiration; decreases intrapulmonary shunting
Pressure support ventilation (PSV)	Clinician-selected amount of positive pressure applied to airway during patient's spontaneous inspiratory efforts; PSV decreases work of breathing caused by demand flow valve, IMV circuit, and narrow inner diameter of ETT
Synchronized IMV (SIMV)	Intermittent ventilator breaths synchronized to spontaneous breaths to reduce competition between ventilator and patient

Guidelines for Ventilatory Support in Patients with Respiratory Failure

RR	>35/min
Pa_{O_2} (mm Hg)	<70 (on supplemental oxygen)
Pa_{CO_2} (mm Hg)	>55
Vital capacity	<15 ml/kg body weight
FEV_1	<10 ml/kg body weight
Negative inspiratory force	<-25 cm H_2O

Data from Pontoppidan H, Geffin B, and Lowenstein E: Acute respiratory failure in the adult, N Engl J Med 287:749, 1972.

in patients with COPD or neuromuscular weakness. In patients with sleep apnea, nocturnal ventilation prevents apneic periods. A face mask or nasal mask can be used for nocturnal positive pressure ventilation.

Complications and Related Nursing Diagnoses

Decreased venous return	Decreased cardiac output
Pulmonary barotrauma	Ineffective breathing pattern Impaired gas exchange
Infection	Ineffective airway clearance Altered body temperature
Fluid/electrolyte imbalance	Fluid volume excess Impaired gas exchange
Tracheal tube obstruction • Mucous plug • Kinked tube • Cuff herniation	Impaired gas exchange
GI bleeding	High risk for injury: stress ulcer
Oxygen toxicity	Impaired gas exchange
Increased ICP	Altered tissue perfusion: cerebral

Patient Care Management Guidelines
Patient assessment
1. Assess placement of the endotracheal tube (ETT): auscultation of breath sounds should be done when intubation has been completed, a minimum of every shift, and with respiratory distress. Auscultate breath sounds bilaterally to assess presence and equality. NOTE: Gurgling heard over the epigastric region on auscultation may

indicate esophageal intubation. Unilateral breath sounds may indicate that the endotracheal tube may be inserted too far into a mainstem bronchus (usually the right mainstem). If the patient coughs repeatedly, one should suspect that the endotracheal tube is placed against the carina. A chest radiograph should be obtained and reviewed to confirm proper placement of the ETT (see Figure 2-4). Once placement is confirmed, document tube placement by using the endotracheal tube markings. EXAMPLES: 25 cm at the lips or 23 cm at the nares. Reconfirm placement each shift and review serial chest radiographs for definitive confirmation.

2. Assess respiratory status: auscultate breath sounds and also note rate and depth of respirations. Check the ventilator settings and monitor peak airway pressure to detect changes in compliance. A change in LOC, tachypnea, tachycardia, or dysrhythmias are all signs of hypoxemia. Cyanosis is a late sign. Obtain ABGs as ordered and analyze results to determine the effectiveness of therapy. NOTE: Breath and heart sounds will be difficult to assess because of the small tidal volumes being delivered and the sound generated by the jet ventilator.

Patient management

1. Continuously monitor oxygen saturation with pulse oximetry (Spo_2). Monitor ventilation with capnography (if available). The $Petco_2$ is 1-4 mm Hg lower than $Paco_2$.

2. Monitor airway cuff pressure to prevent an alteration in tissue integrity resulting from high pressure. Endotracheal tubes have a pilot balloon and port to measure the pressure. A cuff manometer is used to determine that the pressure of the cuff is less than the tracheal capillary pressure; cuff pressure should not exceed 20 mm Hg. A cuff pressure < 15 mm Hg increases the risk of aspiration, although a properly inflated cuff does not prevent aspiration.

3. Prevent pressure ulcers to the lip or tongue by rotating tube placement daily. Caution should be taken so that the tube is not displaced or the patient is inadvertently extubated.

4. Talk with and reassure the patient, or if necessary, sedate the patient when anxious and "fighting" the ventilator. Provide the patient with a communication board to make needs known.

PULM

TABLE 6-5 Summary of Ventilator Alarms

Alarm	Possible causes
High pressure	Secretion build-up, kinked airway tubing, bronchospasm, coughing, fighting the ventilator, decreased lung compliance
Low exhaled volume	Disconnection from ventilator, loose ventilator fittings, leaking airway cuff
Low inspiratory pressure	Disconnection from the ventilator, loose connections, low ventilating pressure
High respiratory rate	Anxiety, pain, hypoxia, fever
Apnea alarm	No spontaneous breath within pre-set time interval

5. Ensure that the ventilator alarms are on and functional. Table 6-5 lists possible causes for ventilator alarming. Manually ventilate the patient's lungs with 100% oxygen if the cause of ventilator malfunction cannot be quickly identified or corrected.

6. Review ABGs at the beginning of the shift and periodically during the shift to ensure that the ventilator settings are appropriate and the patient's lungs are being properly ventilated.

7. Assess fluid balance q8h; note the condition of skin and mucous membranes; and compare serial weights. Ventilated patients are at risk for dehydration as well as increased secretion of ADH and fluid volume excess.

8. If PEEP or CPAP is being used, do not remove the patient from the ventilator to obtain hemodynamic pressure readings; patients may desaturate rapidly when the ventilator is disconnected.

9. Suctioning can lead to airway trauma and infection. To decrease the likelihood of complications, sterile technique is used and suctioning is performed only when rhonchi are auscultated. Ensure that the suction device is not set higher than 120 mm Hg and is applied only when the catheter is being withdrawn. Patients requiring high-frequency jet ventilation will have increased amounts of tracheobronchial and oral secretions. Monitor for possible aspiration and airway plugging. Two

---

Weaning Criteria

Vital capacity > 10-15 ml/kg body weight
Spontaneous tidal volume 2-5 ml/kg
Resting minute ventilation <10 L/min and ability to double during MVV maneuver
Negative (maximal) inspiratory pressure >-20 cm H_2O
Adequate Pao_2 for the patient
RR <25/min
$Paco_2$ 35-45 mm Hg
$P(a/A)o_2$ ratio >0.25

---

nurses will be needed to suction the secretions of patients requiring high-frequency jet ventilation.
10. Administer H_2 antagonists, antacids, or cytoprotective agent as ordered to raise gastric pH.

WEANING AND EXTUBATION

The box lists weaning criteria. There are no criteria that guarantee a successful weaning, since many factors can affect the outcome. The patient's psychological state is important, as well as the circumstances surrounding the respiratory problem, e.g., a longstanding problem versus respiratory failure that has resolved quickly. In addition, malnutrition can adversely affect the diaphragm and other muscles of respiration, making weaning more difficult. Other conditions that have been implicated in failure to wean include hypophosphatemia, hypomagnesemia, and hypothyroidism.

POSTEXTUBATION

Close observation of the patient is essential. Observe for signs of respiratory distress and increased patient effort: diaphoresis, restlessness, respiratory rate > 30/min or < 8/min, or increase of 10 respirations from starting respiratory rate; increase or decrease in HR by 20 beats/min or < 60 beats/min; increase or decrease in BP by 20 mm Hg; PAWP > 20 mm Hg; nasal flaring, recession of suprasternal and intercostal spaces, paradoxical motion of rib cage and abdomen; tidal volume < 250-300 ml; minute ventilation increase of 5 L/min; $Sao_2 < 90\%$, $Pao_2 < 60$ mm Hg, increase in $Paco_2$ with a fall in pH < 7.35.

Critical observation

Consult with the physician for the following:
1. Unequal or absent breath sounds
2. Respiratory distress/increased patient effort

3. Sao_2 <90%, Pao_2 <60 mm Hg, $Paco_2$ >45 mm Hg, or pH <7.35
4. Excessive coughing
5. Persistent cuff leak
6. High peak airway pressures
7. SBP <90 mm Hg
8. Fluid imbalance
9. GI bleeding

EXTRACORPOREAL MEMBRANE OXYGENATION (ECMO)

Clinical Brief

An extracorporeal circuit is used to remove blood from a patient with severe respiratory insufficiency that is unresponsive to conventional therapy, infuse oxygen and extract carbon dioxide, and return the blood to the patient. A venoarterial or venovenous approach can be used; however, the venovenous approach may be a more successful option for an adult with respiratory failure. Generally a perfusionist is responsible for maintaining the ECMO circuit, although the critical care nurse may have this responsibility in some institutions.

▶ Complications and Related Nursing Diagnoses

Thrombus formation	Altered tissue perfusion
Cannula malposition	High risk for injury: hemorrhage Impaired gas exchange
Sepsis	Decreased cardiac output Altered body temperature
Hemorrhage	High risk for injury: hemorrhage Decreased cardiac output Altered tissue perfusion Fluid volume deficit

Patient Care Management Guidelines

Patient assessment

1. Obtain PA, BP, wedge pressures, and CO and calculate CI q1h, more often if titrating pharmacological agents or if patient condition warrants. An increase in PA systolic pressure may be secondary to hypoxia.
2. Assess respiratory status: auscultate breath sounds at least q2h and note rate and rhythm; monitor oxygenation using pulse oximetry (Spo_2) and Svo_2 with fiberoptics (if available). Review serial chest radiographs to assess improvement or worsening in condition.

3. Assess for hemorrhage: obtain vital signs q1h; an increased heart rate may be the first indication. Check cannula site as well as incisions and invasive line sites; observe for changes in LOC, onset of abdominal tenderness or distention; check for bloody sputum, hematuria, or coffee-ground nasogastric drainage. Guaiac-test NG aspirate, urine, and stool. Review serial Hct results for a decreasing trend.
4. Assess peripheral circulation q1h; note skin temperature and color, pulses, and capillary refill.
5. Measure and record hourly urinary output. Decreased urinary output may signify decreased renal perfusion secondary to decreased cardiac output.
6. Assess for signs and symptoms of infection: monitor temperature q4h; assess catheter site for redness, swelling, or drainage; and review serial WBC counts.

Patient management
1. Maintain the ECMO circuit as ordered with the assistance of a perfusionist.
2. Systemic anticoagulants are administered to prevent thrombus formation and are based on ACTs. Activated clotting times are usually maintained between 200-240 sec (normal <180 seconds). An initial heparin dose of 100-200 U/kg followed by a maintenance dose between 20-50 U/kg/hr may be required.
3. Administer fluids and vasoactive drugs as ordered to maintain MAP of at least 80 mm Hg. Carefully monitor the patient for fluid overload or CI < 2.5 L/min/m^2.
4. Provide pulmonary hygiene with gentle suctioning, chest physiotherapy, and turning q2h.
5. Use strict aseptic technique with all procedures: change the cannula dressing daily using a povidone-iodine solution on the site.
6. Administer analgesics, sedatives, and paralytics as ordered.
7. Use pressure-reducing or pressure-relieving devices, since these patients are susceptible to pressure ulcers related to decreased tissue perfusion. Reposition the patient frequently and assist with passive range of motion exercises.

Critical observations
Consult with the physician for the following:
1. Pao$_2$ <60 mm Hg
2. Svo$_2$ <60% or >80%

PULM

3. SBP <90 mm Hg
4. CI <2.5 L/min/m^2
5. Decreased LOC (independent of sedation)
6. Unilateral diminished breath sounds
7. Diminished/loss of pulses in extremity (in arterial cannulation)
8. Obvious bleeding: catheter site, invasive lines, sputum
9. Positive occult blood in NG drainage, urine, or stool
10. u/o <20 ml/hr for 2 hours
11. Decreasing trend in Hct
12. T >38.5° C (101.3° F)
13. Redness, swelling, drainage at catheter site, invasive lines, or incision
14. ACT out of therapeutic range

CHEST DRAINAGE

Clinical Brief

Chest tubes (CT) drain blood, fluid, or air that has accumulated in the thorax to restore negative intrapleural pressure. Intermittent drainage can be accomplished via thoracentesis. A pleural CT is inserted for a pneumothorax, hemothorax, hemopneumothorax, empyema, or pleural effusion. In postop cardiothoracic surgeries, mediastinal tubes may be placed to prevent the accumulation of fluid around the heart, which could lead to cardiac tamponade.

A chest tube drainage system must have two components—a collection container and a water seal. The water seal prevents air from entering the chest on inspiration. A three-bottle system contains a drainage bottle, a water seal bottle, and a third bottle that is attached to a suction and serves as a pressure regulator. Suction is used to increase air flow from the pleural space. Disposable systems are available in either the one-bottle or three-bottle systems (Figure 6-1).

A flutter (Heimlich) valve has been developed that may be used in place of a drainage system to prevent air from entering the chest on inspiration. This valve opens on expiration, allowing air to escape from the chest, and collapses on inspiration to prevent air from entering the thorax (Figure 6-2). The Heimlich valve is useful during patient transport and for increasing patient mobility.

▶ **Complications and Related Nursing Diagnoses**

Pain	Pain related to chest tube
	Ineffective breathing pattern

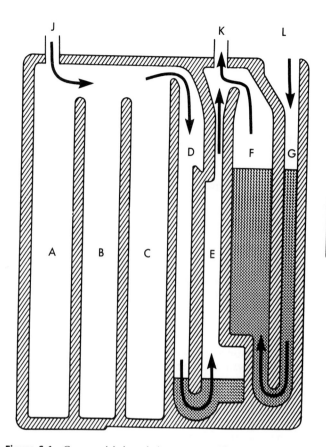

Figure 6-1 Commercial chest drainage system: Pleur-evac. The first chamber provides sections *(A, B, C)* for fluid collection. Air from the patient's pleural space *(J)* moves through the first chamber and into the second chamber *(arrows)*. The second chamber prevents air from being drawn into the pleural cavity. Air leaves pleural cavity and moves from *D* to *E*. The presence of an air leak is ascertained by observing for bubbles in *E*. If the Pleur-evac is established as underwater seal only, air is evacuated to the atmosphere (via *K*). In the third chamber, when Pleur-evac is attached to a vacuum source (via *K*), air is drawn through the vent *(L)* and moves through section *G*, bubbling into section *F* on its way to the vacuum source. The magnitude of negative pressure applied is determined by the depth of water in sections *F* and *G* and not by the vacuum source. (From Bonner JT and Hall JR: Respiratory intensive care of the adult surgical patient, St Louis, 1985, The CV Mosby Co.)

PULM

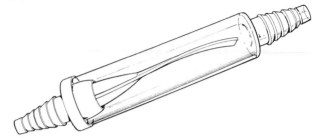

Figure 6-2   Heimlich valve.

| Occluded chest tube | Impaired gas exchange
Ineffective breathing pattern |
| Infection | Impaired skin integrity
Altered body temperature |

Patient Care Management Guidelines
Patient assessment
1. Assess respiratory status: note rate and rhythm and ease of respiration, auscultate breath sounds, and palpate for subcutaneous emphysema. An obstruction or kinked tube can cause a tension pneumothorax; a defect in the system can cause recurrence of hemothorax or pneumothorax.
2. Assess CT drainage on insertion and hourly thereafter until the patient's condition is stabilized. Document the type, color, and amount of drainage. A sudden change in the amount of drainage or a CT output of 200 ml/hr may indicate the need for surgical intervention. Sudden drainage cessation may indicate tube obstruction.

Patient management
1. Ensure that the water seal is at an appropriate level for the system being used and that all connections are tight. Ensure the patency of the tube. The water level should rise on inspiration and fall during expiration. The opposite occurs with mechanical ventilation. Monitor for the development of bubbling in the water seal chamber (see Figure 6-1, *E*), which indicates a leak either at a connection or the tracheobronchial tree. No bubbling or fluctuation should be observed in the water seal chamber when mediastinal CTs are used.
2. To assess for a tracheobronchial leak when the water seal chamber bubbles, clamp the CT close to the pa-

tient's chest; if the bubbling continues, the source is external. Caution must be taken, since a tension pneumothorax can quickly develop when bubbling CTs are clamped. *Do not* clamp CTs with known tracheobronchial leaks.

3. Verify that suction is at the prescribed amount; refill the suction water chamber as needed.
4. If the patient is being transported or if suction is not being used, leave the suction tubing open to air.
5. If the CT becomes disconnected from the drainage system, reconnect the tube—*do not* clamp the CT. If there is an air leak from the lung (e.g., bubbling in the water seal), more air will accumulate in the chest if the tube is clamped. A patient with a mediastinal tube may develop tamponade if the CT is clamped. Keep a 250 ml bottle of sterile saline available; if the chest drainage system breaks, submerge the CT 2-4 cm in sterile saline.
6. Stripping of CTs is a controversial issue because it creates large negative pressures in the thorax. Milking of chest tubes does not create pressures as high as does stripping, so it is more acceptable. Suction applied to the chest drainage system usually makes stripping or milking of chest tubes unnecessary. With large amounts of drainage or clots the physician may still prescribe stripping or milking to prevent an obstruction. A patient with a mediastinal tube may develop tamponade if the CT is obstructed.
7. Should the CT accidentally be pulled out, apply a dressing to the site to prevent air from entering the chest. If an occlusive dressing is used, monitor the patient for the development of a tension pneumothorax. If a three-sided dressing is used, air is allowed to escape on expiration.

Chest tube removal

CTs can be removed when drainage and air leaks have ceased. Trial clamping of the CT may be done before CT removal; closely monitor the patient for respiratory distress. Chest radiographs are reviewed to ensure that the lung is re-expanded. Necessary equipment includes a suture set, plain or petroleum gauze, 4 × 4s, and adhesive tape. The tube is removed quickly on expiration.

Critical observations

Consult the physician for the following:
1. Respiratory rate >28/min
2. Pao_2 <60 mm Hg

PULM

3. Signs of hypoxia: restlessness, ↑ HR, dyspnea
4. CT drainage >200 ml/hr
5. New bubbling in underwater seal chamber not related to loose connections
6. Dislodged/obstructed CT
7. Deviated trachea

THORACIC SURGERY
Clinical Brief
Various procedures are performed to repair or explore abnormalities of the thorax. Indications include congenital or acquired deformities, traumatic injuries, lesions, and drainage of infectious processes (see Table 6-6).

▶ **Complications and Related Nursing Diagnoses**

Pain	Pain related to incision, chest tube
	Ineffective breathing pattern
Hemorrhage	Fluid volume deficit
	Altered tissue perfusion
Dysrhythmias	Decreased cardiac output
Hypoxia	Impaired gas exchange
	Altered tissue perfusion
Infection	High risk for infection
	Altered body temperature

Patient Care Management Guidelines
Patient assessment
1. Obtain BP and HR q15min until stable, hourly for the first 4 hours, then q2h. Hospital protocols may vary. Assess capillary refill (normal < 3 sec) and quality of peripheral pulses. Calculate MAP; a MAP < 60 mm Hg adversely affects cerebral and renal perfusion.
2. Assess oxygenation status: continuously monitor Spo_2, Svo_2, and capnography (if available). Review serial ABGs to evaluate oxygenation and acid-base status. Monitor PA systolic pressure, since hypoxia can increase sympathetic tone and increase pulmonary vasoconstriction. During the weaning process assess the patient for respiratory distress and increased patient effort. (See Weaning, p. 469.)
3. Monitor fluid volume status: record chest drainage, urinary output, and fluid intake hourly; determine fluid balance q8h. PAP and CVP reflect the capacity of the vascular system to accept volume and can be used to

Thoracic procedure	Definition	Indications
Segmental resection	Removal of segment of pulmonary lobe	Chronic, localized pyogenic lung abscess Congenital cyst or bleb Benign tumor Segment infected with pulmonary tuberculosis or bronchiectasis
Wedge resection	Excision of small peripheral section of lobe	Small masses that are close to pleural surface of lung, e.g., subpleural granulomas, small peripheral tumors (benign primary tumors)
Lobectomy	Excision of one or more lobes of lung tissue	Cancer Infections such as tuberculosis Miscellaneous benign tumors
Pneumonectomy	Removal of entire lung	Malignant neoplasms Lung almost entirely infected Extensive chronic abscess Selected unilateral lesions
Decortication of lung	Removal of fibrinous, reactive membrane covering visceral and parietal pleura	Restrictive fibrinous membrane lining visceral and parietal pleura that limits ventilatory excursion; "trapped lung"

From Johanson BC et al: Standards for critical care, St Louis, 1988, The CV Mosby Co.

Continued.

PULM

TABLE 6-6 Thoracic Procedures—cont'd

Thoracic procedure	Definition	Indications
Thoracoplasty	Surgical collapse of portion of chest wall by multiple rib resections to intentionally decrease volume in hemithorax	Closure of chronic cavitary lesions, empyema spaces, recurrent air leaks Reduction of open thoracic "dead space" after large resection
Thymectomy	Removal of thymus gland	Primary thymic neoplasm, myasthenia
Correction of pectus excavatum ("funnel chest")	Depression of sternum and costal cartilage corrected by moving sternum outward and realigning cartilage-sternal junction	Cosmesis and relief of cardiopulmonary compromise
Repair of penetrating thoracic wounds, drainage of hemothorax	Drainage of pleural cavity and control of hemorrhage	Hemorrhage produced by injury to thoracic vessels that causes blood loss as well as compression of lung tissue and mediastinum, resulting in cardiopulmonary compromise
Excision of mediastinal masses	Removal of masses/cysts in upper anterior/posterior mediastinum	Mediastinal tumors (benign or malignant), cysts, abscesses
Tracheal resection	Resection of portion of trachea, followed by primary end-to-end reanastomosis of trachea	Significant stenosis of tracheal orifice, usually related to mechanical pressure of cuffed tracheal tube; pressure produces tracheal wall ischemia, inflammation, and ulceration, leading to formation of granulation tissue and fibrosis, which narrow tracheal orifice; tumors

Esophagogastrectomy	Resection of part of esophagus and at least cardial portion of stomach with primary anastomosis of proximal esophagus to remaining stomach	Carcinoma of esophagus anywhere from neck to esophagogastric junction Severe reflux esophagitis producing hemorrhage Extensive alkali burns of esophagus Failure of medical therapy such as antibiotics and chest physiotherapy to control infection associated with such cysts or pockets
Bullectomy	Removal by excision of cysts or pockets in lung, which result from confluence of many alveoli	Severe compression of tissue adjacent to pulmonary cysts or pockets
Closed thoracostomy	Insertion of chest tube through intercostal space into pleural space; chest tube is attached to water seal system, with or without suction	Provision of continuous aspiration of fluid from pleural cavity Prevention of accumulation of air in chest from leaks in lung or tracheobronchial tree
Open thoracostomy	Partial resection of selected rib or ribs, with insertion of chest tube into infected material to provide for continuous drainage	Drainage of empyemas when pleural space is fixed

From Johanson BC et al: Standards for critical care, St Louis, 1988, The CV Mosby Co.

PULM

monitor for fluid overload and pulmonary edema. PAWP <4 mm Hg, CVP <2 mm Hg, and tachycardia suggest fluid volume deficit. Crackles, S_3, PAWP >20 mm Hg, and CVP >10 mm Hg suggest fluid overload.

4. Continuously monitor ECG to detect dysrhythmias. Hypoxia, acidosis, and electrolyte imbalance are risk factors.
5. Check dressing q1h for bleeding.

Patient management

1. Administer crystalloids or blood products as ordered to replace volume from blood loss.
2. Potassium 10 to 15 mEq/hr may be required to replace depleted levels from blood loss.
3. Reinforce the dressing as needed.
4. Record chest tube drainage q1h. Note the patency of tubes. Milking or stripping of chest tubes may be necessary to maintain patency. (See Chest drainage, p. 472.)
5. Elevate the HOB with the operative side up to facilitate lung expansion. Pneumonectomy patients should be positioned with the "good side" up, since drainage contamination from leaking suture lines or a tension pneumothorax may occur when the operative side is up.
6. Administer analgesics as ordered. Thoracic surgery can cause severe pain, which can result in hypoventilation. Encourage incentive spirometry and C & DB the patient. Provide chest physiotherapy and postural drainage to mobilize secretions.
7. If the patient is intubated and mechanically ventilated, see p. 463.

Critical observations

Consult with the physician for the following:

1. Tracheal deviation
2. Dysrhythmias
3. SBP <90 mm Hg
4. CT drainage >200 ml/hr
5. u/o < 20 ml/hr for 2 hours
6. O_2 sat <90%
7. Pao_2 <60 mm Hg
8. Svo_2 <60% or >80%
9. Potassium <3.5 mEq/L
10. Decreasing trend in Hgb and Hct
11. Development of air leak: bubbling in water seal chamber or subcutaneous emphysema
12. Possible pneumothorax: restlessness, SOB, increased respiratory rate, decreased compliance

Cardiovascular Modalities

AUTOMATIC IMPLANTABLE CARDIOVERTER DEFIBRILLATOR (AICD)

Clinical Brief

The automatic implantable cardioverter defibrillator (AICD) is employed in patients at high risk for sudden death (e.g., cardiac arrest not associated with myocardial infarction). The surgical technique includes a median sternotomy or thoracotomy approach. Electrodes are placed epicardially (ventricle), endocardially (ventricle), and within the superior vena cava. These leads are passed through the diaphragm to the abdomen and a battery-powered defibrillator is placed in the abdomen. This defibrillator is programmed to detect a high end cutoff rate, at which point an electrical shock will be delivered. The device requires 10-35 sec to confirm the rhythm and charge for defibrillation and will recharge and deliver up to three more shocks if needed for each event.

CV

▶ Complications and Related Nursing Diagnosis (for the Implantable Defibrillator)

(See Complications and management guidelines for cardiac surgery)

Malfunction	High risk for injury: dysrhythmias/sudden death
• Inappropriate shock	
• Failure to shock	

Patient Care Management Guidelines

Patient assessment (see Cardiac surgery)

1. Defibrillator function assessment is possible only when defibrillation occurs. The defibrillation is usually interpreted as an artifact on the monitor. If possible, note the time required to deliver the shock when VT/VF was initially detected.
2. Assess the patient's risk factors for a lethal event (e.g., hypoxemia, electrolyte imbalances).

Patient management

1. AICD may be in inactive mode for several days in the post-op period. Therefore, careful, continuous cardiac monitoring for recurrence of lethal dysrhythmias with the prompt initiation of ACLS protocols is warranted.

2. If AICD is in the active mode, up to four shocks can be given. When the AICD discharges, individuals touching the patient can receive up to a 2 joule shock. If VT/VF continues, initiate CPR and countershock. (Use of an external defibrillator does not damage AICD.)

3. Inappropriate discharge of the AICD may occur infrequently (patient shocked while in NSR). Be alert to this complication; countershock and initiate ACLS protocols as indicated. Inactivate the AICD should this occur.

4. Monitor for signs of infection after implantation of the AICD. Monitor temperature q4h. Note any drainage, redness, and increased tenderness at the surgical site.

5. Patient and family teaching must be done to prepare them to live with an AICD. Psychiatric intervention may be required for this adjustment to an altered way of life. The patient should be instructed to avoid 60-cycle interference, because it may temporarily or permanently render the defibrillator nonfunctioning. Magnetic resonance imaging is contraindicated.

Critical observations

Consult with the physician for the following:

1. Inappropriate discharge of AICD
2. Failure to discharge of AICD
3. Evidence of wound infection; T > 38.3° C (101° F), redness, drainage

INTRAAORTIC BALLOON PUMP (IABP) COUNTERPULSATION

Clinical Brief

The purpose of the IABP is to increase coronary artery perfusion and decrease myocardial oxygen consumption. Counterpulsation permits an increased aortic pressure during diastole (balloon inflation), augmenting coronary perfusion, and decreases aortic pressure during systole (balloon deflation), decreasing afterload. Consequently, counterpulsation produces the following effects:

Increased
MAP/SV/CO
Renal perfusion
Cerebral perfusion
Coronary artery perfusion
Decreased
LVEDP (PAWP)
Afterload (SVR)

MVO_2 demand
HR

Indications for IABP include cardiogenic shock related to acute MI or following cardiac surgery, noncardiogenic shock, ventricular septal defect, papillary muscle dysfunction, unstable angina that is unresponsive to medical management, and prophylactically for high-risk CV patients undergoing coronary angiography or general anesthesia.

Contraindications include irreversible brain damage, end-stage cardiac disease, aortic regurgitation, dissecting aortic aneurysm, and significant peripheral vascular disease.

Description

The IABP device consists of a balloon-tipped catheter and power console that permits inflation and deflation of the balloon during diastole and systole, respectively. The patient generally receives anticoagulation therapy. The catheter is inserted in the femoral artery via a percutaneous approach and advanced through the aorta. Correct placement of the catheter should be confirmed in the descending aorta distal to the left subclavian artery and proximal to the renal arteries. The functioning of the IABP is most often triggered according to the ECG (Figure 6-3) and timing adjusted from the arterial waveform (Figure 6-4). The balloon inflation causes an increase in diastolic aortic pressure and coronary artery pressure and improves coronary artery blood flow. This period is called *diastolic augmentation*. Rapid deflation of the balloon is timed to occur just before systole. Proper deflation of the balloon decreases the aortic pressure dramatically and allows the ventricle to empty more completely. Initially, the IABP is usually set to augment every cardiac cycle or every other cycle.

▶ Complications and Related Nursing Diagnoses

Poor IABP augmentation
• Balloon leak
• Incorrect timing
• Mechanical failure

Decreased cardiac output

Balloon migration
• Subclavian artery obstruction
• Renal artery obstruction

Altered tissue perfusion: cerebral, renal

Bleeding
• Thrombocytopenia
• Related to anticoagulation

Decreased cardiac output
Fluid volume deficit

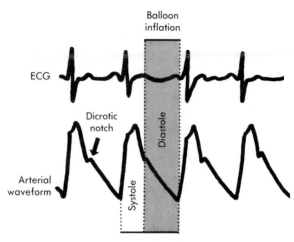

Figure 6-3 IABP period of balloon inflation. Balloon inflation occurs during diastole and should begin at aortic valve closure *(dicrotic notch)*; balloon deflation should occur just before the aortic valve opens. (From Stillwell S and Randall E: Pocket guide to cardiovascular care, St Louis, 1990, Mosby–Year Book, Inc.)

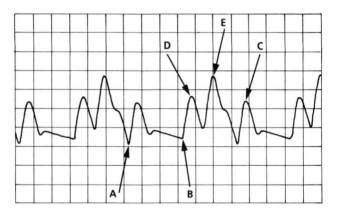

Figure 6-4 IABP timing 1:2 assist mode. *A,* Balloon-assisted aortic end diastolic pressure; *B,* patient aortic end diastolic pressure; *C,* balloon-assisted systole; *D,* patient systole; *E,* peak diastolic augmented pressure.

Hematoma formation at percutaneous access site	Pain in groin area secondary to hematoma Decreased cardiac output
Loss of peripheral pulses related to thrombus formation at access site	Altered tissue perfusion: peripheral Pain in affected extremity
Embolization	Altered tissue perfusion: cerebral, renal, peripheral
Infection	Altered body temperature High risk for injury: sepsis
Aortic dissection	Decreased cardiac output Altered tissue perfusion: peripheral, renal

Patient Care Management Guidelines
Patient assessment

1. The cardiovascular (CV) system should be assessed q30-60min for the first 4-6 hours after IABP insertion and should include VS, CVP, PAP, and cardiac rhythm; u/o should be monitored hourly.

2. A cardiac profile including cardiac output, cardiac index, and systemic vascular resistance (SVR) should be done on admission, q8-12h, and with any significant changes in hemodynamics.

3. Assess peripheral pulses (both pedal and posttibial pulses) for strength and equality q15-30min for 4-6 hours. Radial and brachial pulses in the left arm should also be assessed during these times to check for possible catheter migration, which would result in a diminished or absent pulse in this extremity. Verify that the skin color remains pink, the skin is warm to the touch, and that capillary refill is equally brisk bilaterally. If a change in quality of pulses is noted, a Doppler device should be employed to attempt to identify pulses.

4. Assess the percutaneous insertion site for oozing, ecchymosis, or hematoma formation q15-30min for 4-6 hours after IABP insertion.

5. Augmentation of IABP should be assessed hourly and as needed. Balloon-assisted systolic pressure should be 5-15 mm Hg lower than the patient's diastolic pressure. Balloon migration should be ruled out with the development of poor IABP augmentation, changes in LOC (possible subclavian artery occlusion), a diminished radial pulse in the left arm, or a decrease in urinary output

(possible renal artery occlusion). A stat chest radiograph is crucial to verify placement. The radiopaque catheter tip should be just distal to the aortic arch.

6. If pain occurs at the groin percutaneous access site, assess the area for hematoma formation and administer analgesics as per protocol.

Patient management

1. The inflation of the balloon should be timed to occur at the dicrotic notch and should be timed to deflate just before the next systole (see Figure 6-4). Instruct the patient to keep the affected leg immobilized and do not elevate the HOB > 30 degrees.

2. Inflation and deflation timing are usually adjusted via slide bars. The goal of the adjustment is to achieve maximum diastolic augmentation and minimum aortic end diastolic pressure. Late deflation of the balloon may be a more ominous occurrence by at least partially occluding the left ventricular outflow.

3. If blood is noted in the lumen communicating with the balloon, rupture of the balloon must be ruled out. The balloon should be placed on stand-by and the physician called immediately.

4. A pressure dressing and/or a sandbag may be applied at the insertion site as per unit protocol. A large amount of blood may exsanguinate into the groin and upper thigh without any obvious evidence; therefore close monitoring is warranted. Watch for hematoma formation at the access site. Mark the site carefully with a skin marking pen and assess hourly for the first 4 hr and at least q4h thereafter to determine the magnitude of the hematoma.

5. Maintain proper functioning of the balloon pump according to the manufacturer's guidelines. Maintain airtight seals on all connections between the pump and the patient. Maintain adequate augmentation by setting the timing of inflation and deflation.

Critical observations

Consult with the physician for the following:

1. Inability to maintain adequate augmentation
2. Accidental dislodgment or removal of catheter
3. Migration of balloon tip: decrease in u/o, changes in LOC, decrease or loss of pulse in an extremity
4. Excessive bleeding at access site
5. Balloon rupture
6. Coagulation studies (PTT) out of range

TEMPORARY PACEMAKERS

Clinical Brief

The purpose is to provide an artificial stimulus to the myocardium when the heart is unable to initiate an impulse or the conduction system is defective. Types of pacemakers include temporary (external or internal) or permanent. Pacing modes can be asynchronous, in which the impulse is generated at a fixed rate despite the rhythm of the patient, or synchronous, in which the impulse is generated on demand or as needed according to the patient's intrinsic rhythm.

Indications for pacing include symptomatic type II AV heart block; complete heart block; sick sinus syndrome; bradydysrhythmias and tachydysrhythmias such as SVT, atrial fibrillation, or atrial flutter with rapid ventricular response; and intermittent VT unresponsive to drug therapy.

The external temporary pacemaker (transcutaneous pacemaker) is used to emergently treat symptomatic bradydysrhythmias unresponsive to medications until more definitive treatment can be employed. The external pacemaker includes a pulse generator, pacing cable attached to large external electrodes, and an ECG cable for the demand mode. One electrode is placed at V_3 anteriorly and the other is placed in the left subscapular area. The mA setting ranges from 50 to 210.

Temporary internal pacing can be accomplished via epicardial, transthoracic, or transvenous electrode placement. Epicardial electrodes are placed during cardiac surgery and exit through the chest wall. Transthoracic electrodes are inserted into the right ventricle via a cardiac needle using a subxyphoid approach. Transvenous electrodes are threaded into the right atrium or right ventricle using a venous approach. A version of the PA catheter has a pacing electrode within it. The electrodes are used in the same manner as the transvenous ventricular pacer. All electrodes are attached to the negative and positive poles of the pulse generator.

CV

▶ Complications and Related Nursing Diagnoses

Muscle twitching (external pacer)	Pain
Failure to pace	Decreased cardiac output
Failure to capture	Decreased cardiac output
Failure to sense	Decreased cardiac output
	High risk for injury: life-threatening dysrhythmias

Patient Care Management Guidelines
Patient assessment
1. Monitor ECG for proper pacemaker functioning, e.g., pacing artifact and typical pacing complex.
2. Assess sensorium, skin color and temperature, capillary refill, u/o, HR, and BP.

Patient management
1. Muscle twitching or chest wall discomfort occurs frequently with the use of external pacemakers. Sedation and/or analgesia are usually an effective treatment.
2. Failure to pace:
   a. Check all connections between generator and patient.
   b. If the external pacemaker is in use, check the electrodes for adequate surface contact: excessive hair at the electrode placement should be trimmed; however, shaving may cause nicks and increase chest impedance. A displaced ECG lead, with subsequent flat line, will result in 100% pacing as the pacemaker interprets asystole. If the patient rolls onto the side, poor chest wall contact may result and additional taping may be necessary. The power supply (i.e., the battery) should be changed to rule it out as a source of the problem.
   c. With transvenous or epicardial pacing, lead displacement or fracture may cause failure to pace. If the situation cannot be quickly remedied, prepare to externally pace the patient until more definitive treatment can be rendered.
3. Failure to capture (Figure 6-5):
   a. The problem may arise from any of the problems mentioned in the previous section, and the same interventions are warranted.
   b. The problem may also be low voltage and may be corrected by increasing the mA.
   c. Repositioning the patient to the left side may also correct the problem.
4. Symptomatic hypotension may be a result of too slow a rate and may be corrected by merely increasing the rate.
5. If defibrillation is required, the pulse generator should be disconnected to prevent damage.
6. Failure to sense (transvenous or epicardial pacemakers) (Figure 6-6):
   a. Failure to sense may be a result of catheter tip migration, faulty sensing, or battery failure.

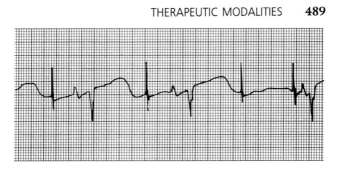

Figure 6-5   Failure to capture. (From Conover M: Pocket guide to electrocardiography, St Louis, 1990, Mosby–Year Book, Inc.)

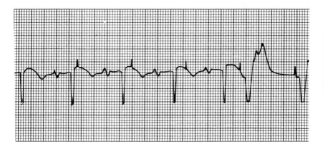

Figure 6-6   Failure to sense. (From Conover M: Pocket guide to electrocardiography, St Louis, 1990, Mosby–Year Book, Inc.)

CV

    b. Turn the patient to the left side, change the power source (battery), or increase the sensitivity of the generator.
    c. If failure to sense is creating extra impulses that are dangerously close to R on T phenomenon, then prepare to externally pace the patient and turn off the pacer.
    d. Sustained dysrhythmias should be treated as per ACLS protocol.

Critical observations

Consult with the physician for the following:
1. Failure to capture despite nursing interventions
2. Failure to pace despite nursing interventions
3. Failure to sense despite nursing interventions

VENTRICULAR ASSIST DEVICES (VAD)
Clinical Brief
The purpose of a VAD is to maintain systemic circulation and improve tissue perfusion in patients with severe ventricular dysfunction while allowing the ventricle(s) to recover. Roller, vortex, or pneumatic devices can be used to reroute blood from the ventricle(s) to reduce preload and afterload and thus decrease the workload of the heart. Both right and left VADs can be used if needed to support ventricular function. Improvement is generally observed within 48 hours.

Indications include patients with profound cardiogenic shock refractory to medications, counterpulsation, and those patients who are unable to be weaned from cardiopulmonary bypass. A VAD can also be used while the patient awaits cardiac transplantation. Contraindications include irreversible disease processes from which recovery is unlikely.

▶ Complications and Related Nursing Diagnoses

Significant postoperative bleeding	Decreased cardiac output
• Anticoagulation	Fluid volume deficit
• Hemolysis	
Air embolus and thrombus	Altered tissue perfusion
• Cerebral	
• Peripheral	
• Renal	
• GI	
Right ventricular failure with LVAD implanted	Decreased cardiac output
Sepsis	High risk for infection
Mechanical failure	Decreased cardiac output

(Also see Complications following cardiac surgery.)

Patient Care Management Guidelines
NOTE: Follow the guidelines detailed under Cardiac surgery (p. 501), as appropriate, in addition to the following.
Patient assessment
1. A thorough assessment should be completed on the patient on arrival to the recovery area. The patient should be frequently assessed because of the instability often present in the early postoperative period. Careful assessment of patient, tubing, LVAD, and blood flow should be performed on initial examination and q1h thereafter.
2. The cardiovascular system should be assessed q15-30min for the first 6-8 hours and include VS, CVP, PAP, car-

diac rhythm, incision-dressing appearance, hourly chest tube drainage, quality of the peripheral pulses, and hourly u/o.

3. A cardiac profile including CO, CI, and SVR should be done on admission, q8-12h, and with any significant changes in hemodynamic status.

4. Monitor serial Hgb and Hct and coagulation profiles as ordered for evidence of bleeding and/or coagulopathy.

5. Monitor temperature q2h.

Patient management

1. Keep patient supine; partially turn as necessary. Keep the patient sedated with intravenous diazepam (Valium) or midazolam (Versed) and restrain the patient to decrease risk of exsanguination.

2. Avoid tension in the tubes; eliminating kinks in tubing will assist in preventing emboli or thrombi formation. The use of heparin via a continuous IV infusion may be necessary, especially with continuous flow devices.

3. Monitor PAP and hemodynamics to maintain filling pressures. Maintain MAP > 70 mm Hg and LAP 10-20 mm Hg.

4. RV failure may occur after initiation of LVAD use and may necessitate RVAD.

5. Chest tube drainage in excess of 150 ml/hr for 2 hours may indicate increased bleeding and may require emergent thoracic reexploration. Excess bleeding may also be a result of coagulopathy. Serum coagulation profiles (e.g., PT, PTT, platelet count, fibrinogen) may reveal deficits requiring replacement with fresh frozen plasma, platelets, cryoprecipitate, and clotting factors. Anemia associated with excess bleeding can lead to relative hypoxemia and requires prompt replacement with packed RBCs.

6. Prophylactic antibiotic therapy may be ordered.

7. If cardiac arrest occurs, internal cardiac massage and internal defibrillation should be substituted in the ACLS protocol.

Critical observations

Consult with the physician for the following:

1. Dislodgment of cannulas in chest
2. Tubing obstruction
3. Inability to maintain MAP
4. Evidence of infection

CV

PERCUTANEOUS TRANSLUMINAL CORONARY ANGIOPLASTY (PTCA)

Clinical Brief

The purpose of PTCA is to restore adequate blood supply to the myocardium by restoring the lumen diameter of a coronary artery. Indications for PTCA include documented myocardial ischemia unresponsive to medical management and emergently in the treatment of acute myocardial infarction.

Patient selection

In general, patients who are candidates for PTCA include individuals with discrete lesions, preferably involving one or two vessels, and not at vessel bifurcations. The patient also should be a candidate for coronary artery bypass graft (CABG) surgery. Contraindications include patients who are not surgical candidates, patients who have nonviable myocardium distal to the stenotic lesion, and patients with tortuous coronary arteries.

The procedure is similar to a cardiac catheterization. Once a percutaneous access is established, a specially equipped catheter with a balloon tip is advanced to the affected coronary artery. The lesion is crossed with the catheter and the balloon is inflated, compressing the atherosclerotic plaque in an effort to increase the lumen diameter. Because the coronary artery distal to the balloon is occluded during inflation, the patient may experience angina. The patient receives anticoagulation therapy during the procedure with intravenous heparin. Intracoronary thrombolytic therapy may be administered to treat acute thrombus formation local to the culprit lesion. Intracoronary nitroglycerin may also be administered to prevent or treat vasospasm.

▶ Complications and Related Nursing Diagnoses

Acute restenosis	Pain
Reaction to contrast dye	Decreased cardiac output Fluid volume excess Ineffective breathing pattern
Vasovagal reaction	High risk for injury: bradycardia
Reperfusion dysrhythmias	High risk for injury: heart blocks, ventricular ectopy/tachycardia, and/or accelerated idioventricular rhythm
Bleeding related to anticoagulation	Decreased cardiac output High risk for injury: bleeding

Hematoma formation at percutaneous access site	Pain in groin area secondary to hematoma Decreased cardiac output
Loss of peripheral pulses	Altered tissue perfusion: peripheral Pain in affected extremity

Patient Care Management Guidelines
Patient assessment

1. Assess cardiovascular status (i.e., HR and BP) for evidence of restenosis q1h for 6-12 hours. ECGs should be performed q4-6h for 12-24 hours and prn with any complaint of angina or SOB. Anginal pain, SOB, and/or ST segment changes represent potential acute restenosis. The patient should also be monitored for dysrhythmias, which can signal successful reperfusion. These reperfusion dysrhythmias are usually not treated unless the patient is symptomatic (e.g., acute drop in SBP, acute change in sensorium, and/or cool, pale, diaphoretic skin).
2. Assess access site for oozing, ecchymosis, or hematoma formation q15-30min for 4-6 hours. If a hematoma develops at the groin access site, the size should be monitored by outlining the borders with a skin marking pen. A large amount of blood may exsanguinate into the groin and upper thigh without necessarily an early drop in SBP or an increase in HR; therefore close observation of the access site is warranted.
3. Assess for comfort level q1-2h for 12-24 hours. If pain develops at the groin access site, assess for local hematoma formation.
4. Assess peripheral pulses (pedal and posttibial pulses) for strength and equality q15-30min for 4-6 hours. A Doppler device may be helpful in identifying peripheral pulses, especially if the patient is cool.
5. Monitor coagulation studies, specifically PT and PTT. The normal value for the PT is < 14 sec and the normal value for the PTT is < 37 sec.

Patient management

1. The patient should be instructed to promptly report any chest pain or SOB.
2. Low-flow oxygen therapy should be administered as per protocol.

CV

3. The HOB should be kept less than 30 degrees to prevent dislodgment of groin access catheter.
4. Maintain hypercoagulated state as per protocol.
5. If the patient was sedated during the procedure and remains sedated, institute aspiration precautions until the patient is fully alert.
6. If the patient reports chest pain, intravenous or sublingual nitroglycerin may be effective in relieving discomfort: sublingual, 1 tablet q5min × 3; IV, start with an infusion of 5 μg/min; titrate to desired response or to maintain SBP > 90 mm Hg. Increase dosage q5-10min by 5-10 μg/min. If hypotension occurs, raise the patient's legs and stop the infusion.
7. If the patient becomes hypotensive, place the patient flat. Fluid challenges may be ordered. If the patient is also bradycardic, administer atropine as per ACLS protocol.
8. If pain occurs at the groin access site, administer analgesics as per protocol.
9. If a hematoma forms at the access site, a pressure dressing should be applied.
10. If nausea and/or vomiting occur, administer antiemetics as per protocol.

SHEATH REMOVAL
1. Once the physician has ordered the catheter(s) removed, the patient should be informed of the forthcoming procedure.
2. The access site should be prepared as per protocol (local anesthesia, betadine prep, suture removal).
3. The catheters should be removed and direct pressure applied until hemostasis is achieved.
4. Once the site is stable, a pressure dressing should be applied and the site and peripheral pulses should be monitored frequently.

Critical observations:
Consult with the physician for the following:
1. Increase or onset of chest pain or angina symptoms
2. Hypotension and bradycardia
3. Significant groin site hematoma formation
4. Significant oozing or bleeding at groin site
5. A change in quality or loss of peripheral pulses
6. Increased times in coagulation studies
7. The onset of dysrhythmia formation

OTHER PERCUTANEOUS CARDIOVASCULAR MODALITIES

Clinical Brief

Lasers, atherectomies, and stents may be treatment options to improve blood supply to the myocardium by restoring the lumen diameter of a coronary artery in patients with CAD. These procedures are used with PTCA to treat complications of dilation and prevent restenosis. A catheter equipped with a laser, atherectomy device, or a loaded wire stent is used to vaporize or shave the atheromatous plaque or to mechanically support the coronary artery. Lasers may be used alone or in combination with balloon angioplasty.

The laser may be used to burn a hole in the center of the plaque so that balloon angioplasty can be employed or the laser can be used to thermally seal the artery following angioplasty. Arterial perforation, embolization, and spasm are laser-related complications.

Transluminal atherectomy involves positioning the device toward the lesion and shaving away the plaque. A balloon is inflated to stabilize the catheter, and the excised plaque is collected in a housing compartment and removed. Restenosis of the artery can occur following the atherectomy.

The intracoronary stent is a wire device designed to support the coronary artery and prevent acute stenosis following PTCA. A delivery system positions the stent at the lesion site and is released. The stent expands and improves the vessel's intraluminal diameter. However, acute closure secondary to thrombosis may occur; aggressive heparinization is required.

Patient selection

In general, patients who are candidates for PTCA will be candidates for these new interventional procedures. Clinical studies are investigating the types of devices and techniques, as well as the safety and efficacy of the procedures.

Complications and Related Nursing Diagnoses

See PTCA, p. 492.

Patient Care Management Guidelines

See PTCA, p. 493.

PERIPHERAL ANGIOPLASTY OR LASER THERAPY

Clinical Brief

The purpose of angioplasty or laser therapy is to restore blood flow distal to the lesion. This is accomplished in the same manner as with PTCA or coronary artery laser therapy.

▶ **Complications and Related Nursing Diagnoses**
See PTCA, p. 492.

Ischemia to organ system with reduced blood supply	Altered tissue perfusion: renal, GI, and/or peripheral

Patient Care Management Guidelines
Patient assessment
See PTCA, p. 493.
1. Monitor affected organ system for return of functioning or acute loss of function.

Patient management
See PTCA, p. 493.

Critical observations
See PTCA, p. 494.

PERCUTANEOUS VALVULOPLASTY (PV)

Clinical Brief

The purpose of PV is to restore normal blood flow through a previously stenotic cardiac valve. The procedure is similar to a cardiac catheterization. Percutaneous access is established and the patient receives anticoagulation therapy. For tricuspid, pulmonic, or mitral PV a right-sided (venous) approach is used. Mitral PV requires an atrial transseptal approach and creates an increased risk for complications. For aortic PV, the most common form, a left-sided (arterial) approach is used. Regardless of which valve is involved, a specially equipped balloon-tip catheter is used. Once the valve is crossed with the catheter, the balloon is inflated and the commissures are split or the calcium nodules are fractured. Indications for PV include a documented (via an echocardiogram or a ventriculogram) critical flow gradient across a valve. Because of the high restenosis rate, the procedure is used for patients who are high surgical risks. Contraindications include heavy calcification associated with the stenosis.

▶ **Complications and Related Nursing Diagnoses**

Leaflet tearing, fragmentation of leaflets, annulus disruption	Decreased cardiac output Impaired gas exchange: pulmonary edema
Embolization to brain	Altered tissue perfusion: cerebral
Cardiac tamponade	Decreased cardiac output
Dysrhythmias secondary to local edema resulting from balloon manipulation	Decreased cardiac output

Left to right shunt related to transseptal approach	Decreased cardiac output
Reaction to contrast dye	Decreased cardiac output Fluid volume excess Ineffective breathing pattern
Vasovagal reaction	High risk for injury: symptomatic bradycardia
Reperfusion dysrhythmias	High risk for injury: symptomatic heart blocks and/or ventricular ectopy/ tachycardia
Bleeding related to anticoagulation therapy	High risk for injury: bleeding
Hematoma formation at percutaneous access site	Pain in groin area secondary to hematoma
Loss of peripheral pulses related to thrombus formation at access site	Altered tissue perfusion: peripheral Pain in affected extremity

CV

Patient Care Management Guidelines
Patient assessment
1. Assess cardiovascular status every half hour for 4-6 hours. The patient will most likely have central venous pressure (CVP) and pulmonary artery (PA) catheters in place, and these readings should be included in the cardiovascular assessment. Changes in CVP readings, PAP readings, and/or heart sounds may indicate acute valvular failure, cardiac tamponade, or exacerbation of left to right shunt resulting from the transseptal approach, requiring emergency surgery. Heart sounds should be auscultated and murmurs graded. Diastolic murmurs may develop as the procedure corrects the stenotic valve. The patient should also be monitored for dysrhythmias.
2. Assess access site for oozing, ecchymosis, or hematoma q15-30min for 4-6 hours. If a hematoma develops at the groin access site, the size should be monitored by outlining the borders with a skin marking pen. A large amount of blood may exsanguinate into the groin and upper thigh without an early drop in SBP or an increase in HR; close observation of the access site is warranted.
3. Assess for comfort level q1-2h for 12-24 hours. If pain develops at the groin access site, assess for local hematoma formation.

4. Assess peripheral pulses (pedal and posttibial pulses) for strength and equality q15-30min for 4-6 hours. A Doppler device may be helpful in identifying peripheral pulses especially if the patient is cool.
5. Monitor coagulation studies.

Patient management

1. Low-flow oxygen therapy should be administered.
2. The HOB should be kept less than 30 degrees to prevent dislodgement of the groin access catheter.
3. Maintain the hypercoagulated state as per protocol.
4. If the patient was sedated during the procedure and remains sedated, institute aspiration precautions until the patient is fully alert.
5. If the patient becomes hypotensive, place the patient flat and administer fluid challenges as ordered. If the patient is also bradycardic, administer atropine as per ACLS protocols.
6. If pain occurs at the groin access site, administer analgesics as per protocol.
7. If a hematoma forms at the access site, a pressure dressing should be applied.
8. If nausea and/or vomiting occur, administer antiemetics as per protocol.

SHEATH REMOVAL

1. Once the physician has ordered the catheter(s) removed, the patient should be informed of the forthcoming procedure.
2. The access site should be prepared as per protocol (e.g., local anesthesia, betadine prep, suture removal).
3. The catheters should be removed and direct pressure applied.
4. Once the site is stable, a pressure dressing should be applied.
5. The site and peripheral pulses should be monitored frequently.

Critical observations

Consult with the physician for the following:
1. Significant changes in BP, CVP, and PAP readings
2. Muffling of heart sounds or development or changes in the quality of a murmur
3. Significant groin site hematoma formation
4. Significant oozing or bleeding at the groin site
5. A change in quality or loss of peripheral pulses

THROMBOLYTIC THERAPY

Clinical Brief

The purpose of thrombolytic therapy is to lyse acutely formed thrombi in the coronary artery and restore blood flow to the myocardium. Thrombolytic agents act as plasminogen activators and have an affinity for circulating plasminogen (non-clot-specific) or fibrin-bound plasminogen (clot-specific). Alteplase (activase) is clot specific. Streptokinase (SK) and anisoylated plasminogen streptokinase activator complex (APSAC) are non-clot-specific. In lower doses, APSAC is more clot-specific than SK. The half-life of SK and APSAC are 25 and 90 minutes, respectively.

Indications for thrombolytic therapy include patients with ongoing angina unresolved by nitroglycerin, lasting more than 30 minutes but less than 6 hours, who have evidence of S-T elevation, who are younger than 75 years old, and have no contraindications.

Contraindications include active internal bleeding, a history of cerebrovascular disease, uncontrolled hypertension (SBP >200 or DBP >110), recent major surgery, recent trauma, history of intracranial or intraspinal surgery, pregnancy, diabetic hemorrhagic retinopathy, or intracranial disorders.

CV

▶ Complications and Related Nursing Diagnoses

Hematoma formation	High risk for injury: bleeding Decreased cardiac output Pain at puncture site
Acute reocclusion	Altered tissue perfusion: myocardial ischemia Pain: chest discomfort
Reperfusion dysrhythmias	Decreased cardiac output
Bleeding	Decreased cardiac output Fluid volume deficit Altered tissue perfusion: peripheral and/or cerebral Pain: abdominal pain, back pain, headache, and/or puncture site pain

Patient Care Management Guidelines

NOTE: Refer to policy/procedure and pharmacy protocol.

Patient assessment

1. The cardiovascular (CV) system should be assessed on patient's arrival to the unit and hourly thereafter until

the patient's condition is stable. This assessment should include P, RR, and BP and cardiac rhythm strip assessment. Urinary output should be monitored hourly.

2. Obtain a baseline ECG and compare with prior ECGs to determine the effectiveness of therapy. Mark lead placement sites with a skin marking pen to ensure proper lead placement. Monitor serial ECGs as ordered by the physician and compare each new ECG to prior ECGs to determine the efficacy of therapy as evidenced by normalization of ST segments and T waves. Although the patient may continue to experience minimal residual discomfort, any change in the quality of pain should be investigated with an ECG.

3. Assess the patient for bleeding. All recent puncture sites should be monitored for oozing or hematoma formation. Test all stools and emesis and dipstick urine for occult blood. Assess for headache or change in LOC.

Patient management

1. Before the initiation of thrombolytic therapy, noncompressible IV sites should be avoided. If feasible, use double-lumen peripheral intravenous catheters and place a heparin lock before thrombolytic administration for blood sampling. Avoid IM injections and unnecessary trauma (e.g., continuous-use automatic blood pressure cuffs). Insertion of a Foley catheter after therapy is initiated should be avoided.

2. Nitroglycerin and/or morphine sulfate should be administered to treat angina. Recurrence of angina with documented ECG changes represents possible reocclusion, and the patient should be prepared for possible emergent cardiac catheterization, PTCA, or CABG surgery.

3. A wide variety of dysrhythmias occurs with thrombolytic therapy, including nonsustained VT, bradydysrhythmias, junctional escape rhythms, and idioventricular rhythms. Most of these rhythms do not require intervention despite their lethal appearance. However, sustained rhythms should be treated as per ACLS protocol.

4. All puncture sites should be compressed until hemostasis is assured.

5. Prophylactic antiulcer medication, such as IV cimetidine or ranitidine, and/or PO antacids may be ordered.

6. Monitor PTT and hemograms for acute changes. PTT is generally kept 2½ times greater than normal during heparin therapy to prevent thrombus reformation.

Critical observations

Consult with the physician for the following:

1. Inability to achieve ordered PTT value
2. Signs of bleeding
3. Significant hematoma formation
4. New onset of chest pain
5. New changes in ECG after initial improvement
6. No change in ECG/pain level despite thrombolytic therapy
7. Neurological changes

CARDIAC SURGERY

Clinical Brief

Generally, the purpose of cardiac surgery is to optimize cardiac function. Cardiac surgery is employed when medical management and less invasive interventions fail or no longer control symptoms. For all of the cardiac surgeries detailed in this section, general anesthesia and a sternotomy (vertical midsternal incision) approach is used. The anterior surface of the heart is accessed and the patient is placed on cardiopulmonary bypass (CPB) via cannulation of the aortic root and vena cava or right atrium. Proximal to the cannulation, the aortic root is clamped in order to ensure a bloodless environment. A cold, potassium-rich solution is instilled in and around the heart to create a motion-free environment and to dramatically reduce myocardial oxygen demand. Once the surgical procedure is complete, the aorta is unclamped and the heart is warmed. The heart is defibrillated to restore normal electrical function and the patient is then weaned from the CPB machine. Epicardial pacing wires are placed in the event of bradycardia and chest tubes are inserted to drain the mediastinum and thoracic cavity.

The purpose, indications, and description of the various cardiac surgeries are detailed in the box on pp. 502-503. Contraindications for cardiac surgery are limited to patients who are not surgical candidates or whose conditions are terminal in the short term.

► Complications and Related Nursing Diagnoses

(Common following cardiac surgery)

Perioperative myocardial infarction	Decreased cardiac output
Excess bleeding	Decreased cardiac output Altered tissue perfusion Fluid volume deficit

CV

Cardiovascular Surgeries

Type: Coronary artery bypass graft surgery (CABG)

Purpose: To restore adequate blood flow to the myocardium distal to the coronary artery stenosis.

Indications: Myocardial ischemia refractory to medical management. Lesions must be discrete and not amenable to PTCA (e.g., triple vessel disease, diffuse disease, proximal lesions with a large amount of myocardium at risk).

Description: Saphenous vein grafts (SVG) are harvested from the lower extremities, and/or the internal mammary artery (IMA) is stripped down from the anterior chest wall. The SVG are anastomosed to the aortic root at one end and the other end of the graft is anastomosed to the coronary artery distal to the stenosis. If the IMA is used, the distal end is anastomosed to the coronary artery distal to the stenosis.

Type: Valvular repair/replacement (VR)

Purpose: To restore normal or near-normal function to a valve that is stenotic and/or incompetent.

Indications: Critical tricuspid, pulmonic, mitral, or aortic stenosis and/or incompetence. The patient must also be a candidate for major surgery.

Description: Access is gained by an atrial incision or aortic/pulmonic artery root incision. During valvuloplasty the fused commissures may be split via incision. Leaflets may be sewn to repair tears or stretching. A prosthetic annulus may be installed to restore normal shape. During VR the dysfunctional valve is removed and replaced with a mechanical or bioprosthetic (tissue) valve.

Type: Atrial/ventricular septal defect repair

Purpose: To repair left to right shunts that are a result of congenital defects or septal perforation related to acute myocardial infarction.

Indications: Congenital septal defects or acute septal perforation related to myocardial infarction. Surgical repair is reserved for hemodynamic instability secondary to the defect.

Description: An incision is made in the atrium or ventricle. The defect is patched with a synthetic graft; the incision is closed.

Type: Ventricular aneurysm repair

Purpose: To remove scar tissue that has formed as a result of myocardial infarction.

Indications: Ventricular aneurysm. Surgical repair is performed when the aneurysm is large enough to put the patient at high risk for ventricular rupture or there is evidence of significant thrombus formation.

Description: The aneurysm is excised and the ventricle is surgically repaired.

Cardiovascular Surgeries—cont'd

Type: Myotomy/myomectomy
Purpose: To restore an adequate left ventricular outflow tract.
Indications: Symptomatic obstructive hypertrophic cardiomyopathy.
Description: Access to the left ventricle is gained via the aortic valve orifice or a ventricular incision. Excess myocardium is shaved from the surface to create an adequate outflow tract. The aortic or mitral valve may be replaced as necessary.

Cardiac tamponade	Decreased cardiac output Altered tissue perfusion
Increased afterload/hypertension	High risk for injury Pain
Decreased preload/hypovolemia	Decreased cardiac output Fluid volume deficit
Dysrhythmias	Decreased cardiac output: bradycardia/SVT/VT/ asystole/atrial fibrillation
Fluid and electrolyte imbalance	Fluid volume excess Fluid volume deficit
Acid/base imbalance	Impaired gas exchange Altered tissue perfusion
Renal failure	Altered tissue perfusion Fluid volume excess
Respiratory failure	Impaired gas exchange
Cerebral vascular accident	Altered tissue perfusion: cerebral

CV

Patient Care Management Guidelines
Patient assessment
1. A thorough assessment should be completed on the patient on arrival in the recovery area. The patient should be assessed frequently because of the instability often present in the early postoperative period.
2. The cardiovascular system should be assessed q15-30min for the first 6-8 hours and include VS, CVP, PAP, cardiac rhythm, incision dressing appearance, hourly chest tube drainage, quality of peripheral pulses, and hourly

urinary output. Heart sounds should be assessed for changes in quality and intensity of murmurs (VR and VSD/ASD repairs) and muffled tones.

3. A cardiac profile including CO, CI, and SVR should be done on admission, q8-12h, and with any significant changes in hemodynamic status.

Patient management

1. Restlessness as the patient is waking up from anesthesia is often associated with profound hypertension and hemodynamic instability. Restlessness may require the use of IV diazepam (Valium) or midazolam (Versed). Pain can be managed with intravenous morphine sulfate; give IVP in 2 mg increments q5min to relieve symptoms. Dilute with 5 ml NS and administer over 4-5 min.

2. It is recommended to keep systolic blood pressure less than 140 mm Hg to prevent damage to the anastomoses or the fresh suture lines in patients who have had CABG surgery. Furthermore, a MAP of > 70 mm Hg is desirable in these patients to prevent the acute collapse of the grafts.

3. Increased afterload occurs often postoperatively and is usually managed via intravenous administration of sodium nitroprusside and/or nitroglycerin. Nitroglycerin may be administered IV to gain desired response: start with an infusion of 5 μg/min; titrate to desired response or to maintain SBP > 90 mm Hg. Increase dosage q5-10min by 5-10 μg/min. If hypotension occurs, raise the patient's legs and stop the infusion. Sodium nitroprusside may be administered by IV infusion to maintain systolic BP to 100 mm Hg. Dose may range from 0.5-10 μg/kg/min. Do not administer more than 10 μg/kg/min or the patient may exhibit signs and symptoms of cyanide toxicity: tinnitus, blurred vision, delirium, and muscle spasm. (See Chapter 7, Pharmacology, for more information.)

4. Decreased preload occurs often postoperatively and is usually secondary to hypovolemia. This relative hypovolemia is usually the result of CPB, diuretics administered while weaning from CPB, postoperative bleeding, and postoperative warming of the patient.

   Blood products and colloid fluids are usually the most effective in correcting hypovolemia due to their longer intravascular half-life.

5. Myocardial ischemia and/or infarction is suspected when ECG reveals ST elevation, ST depression, or inverted T waves resulting in potential decreased CO with subsequent hypotension and increased dysrhythmias. Ensuring adequate oxygenation, administration of topical or intravenous nitroglycerin, and administration of sublingual nifedepine as per protocol may prove effective in relieving ischemia. Serial ECGs will reveal effectiveness of interventions. Decreased CO can be treated with inotropic agents such as dobutamine or amrinone administered as per protocol. Dobutamine can be administered via continuous IV infusion. Infuse initially at 0.5 μg/kg/min. Doses of 2.5-10 μg/kg/min are normal. Amrinone is typically administered via initial IV bolus followed by a maintenance drip. Initial IV bolus should be given as 0.75 mg/kg over 2-3 min. Titrate infusion at 5-10 μg/kg/min. Total 24-hour dose should not exceed 10 mg/kg. (See Chapter 7 for more information.)

6. Chest tube drainage in excess of 150 ml/hr for 2 hours may indicate bleeding at graft anastomoses and may require emergent thoracic reexploration. Excess bleeding may also be a result of coagulopathy. Serum coagulation profiles (e.g., PT, PTT, platelet count, fibrinogen) may reveal deficits requiring replacement with fresh frozen plasma, platelets, cryoprecipitate, and clotting factors. Anemia associated with excess bleeding can lead to relative hypoxemia and requires prompt replacement with packed RBCs.

7. While the patient's lungs are being mechanically ventilated, the use of positive end-expiratory pressure (PEEP) may be helpful in reducing bleeding at anastomosed sites in the thoracic cavity.

8. Dysrhythmias are common occurrences and can include atrial fibrillation, SVT, VT, junctional tachycardia, complete heart block, asystole, and ventricular standstill. Dysrhythmias should be treated as per ACLS protocol. Postoperatively, patients are prone to hypokalemia; therefore the dysrhythmia breakthrough threshold is decreased. Hypokalemia should be treated promptly and serum potassium levels monitored frequently. A temporary pacemaker should be available to use with epicardial pacing leads in the event of asystole, ventricular standstill, or hemodynamically unstable bradycardia.

CV

9. Cardiac tamponade usually occurs as a result of excessive intrathoracic bleeding and/or ineffective draining of chest tubes. Signs of cardiac tamponade include narrowing pulse pressure, increasing PAP and CVP, increase in size of cardiac silhouette on chest radiograph, and muffled heart sounds. Treatment of related decrease in cardiac output includes inotropic agents and increasing intravascular volume replacement until thoracic reexploration can be performed.

Critical observations

Consult with the physician for the following:

1. Acute drop in or trend of decreasing cardiac output
2. Inability to control blood pressure (sustained hypotension or hypertension)
3. Sudden cessation of chest tube drainage
4. Excessive chest tube drainage
5. New onset of ECG S-T changes
6. Muffling of heart sounds

PERIPHERAL VASCULAR SURGERY (PVS)

Clinical Brief

Peripheral arterial occlusive disease applies to any disease involving the aorta, its major branches, and the arteries. The cause of occlusive arterial disease may be (1) vasospastic, as in Raynaud's phenomenon; (2) inflammatory, as in thromboangiitis obliterans (Buerger's disease); or (3) atherosclerotic (arteriosclerosis obliterans), whereby the atheroma obliterates part of the lumen of the vessel, thereby obstructing blood supply. These conditions cause ischemia of the peripheral tissues that may result in pain, or a gangrenous extremity that requires amputation.

Aortic aneurysms occur when there is an abnormal widening of the three layers of the aorta, resulting in increased aortic wall tension at the site. Rupture of this segment can occur. Aneurysms may be either fusiform, in which the entire circumference of the diseased segment has expanded, or saccular, in which there exists an outpouching at the site of the diseased segment. The cause of aortic aneurysms may be ASCVD, cystic medial necrosis, trauma, or syphilis.

The purpose of PVS is to bypass and/or remove occlusion and restore blood flow distal to the lesion. Common surgical procedures (see box) include thoracic aortic aneurysm repair, abdominal aortic aneurysm repair, aortofemoral bypass, iliofemoral bypass, or femoropopliteal bypass.

Peripheral Vascular Surgeries

Type: Thoracic aortic aneurysm repair

Indications: Aneurysms greater than 6 cm in diameter, dissecting aneurysms, or leaking aneurysms.

Description: Requires a sternotomy approach and may require cardiopulmonary bypass (CPB). The aneurysm is excised and replaced by a synthetic graft. Any vessels that arise from the aneurysm are reanastomosed to the graft.

Type: Abdominal aortic aneurysm repair

Indications: Same as above.

Description: Requires a large midline vertical incision and groin incisions for distal anastomosis. Although CPB is not required, the surgical procedure is similar to thoracic repair.

Type: Peripheral bypass surgery

Indications: Rapid onset of decreasing ability to walk and peripheral ischemia resulting in ulcerative or gangrenous lesions.

Description: Requires abdominal, groin, or lower extremity incision according to location of proximal and distal anastomosis sites. Areas of occlusion are either excised or bypassed and a synthetic graft is anastomosed in place.

CV

▶ **Complications and Related Nursing Diagnoses**

Increased afterload (relative)	High risk for injury: hypertension
	Altered tissue perfusion
Acute graft occlusion	Altered tissue perfusion
	Pain
Graft leakage	Decreased cardiac output
Respiratory insufficiency	Impaired gas exchange
	Ineffective breathing pattern
GI ileus	Altered tissue perfusion

Patient Care Management Guidelines

See Cardiac surgery, p. 501, for procedures requiring CPB.

Patient assessment

1. A thorough, complete physical should be completed upon patient arrival to the recovery area. The patient should be frequently assessed because of the instability often present in the early postoperative period. (CVP and PA lines and chest tubes may or may not be present according to the type of PV surgery performed.)

2. The cardiovascular (CV) system should be assessed q15-30min for the first 6-8 hours or as appropriate after returning to the recovery area. The CV assessment should include VS, CVP, PAP, cardiac rhythm, and incisional dressing monitoring. Chest tube drainage and u/o should be monitored hourly. Hourly monitoring of peripheral pulses for presence and quality is necessary to detect early onset of graft occlusion. Adjunctive devices such as Dopplers are useful in detecting faint pulses. Mark pulse sites with a skin marking pen. Warming the extremity with thermal blankets may increase peripheral pulse amplitude.

3. A cardiac profile including CO, CI, and SVR should be done on admission, q8-12h, and with any significant changes in hemodynamics.

4. Compare serial hemograms to detect significant blood loss requiring replacement with PRBCs.

5. Assess the patient's ability to take a deep breath. Auscultate lung sounds q4h and as clinically indicated for adventitious sounds that may indicate atelectasis/pneumonia.

6. Assess for return of bowel sounds postoperatively and check abdominal girth daily, if distention is a concern, for an increase in size. Mark the sites of measurement with a skin marking pen for consistency in assessments. Ileus is a common complication of PVS.

7. Assess comfort level via interview, monitoring facial expression, and ability to take a deep breath.

Patient management

1. Nitroprusside may be ordered to maintain SBP <130 mm Hg, DBP <70 mm Hg, and SVR in the normal range (700-1200) to prevent leaking or rupture of anastomoses. Monitor MAP; a MAP of 70 is critical in preventing acute graft occlusion. Titrate by IV infusion to maintain systolic BP to 100 mm Hg. Dose may range from 0.5-10 μg/kg/min. Do not administer more than 10 μg/kg/min or patient may exhibit signs and symptoms of cyanide toxicity: tinnitus, blurred vision, delirium, and muscle spasm (see Chapter 7).

2. Pain management is crucial in blood pressure control and the patient's ability to C & DB. Intravenous morphine sulfate or epidural analgesia is usually ordered in

the immediate postoperative period. If managing pain with intravenous morphine sulfate, give IVP in 2 mg increments q5min to relieve symptoms. Dilute with 5 ml NS and administer over 4-5 minutes. Intramuscular and oral analgesia will be helpful later in postoperative course.

3. Encourage the patient to use the spirometry device and to C & DB. Instruct the patient on splinting with a pillow while coughing. IPPB may be helpful in preventing atelectasis.

4. Leave the NG tube in place until bowel sounds return to prevent vomiting and reduce the risk of aspiration. Early postoperative mobility may be the most important intervention in preventing an ileus. Metoclopramide may be used to stimulate return of gastric motility. Administer 10-20 mg IV over 1-2 minutes as ordered.

Critical observations

Consult with the physician for the following:

1. Inability to control hypertension
2. Changes in intensity or quality of peripheral pulses
3. Signs of bleeding (hypotension)

TRANSPLANTATION

Clinical Brief

Cardiac transplantation is reserved for patients with end-stage cardiac disease who are unresponsive to medical or interventional therapy. Contraindications include age >55 years old, severe pulmonary hypertension, irreversible hepatic or renal failure, IDDM, active peptic ulcer, any condition with poor short-term survival, active or potential infection, or a patient prone to noncompliance (e.g., active substance abuse). The surgical procedure involves a sternotomy incision, hypothermia induction, and invitation of CPB. The recipient's heart is removed leaving the posterior walls of the atria; the inferior and superior vena cava and pulmonary veins are left intact. The donor's atria are anastomosed to the recipient's atria walls, and pulmonary artery and aorta are then anastomosed. Epicardial pacing wires are placed in the event of bradycardia and the chest tube inserted to drain the mediastinum. As a result of this procedure the heart is denervated and does not respond to ANS stimulation (heart rate changes in response to stressors).

▶ **Complications and Related Nursing Diagnoses**

Organ rejection	Decreased cardiac output
	Altered tissue perfusion: cardiac, pulmonary, renal, cerebral
	Impaired gas exchange
	Altered urinary elimination: decreased
	Activity intolerance
	Altered body temperature
Infection	Altered body temperature
Adverse effects of immuno-suppressive therapy	High risk for infection
	Altered body image
	Altered urinary elimination: decreased
	High risk for injury: GI bleeding

See Cardiac surgery for other complications and nursing diagnoses.

Patient Care Management Guidelines

See Cardiac surgery, p. 501, for guidelines for the general cardiac surgery client.

Patient assessment

1. Assess for signs of infection secondary to immunosuppression. Assess wound sites, IV, and invasive monitoring access sites for redness, tenderness, or drainage each shift and as clinically indicated. Assess lung sounds q4h and as clinically indicated for new onset or changes in adventitious sounds. Monitor temperature q4h and as clinically indicated for T >101° F (38.3° C) or <97.5° F (36.4° C).

2. Obtain P, RR, BP q1h and as clinically indicated. Measure hemodynamic pressures: PAP and CVP (RA) q1h or more frequently if titrating pharmacological agents. Obtain CO as patient condition indicates; note trends and the patient's response to therapy. Calculate CI, PVR, and SVR and note trends and the patient's response to therapy. Calculate LVSWI and RVSWI to evaluate contractility.

3. Chronic hypoperfusion renders poorly functioning kidneys, and cyclosporin is nephrotoxic. Renal function should be carefully monitored via serum chemistries (BUN > 20, Cr > 1.5 are elevated above normal) and

serial 24-hour creatinine clearances; u/o should be > 0.5 ml/kg/hr.

4. Coagulopathies are often the result of hepatic hypoperfusion. Note any evidence of sanguineous oozing at wound sites or IV access sites. Note elevation of coagulation studies: PT > 14 sec, PTT > 37 sec.

Patient management

1. The patient is at high risk for infection secondary to immunosuppressive therapy and therefore must be kept in strict isolation. Isolation protocols should be followed. All dressing changes should be completed with strict sterile technique. All intravenous access should be changed frequently according to institutional protocol. Vigorous pulmonary toilet should be initiated and maintained at least q4h. The patient should be taught a technique for proper administration of antiseptic mouthwashes.

2. Monitor fingerstick serum glucose q6h or more frequently as needed for evidence of hyperglycemia as an adverse effect of immunosuppression. Administer prophylactic IV cimetidine or ranitidine and oral antacids as ordered to prevent GI bleeding, which can also result from immunosuppression. Test all stools and emesis for evidence of occult blood.

3. Cardiac function may be hampered postoperatively. Hemodynamic monitoring and cardiac profiles should be used to evaluate cardiac function. Hemodynamic instability may be treated with isoproterenol, nitroprusside, prostaglandins, and dopamine. Isoproterenol is used to enhance contractility and heart rate. Titrate the infusion to achieve desired hemodynamic response. Common dose is 5 μg/min. Nitroprusside is used to control SVR and blood pressure. Titrate infusion to maintain systolic BP at 100-120 mm Hg. Dose may range from 0.5-10 μg/kg/min. Do not administer more than 10 μg/kg/min, or the patient may exhibit signs and symptoms of cyanide toxicity: tinnitus, blurred vision, delirium, and muscle spasm. Prostaglandins may be used to decrease elevated pulmonary vascular resistance. Renal dose dopamine is often used to enhance renal output. Titrate at 2-5 μg/kg/min for the desired renal response. (See Chapter 7, Pharmacology, for more information.)

4. Coagulopathies are often the result of hepatic hypoper-

CV

fusion. Review coagulation studies frequently. FFP, platelets, vitamin K, and other clotting factors to correct coagulation abnormalities may be required. To prevent blood reactions, autotransfused blood is preferred (if available).

Critical observations

Consult the physician for the following:

1. Signs and symptoms of rejection
2. Signs and symptoms of adverse effects of immunosuppression: GI bleeding, hyperglycemia
3. Early signs of acute renal failure (increased serum BUN and creatinine, decreased urine output)

Gastrointestinal Modalities

GI SURGERY

Clinical Brief

Surgical intervention may be required to control gastric bleeding if conservative medical therapy fails. Peptic ulcer disease (PUD) will require surgery if gastric perforation occurs. Common surgical procedures may include antrectomy accompanied by gastroduodenostomy with or without vagotomy. Common surgical procedures to treat duodenal ulcers may include vagotomy with pyloroplasty or gastroenterostomy, or vagotomy with antrectomy and either a gastroduodenostomy (Bilroth I) or gastrojejunostomy (Bilroth II). These procedures partially neutralize gastric acid and remove stimuli for acid secretion.

Esophageal varices can be corrected with (1) portacaval, (2) mesocaval, and (3) splenorenal shunts. These procedures decrease venous blood flow through the portal system and consequently reduce portal hypertension.

▶ Complications and Related Nursing Diagnoses

Gastric surgery

Hemorrhage	Decreased cardiac output
	Fluid volume deficit
	Altered tissue perfusion
Paralytic ileus/obstruction	Pain
	Ineffective breathing pattern
Respiratory distress	Ineffective breathing pattern
	Altered tissue perfusion
	Impaired gas exchange
Stump leakage/peritonitis	Altered body temperature
	Pain
Wound infection	Altered body temperature
	Impaired skin integrity
Dumping syndrome	Altered nutrition: less than body requirements
Fluid and electrolyte loss	High risk for injury
	Fluid volume deficit

GI

513

Dehiscence	High risk for infection
	Pain
Acute gastric dilation	Ineffective breathing pattern
	Pain
	Constipation
Fistula	Alteration in nutrition
	Diarrhea

Shunt

Encephalopathy	Altered thought process
	Altered protection
GI bleed	Decreased cardiac output
	Altered tissue perfusion
Ascites	Ineffective breathing pattern
	Fluid volume deficit

Patient Care Management Guidelines
Patient assessment
1. Assess hemodynamic status: A HR >100 beats/min, SBP <90 mm Hg, CVP <2 mm Hg, and a PAWP <4 mm Hg are signs of hypovolemia. A MAP <60 mm Hg reflects inadequate tissue perfusion. Assess the surgical dressing for excessive bleeding or drainage. Review serial hemoglobin and hematocrit levels. Measure I & O hourly, including drainage from all tubes and drains. Urine output should be > 30ml/hr; 50ml/hr is more desirable. Determine fluid balance q8h: output should approximate intake. Compare serial weights to evaluate rapid changes (0.5-1 kg/day indicates fluid imbalance; 1 kg ~ 1000 ml fluid). Note skin turgor on the inner thigh or forehead, the condition of buccal membranes, and development of edema or crackles. Gastric surgery: NG drainage may be bright red postoperatively but should become dark red or brown within 12 hours after surgery; drainage should normalize to green-yellow within 24-36 hours postoperatively.
2. Continuously monitor ECG for lethal dysrhythmias that may result from electrolyte imbalance, hypoxemia, hemorrhage.
3. Assess respiratory status: Note depth, rate, and skin color q15min postoperatively until stable, then every 1 to 2 hours. Patients with abdominal surgery tend to take shallow breaths secondary to incisional pain.

4. Assess GI function: epigastric pain, tachycardia, and hypotension may signal gastric dilation; distention, rebound tenderness or rigidity may signal internal bleeding. Note any hiccups or complaints of fullness or gagging and auscultate abdomen for return of bowel sounds.
5. Determine level of comfort by using a visual acuity scale (VAS) or other pain-measuring tool (see Figure 1-1).
6. Record temperature and monitor for development of infection: assess incision, IV sites, and drain sites. Consider the urinary tract and lungs as potential sites of infection. Review serial WBC and culture reports (if available).
7. Assess neurological status, development of GI bleeding, and onset of ascites in patients undergoing portacaval shunts.

Patient management

1. Provide supplemental oxygen as ordered. If the patient is intubated and lungs are mechanically ventilated, see p. 463.
2. Administer IV fluids and/or blood products as ordered to correct intravascular volume and replace blood loss.
3. Monitor serum electrolytes and replace as ordered.
4. Use sterile procedure when manipulating gastrointestinal tubes, surgical dressings, and indwelling lines. Protect the integrity of the skin during frequent dressing changes by using Montgomery straps. Use an abdominal binder to protect against wound dehiscence.
5. Maintain patency of the NG tube to prevent undue pressure on suture line. Do not irrigate or reposition tubes without the physician's order. Provide good care of the nares and mouth. Test gastric secretions for blood and pH. Generally, gastric pH is maintained between 3.5 and 5 to prevent further development of stress ulcers. Antacids may be prescribed.
6. Administer antiemetics to prevent vomiting and preserve the integrity of the suture line.
7. Administer nutritional supplements or support as ordered. Vitamin B_{12} will be ordered for patients undergoing a total gastrectomy to prevent pernicious anemia. Oral feedings may not be instituted until bowel sounds have returned.
8. Administer analgesics as indicated, since abdominal pain

GI

may interfere with adequate ventilation; note RR before and after medication administration. If RR is <12/min, do not administer narcotics. Evaluate effectiveness of pain medication.

Critical observations

Consult with the physician for the following:

1. Signs of hypovolemia: increasing trend in heart rate; decreasing trend in u/o, CVP, PAP, and BP
2. Respiratory distress
3. Temperature elevation or signs of infection
4. An unusual amount of bright red blood that appears 24 hours after surgery, either through the NG/NI tube or on the dressings
5. Increasing abdominal distention
6. Absence of drainage from the NG/NI tube
7. u/o less than 30 ml/hr
8. Wound dehiscence
9. Abnormal laboratory data
10. Uncontrolled pain

GI INTUBATION

Clinical Brief

GI tubes are used to evacuate gastric contents, to decompress the stomach and intestines, to instill irrigants and/or medications, and to feed the patient. GI tubes are summarized in Table 6-7.

Contraindications for nasogastric tubes include patients with aneurysms or obstructive diseases of the throat or who have had a recent MI. Nasointestinal tubes should not be placed in patients with decreased intestinal motility or an obstruction of any kind, unless the tube is being used to decompress the intestines.

In addition to nasogastric and nasointestinal tubes, several types of tubes are available to tamponade (compress) the stomach and esophagus to temporarily control bleeding.

▶ Complications and Related Nursing Diagnoses

General

Excessive removal of body fluids and electrolytes	High risk for injury: dysrhythmias
	Fluid volume deficit
Nares breakdown	Impaired skin integrity
Esophageal ulceration	Altered tissue perfusion

TABLE 6-7 Summary of Gastrointestinal Tubes

Tube	Description
Nasogastric	
Levin	Single-lumen, no air vent; rubber or plastic; risk of mucosal damage when applied to suction
Salem sump	Double-lumen; air vent reduces risk of mucosal damage; clear plastic
Nutriflex	Feeding tube, weighted tip
Ewald	Large bore used to lavage clots or substances from the stomach; used for emergencies only
Esophageal	
Sengstaken-Blakemore	Triple-lumen, double balloon: one for esophageal compression and one for gastric compression; allows for gastric aspiration but not esophageal suction
Minnesota	Quadruple-lumen, double balloon for esophageal and gastric compression as well as gastric and esophageal suctioning
Linton	Triple-lumen, single balloon for gastric compression allows for gastric and esophageal suctioning
Nasointestinal	
Miller-Abbott	Double-lumen, one for suctioning, one to fill the distal balloon with mercury or air after insertion to decompress the small bowel
Cantor	Weighted with mercury before insertion; single-lumen, largest NI tube
Harris	Weighted, single-lumen
Duotube (Entriflex, Dobhoff)	Feeding tubes, weighted, single-lumen; guidewire used to facilitate insertion

GI

Esophageal rupture	Decreased cardiac output
Otitis media or parotitis	Pain
Incompetent gastroesophageal sphincter	High risk for aspiration
Inadequate airway clearance	Ineffective breathing pattern Impaired gas exchange

Nasogastric

Pharyngeal obstruction with Sengstaken-Blakemore tube	Ineffective breathing pattern
Esophageal/gastric erosion	Pain Decreased cardiac output Fluid volume deficit

General Patient Care Management Guidelines
Patient assessment
1. Assess level of consciousness; patients with altered mentation may inadvertently remove the NG or NI tube.
2. Examine the nares daily for redness or skin breakdown.
3. Be alert for complications related to nasoenteric intubation.

Patient management
1. Secure the tube once the tube has reached its proper placement. The skin should be prepared with tincture of benzoin or an equivalent solution. Hypoallergenic tape is then applied. The tube is positioned over this tape and secured with another piece. Op-site dressings can be used to secure tubes as well as allow visualization of the skin condition. Avoid movement at the naris to avoid skin irritation.
2. Attach to appropriate amount and type of suction as prescribed by the physician.
3. Provide meticulous mouth care: teeth brushing, mouthwash, lozenges if permitted. Mucous membranes should be kept moist; apply lip balm as needed.
4. Keep HOB elevated to prevent the possibility of aspiration.
5. Irrigate the tube as ordered to ensure patency. Validate tube irrigation with physician if the patient has undergone gastric surgery.
6. Check placement of the tube before administering anything down the tube. Clamp tube for 30 minutes after the instillation of medications.

7. To obtain a gastric pH reading, have the patient lie on the left side; stop NG suction, and withdraw 10-15 ml discard fluid; use a second syringe to withdraw a sample for testing. Use pH paper with appropriate pH range. Do not use the syringe used for antacid administration to obtain the gastric sample. Generally, gastric pH should be kept above 3.5 to decrease the chance for stress ulcers. An inability to raise pH >4 may indicate sepsis.

8. Record color, consistency, and amount of drainage.

Nasogastric-tube patient care management

1. Check placement of tube in the stomach by aspirating with a syringe: stomach contents should be present in the tube. Instill 10-30 ml of air into the tube and auscultate the gastric area: air rushing or gurgling will be heard if the tube is in the proper position.

Nasointestinal-tube patient care management

1. When inserting an NI tube that uses a stylet to facilitate placement, place the proximal end of the tube in a glass of water periodically during placement and watch for bubbling in the water. The bubbling is indicative of endotracheal intubation and the tube should be removed immediately. (Never reinsert the stylet into the tube once it is placed in the patient.)

2. Feeding tubes require radiographic verification of position before feedings can begin. Placing the patient in a right side-lying position may enhance tube advancement.

3. See Nutrition (p. 521) for enteral feedings.

Sengstaken-Blakemore type–tube patient care management

1. Intubation and sedation are recommended before insertion of a Sengstaken-Blakemore (Figure 6-7) or Minnesota tube.

2. Tube placement is verified by air injection into the stomach or aspiration of gastric contents. A radiograph confirms the position of the gastric balloon against the cardia of the stomach.

3. After radiographic verification, the gastric balloon is inflated with 200-500 ml of air. Many institutions require a football helmet to be placed on the patient's head to secure the tractioned tube to the helmet. Be sure the helmet is a proper fit. A Salem sump is inserted into the esophagus to remove secretions if a Sengstaken-

GI

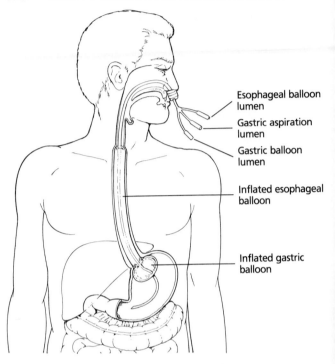

Esophageal balloon
lumen

Gastric aspiration
lumen

Gastric balloon
lumen

Inflated esophageal
balloon

Inflated gastric
balloon

Figure 6-7 Sengstaken-Blakemore tube.

Blakemore tube is used, since the patient will not be able to swallow. A gastric aspirate port and Salem sump (or esophageal aspirate port) are connected to low suction.

4. The esophageal balloon is inflated only after radiographic confirmation of the position of the gastric balloon and if bleeding continues. Pressure in the esophageal balloon (usually 2-25 mm Hg) should be checked q2h to be sure it does not exceed 40 mm Hg. Esophageal balloon deflation should be done q4h for 10 minutes by physician's order only. The gastric balloon is never deflated while the esophageal balloon is inflated. Generally, the tube is not left inflated for more than 48 hours.

5. Scissors should be kept at the bedside to cut the balloon

ports in case of airway obstruction from upward migration of the tube.

6. All ports of the tube should be clearly labeled. Never inject fluids in the esophageal port. Normal saline irrigation may be needed to keep the gastric aspirate port patent.

7. If bleeding appears to have stopped, the esophageal balloon is slowly deflated. Traction is relaxed on the gastric balloon and gastric aspirate is monitored for recurrence of bleeding. All air from the esophageal and gastric balloon is aspirated before the tube is removed.

8. Hgb and Hct are usually monitored every 2-4 hours. A drop in hematocrit by 3 indicates 1 unit of blood lost.

9. An acute onset of abdominal or back pain may indicate esophageal rupture.

Critical observations

Consult with the physician for the following:

1. Fluid or electrolyte imbalance from prolonged gastric suctioning

2. Possible esophageal or gastric rupture and patient showing signs of shock

3. Respiratory distress from tube displacement or aspiration

4. Complaints of ear or neck pain associated with otitis media or parotitis

5. Increasing abdominal distention

6. Obstructed tube that will not irrigate

7. Inability to remove the tube

8. Gastric pH less than 3.5 or value specified by the physician

GI

NUTRITION: ENTERAL FEEDINGS

Clinical Brief

Enteral feedings include liquid formula diets that are provided orally or via a tube placed down the esophagus into either the stomach or the intestines when the patient's voluntary intake does not meet at least two thirds of the patient's needs. Intermittent feedings are recommended when feedings are instilled into the stomach. If feedings are entering the duodenum or jejunum, continuous feeding is recommended, which usually results in less bowel distention, less fluid and electrolyte imbalance, less aspiration, and improved patient tolerance of the product. When tube feedings are considered for long-term nutritional therapy (greater than 4 weeks), the tube is surgically placed in the patient, e.g., gastrostomy or jejunostomy. Blenderized feedings and commercially prepared dietary formulations are ordered by the physician based on GI tract ability to digest and absorb nutrients, the nutrient needs of the patient, and fluid and electrolyte restrictions.

Preparations

Dietary formulations can be milk based, lactose, or protein free; contain high quantities of branched-chain amino acids (BCAAs); or specially designed to include nutrients specific to the needs and illness state of the patient.

A specialized formula for patients with hepatic encephalopathy may include Travasorb-Hepatic or Hepatic Aid II, since they contain high quantities of BCAAs. Amin-Aid or Travasorb-Renal may be prescribed for patients in renal failure, since these formulas attempt to decrease the urea production. Patients who are burned or septic may be prescribed Stresstein, Criticare, or Traum-Aid, which attempt to stimulate protein synthesis and reduce proteolysis. Patients in respiratory failure having difficulty weaning from the ventilator may be prescribed Pulmocare or formulas with increased fat content, which attempt to reduce CO_2 production, oxygen consumption, and ventilatory requirements.

Most formulas are isotonic and provide about 45 g of protein per liter although hypertonic formulas are available. High-fiber (Jevity) and low-residue (Resource, Fortison) formulas are available, as are supplements that provide extra calories (Microlipid, Promod, MCT oil).

Contraindications

Enteral feedings are not recommended in patients with vomiting, severe ileus, intestinal obstruction, and upper GI bleeding.

▶ Complications and Related Nursing Diagnoses

Aspiration	Ineffective airway clearance Impaired gas exchange
Diarrhea	Impaired skin integrity
Abdominal distention	Pain
Hyperglycemic hyperosmolar nonketotic coma	Decreased cardiac output Fluid volume deficit High risk for injury: seizures
Hyponatremia/hypokalemia	High risk for injury

Patient Care Management Guidelines
Patient assessment

1. Assess nutritional status: prealbumin is considered the best indicator of nutrition status. Serum albumin <3.5 g/dl, transferrin <180 mg/dl, and lymphocyte <1500/μl are indications of malnourishment. Skin anergy testing (negative response to antigen) represents malnutrition. Twenty-four-hour urinary urea nitrogen study measures nitrogen balance by subtracting the amount of nitrogen lost from the daily intake in either enteral or parenteral sources. Creatinine-height index measures the amount of creatinine excreted in a 24-hour period proportionately to the height of the patient and reflects muscle wasting. Anthropometric measurements of body size can be taken; tricep skinfold thickness < 3 mm indicates severely depleted fat stores; a midarm circumference < 15 cm means muscle wasting. Measure height and weight and compare with desired-weight tables. A decrease of 15% from ideal weight indicates impaired nutrition.
2. Assess GI tolerance: note nausea, vomiting, diarrhea or cramping, and any abdominal distention or absence of bowel sounds; the infusion rate may need to be reduced if these symptoms appear.
3. Monitor flow rates and volumes to ensure that the patient is actually receiving the prescribed amount of calories, since continuous feedings are often interrupted.

Patient management

1. Insufflation of air and aspiration of gastric contents do not confirm placement of nasoenteric tubes. Confirmation with radiography is necessary before feedings are initiated.
2. With continuous feedings, elevate the HOB 30 degrees at all times to reduce the risk of aspiration. If the patient needs to be supine, turn off the feeding.
3. Small bowel feedings are generally initiated at 50 ml/hr with full-strength isotonic solution. A hypertonic formula can be diluted to quarter-strength or half-strength. Gradually increase the rate, usually 25 ml q8h, and strength of the formula; and evaluate patient tolerance.
4. For intragastric feedings, generally, tube feedings are initiated with an isotonic formula and the nutrient requirements are achieved by increasing the rate over 1-2 days.

GI

5. A small amount of food dye added to the formula will help assess the patient for possible aspiration. When suctioning or coughing produces sputum that matches the color of the formula, turn the feeding off. Check the sputum or tracheal aspirate for glucose with a glucose reagent strip if aspiration of formula is suspected. Have the placement of the feeding tube confirmed.

6. Check residual at least q4h for patients receiving continuous gastric feedings. If more than 100 ml or greater than 50% of the hourly rate, hold the feedings. Metoclopramide (Reglan) may be ordered to increase gastric motility. Small-bore feeding tubes often collapse when the nurse is aspirating for residuals. Observe the patient for the development of abdominal distention.

7. Administer the feeding as ordered, slowly and consistently. A feeding pump is recommended for more accurate administration. Time tape the bag if a pump is not readily available.

8. Irrigate the feeding tube with 50-150 ml of water or carbonated beverage q4h, before and after each intermittent feeding, or once a shift for continuous feeding. Irrigate the tube if the feeding has been stopped for any reason and after administration of medications via the tube. Carbonated beverages have been shown to unclog feeding tubes. Use a clear beverage (not colas) to accurately assess the gastric residual if GI bleeding is suspected. Other substances that have been used successfully to clear an obstructed tube include cranberry juice, meat tenderizer, and pancreatic enzymes.

9. Have medications changed to elixirs. If medications must be crushed, be certain they are finely ground and dissolved in water to prevent obstruction of the feeding tube. Sustained-release and enteric-coated medications must not be crushed. Irrigate the tube before and after medication administration.

10. Provide good oral care, since mouth breathing is common in patients who have a nasal tube present.

11. Limit bacterial growth by changing tube-feeding containers q24h or per hospital policy; generally, formula should not hang longer than 4 hours.

12. Administer free-water supplements as ordered by the physician to prevent dehydration; as much as 0.5 ml for every 1 ml of feeding can be ordered.

13. When irrigating small-bore tubing, use the syringe size

recommended by the manufacturer. A small syringe can exert greater pressure with minimal effort and may rupture the tube.

Critical observations

Consult with the physician for the following:

1. Gastric residual > 50% of hourly delivery rate
2. Uncontrolled diarrhea
3. Increasing abdominal distention, N/V, absent bowel sounds
4. Elevated serum glucose
5. Dehydration: dry buccal membranes, nonelastic skin turgor, specific gravity > 1.035
6. Tube displacement
7. Possible aspiration/respiratory distress
8. Mucosal damage from tube

PARENTERAL NUTRITION

Clinical Brief

In the event the patient does not receive sufficient nutrition with enteral feedings or cannot functionally take substances through the stomach or bowel or when it is necessary to put the GI system to rest, parenteral nutrition (PN) containing all the water, nutritional, vitamin, and mineral requirements may be initiated. A hypertonic solution of as much as 50% dextrose, amino acids, electrolytes, vitamins, and minerals can be tailored to meet the needs of the patient. Daily laboratory assessment (nutritional panel) and anthropometric measurements provide information to guard against underfeeding or overfeeding, conditions that can adversely affect pulmonary, renal, and hepatic functioning.

Peripheral parenteral nutrition can be initiated when the objective is to prevent starvation and not to treat malnutrition or when central venous access cannot be obtained. The glucose concentration is limited to 10% in peripheral parenteral nutrition, since sclerosis of the vein can occur with more hypertonic solutions. Other components include amino acids, vitamins, electrolytes, and trace elements. The prescribed solution is transfused through a dedicated peripheral line, eliminating the complications of central line insertion and maintenance.

Lipids

To avoid the excessive production of carbon dioxide that results when carbohydrates are used as the sole caloric source and to prevent essential endogenous fatty acid deficiency,

GI

lipids are administered in addition to PN. Lipids supply the essential fatty acids necessary for protein metabolism and cell function. Usually a 10% emulsion (500 ml) is administered 2-3 times a week.

▶ **Complications and Related Nursing Diagnoses**

Sepsis	Decreased cardiac output
	Altered tissue perfusion
Glucose intolerance/	Altered thought processes
hyperglycemia	High risk for infection
Electrolyte imbalance	High risk for injury
Dehydration	Fluid volume deficit

Catheter-related complications can be found on p. 445.

Patient Care Management Guidelines

Patient assessment

1. Monitor temperature at least once each shift to evaluate the onset of infection. Unexplained fever may be related to central venous catheter sepsis.
2. Assess IV catheter insertion site for redness, drainage, or tenderness.
3. Check serum glucose as ordered to identify onset of hyperglycemia. Glucose homeostasis should be 120-180 mg/dl. Levels > 220 mg/dl can impair phagocyte function. Acute hyperglycemia may signal sepsis.
4. Review laboratory results for metabolic abnormalities associated with PN therapy: serum glucose, potassium, phosphate, calcium, magnesium, BUN, alkaline phosphatase, bilirubin, and AST (SGOT).
5. Monitor total lymphocyte count, serum albumin, and transferrin to determine efficacy of PN.
6. Assess fluid volume status: compare daily weights and record intake and output. Note signs and symptoms of dehydration or fluid overload.

Patient management

1. Do not administer medications or blood products through the nutrition-dedicated line. If long-term parenteral nutrition is necessary, a Broviac catheter may be required.

2. To prevent infection, use aseptic technique when performing dressing changes or tubing changes. Change dressing and tubing per hospital guidelines or if dressing becomes soiled or nonocclusive. Keep all solutions refrigerated, check expiration dates, and administer within 24 hours of preparation. Do not use the PN if the solution is cloudy or contains particulates. Luer lock all tubing connections to prevent inadvertent disconnection and a possible air embolus.

3. Validate correct nutritional components and infuse as ordered. Initial rate is usually 50-100 ml/hr and increased 25-50 ml/hr/day, depending on cardiovascular and renal status.

4. Do not stop PN abruptly, since hypoglycemia can result. If PN is not available, administer $D_{10}W$ at the PN rate until the solution is available. To avoid inconsistent delivery rates that may precipitate rebound hypoglycemia or hyperglycemia reactions, use an infusion pump to administer PN.

5. Insulin on a sliding scale is usually required to control hyperglycemia. Check glucose levels q6h.

6. Phytonadione may be given weekly to prevent coagulopathy associated with vitamin K deficiency.

7. Fat supplements may be prescribed. Initial therapy requires a slow infusion rate for the first 15-30 minutes (1 ml/min for a 10% emulsion; 0.5 ml/min for a 20% emulsion); monitor the patient for respiratory distress associated with hypoxemia and cyanosis. If no adverse effects occur, resume the prescribed infusion rate. Blood samples to measure serum triglyceride may be obtained to determine the patient's ability to utilize lipids.

Critical observations

Consult with physician for the following:

1. Temperature elevation
2. Catheter displacement or thrombosis
3. Fluid overload or dehydration
4. Hyperglycemia
5. Electrolyte imbalances
6. Adverse effects with lipid administration

Renal Modalities

DIALYSIS
Clinical Brief
Dialysis is a process of filtering plasma to remove toxic metabolites and to normalize the concentration of fluids and electrolytes. Dialysis is indicated in both acute and chronic renal failure and can also be used to remove substances in cases of poisoning.

In all forms of dialysis an exchange of solutes occurs across a semipermeable membrane with blood perfusing on one side of the membrane. Commonly, dialysate (a physiological salt solution) is utilized on the opposite side of the membrane to improve removal of fluid and waste products. There are three types of dialysis, each having different advantages and disadvantages (see Table 6-8). The three forms are hemodialysis, peritoneal dialysis, and continuous arteriovenous hemofiltration.

Hemodialysis involves pumping the patient's heparinized blood through an extracorporeal filter composed of semipermeable membranes. Blood is removed from and returned to the body through a venous or an arteriovenous access in the form of femoral lines, a subclavian catheter, arteriovenous (AV) shunt, AV fistula, or AV graft.

Peritoneal dialysis involves introducing a hypertonic glucose solution (dialysate) into the peritoneal cavity through an abdominal catheter. The dialysate is left to dwell in the abdomen, allowing the exchange of solutes across the peritoneal membrane. The solution is then drained from the abdominal cavity.

Continuous arteriovenous hemofiltration (CAVH) is a continuous, slow form of dialysis that requires arteriovenous blood flow and extracorporeal filtration but does not use a blood pump or air detector as is done in hemodialysis (Figure 6-8). Blood flow through the CAVH circuit is primarily determined by the patient's mean arterial blood pressure, and an ultrafiltrate of plasma is removed (urea clearance is limited). Hypertonic dialysate can also be run countercurrent to the blood flow in a form of hemofiltration called *con-*

TABLE 6-8 Comparison of Three Forms of Dialysis

	Peritoneal dialysis	Hemodialysis	Continuous hemofiltration
Access	Peritoneal catheter	Arteriovenous or venous access	Arteriovenous or venous access
Membrane	Peritoneal	Extracorporeal filter	Extracorporeal filter
Advantages	Continuous, gentle fluid removal	Rapid, efficient fluid and waste removal	Continuous; slow, gentle fluid removal
Disadvantages	Protein loss, poor potassium removal	Hemodynamic instability, heparinization	Heparinization
Contraindications	Abdominal surgery, adhesions, or an undiagnosed acute condition of the abdomen; respiratory insufficiency	Hypotension, bleeding	Bleeding

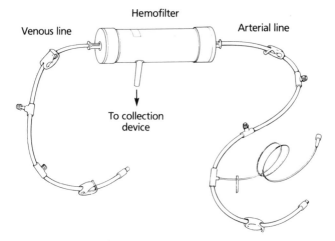

Figure 6-8   CAVH system. Venous blood flows through the hemofilter and returns through the arterial line. Various ports are available for fluid replacement, blood drawing, and heparinizing the system.

tinuous arteriovenous hemodialysis (CAVHD). CAVHD combines the advantages of CAVH with the clearance of BUN.

▶ **Complications and Related Nursing Diagnoses**

All forms of dialysis

Hypotension	Decreased cardiac output Fluid volume deficit Altered tissue perfusion
Infection	High risk for infection Altered body temperature
Electrolyte imbalances	High risk for injury

Hemodialysis

Disequilibrium syndrome	High risk for injury
Air embolus	Decreased cardiac output Impaired gas exchange Pain
Hemolysis	Impaired gas exchange Altered tissue perfusion
Hemorrhage	Altered tissue perfusion Fluid volume deficit Decreased cardiac output

RENAL

Continuous hemofiltration

Hemorrhage	Altered tissue perfusion
	Fluid volume deficit
	Decreased cardiac output
Clotting of filter	High risk for injury: throm-boembolism

Peritoneal dialysis

Respiratory insufficiency	Ineffective breathing pattern
	Impaired gas exchange
Peritonitis	High risk for infection
	Altered body temperature

Patient Care Management Guidelines
HEMODIALYSIS
Patient assessment

1. Assess arteriovenous (AV) shunt, fistula, or graft for bruit and thrill each shift.
2. Assess for signs of infection, including redness, swelling, increased tenderness, and drainage at access site. Obtain temperature q4h and note any increase.
3. Assess hemodynamic and fluid volume status by monitoring:
   a. Hourly I & O.
   b. Vital signs and hemodynamic parameters (if available) q15min at the onset of treatment until stable, every half-hour during treatment once stable, and q4h when not being dialyzed.
   c. Breath sounds and heart sounds q4h.
   d. Weights daily if no dialysis is done; weights before, during, and after hemodialysis.

Patient management

1. Prevent infection by using good handwashing; initiating good hygiene; separating the patient from other patients with infections; aseptically caring for wounds and all invasive catheters, including the Foley; having the patient turn and C & DB; encouraging early ambulation; and providing good nutrition.
2. Post a sign in the patient's room informing all personnel not to draw blood or check blood pressure in limb with permanent vascular access device.
3. Keep two cannula clamps next to AV shunt at all times. If shunt becomes disconnected, apply clamps or direct pressure. Reconnect and assess for blood loss.

4. Aseptically clean insertion sites daily and before initiating dialysis. Change wet or soiled dressings immediately.
5. Consult with the physician regarding administration of antihypertensive, antiemetic, or narcotic agents before hemodialysis, since these agents induce hypotension.
6. Adjust schedule for administration of medications based on dialyzability of drug and time of dialysis (see box for common dialyzable medications). Consult with the physician about administering a postdialysis supplemental dosage of any medication that is dialyzed out. Consult with the physician about obtaining drug levels of dialyzable medications to increase accuracy of dosing.
7. If the patient becomes hypotensive (SBP < 90 mm Hg), place the patient flat. If SBP remains low, raise the patient's legs. Administer normal saline, replacement solution, or vasoactive medications as ordered. Assess for dysrhythmias and chest pain during hypotension.

Common Dialyzable Medications

Aminoglycosides: Amikacin, gentamycin, kanamycin, neomycin, streptomycin, tobramycin

Cephalosporins: Cefazolin, cefuroxime, cefoxitin, ceftazidime, cephalothin, cephaloridine, cephalexin, cephapirin

Penicillins: Amoxicillin, ampicillin, carbenicillin, oxacillin, piparacillin, penicillin G, ticarcillin

Other antibiotics: Chloramphenicol, sulfonamides, trimethoprim

Cardiovascular agents: Procainamide, bretylium, nitroprusside, captopril

Immunosuppressives/antineoplastics: Azathioprine, methylprednisolone, methotrexate

Miscellaneous: Acetaminophen, acetylsalicylic acid, cimetidine, antituberculous drugs, librium, theophylline, phenobarbital, phenytoin

---

These medications often require increased dosing during dialysis or supplemental dosing after dialysis.
NOTE: Digoxin, propranolol, quinidine, lidocaine, furosemide, and heparin are not removed by hemodialysis.

RENAL

8. If the patient experiences cramping in extremities, administer normal saline or hypertonic saline as ordered and decrease the rate of dialysis.

9. If the patient complains of popping or ringing in ears, dizziness, chest pain, and coughing or if the air is visible entering the patient's vascular return, suspect air embolus. Clamp all blood lines and place the patient in Trendelenberg position and on left side; administer oxygen.

10. If the patient develops nausea, vomiting, confusion, headache, hypertension, or seizures, suspect disequilibrium syndrome. Reduce the dialysis rate and treat the symptoms.

11. If the patient's blood takes on a "cherry pop" appearance and the patient develops chest pain, dyspnea, burning at the access site, and cramping, suspect acute hemolysis. Clamp the blood line, monitor vital signs, and observe for dysrhythmias. Be prepared to manage a shock state.

Critical observations
Consult with the physician for the following:

1. Absent bruit or thrill
2. Infected dialysis access site
3. Suspected air embolus
4. Disequilibrium syndrome
5. Acute hemolysis
6. Shock

PERITONEAL DIALYSIS

Patient assessment

1. Assess for signs of infection, including redness, swelling, increased tenderness, and drainage at peritoneal access site. Obtain temperature q4h and note any increase.
2. Assess fluid volume status by monitoring:
   a. Weight
   b. Vital signs
   c. I & O (including dialysate infused and effluent drained) q4h or with each exchange
3. Assess the patient for abdominal pain and assess effluent for cloudiness, blood, and/or fibrin clots with each exchange.

Patient management

1. Prevent infection by using good handwashing; initiating good hygiene; separating patient from other patients with infections; aseptically caring for wounds

and all invasive catheters including Foley; having patient turn, C & DB; encouraging early ambulation; and providing good nutrition.

2. Until the catheter exit site is healed, use sterile technique to clean around the exit site and change the dressing around catheter once per day or when wet. Once the exit site is healed, the patient may shower and should clean with betadine or should apply a topical antibiotic ointment around the exit site at the end of the shower.

3. Use strict aseptic technique during exchanges. If the effluent is cloudy and peritonitis is suspected, obtain a sample of effluent before administration of antibiotics.

4. Before an exchange, warm the dialysate solution to body temperature.

5. If ordered, add medications to the dialysate and label the dialysate appropriately (heparin is often used to prevent catheter obstructions by fibrin or blood clots; insulin is often used to control glucose in the diabetic patient; antibiotics may be administered in the dialysate to patients with peritonitis).

6. Instill the ordered amount and concentration of dialysate with medications (over 10 minutes) via the peritoneal catheter using aseptic technique. Allow fluid to dwell in the abdomen for physician-ordered time period. When dwell-time is over, drain the effluent from the abdomen by gravity over a 20- to 30-minute period.

7. Measure effluent volume by weighing or draining.

8. If difficulty is encountered in draining, check for kinks or clamps on tubing, turn the patient from side to side, sit the patient up in bed, reposition the drainage bag to the lowest possible position, and apply gentle pressure to the abdomen.

9. If the patient develops tachypnea and dyspnea, place the patient in semi-Fowler's position and encourage deep breathing.

10. If a tubing spike becomes contaminated by touching a nonclean surface, soak the spike in betadine for 5 minutes. If the spike becomes grossly contaminated (e.g., by touching clothing, the floor), clamp tubing; do not continue exchanges.

11. Change peritoneal dialysis tubing monthly using sterile technique.

Critical observations

Consult with the physician for the following:

1. Symptoms of peritonitis
2. Blood or fibrin clots noted in peritoneal effluent
3. Inability to drain effluent
4. Respiratory distress
5. Grossly contaminated tubing spike

CONTINUOUS ARTERIOVENOUS HEMOFILTRATION (CAVH)

Patient assessment

1. Assess for signs of infection, including redness, swelling, increased tenderness, and drainage at access site. Obtain a temperature q4h and note any increase.
2. Assess hemodynamic and fluid volume status by monitoring:
   a. Hourly I & O
   b. Vital signs and hemodynamic parameters (if available) q15min at onset of treatment until stable, every half-hour during treatment once stable, and q4h when not being dialyzed.
   c. Breath sounds and heart sounds q4h
   d. Weights three times per day
   e. Ultrafiltrate rate q15min until stable and then qh
   f. Activated clotting time (ACT) q15min until stable and then q4h.

Patient management

1. Prime filter and blood circuit with heparinized saline and administer a physician-ordered heparin bolus to the patient at the onset of CAVH. Connect the hemofilter circuit to the patient's arterial and venous access, ensuring that all connections are secure.
2. For CAVHD, administer dialysate through the filter, countercurrent to blood flow.
3. Infuse a heparin drip through the arterial side of the circuit and titrate the heparin infusion to achieve the desired ACT.
4. If ordered, infuse replacement solution, usually hourly, via the arterial side (predilutional) or the venous side (postdilutional) of the circuit. Adjust amount of replacement solution to obtain desired fluid balance. Replacements are based on ultrafiltration rate (UFR). If the UFR is high, volume depletion may occur.

5. If using a gravity drainage bag, keep the bag at least 16 inches below the filter. The ultrafiltration rate can be increased by lowering the bag or can be decreased by raising the collection bag.

6. If collecting ultrafiltrate using vacuum suction, keep suction set between 80 and 120 mm Hg.

7. If SBP <90, place the patient flat or in Trendelenberg position. Reduce the ultrafiltrate rate by lowering the bed, raising the collection bag, or decreasing suction. Administer normal saline, replacement solution, or vasoactive medications as ordered. If hypotension continues or becomes extreme, clamp ultrafiltrate line.

8. If the amount of ultrafiltrate is reduced, check for kinks or clamps in the access site or tubing; check for changes in the blood flow rate (e.g., decreased cardiac output, hypovolemia); raise the bed, lower the collection bag, or increase the suction; and assess for a clotted filter.

9. Hematest ultrafiltrate q4h.

10. If the ultrafiltrate appears pink-tinged or the hematest result is positive, suspect a blood leak. Clamp the ultrafiltrate line.

11. If the ultrafiltrate rate decreases and the blood in the circuit is darkened, suspect clotting in the filter. Adjust heparinization; be prepared to replace the circuit.

Critical observations

Consult with the physician for the following:

1. Cardiovascular collapse
2. Blood in ultrafiltrate
3. Clotted filter

RENAL TRANSPLANTATION

Clinical Brief

Renal transplantation is indicated as a treatment for chronic renal failure. The procedure involves transplanting a tissue-matched kidney from a living-related or a cadaveric donor into the recipient's iliac fossa. Success of the transplant depends on avoiding rejection through the use of immunosuppressive medications. Transplants are contraindicated if the patient has an underlying disease process that could be aggravated by immunosuppression, such as chronic infection or malignancy.

RENAL

▶ Complications and Related Nursing Diagnoses

Rejection	Altered urinary elimination High risk for fluid volume excess
Acute tubular necrosis (ATN)	Altered urinary elimination High risk for fluid volume excess
Infection	High risk for infection
Fluid overload	Fluid volume excess
Dehydration	Fluid volume deficit Decreased cardiac output
Hematoma/bleeding	High risk for fluid volume deficit Altered tissue perfusion

Patient Care Management Guidelines
Patient assessment

1. Monitor BP, HR, CVP q15min postoperatively until stable, then every hour.
2. Monitor urine flow q15min postoperatively until stable, then hourly. Diuresis is induced following the cold ischemic period; u/o as great as 600 ml/hr can result.
3. Assess for signs of hemorrhage or hematoma at the incisional site every hour for the first 8 hours postoperatively and then every shift. Monitor Hgb and Hct.
4. Assess for signs of urinary leak by assessing for urinary drainage from incisional site, decreased urine output, and for edema of the scrotum, labia, or thigh near the transplant site every hour for the first 8 hours postoperatively and then every shift.
5. Assess I & O hourly and weights each day to determine fluid volume status. Assess fluid volume status and cardiac output to ensure adequate renal perfusion and to avoid fluid volume excess.
6. Monitor electrolytes frequently and assess the patient for signs of electrolyte imbalances, especially cardiac dysrhythmias related to hypokalemia during large diuresis or hyperkalemia related to allograft dysfunction.
7. Assess weight, BUN, and creatinine daily to determine renal functioning.
8. Monitor for temperature elevation q4h and each shift for signs of infection. Assess lung sounds q4h; apnea monitoring may be used in the immediate postoperative period to continuously monitor respiratory status.

9. Monitor for signs of rejection, which include decreased urine output, weight gain, increased creatinine, hypertension, general malaise, fever, and graft pain, tenderness, or swelling.

Patient management

1. Anticipate diuresis in living-related donor transplants and cadaver-donor transplants with a short ischemic time.

2. Anticipate acute tubular necrosis in cadaveric donor transplants.

3. If ATN develops, educate the patient on clinical course of ATN, the need for dialysis, difference between ATN and rejection. Frequently reinforce to the patient that ATN does not predict or affect graft survival.

4. Replace fluids according to urine output (usually milliliter for milliliter, based on the previous-hour urine output) and CVP to maintain normal fluid and electrolyte balance.

5. Anticipate blood in urine for first 24 to 48 hours.

6. If ordered, irrigate the bladder to prevent Foley catheter occlusion by blood clots.

7. If urine output suddenly drops, suspect Foley catheter obstruction by a blood clot and gently irrigate the catheter using sterile technique. If the catheter is not obstructed, assess the patient for signs of dehydration and rejection.

8. Once the Foley catheter is removed, encourage frequent urination. Recatheterization may be required if the patient is unable to void within 6 hr.

9. Prepare the patient for a renal scan or biopsy if ordered.

10. Administer immunosuppressive medications as ordered. Corticosteroids (prednisone, methylprednisolone), azathioprine (Imuran), and cyclosporine (Sandimmune) are most frequently used. Administer oral cyclosporine before meals by diluting it in juice or milk. Monitor for side effects of immunosuppressive medications. Monitor cyclosporine drug levels to ensure adequate immunosuppression without causing toxic damage to the kidney. Hold azathioprine if WBC count is $< 3 \times 10^3/\mu l$.

11. Prevent infection by using good handwashing technique; initiating good hygiene; preventing contact with patients, staff, or visitors who have infectious diseases;

RENAL

aseptically caring for wound and all invasive catheters, including meticulous care of the Foley; having the patient turn, C & DB; encouraging early ambulation; and providing good nutrition.

12. Encourage the physician to remove invasive lines at the earliest possible date to minimize the risk of infection.

13. During acute rejection, muromonab-CD3 (Orthoclone OKT3) may be administered. Ensure that the patient is not fluid overloaded before receiving Orthoclone OKT3. If it is ordered, premedicate the patient before the first dose with methylprednisolone and acetaminophen. If ordered, administer hydrocortisone after administering Orthoclone OKT3. Anticipate fever, chills, dyspnea, and malaise within the first 6 hours after the first dose of Orthoclone OKT3. With first dose of Orthoclone OKT3, monitor VS q15min for 2 hours and then q30min until the patient is stable; monitor closely for pulmonary edema, especially in patients who are fluid overloaded.

14. Antilymphocyte globulin (ALG) and antithymocyte globulin (ATG) can also be used in acute rejection. Local or systemic allergic responses should be anticipated when administering these medications. If ordered, skin testing should be done before administering the first dose and premedication with acetaminophen and diphenhydramine hydrochloride (Benadryl) should be provided before each dose. Administration through a central line is preferred; if administration is through a peripheral line, monitor for signs of thrombophlebitis.

15. Maintain stringent infection control interventions during treatment with antirejection medications.

Critical observations

Consult with the physician for the following:

1. Sudden increase in drainage from incision site
2. Hematoma formation at surgical site
3. Urinary drainage noted at the incision site or edema development in the scrotum, labia, or thigh areas
4. Decreased urine output despite nursing interventions
5. Signs of infection
6. WBC count below $3 \times 10^3/\mu l$
7. Onset of dyspnea during Orthoclone OKT3 infusion

BIBLIOGRAPHY

1. Alspach JG and Williams SM: Core curriculum for critical care nursing, ed 3, Philadelphia, 1985, WB Saunders Co.
2. Anderson RJ and Schrier RW: Clinical use of drugs with kidney and liver disease, Philadelphia, 1983, WB Saunders Co.
3. Anderson WD and George R: Techniques for bedside pulmonary assessment in the ICU, J Crit Illness 2(10):57-64, 1987.
4. Barker E: Brain tumor: frightening diagnosis, nursing challenge, RN 46(9):53, 1990.
5. Bell GC: Tracheal intubation and airway management. In Kirby RR and Taylor RW, editors: Respiratory failure, Chicago, 1986, Year Book Medical Publishers, Inc.
6. Bevan NE: Nursing care of the patient with unilateral lung injury, Crit Care Nurse 10(7):85-88, 1990.
7. Blansfield J: Emergency autotransfusion in hypovolemia, Crit Care Nurs Clin North Am 2(2):195-199, 1990.
8. Bonner JT and Hall JR: Respiratory intensive care of the adult surgical patient, St Louis, 1985, The CV Mosby Co.
9. Bragg C: Practical aspects of epidural and intrathecal narcotic analgesia in the intensive care setting, Heart Lung 18:599-608, 1989.
10. Broughton W et al: Nasoenteric tube placement user's guide to possible complications, J Crit Illness 15(10):1085-1101, 1990.
11. Broughton W et al: The technique of placing a nasoenteric tube, J Crit Illness 15(10):1101-1108, 1990.
12. Brown LH: Pulmonary oxygen toxicity, Focus Crit Care, 17(1):68-75, 1990.
13. Burns S: Advances in ventilator therapy, Focus Crit Care 17(3):227-237, 1990.
14. Clinical Practice Committee: Outcome criteria and nursing diagnosis in ESRD patient care planning. II. Peritoneal dialysis, ANNA J 14:131, 1987.
15. Clinical Practice Committee: Outcome criteria and nursing diagnosis in ESRD patient care planning. III. Renal transplantation, ANNA J 14:197, 1987.
16. Clinical Practice Committee: Outcome criteria and nursing diagnosis in ESRD patient care planning. IV. Hemodialysis, ANNA J 14:213, 1987.
17. Comty CM and Collins AJ: Dialytic therapy in the management of chronic renal failure, Med Clin North Am 68:399, 1984.
18. Cunha BA and Friedman PE: Antibiotic dosing in patients with renal insufficiency or receiving dialysis, Heart Lung 17:612, 1988.
19. Delaney CW and Lauer ML: Intravenous therapy: a guide to quality care, Philadelphia, 1988, JB Lippincott Co.

RENAL

20. DeVault G: Nutritional support of the critically ill: writing the TPN prescription, J Crit Illness 4(10):54-69, 1989.
21. Drummond BL: Preventing increased intracranial pressure: nursing care can make the difference, Focus Crit Care 116(2):17, 1990.
22. Eisenberg HM et al: High-dose barbiturate control of elevated intracranial pressure in patients with severe head injury, J Neurosurg 15:69, 1988.
23. Eisenberg P: Enteral nutrition indications, formulas, and delivery techniques. Nurs Clin North Am 24(2):315-338, 1989.
24. Eisenberg P: Monitoring gastric pH to prevent stress ulcer syndrome, Focus Crit Care 17(4):316-322, 1990.
25. Emde KL and Searle LD: Current practices with thrombolytic therapy, J Cardiovasc Nurs 4(1):11-21, 1989.
26. Enright T and Hill MG: Treatment of fever, Focus Crit Care 16(2):96-102, 1989.
27. Erickson RS: Mastering the ins and outs of chest drainage, Nurs 89 19(5):36-43; 19(6):47-49, 1989.
28. Farley JM: Current trends in enteral feeding, Crit Care Nurse 8(4):23, 1988.
29. Farrell ML: Orthoclone OKT3: a treatment for acute renal allograft rejection, ANNA J 14:373, 1987.
30. Foster JK: Dialysis: a treatment modality in renal failure, Crit Care Q 1(2):25, 1978.
31. Futterman L: Cardiac transplantation: a comprehensive nursing perspective, Heart Lung 17(5):499-510, 1988.
32. Gharbieh PA: Renal transplant: surgical and psychologic hazards, Crit Care Nurse 8(6):58, 1988.
33. Hanson P: Current concepts in renal transplantation, ANNA J 14:367, 1987.
34. Harasyko C: Kidney transplantation, Nurs Clin North Am 24:851, 1989.
35. Holder C and Alexander J: A new and improved guide to IV therapy, Am J Nurs 90(2):43-47, 1990.
36. Holmes D et al: Advances in interventional cardiology, Mayo Clinic Proc 65(4):565-583, 1990.
37. Johanson B et al: Standards for critical care, ed 3, St Louis, 1988, The CV Mosby Co.
38. Kim M, McFarland G, and McLane A: Pocket guide to nursing diagnoses, St. Louis, 1990, The CV Mosby Co.
39. Konopad E and Noseworthy T: Stress ulceration: a serious complication in critically ill patients, Heart Lung 17:339-345, 1988.
40. Kruse DH: Postoperative hypothermia, Focus Crit Care 10(2):48-50, 1983.
41. La Rocca JC and Otto SE: Pocket guide to intravenous therapy, St Louis, 1989, The CV Mosby Co.

42. Lawyer LA and Velasco A: Continuous arteriovenous hemodialysis in the ICU, Crit Care Nurse 9(1):29, 1989.

43. Lerb RA and Hurtig JB: Epidural and intrathecal narcotics for pain management, Heart Lung 14:164-174, 1985.

44. Maher JF: Principles of dialysis and dialysis of drugs, AJM 62:475, 1977.

45. Manifold SL: Aneurysmal SAH: cerebral vasospasm and early repair, Crit Care Nurse 62(8):10, 1990.

46. Marchetto S and Stennis E: Ventricular assist devices: application for critical care, J Cardiovasc Nurs 2(2):39-55, 1990.

47. Martin E and others: Autotransfusion systems (ATS), Crit Care Nurse 9(7):65-73, 1989.

48. Marvin JA: Nutritional support of the critically injured patient, Crit Care Q 11(2):21-34, 1988.

49. McCrum AL and Tyndall A: Nursing care of patients with implantable defibrillators, Crit Care Nurse 9(4):48-68, 1989.

50. Mitchell P et al: AANN's neuroscience nursing: phenomena and practice, Norwalk, Conn, 1988, Appleton & Lange.

51. Munoz S and Maddrey W: Major complications of acute and chronic liver disease. Gastroenterol Clin North Am 17(2):265-288, 1988.

52. Newman LN: A side by side look at two venous access devices, Am J Nurs 89(6):826-833, 1989.

53. Nova G: Dialyzable drugs, Am J Nurs 87(7):933, 1987.

54. Ohler L, Fleagle D, and Lee B: Aortic valvuloplasty: medical and critical care nursing perspectives, Focus 16(4):275-287, 1989.

55. Olson GL, Leddo CO, and Wild L: Nursing management of patients receiving epidural narcotics, Heart Lung 18:130-138, 1989.

56. Persenti A, Kolobow T, and Gattinoni L: Extracorporeal respiratory support in the adult, Transamerican Society of Artificial and Internal Organs 34:1006-1008, 1988.

57. Peterson K and Brown MM: Extracorporeal membrane oxygenation in adults: a nursing challenge, Focus Crit Care 17(1):41-49, 1990.

58. Petrosino BM et al: Implications of selected problems with nasoenteral tube feedings, Crit Care Q 12(3):1-18, 1989.

59. Petty TL: Adult respiratory distress syndrome. In Mitchell RS and Petty TL, editors: Synopsis of clinical pulmonary disease, ed 4, St Louis, 1989, The CV Mosby Co.

60. Phillips R and Skov P: Rewarming and cardiac surgery: a review, Heart Lung 17(5):511-519, 1988.

61. Pierce AK: Acute respiratory failure. In Guenter CA and Welch MH, editors: Pulmonary medicine, ed 2, Philadelphia, 1982, JB Lippincott Co.

62. Pierson D: Overcoming nonrespiratory causes of weaning failure, J Crit Illness 5(3):267-283, 1990.

63. Prewit D: Post-operative complications—an overview, Nephrol Nurse 5(4):27, 1983.
64. Price CA: Continuous arteriovenous ultrafiltration: a monitoring guide for ICU nurses, Crit Care Nurse 9(1):12, 1989.
65. Purcell JA, Kloosterman N, and Miller L: Care of the hospitalized patient undergoing pacemaker therapy. In Riegel B et al, editors: Dreifus' pacemaker therapy: an interprofessional approach, Philadelphia, 1986, FA Davis.
66. Quaal S: Comprehensive intra-aortic balloon pumping, St Louis, 1984, The CV Mosby Co.
67. Rabetoy GM et al: Continuous arteriovenous hemofiltration (CAVH), Dialysis Transplant 18:120, 1989.
68. Rao KV: Status of renal transplantation: a clinical perspective, Med Clin North Am 68:427, 1984.
69. Rikkers L: Variceal hemorrhage. Gastroenterol Clin North Am 17(2):289-302, 1988.
70. Rolandelli R et al: Enteral nutrition: advantages, limitations, and formula selection, J Crit Illness 3(10):93-106, 1988.
71. Rolandelli R et al: Techniques for administering enteral nutrition in the ICU, J Crit Illness 3(10):107-112, 1988.
72. Rosen P et al: Emergency medicine: concepts and clinical practice, St Louis, 1988, The CV Mosby Co.
73. Rosenblum B: Long term venous access for home infusion therapy, Infusion 10(2):39, 1986.
74. Ruppel G: Manual of pulmonary function tests, ed 4, St Louis, 1986, The CV Mosby Co.
75. Rutherford C: The technique of selecting and administering blood components, J Crit Illness 5(5):487, 1990.
76. Sahn SA: Pneumothorax and pneumomediastinum. In Mitchell RS and Petty TL, editors: Synopsis of clinical pulmonary disease, ed 4, St Louis, 1989, The CV Mosby Co.
77. Sanders MH and Kern N: Obstructive sleep apnea treated by independently adjusted inspiratory and expiratory positive airway pressures via nasal mask, Chest 98(2):317-324, 1990.
78. Sassoon C, Mahutte K, and Light R: Ventilator modes: old and new, Crit Care Clin 6(3):605-626, 1990.
79. Sheldon RL: Clinical application of the chest radiograph. In Wilkins RL, Sheldon RL, and Krider SJ, editors: Clinical assessment in respiratory care, St Louis, 1990, The CV Mosby Co.

80. Sherman DW: Managing an acute head injury, Nurs 90, 46(4):20, 1990.
81. Smith S: Concepts in renal transplantation, Crit Care Q 1(2):53, 1978.
82. Strumpf DA et al: An evaluation of the Respironics Bi-Pap bi-level CPAP device for delivery of assisted ventilation, Resp Care 35(5):415-422, 1990.
83. Sullivan L: Administering medications on hemodialysis, Nephrol Nurse 4(5):46, 1982.
84. Talbot L and Meyers-Marquardt M: Pocket guide to critical care assessment, St Louis, 1989, The CV Mosby Co.
85. Taylor J and Taylor J: Vascular access devices: uses and after-care, JEN 13(3):160-167, 1987.
86. Technical manual, ed 10, Arlington, Va, 1990, American Association of Blood Banks.
87. Thelan LA, Davie JK, and Urden LD: Textbook of critical care nursing, St Louis, 1990, The CV Mosby Co.
88. Thompson JM et al: Mosby's manual of clinical nursing, St Louis, 1989, The CV Mosby Co.
89. Tobin M: Respiratory parameters predict successful weaning, J Crit Illness 5(8):819-837, 1990.
90. Underhill S et al: Cardiac nursing, ed 2, Philadelphia, 1989, JB Lippincott Co.
91. Vitello-Cicciu J: Aortic and mitral valvuloplasty, J Cardiovasc Nurs 1(3):70-78, 1987.
92. Warren H: Changes in peritoneal dialysis nursing, ANNA J 16:237, 1989.
93. Wasserman A and Ross RC: Coronary thrombolysis, Curr Prob Cardiol 43:12-19, 1987.
94. Weilitz PB: New modes of mechanical ventilation, Crit Care Nurs Clin North Am 1(4):689-695, 1989.
95. Wetmore NE et al: Extracorporeal membrane oxygenation (ECMO): a team approach in critical care and life-support research, Heart Lung 8:288-295, 1979.
96. Worthington PH and Wagner BA: Total parenteral nutrition, Nurs Clin North Am 24(2):355-372, 1989.
97. Young ME: Fever in the postoperative patient, Focus Crit Care 14(2):13-18, 1987.
98. Zimmerman R, Spetzler R, and Zabramski J: Cerebral arterial vasospasm: an update, BNIQ 6(3):2-9, 1990.

RENAL

CHAPTER 7

Pharmacology: Emergency Drugs

ADENOSINE (ADENOCARD)

Classification
Antidysrhythmic

Effects
Adenosine restores normal sinus rhythm by slowing conduction time through the AV node.

Indications
Paroxysmal supraventricular tachycardia (PSVT), including PSVT associated with Wolff-Parkinson-White (W-P-W) syndrome

Contraindications
Hypersensitivity to adenosine, second- or third-degree AV heart block, sick sinus syndrome (unless functioning artificial pacemaker is present); not recommended in the treatment of atrial fibrillation, atrial flutter, and ventricular tachycardia (VT)

Administration

Dose

Administer 6 mg IV bolus over 1 to 2 seconds; follow with a saline flush to ensure that the drug reaches the circulation. Give 12 mg rapid IV bolus if the first dose fails to eliminate the PSVT within 1 to 2 minutes. Repeat the 12 mg dose a second time if needed. Doses greater than 12 mg are not recommended; the unused solution should be discarded.

Precautions

Use cautiously in patients with asthma because inhaled adenosine causes bronchoconstriction in this population. A short-lasting first-, second-, or third-degree heart block may result. Patients developing high-level block after one dose of adenosine should not be given additional doses. New dysrhythmias may develop during conversion, e.g., PVCs, PACs, sinus bradycardia, sinus tachycardia, and AV blocks, but are generally self-limiting because the half life of adenosine is <10 seconds. Higher degrees of heart block may result in patients taking carbamazepine. Smaller doses of adenosine may be required in patients taking dipyridamole, since dipyridamole potentiates the effects of adenosine. Larger doses may be required in patients taking theophylline or other methylxanthine products, since the effects of adenosine are antagonized by methylxanthines.

Patient Management

- Check patency of IV and flush IV after adenosine administration to ensure that the drug reaches the circulation.
- Evaluate heart rate (HR) and rhythm 1 to 2 minutes after administering adenosine and monitor for dysrhythmias during conversion; blood pressure (BP) is not adversely affected with the usual dose of adenosine, but larger doses may result in hypotension.
- Measure PR interval for development of AV block.
- Observe for adverse effects: nonmyocardial chest discomfort, hypotension, and dyspnea. Patients may complain of facial flushing, sweating, headache, lightheadedness, tingling in the arms, blurred vision, heaviness in arms, burning sensation, neck and back pain, numbness, metallic taste, tightness in throat, and pressure in groin.
- Individualize treatment for prolonged adverse effects.

AMINOPHYLLINE/THEOPHYLLINE

Classification
Bronchodilator

Effects
Aminophylline/theophylline dilates bronchioles. It also increases cardiac output (CO), HR, and myocardial contractility. It decreases BP, increases urine output, and stimulates the CNS.

Indications
Prevention and treatment of bronchospasm; not very useful in treating an acute asthma attack; possible use as an adjunct in the treatment of Cheyne-Stokes respiration and pulmonary edema

Contraindications
Hypersensitivity to xanthine preparations such as caffeine

Administration
Dose

The dose must be individualized because it has a narrow therapeutic window. The loading dose of theophylline is 5 mg/kg. Aminophylline is 80% theophylline. If levels are not immediately obtainable, 2.5 mg/kg may be administered.

Lean body weight should be used for dosage determination in obese patients. Serum theophylline levels will increase by 2 µg/ml for every 1 mg/kg of loading dose administered.

IV administration should not exceed a rate greater than 20 mg/min. Rapid infusion can cause ventricular fibrillation (VF) or cardiac arrest. IV infusion of theophylline is usually 0.4 to 0.5 mg/kg/hr.

Precautions

Adjust dose for patients with hepatic disease because the drug is metabolized in the liver. Use cautiously in patients with congestive heart failure, preexisting cardiac dysrhythmias, and hyperthyroidism. Side effects are related to theophylline serum levels.

Patient Management

- Check serum theophylline levels; therapeutic drug level is 10 to 20 µg/ml.
- Monitor vital signs; tachycardia and hypotension can occur with rapid administration.
- Assess lungs for adventitious sounds, evaluating patient response to therapy.
- Maintain the ordered infusion rate, using an IV volume infusion-control pump.
- Observe for adverse effects: restlessness, dizziness, insomnia, convulsions, palpitations, tachycardia, hypotension, dysrhythmias, nausea and vomiting, anorexia, and epigastric pain.

AMRINONE (INOCOR)

Classification

Inotrope/vasodilator

Effects

Amrinone increases myocardial contractility and CO. It decreases afterload, preload, pulmonary artery wedge pressure (PAWP), diastolic blood pressure (DBP), and mean arterial pressure (MAP).

Indications

Congestive heart failure refractory to traditional therapies

Contraindications

Hypertrophic obstructive cardiomyopathy and aortic or pulmonic valvular disease

Administration

Dose

The IV loading dose is 0.75 mg/kg over 2 to 3 minutes. Loading dose may be repeated in 30 minutes. The drug can be given undiluted. As an infusion, administer at 2 to 20 µg/kg/min.

Precautions

Avoid administration with disopyramide. Use cautiously in patients who have hepatic or renal disease. Thrombocytopenia may occur.

Patient Management

- Monitor BP, PAWP, MAP, systemic vascular resistance (SVR), pulmonary vascular resistance (PVR), HR, and CO during infusion.
- Observe for adverse effects: thrombocytopenia, hypotension, dizziness, dysrhythmias, chest pain, hypokalemia, nausea and vomiting, abdominal pain, anorexia, hepatic toxicity, and fever.

ATROPINE

Classification

Anticholinergic

Effects

Atropine increases conduction through the AV node and increases the HR.

Indications

Symptomatic bradycardia and asystole

Contraindications

Adhesions between the iris and lens, advanced renal and hepatic impairment, asthma, narrow-angle glaucoma, obstructive disease of the GI and urinary tract, myasthenia gravis, and paralytic ileus

Administration

Dose

For bradycardia, administer 0.5 mg IV bolus every 5 minutes until adequate response or a total dose of 2 mg is given. Doses of less than 0.5 mg can cause bradycardia. For asystole, administer 1 mg IV; repeat once if needed.

Atropine can be given undiluted IV push in emergency situations. Atropine may also be given via the endotracheal tube by diluting 1 to 2 mg in 10 ml sterile water or normal saline (NS) and followed by five forceful inhalations.

Precautions

In the presence of an acute infarction, atropine can increase cardiac irritability.

Patient Management

- Monitor HR for response to therapy (>60 is desirable); be alert for development of VF or VT.

- Excessive doses can result in tachycardia, flushed hot skin, delirium, coma, or death.
- Antidote for overdose is physostigmine salicylate.

BRETYLIUM (BRETYLOL)

Classification
Antidysrhythmic

Effects
Bretylium increases the refractory period without increasing HR. Initially, it causes an increase in BP, HR, and myocardial contractility as a result of the norepinephrine release. This response is followed by hypotension, which is caused by neuronal blockade.

Indications
VF and VT, currently the second drug of choice (after lidocaine) in the treatment of refractory or recurrent VF.

Contraindications
Digitalis-induced dysrhythmias, not effective in abolishing atrial dysrhythmias

Administration
Dose

Administer 5 mg/kg IV followed by 10 mg/kg every 15 to 30 minutes if necessary. A maximum total dose of 30 mg/kg may be given. A continuous infusion of 1 to 4 mg/min may be required (see drug dosage chart, p. 582).

Precautions

Postural hypotension occurs regularly following administration of bretylium. Correct hypovolemia before administration. The dosage should be adjusted accordingly for patients with renal impairment.

Patient Management
- Keep patient supine and monitor BP during infusion.
- Evaluate dysrhythmia control and CO.
- Evaluate patient receiving digitalis for digitalis toxicity.
- Observe for adverse effects: hypotension, vertigo, dysrhythmias, angina, syncope, and nausea and vomiting.

BUMETANIDE (BUMEX)

Classification
Diuretic

Effects
Bumetanide promotes the excretion of fluid and electrolytes and reduces plasma volume. It is 40 times more potent than furosemide (Lasix).

Indications

Edematous states: congestive heart failure, pulmonary edema, and hepatic and renal disease

Contraindications

Hepatic coma, anuria, and hypersensitivity to sulfonamides

Administration

Dose

Administer 500 µg to 2 mg orally per day as a single dose. If a diuretic response is not achieved, a second or third dose may be given at 4 to 5 hour intervals. Maximum is 10 mg. IV dose is 500 µg to 1 mg given undiluted over 1 to 2 minutes. May repeat at 2 to 3 hour intervals.

Precautions

Profound electrolyte and water depletion can occur. Concurrent use with aminoglycosides may increase the risk for ototoxicity.

Patient Management

- Assess potassium level before administration; hypokalemia should be corrected before administration.
- Monitor for signs of electrolyte and water depletion.
- Monitor BP and HR during increased diuresis period.
- Assess serial weights and I & O to evaluate fluid loss (1 kg = 1000 ml fluid).
- Monitor patient receiving digitalis for digitalis toxicity secondary to diuretic-induced hypokalemia.
- Evaluate hearing and assess for ototoxicity.
- Monitor serial BUN and creatinine levels to assess renal function.
- Observe for adverse effects: volume depletion (e.g., dryness of the mouth, increased thirst, dizziness, and orthostatic hypotension), headache, muscle cramps, nausea, transient deafness, glucose intolerance, and hepatic dysfunction.

CALCIUM CHLORIDE

Classification

Electrolyte replenisher

Effects

Calcium chloride replaces and maintains calcium in body fluids.

Indications

Hypocalcemia, hyperkalemia, magnesium toxicity, and calcium channel–blocker overdose; possibly indicated during a cardiac resuscitation

Contraindications
VF, hypercalcemia, renal calculi, and digitalis toxicity
Administration
Dose
Give 500 mg to 1 g slowly IV, not to exceed 50 to 100 mg/min. When adding to parenteral fluids, monitor for a precipitate. One gram of calcium chloride is equivalent to 13.6 mEq of calcium.
Precautions
The dosage of calcium may need to be adjusted in patients with renal or cardiac disease. Cardiac dysrhythmias may be evidenced when calcium is administered to patients who are receiving digitalis glycosides or who have been digitalized. Severe necrosis and sloughing of tissues will occur with infiltration.
Patient Management
- Administer calcium through a central line.
- Assess patency of IV; note any precipitate.
- Monitor BP, since peripheral vasodilation will occur.
- Monitor serial serum calcium levels.
- Continuously monitor ECG for onset of dysrhythmias.
- Monitor for electrolyte imbalances.
- Observe for adverse effects: bradycardia, cardiac arrest, constipation, fatigue, venous irritation, depression, loss of appetite, and tingling.

DEXAMETHASONE (DECADRON)
Classification
Adrenocortical steroid
Effects
Dexamethasone decreases inflammation, suppresses the immune response, stimulates bone marrow, and influences protein, fat, and carbohydrate metabolism.
Indications
Cerebral edema, inflammatory conditions, and allergic reactions
Contraindications
Systemic fungal infections
Administration
Dose
Initially, administer 10 mg IV, then 4 to 6 mg IV or IM. It can be given undiluted over 1 minute. Oral dose is 0.25 to 4 mg, which is administered two, three, or four times daily.

Precautions

Use cautiously in patients with GI ulceration or renal disease, hypertension, osteoporosis, varicella, diabetes mellitus, or myasthenia gravis. The drug may mask or exacerbate infections. The drug should be gradually reduced after long-term therapy.

Patient Management

- Administer single dose before 9 AM.
- Observe for signs and symptoms of hyperglycemia, especially in patients with diabetes.
- Monitor serial serum electrolyte levels.
- Observe for adverse effects: euphoria, insomnia, congestive heart failure, peptic ulcer, possible hypokalemia, hyperglycemia, and carbohydrate intolerance. Depression may occur after tapering.

DIAZEPAM (VALIUM)

Classification

Antianxiety agent, anticonvulsant, skeletal muscle relaxant

Effects

Diazepam depresses the CNS, suppresses the spread of seizure activity, and relaxes skeletal muscle.

Indications

Anxiety, status epilepticus, and preprocedure sedation

Contraindications

Shock, coma, acute alcohol intoxication, acute glaucoma, psychoses, and myasthenia gravis

Administration

Dose

Administer 2 to 10 mg orally three or four times daily. IV dose is 5 to 10 mg initially, with a maximum of 30 mg in 8 hours. The drug may be given IV push at a rate of 2 to 5 mg/min.

In status epilepticus, administer 5 to 10 mg IV; can be repeated every 5 to 10 minutes, up to 30 mg in 1 hour. Do not mix diazepam with other drugs.

Precautions

Dosage should be reduced in the elderly. Use cautiously in patients with blood dyscrasias, hepatic or renal damage, or depression and in those with diminished pulmonary function.

Patient Management

- Monitor respirations frequently before and after the IV dose.

- Evaluate patient's response (e.g., decreased anxiety, absence of seizures).
- Observe for adverse effects: drowsiness, cardiovascular collapse, pain, phlebitis at injection site, and respiratory depression.

DIGOXIN (LANOXIN)
Classification
Cardiac glycoside
Effects
Digoxin increases myocardial contractility, decreases HR, and enhances CO, which improves renal blood flow and increases urinary output.
Indications
Patients with congestive heart failure, cardiogenic shock, and atrial dysrhythmias such as atrial fibrillation, atrial flutter, and paroxsysmal atrial tachycardia
Contraindications
Patients who demonstrate signs and symptoms of digitalis toxicity
Administration
Dose
Digitalizing and maintenance doses must be individualized. Usual loading dose is 1 to 1.25 mg IV or orally in divided doses over 24 hours. Maintenance dose is 0.125 to 0.5 mg IV or PO daily. IV dose may be given undiluted over at least 5 minutes.
Precautions
Use cautiously in the elderly and in patients with acute infarction or renal impairment. Administer IV digoxin with caution in the hypertensive patient because a transient increase in BP may occur. Patients with partial AV block may develop complete heart block. Patients with W-P-W may experience fatal ventricular dysrhythmias.
Patient Management
- Check potassium level before administration, since hypokalemia is associated with increased risk of digitalis toxicity.
- Take apical pulse before administration; if <60, consult with physician.
- Measure serial PR intervals for development of heart block.
- Evaluate patient for controlled dysrhythmia (decreased ventricular response to atrial fibrillation or atrial flutter).

Digibind

The dose of Digibind varies according to the amount of digoxin to be neutralized. Each vial (40 mg) will bind with 0.6 mg of digoxin. An average dose is 10 vials, administered over 30 minutes through a 0.22 μm filter. If the toxicity has not been reversed after several hours, readministration may be required. Monitor potassium levels because digibind can cause a rapid drop in potassium secondary to reversing the effects of digitalis. Monitor HR because the withdrawal of digoxin effects in patients with atrial fibrillation or atrial flutter may cause a return of rapid ventricular rate. Heart failure may worsen secondary to withdrawal of the inotropic effects of digitalis.

- Evaluate patient for resolution of heart failure.
- Be prepared to treat overdose with IV magnesium sulfate or digoxin immune fab (Digibind) if patient has severe, life-threatening refractory dysrhythmias (see box).
- Observe for digitalis toxicity: nausea and vomiting, anorexia, epigastric pain, unusual fatigue, diarrhea, dysrhythmias, blurred or yellow vision, irritability or confusion, ST segment sagging, or prolonged PR interval.

DOBUTAMINE (DOBUTREX)
Classification
Inotrope, adrenergic-stimulating agent
Effects
Dobutamine increases myocardial contractility and increases CO without significant change in BP. It increases coronary blood flow and myocardial oxygen consumption.
Indications
Heart failure and cardiogenic shock
Contraindications
Idiopathic hypertrophic stenosis
Administration
Dose
IV infusion is 2.5 to 20 μg/kg/min titrated to desired patient response. A dose of 250 mg/250 ml 250 D_5W yields 1 mg/ml. Concentration of solution should not exceed 5 mg/ml of dobutamine (see drug dosage chart, p. 580).

Precautions
Hemodynamic monitoring is recommended for optimal benefit when dobutamine is administered. Fluid deficits should be corrected before infusion of dobutamine. At doses greater than 20 µg/kg/min, an increase in HR may occur. Dobutamine facilitates conduction through the AV node and can cause a rapid ventricular response in patients with inadequately treated atrial fibrillation. Concurrent use with general anesthetics may increase the potential for ventricular dysrhythmias.

Patient Management
- Use large veins for administration; an infusion pump should be used to regulate flow rate.
- Check BP and HR every 2 to 5 minutes during initial administration and during titration of the drug.
- Monitor CO, PAWP, and urine output continuously during administration.
- Observe for adverse effects: tachycardia, hypertension, chest pain, and cardiac dysrhythmias.

DOPAMINE (INTROPIN)

Classification
Sympathomimetic, vasopressor

Effects
Dopamine in low doses (3-5 µg/kg/min) increases blood flow to the kidneys, glomerular filtration rate, urine flow, and sodium excretion. In low to moderate doses (5-10 µg/kg/min), it increases myocardial contractility and CO. In high doses (10-20 µg/kg/min), it increases peripheral resistance and renal vasoconstriction.

Indications
Shock states, septicemia, myocardial infarction, and renal failure

Contraindications
Uncorrected tachydysrhythmias, pheochromocytoma, VF

Administration
Dose
For IV infusion, administer 2 to 20 µg/kg/min up to 50 µg/kg/min, titrated to effect and/or renal response. A dose of 400 mg/500 ml D_5W yields 800 µg/ml (see drug dosage chart, p. 581).

Precautions
Concurrent use with β blockers may antagonize the effect of dopamine. Use with caution in patients receiving mono-

amine oxidase (MAO) inhibitors because the drug may cause a hypertensive crisis. Use cautiously in patients with occlusive vascular disease, arterial embolism, and diabetic endarteritis.

Patient Management

- Use large vein; check vein frequently for blanching/pallor, which may indicate extravasation.
- Notify physician if extravasation occurs. Treat with phentolamine (5 to 10 mg in 10 to 15 ml NS) via local infiltration as soon as possible.
- Do not use the proximal port of a pulmonary artery (PA) catheter to infuse the drug if CO readings are being obtained.
- Monitor BP and HR every 2 to 5 minutes initially and during titration of the drug.
- Measure urine output hourly to evaluate renal function.
- Determine pulse pressure, since a decrease indicates excessive vasoconstriction.
- Taper infusion gradually to avoid sudden hypotension.
- Observe for adverse effects: tachycardia, headache, dysrhythmias, nausea and vomiting, hypotension, chest pain, shortness of breath, and vasoconstriction (numbness, tingling, pallor, cold skin, decreased pulses, decreased cerebral perfusion, and decreased urine output).
- Report the drug's inability to maintain a desired response despite increased dosage.

EDROPHONIUM (TENSILON)

Classification
Cholinesterase inhibitor

Effects
Edrophonium produces vagal stimulation, which results in a decreased HR.

Indications
Diagnosis of myasthenic crisis and treatment of PSVT

Contraindications
Hypersensitivity to anticholinesterase agents, bronchial asthma, or intestinal or urinary obstruction

Administration
Dose

For patients with myasthenia gravis, administer 1 mg IV; if no response, repeat dose in 1 minute. Increased muscular strength confirms myasthenic crisis, and no increase confirms cholinergic crisis, at which point atropine sulfate (0.4 to 0.5

mg) needs to be given. For patients with supraventricular tachyarrhythmias, administer 5 to 10 mg IV; repeat in 10 minutes if needed. The drug is administered undiluted.

Precautions

Use cautiously in patients with cardiac dysrhythmias, those who are receiving digitalis, and those with hypotension and bradycardia.

Patient Management

- Have atropine available to counteract cholinergic reactions.
- Monitor HR and respirations; observe for signs of respiratory distress and bradycardia.
- Observe for adverse effects: muscle weakness, shortness of breath, bradycardia, fatigue and weakness, bronchospasm, cardiac arrest, convulsions, diarrhea, increased lacrimation, laryngospasm, ptosis, urinary frequency, vomiting, and perspiration.

EPINEPHRINE (ADRENALINE)

Classification

Bronchodilator, vasopressor, cardiac stimulant

Effects

Epinephrine increases myocardial contractility, HR, systolic BP, and CO. It also relaxes bronchial smooth muscle.

Indications

Cardiac arrest, hypersensitivity reactions, anaphylaxis, and acute asthma attacks

Contraindications

Acute narrow-angle glaucoma and coronary insufficiency

Administration

Dose

For patients in cardiac arrest, give 0.5 to 1.0 mg IV or endotracheally of a 1:10,000 solution every 5 minutes. With an IV infusion, administer 2 μg/min and titrate to desired response; 1 mg/250 ml D_5W yields 4 μg/ml (see drug dosage chart, p. 582).

For bronchospasm/anaphylaxis, give 0.1 to 0.5 ml of 1:1000 solution subcutaneously and repeat every 10 to 20 minutes. If using an IV route, give 0.1-0.25 ml of 1:1000 solution.

Precautions

Use cautiously in elderly patients and patients with angina, hypothyroidism, hypertension, psychoneurosis, and diabetes. Epinephrine should be administered cautiously in patients with long-standing bronchial asthma and emphysema who have developed degenerative heart disease. Do not administer concurrently with isoproterenol—death may result. Repeated local injections can cause necrosis at the site.

Patient Management

- Monitor BP and HR every 2 to 5 minutes during the initial infusion and during drug titration.
- Use an infusion device; validate correct drug and infusion rate.
- Do not use the proximal port of a PA catheter for infusing epinephrine if CO readings are being obtained.
- Evaluate patient's response; monitor CO.
- Observe for adverse effects: chest pain, dysrhythmias, headache, restlessness, dizziness, nausea and vomiting, weakness, and excessive vasoconstriction.
- Report the drug's inability to maintain a desired effect despite increased doses.

ESMOLOL (BREVIBLOC)

Classification
β-Adrenergic blocking agent

Effects
Esmolol decreases HR, BP, contractility, and myocardial oxygen consumption.

Indications
Supraventricular tachycardia and hypertension

Contraindications
Sinus bradycardia, heart block greater than first degree, cardiogenic shock, and overt heart failure

Administration
Dose

Administer 500 μg/kg/min IV for 1 minute; give 50 μg/kg/min for 4 minutes. Repeat loading dose and increase infusion to 100 μg/kg/min if desired response is not achieved in 5 minutes. Continue same loading dose but increase maintenance dose by 50 μg/kg/min until desired response is achieved or hypotension occurs. Do not exceed 200 μg/kg/min. A dose of 5 g/500 ml D_5W yields 10 mg/ml.

Discontinue infusion: Infusion dose can be reduced by 50% 30 minutes after the first dose of an alternate antidysrhythmic agent is given. If patient remains stable an hour after the second dose of the alternative agent is administered, esmolol may be discontinued.

Precautions

Use cautiously in patients with impaired renal function, diabetes, or bronchospasm.

Patient Management

- Monitor BP every 2 minutes during titration. Hypotension can be reversed by decreasing the dose or by discontinuing the infusion.
- Evaluate dysrhythmia control.
- Monitor ECG for bradycardia or heart block.
- Evaluate patient for heart failure.
- Monitor glucose levels closely, especially in patients with diabetes.
- Observe for adverse effects: hypotension, pallor, lightheadedness, paresthesias, urinary retention, nausea and vomiting, bronchospasm, and inflammation at the infusion site.
- Report signs of overdose: tachycardia/bradycardia, dizziness/fainting, difficulty in breathing, bluish color on palmer surface of hands, seizures, cold hands, fever, sore throat, or unusual bleeding.

FUROSEMIDE (LASIX)

Classification

Diuretic

Effects

Furosemide promotes the excretion of fluid and electrolytes and reduces plasma volume.

Indications

Edematous states: congestive heart failure, pulmonary edema, hepatic and renal disease, and hypertension

Contraindications

Sensitivity to furosemide or sulfonamides

Administration

Dose

Oral dose is 20 to 80 mg in the morning, followed by a second dose 6 to 8 hours later if necessary. IV dose is 20 to 40 mg given undiluted over 1 to 2 minutes; additional doses may be given until the desired outcome is achieved.

Precautions

Profound electrolyte and water depletion can occur.

Patient Management

- Check potassium level before administering furosemide; hypokalemia should be corrected before administering the drug.

- Evaluate hearing and assess for ototoxicity.
- Monitor urine output to evaluate drug effectiveness.
- Monitor serial BUN and creatinine levels to assess renal function.
- Assess patient for volume depletion and electrolyte imbalance.
- Monitor BP and I & O and assess serial weights (1 kg = 1000 ml fluid) to evaluate fluid loss.
- Monitor patient receiving digitalis for digitalis toxicity secondary to diuretic-induced hypokalemia.
- Advise patient to report ringing in ears, severe abdominal pain, or sore throat and fever. These symptoms may indicate furosemide toxicity.
- Observe for adverse effects: volume depletion, orthostatic hypotension, electrolyte imbalance, transient deafness, glucose intolerance, and hepatic dysfunction.

HYDROCORTISONE (SOLU-CORTEF)

Classification
Steroid

Effects
Hydrocortisone decreases inflammation, suppresses the immune response, stimulates bone marrow, and influences protein, fat, and carbohydrate metabolism.

Indications
Inflammatory diseases, adrenal insufficiency, and shock states

Contraindications
Systemic fungal infections and septic shock

Administration
Dose

For inflammation and adrenal insufficiency, IV or IM doses of 100 to 250 mg may be given initially, then 50 to 100 mg IM. In shock states, 500 mg to 2 g is given every 2 to 6 hours if indicated.

Hydrocortisone is administered undiluted. The IM dose should be given deep into the gluteal muscle.

Subcutaneous injections should be avoided because atrophy and sterile abscesses may occur.

Precautions
Use with indomethacin and aspirin can result in an increased risk of GI distress and bleeding. Use cautiously in patients with GI ulceration or renal disease, hypertension, osteoporosis, varicella, diabetes mellitus, Cushing's syndrome, thromboembolic disorders, seizures, myasthenia gravis, metastatic

cancer, congestive heart failure, ocular herpes simplex, and hypoalbuminemia.

The drug can cause an increase in BP and fluid retention and may mask signs of infection.

Patient Management

- Administer the drug before 9 AM to limit suppression of adrenocortical activity.
- Monitor weight, serum electrolyte levels, and BP.
- Observe for adverse effects: euphoria, insomnia, congestive heart failure, peptic ulcer, hypokalemia, hyperglycemia, and Cushing's syndrome

ISOPROTERENOL (ISUPREL)

Classification

Sympathomimetic, β-adrenergic agonist

Effects

Isoproterenol increases CO, coronary blood flow, and stroke volume; decreases MAP; and relaxes bronchial smooth muscle.

Indications

Bronchial asthma, obstructive pulmonary disease, bronchospasm, heart block, atropine refractory bradycardia, and shock states

Contraindications

Digitalis-induced tachycardia or patients receiving β blockers

Administration

Dose

The IV infusion rate is 2 to 20 µg/min; titrate to desired response. A dose of 1 mg/250 ml D_5W yields 4 µg/ml (see drug dosage chart, p. 582).

Precautions

Volume deficit should be corrected before initiating isoproterenol. Administer cautiously in patients with hypertension, coronary artery disease, hyperthyroidism, and diabetes. The drug is not indicated in cardiac arrest. Do not use concurrently with epinephrine. VF and VT may develop.

Patient Management

- If the HR exceeds 110 bpm, the dose may need to be decreased. If the HR exceeds 130 bpm, ventricular dysrhythmias may be induced.
- Monitor BP, MAP, central venous pressure (CVP), and urinary output.
- An infusion pump should be used to administer the infusion.

- Observe for adverse effects: headache, tachycardia, anginal pain, palpitations, flushing of the face, nervousness, sweating, hypotension, and pulmonary edema.

LABETALOL (NORMODYNE, TRANDATE)

Classification
β-Adrenergic blocking agent

Effects
Labetalol decreases BP and renin secretion and can decrease HR and CO.

Indications
Hypertension

Contraindications
Bronchial asthma, cardiac failure, heart block, cardiogenic shock, and bradycardia

Administration

Dose
Oral dose is 100 mg twice daily. IV dose is 20 mg given undiluted over 2 minutes, and additional doses of 40 to 80 mg every 10 minutes up to 300 mg may be required for the desired effect. IV infusion is 2 mg/min titrated to desired response; 200 mg/160 ml D_5W yields 1 mg/ml.

Precautions
Use cautiously in patients with congestive heart failure, hepatic impairment, chronic bronchitis, emphysema, preexisting peripheral vascular disease, and pheochromocytoma.

Patient Management
- Check HR and BP before administering labetalol and 10 minutes after an IV dose.
- Monitor BP every 5 minutes during infusion; avoid rapid BP drop because cerebral infarction or angina can occur.
- Have patient remain supine immediately following injection.
- Assess patient for congestive heart failure development.
- Monitor blood glucose levels closely in patients with diabetes.
- Observe for adverse effects: dizziness, orthostatic hypotension, fatigue, nasal stuffiness, edema, and paresthesias.

LIDOCAINE

Classification
Antidysrhythmic

Effects
Lidocaine suppresses the automaticity of ectopic foci.

NIFEDIPINE (ADALAT, PROCARDIA)

Classification
Calcium channel blocker

Effects
Nifedipine dilates coronary arteries and arterioles. It has less effect on decreasing HR and myocardial contractility than other calcium channel blockers.

Indications
Chronic angina and hypertension

Contraindications
Aortic stenosis, cardiogenic shock, and acute angina attacks

Administration
Dose
Give 10 mg orally three times daily. Maximum is 180 mg. Single doses should not exceed 30 mg. Nifedipine should be decreased gradually if it is to be discontinued. The liquid in the oral capsule can be withdrawn by puncturing the capsule with a needle and administering 10 to 20 mg sublingually or bucally. Maximal effects can be achieved by chewing and swallowing the capsules. The extended-release preparation (Procardia XL) should never be crushed, chewed, or administered sublingually.

Precautions
Use with β blockers may cause profound hypotension and heart failure. Use cautiously in elderly patients, patients with congestive heart failure or hypotension, and patients with impaired renal or hepatic function.

Patient Management
- Measure serial PR intervals.
- Check HR and BP before administration; if systolic blood pressure (SBP) <90 or HR <50, notify physician.
- Monitor CO and assess patient for development of heart failure.
- Monitor serum potassium levels frequently.
- Assess for signs of peripheral edema (pedal edema is dose related).
- Observe for adverse effects: dizziness, lightheadedness, flushing, headache, and nausea.

NITROGLYCERIN (TRIDIL, NITROL)

Classification
Vasodilator

Effects

Nitroglycerin decreases venous return, preload, myocardial oxygen demand, BP, MAP, CVP, PAWP, PVR, and SVR. It improves coronary artery blood flow and oxygen delivery.

Indications

Angina, hypertension, and congestive heart failure in acute myocardial infarction

Contraindications

Patients with hypersensitivity to nitrites; patients with head trauma, cerebral hemorrhage, severe anemia, pericardial tamponade, or constrictive pericarditis; and those with hypertrophic cardiomyopathy who are experiencing chest pain

Administration

Dose

IV infusion is 5 μg/min; increase by 5 μg every 3 to 5 minutes and titrate to desired response. A dose of 50 mg/500 ml D_5W yields 100 μg/ml. No fixed maximum dose has been established (see drug dosage chart, p. 582).

Precautions

Use with tricyclic antidepressants may result in additive hypotension. Orthostatic hypotension may be potentiated with antihypertensives or vasodilators. Correct volume deficit to prevent profound hypotension. Tolerance may develop with prolonged use of nitroglycerin.

Patient Management

- Monitor HR; a 10 bpm increase suggests adequate vasodilation.
- Monitor BP every 2 to 5 minutes while titrating.
- Stop infusion and lift patient's lower extremities if SBP <90 or if patient complains of dizziness/lightheadedness.
- Calculate coronary perfusion pressure (CPP); monitor PAWP, SVR, and PVR; and evaluate CO.
- Observe for adverse effects: headache, dizziness, dry mouth, blurred vision, orthostatic hypotension, tachycardia, angina, flushing, palpitations, nausea, and restlessness.
- Report unrelieved angina and signs and symptoms of overdose: cyanotic lips and palmar surface of hands, extreme dizziness, pressure in head, dyspnea, fever, seizure, and weak/fast HR.

NITROPRUSSIDE (NIPRIDE)

Classification

Vasodilator, antihypertensive

Effects

Nitroprusside decreases BP and peripheral resistance and usually increases CO.

Indications

Hypertension

Contraindications

Coarctation of aorta

Administration

Dose

IV infusion is 0.5-10 μg/kg/min. Maximum is 10 μg/kg/min. A dose of 50 mg/250 ml D_5W yields 200 μg/ml (see drug dosage chart, p. 583).

Precautions

Use cautiously in patients with hypothyroidism or hepatic or renal disease and in those receiving antihypertensive agents.

Patient Management

- Monitor BP every 2 to 5 minutes; if hypotension develops, discontinue IV nitroprusside.
- Use an IV infusion device; validate concentration/dosage.
- Protect solution from light; it normally is brownish.
- Assess patient for chest pain, dysrhythmias, and fluid retention.
- Observe for adverse effects: headache, dizziness, excessive sweating, nervousness, restlessness, ataxia, delirium, loss of consciousness, and ringing in the ears.
- Tolerance to nipride may indicate toxicity. Thiocyanate levels of greater than 100 μg/ml indicate toxicity.
- Assess for signs of toxicity: profound hypotension, metabolic acidosis, dyspnea, headache, loss of consciousness, and vomiting.

NOREPINEPHRINE (LEVOPHED)

Classification

Sympathomimetic, vasopressor

Effects

Norepinephrine produces vasoconstriction, increases myocardial contractility, and dilates coronary arteries.

Indications

Hypotensive states caused by trauma, shock, and myocardial infarction

Contraindications

Mesenteric or peripheral vascular thrombosis, pregnancy, profound hypoxia, hypercarbia, hypotension from volume deficit, or with cyclopropane or halothane anesthesia

Administration

Dose

IV infusion is 2 μg/min; titrate to desired BP. A dose of 4 mg/250 ml D_5W yields 16 μg/ml (see drug dosage chart, pp. 584, 585).

Precautions

Concurrent administration with MAO inhibitors increases the risk of hypertensive crisis. When the drug is administered with tricyclic antidepressants, severe hypertension may result. Use cautiously in patients with hypertension, hyperthyroidism, and severe cardiac disease.

Patient Management

- Monitor BP every 2 to 5 minutes.
- Evaluate CO.
- Assess patency of IV site and observe for extravasation; blanching may indicate extravasation. If extravasation occurs, stop the infusion and call the physician. Be prepared to infiltrate the area with phentolamine 5 to 10 mg in 10 to 15 ml NS.
- Use an infusion pump to regulate flow.
- Assess for signs and symptoms of excessive vasoconstriction: cold skin, pallor, decreased pulses, decreased cerebral perfusion, and decreased pulse pressure.
- Report decreased urinary output.
- Taper medication gradually and monitor vital signs.
- Observe for adverse effects: headache, VT, bradycardia, VF, decreased urinary output, metabolic acidosis, restlessness, and hypertensive state.

PANCURONIUM (PAVULON)

Classification

Neuromuscular blocking agent

Effects

Pancuronium causes skeletal muscle paralysis but has no effects on consciousness or pain.

Indications

Facilitation of controlled mechanical ventilation

Contraindications

Hypersensitivity to bromides, preexisting tachycardia, and conditions in which an increase in HR is undesirable

Administration

Dose

A dose of 0.04 to 0.1 mg/kg IV may be given undiluted; a single dose may be given over 1 to 2 minutes. Subsequent doses are repeated as required and usually start at 0.01 mg/kg for continued muscle relaxation. As a constant infusion, titrate the dose to patient response.

Precautions

The dose needs to be adjusted when aminoglycosides are being administered. Use with quinidine can result in increased neuromuscular blockage. Use cautiously in elderly or debilitated patients and those with renal, hepatic, or pulmonary impairment; myasthenia gravis; dehydration; thyroid disorders; collagen disease; electrolyte disturbances; hyperthermia; and cardiac dysrhythmias.

Patients must have a patent airway and be artificially ventilated. Patients are conscious but unable to communicate and should be sedated.

Patient Management

- Ensure patent airway and controlled mechanical ventilation.
- Analyze arterial blood gases (ABGs) for adequate oxygenation.
- Monitor serial serum electrolyte levels because potassium disturbances can potentiate pancuronium.
- Use adjunctive therapy for pain control and sedation when administering pancuronium.
- Have emergency respiratory equipment readily available in case of accidental extubation or lack of endotracheal tube patency.
- Observe for adverse effects: respiratory depression, apnea, and tachycardia.

PHENOBARBITAL

Classification

Anticonvulsant, sedative, hypnotic

Effects

Phenobarbital depresses the CNS and increases the threshold for seizure activity.

Indications

Seizures and need for sedation

Contraindications

Barbiturate hypersensitivity, porphyria, hepatic dysfunction, respiratory disease, nephritis, and lactation

Administration

Dose

Oral or IV dose is 1 to 3 mg/kg/day. IV loading dose of 15 to 20 mg/kg is recommended for the treatment of patients with status epilepticus. Do not give faster than 60 mg/min intravenously.

Precautions

Use with other CNS depressants can result in excessive CNS depression. There may be a potentiated barbiturate effect when the drug is given concurrently with MAO inhibitors. Rifampin may decrease the barbiturate levels. Primidone and valproic acid may cause phenobarbital levels to be elevated. Diazepam and phenobarbital given together may result in an increased effect of both drugs and should be used cautiously. Use cautiously in patients with hyperthyroidism, diabetes mellitus, or anemia and in elderly or debilitated patients.

Rapid infusion of phenobarbital may cause respiratory depression.

Patient Management

- Monitor vital signs hourly, including respiratory rate; ensure patent airway.
- Check phenobarbital level; therapeutic level is 15 to 40 μg/ml.
- Evaluate patient response, e.g., absence of seizure activity and degree of sedation.
- Observe for adverse effects: drowsiness, lethargy, nausea and vomiting, hypotension, apnea, and hypothermia.

PHENYTOIN (DILANTIN)

Classification

Anticonvulsant

Effects

Phenytoin depresses seizure activity.

Indications

Generalized seizure control and digitalis-induced dysrhythmias

Contraindications

Bradycardia, SA and AV block, and Adams-Stokes syndrome

Administration

Dose

Anticonvulsant IV loading dose is 15 to 18 mg/kg followed by a maintenance dose of 5 to 7 mg/kg/day; 150 to 250 mg may be given, followed by 100 to 150 mg after 30 minutes if necessary.

Antidysrhythmic dose is 50 to 100 mg IV every 10 to 15 minutes, until desired effects are obtained. The dose should not exceed a total dose of 15 mg/kg. Do not exceed a rate of 50 mg/min. An in-line filter is recommended to administer the diluted phenytoin. Before and after each dose of phenytoin, the line should be flushed with normal saline.

Precautions

The effects of phenytoin may be decreased with barbiturates and folic acid. The effects of phenytoin can be increased when used with chloramphenicol, cimetidine, disulfiram, isoniazid, or sulfonamides. Use with antidysrhythmics may result in an additive cardiac depressant effect. Oral contraceptives and phenytoin may result in decreased contraceptive reliability and/or loss of seizure control. Use cautiously in patients with hepatic or renal dysfunction, hypotension, myocardial insufficiency, or respiratory depression and in elderly or debilitated patients.

Patient Management

- Assess patency of IV; follow each injection with NS. Extravasation of phenytoin is damaging to the tissues.
- Monitor BP, HR, and respiratory rate with administration of IV phenytoin; bradycardia, cardiac arrest, and respiratory arrest can occur.
- Monitor blood levels; therapeutic level is 10 to 20 µg/ml.
- Observe for adverse effects: nystagmus, skin rash, blurred vision, double vision, unusual bleeding, jaundice, drowsiness, gum hyperplasia, and hypotension.

PROCAINAMIDE (PRONESTYL)

Classification

Antidysrhythmic

Effects

Procainamide depresses cardiac automaticity, excitability, and conductivity.

Indications

Premature ventricular complexes, ventricular tachycardia, and atrial dysrhythmias

Contraindications

Second- or third-degree heart block, hypersensitivity to procaine, and myasthenia gravis

Administration

Dose

Administer 25 to 50 mg IV every 5 minutes until the dysrhythmia is abolished, hypotension occurs, QRS widens by 50%, or a total of 1 g has been given. Administer at a rate of

20 mg over 1 minute. IV infusion is 1 to 4 mg/min; a dose of 2 g/500 ml D_5W yields 4 mg/ml (see drug dosage chart, p. 582).

Precautions

Concurrent administration with cimetidine or amiodarone may result in increased procainamide blood levels. Use cautiously in patients with conduction delays, hepatic or renal insufficiency, and congestive heart failure. Patients with atrial fibrillation and atrial flutter may develop tachycardia.

Patient Management

- Monitor BP and ECG every 2 to 5 minutes during IV titration.
- Measure PR, QT, and QRS intervals.
- Assess for heart failure development.
- Evaluate CO.
- Observe for adverse effects: hypotension, agranulocytosis, neutropenia, joint pain, fever, chills, bradycardia, VT, VF, nausea and vomiting, anorexia, diarrhea, bitter taste, maculopapular rash, and lupus erythematosus-like syndrome.

PROPRANOLOL (INDERAL)

Classification

β-Adrenergic blocking agent, antidysrhythmic

Effects

Propranolol decreases cardiac oxygen demand, HR, BP, and myocardial contractility.

Indications

Angina, cardiac dysrhythmias, hypertension, migraine or vascular headache, and pheochromocytoma

Contraindications

Diabetes mellitus, asthma, chronic obstructive pulmonary disease (COPD), allergic rhinitis, sinus bradycardia, heart block greater than first degree, cardiogenic shock, and right ventricular failure secondary to pulmonary hypertension

Administration

Dose

Oral dose is 10 to 60 mg three or four times daily. IV dose is 1 to 3 mg; drug may be given undiluted at a rate of 1 mg/min. After 3 mg have been administered, wait 2 minutes and give 3 mg (1 mg at a time, if needed). Subsequent doses may not be given for at least 4 hours, regardless of route to be administered.

Precautions

Additive effects may result when the drug is administered with diltiazem or verapamil. Use with digoxin may result in excessive bradycardia with potential for heart block. Concurrent use with epinephrine may result in significant hypertension and excessive bradycardia. Propranolol may mask certain symptoms of developing hypoglycemia. Use cautiously in patients with congestive heart failure or respiratory disease and in patients taking other antihypertensive drugs. The dosage should be adjusted in elderly patients.

Patient Management

- Continuously monitor ECG with IV administration; if bradycardia develops, do not administer propranolol.
- Monitor BP and other hemodynamic parameters (e.g., CVP, PAWP) frequently during IV administration; if SBP <90, notify physician.
- Assess patient for development of congestive heart failure.
- Monitor blood glucose levels, especially in patients with diabetes.
- Do not abruptly withdraw medication.
- Observe for adverse effects: bradycardia, congestive heart failure, intensification of AV block, nausea and vomiting, abdominal cramps, hypoglycemia, and difficulty in breathing.

SODIUM BICARBONATE

Classification

Alkalizer, antacid, electrolyte replenisher

Effects

Sodium bicarbonate increases the plasma bicarbonate, buffers excess hydrogen ion concentration, and increases blood pH.

Indications

Metabolic acidosis and need to alkalinize the urine

Contraindications

Metabolic or respiratory acidosis, hypocalcemia, not recommended in cardiac arrest unless other interventions have been instituted and specific clinical circumstances exist (e.g., preexisting metabolic acidosis)

Administration

Dose

If used in cardiac arrest, the IV dose is 1 mEq/kg initially, then 0.5 mEq/kg in 10 minutes if indicated by arterial pH and Pco_2. IV infusion is 2 to 5 mEq/kg; drug may be administered over 4 to 8 hours in less acute acidosis.

Precautions

Rapid administration of sodium bicarbonate may result in severe alkalosis. Tetany or hyperirritability may occur with increased alkalosis.

Patient Management

- Assess patency of IV; extravasation may cause necrosis or sloughing of tissue.
- Obtain arterial blood pH, Po_2, and Pco_2 results before administering sodium bicarbonate.
- Flush line before and after administration of sodium bicarbonate.
- Observe for adverse effects: restlessness, tetany, hypokalemia, alkalosis, and hypernatremia.

VECURONIUM (NORCURON)

Classification

Neuromuscular blocking agent

Effects

Vecuronium produces skeletal muscle paralysis but has no effect on consciousness or pain.

Indications

Facilitation of endotracheal intubation, need for skeletal muscle relaxation during surgery or mechanical ventilation, and adjunct to general anesthesia

Contraindications

Hypersensitivity to bromides

Administration

Dose

Administer 0.08 to 0.10 mg/kg IV; the drug may be given over 1 minute. Maintenance doses of 0.010 to 0.015 mg/kg may be required to prolong the muscle relaxant effects. Maintenance doses may be repeated as necessary.

Precautions

Neuromuscular blockade may be potentiated by administration of aminoglycoside antibiotics. Patients must have a patent airway and be mechanically ventilated. Patients are conscious but unable to communicate.

Patient Management

- Ensure patent airway and controlled mechanical ventilation.

- Analyze ABGs for adequate oxygenation.
- Use adjunctive therapy for pain control and sedation.
- Have emergency respiratory support available in case of accidental extubation or lack of endotracheal tube patency.
- Observe for adverse effects: respiratory depression, apnea.

VERAPAMIL (CALAN, ISOPTIN)

Classification
Calcium channel-blocking agent

Effects
Verapamil decreases myocardial contractility, dilates coronary arteries and arterioles, decreases BP, and decreases HR.

Indications
Angina, atrial dysrhythmias, hypertension, and migraine headache prophylaxis

Contraindications
Advanced heart failure, heart block, cardiogenic shock, aortic stenosis, W-P-W syndrome, and severe hypotension

Administration
Dose

IV dose is 0.075 to 0.15 mg/kg given undiluted over 2 minutes. Repeat in 30 minutes if no response.

Precautions

Concurrent administration with β blockers, disopyramide, or verapamil may produce profound cardiac depressant effects. Use caution in patients with myocardial infarction, advanced heart block, heart failure, and atrial tachydysrhythmias.

Patient Management
- Monitor ECG continuously in patients receiving verapamil intravenously.
- Measure serial PR intervals and HR.
- Assess for development of congestive heart failure.
- Monitor BP and HR before administration; if SBP <90 or HR <50, notify the physician.
- Evaluate CO and efficacy of therapy (e.g., BP control, dysrhythmia control, angina control).
- Observe for adverse effects: transient hypotension, dizziness, heart failure, and constipation.

DRUG DOSAGE CHARTS

Dobutamine: 250 mg/250 ml*
CONCENTRATION: 1000 µg/ml

Weight (kg)	45	50	55	60	65	70	75	80	85	90	95	100
µg/kg/min	Flow rate (ml/hr)											
5	14	15	17	18	20	21	23	24	26	27	29	30
7.5	20	23	25	27	29	32	34	36	38	41	43	45
10	27	30	33	36	39	42	45	48	51	54	57	60
12.5	34	38	41	45	49	53	56	60	64	68	71	75
15	41	45	50	54	59	63	68	72	77	81	86	90
17.5	47	53	58	63	68	74	79	84	89	95	100	105
20	54	60	66	72	78	84	90	96	102	108	114	120

*Dobutamine—ACLS: Multiply patient weight in kg × 15 to determine the amount of dobutamine (mg) to be added to 250 ml of IV fluid. The rate set on the infusion pump = µg/kg/min.

Dopamine: 400 mg/500 ml*
CONCENTRATION: 800 μg/ml

Weight (kg)	45	50	55	60	65	70	75	80	85	90	95	100
μg/kg/min	Flow rate (ml/hr)											
1	3	4	4	5	5	6	6	6	6	7	7	8
2	7	8	8	9	10	11	11	12	13	14	14	15
3	10	11	12	14	15	16	17	18	19	20	21	23
5	17	19	21	23	24	26	28	30	32	34	36	38
7	24	26	29	32	34	37	39	42	45	47	50	53
10	34	38	41	45	49	53	56	60	64	68	71	75
13	44	49	54	59	63	68	73	78	83	88	93	98
15	51	56	62	68	73	79	84	90	96	101	107	113
20	68	75	83	90	98	105	113	120	128	135	143	150
25	84	94	103	113	122	131	141	150	159	167	178	188
30	101	113	124	135	146	158	169	180	191	203	214	225

*Dopamine—ACLS: Multiply patient weight in kg by 15 to determine the amount of dopamine (mg) to be added to 250 ml of IV fluid. The rate set on the infusion pump = μg/kg/min.

Lidocaine, Bretylium, Procainamide: 2 g/500 ml
CONCENTRATION: 4 mg/ml

Dose (mg/min)	Rate (ml/hr)
1	15
2	30
3	45
4	60

Isoproterenol, Epinephrine: 1 mg/250 ml
CONCENTRATION: 4 μg/ml

Dose (μg/min)	Rate (ml/hr)
1	15
2	30
3	45
4	60

Nitroglycerin: 50 mg/500 ml
CONCENTRATION: 100 μg/ml

Dose (μg/min)	Rate (ml/hr)
5	3
10	6
15	9
20	12
25	15
30	18
35	21
40	24
45	27
50	30

Nitroprusside: 50 mg/250 ml
CONCENTRATION: (200 µg/ml)

Weight (kg)	45	50	55	60	65	70	75	80	85	90	95	100
µg/kg/min	Flow rate (ml/hr)											
1	14	15	16	18	20	21	23	24	26	27	29	30
2	27	30	33	36	39	42	45	48	51	54	57	60
4	54	60	66	72	78	84	90	96	102	108	114	120
6	81	90	99	108	117	126	135	144	153	162	171	180
8	108	120	132	144	156	168	180	192	204	216	228	240

Norepinephrine: 4 mg/250 ml
CONCENTRATION: 16 µg/ml

Weight (kg)	45	50	55	60	65	70	75	80	85	90	95	100
µg/kg/min	Flow rate (ml/hr)											
0.1	17	19	21	23	24	26	28	30	32	34	36	38
0.2	34	38	41	45	49	53	56	60	64	68	71	75
0.3	51	56	62	68	73	79	84	90	96	101	107	113
0.4	68	75	82	90	98	105	112	120	128	135	142	150
0.5	85	94	103	113	122	132	141	150	160	169	178	188
0.6	101	113	124	135	146	158	168	180	191	203	214	225
0.7	118	132	144	158	171	184	197	210	223	237	249	263
0.8	135	150	165	180	195	210	225	240	255	270	285	300
0.9	152	169	185	203	220	237	253	270	287	304	320	338
1.0	169	188	206	225	244	263	281	300	319	338	356	375

Norepinephrine: 4 mg/250 ml
CONCENTRATION: 16 μg/ml

Dose (μg/min)	Rate (ml/hr)
1	4
2	8
3	12
4	16
5	20

CALCULATIONS

The critical care environment requires that nurses be able to calculate infusion drips to determine the amount of drug that is being administered. Medications are frequently administered as continuous IV infusions and titrated to achieve the desired response.

Drug Concentration in mg/ml or μg/ml

$$1 \text{ mg} = 1000 \text{ μg}$$

$$1 \text{ g} = 1000 \text{ mg}$$

To determine the amount of drug in one ml, divide the amount of drug in solution by the amount of solution (ml).

Example: 200 mg of drug in 500 ml
Determine mg/ml:

$$\frac{200 \text{ mg}}{500 \text{ ml}} = 0.4 \text{ mg/ml}$$

Determine μg/ml:
First change mg to μg:

$$200 \text{ mg} \times 1000 \text{ μg/mg} = 200,000 \text{ μg}$$

Then divide μg by ml of solution:

$$\frac{200,000 \text{ μg}}{500 \text{ ml}} = 400 \text{ μg/ml}$$

Calculating μg/kg/min

Drug dosages are often expressed in μg/kg/min. Three parameters must be known to determine the amount of medication the patient is receiving:
1. Patient weight in kg (1 kg = 2.2 lb)

2. Infusion rate (ml/hr)
3. Drug concentration

The drug concentration is multiplied by the infusion rate and divided by the patient weight $\times$ 60 min/hr:

$$\mu g/kg/min = \frac{\mu g/ml \times ml/hr}{kg \times 60 \ min/hr}$$

Example: A patient weighing 75 kg is receiving dobutamine at 20 ml/hr. There is 250 mg of dobutamine in 250 ml D_5W.
1. The patient weight is 75 kg
2. The infusion rate is 20 ml/hr
3. The drug concentration needs to be determined in $\mu g/ml$:

First change mg to μg:

$$250 \ mg = 250{,}000 \ \mu g$$

Next, divide the dosage by the amount of solution:

$$\frac{250{,}000 \ \mu g}{250 \ ml} = 1000 \ \mu g/ml$$

Since all three parameters are known, now determine $\mu g/kg/min$:

$$\mu g/kg/min = \frac{\mu g/ml \times ml/hr}{kg \times 60 \ min/hr}$$

$$= \frac{1000 \times 20}{75 \times 60}$$

$$= \frac{20{,}000}{4500}$$

$$= 4.44 \ \mu g/kg/min$$

Calculating the Amount of Fluid to Infuse (ml/hr)

Three parameters must be known to determine the infusion rate for the IV pump:
1. The patient weight in kg (1 kg = 2.2 lb)
2. The dose ordered by the physician in $\mu g/kg/min$
3. The drug concentration in $\mu g/min$

Multiply the dose ordered by the patient weight $\times$ 60 min. and divide by the drug concentration:

$$ml/hr = \frac{\mu g/kg/min \ ordered \times kg \times 60 \ min}{\mu g/ml}$$

Example: A patient weighing 70 kg is to receive dopamine at 6 μg/kg/min. There is 400 mg of dopamine in 250 ml D_5W.

1. The patient weight is 70 kg
2. The dose ordered is 6 μg/kg/min
3. The drug concentration needs to be determined in μg/ml:

First change mg to μg:

$$400 \text{ mg} \times 1000 \text{ μg/mg} = 400,000 \text{ μg}$$

Next, divide the dosage by the amount of solution:

$$\frac{400,000 \text{ μg}}{250 \text{ ml}} = 1600 \text{ μg/ml}$$

Since all three parameters are known, determine ml/hr:

$$\text{ml/hr} = \frac{\text{μg/kg/min ordered} \times \text{kg} \times 60 \text{ min}}{\text{μg/ml}}$$

$$= \frac{6 \times 70 \times 60}{1600}$$

$$= \frac{25,200}{1600}$$

$$= 16 \text{ ml/hr}$$

BIBLIOGRAPHY

1. American Hospital Formulary Service: Drug information 90, Bethesda, Md, 1990, American Society of Hospital Pharmacists.
2. Eisenberg MS, Cummins RO, and Ho MT: Code blue: cardiac arrest and resuscitation, Philadelphia, 1987, WB Saunders Co.
3. Gahart BL: Intravenous medications, ed 7, St Louis, 1990, Mosby–Year Book, Inc.
4. Govoni LE and Hayes JE: Drugs and nursing implications, ed 3, New York, 1987, Appleton-Century-Crofts.
5. Grauer K and Cavallaro D: ACLS certification preparation and a comprehensive review, ed 2, St Louis, 1987, The CV Mosby Co, pp 23-51.
6. Kinney MR, Packa DR, and Dunbar SB: AACN's clinical reference for critical-care nursing, New York, 1988, McGraw-Hill Book Co, pp 1640-1720.
7. Nursing 90: Drug handbook, Springhouse, Pa, 1990, Springhouse Corporation.
8. Textbook of advanced cardiac life support, Dallas, 1987, American Heart Association, pp 97-125.

CHAPTER 8

Nursing Care Modifications for the Child in the Adult ICU

To facilitate a smooth and optimal modification of the adult intensive care unit (ICU) for the care of the critically ill child, "PEDS," a framework categorizing the essential elements, will be presented.[34] The proposed framework not only encompasses physical assessment adaptations but also includes other required clinical skills as well as environmental and equipment needs and safety measures. The "PEDS" framework includes the following components:

Psychosocial and physical assessment skills
Environment and equipment
Delivery of fluids, blood components, and medications
Safety issues

PSYCHOSOCIAL ASSESSMENT SKILLS

The typical child admitted to the adult ICU is in the presence of an unfamiliar and threatening ICU environment. The timing and importance of psychosocial skills is heightened and cannot be overemphasized. The nurse does not have to meet the child and family to begin the assessment phase; data may be derived by knowing only the cognitive and physical age of the child. Proactive assessment and planning of the child's and family's psychosocial and developmental needs are prerequisites to therapeutically approaching and effectively communicating with the child and family. Important psychosocial skills include the following:

1. Integrating therapeutic communication skills and behavioral assessment techniques into the nursing care of the child and family
2. Recognizing developmental differences, common fears of children, and the methods of supporting their coping mechanisms
3. Identifying concepts regarding family-centered care and methods of incorporating these concepts into the care of the child and family

Communication

Therapeutic communication skills are essentially the same for the care of the pediatric patient and family as they are for the care of the adult patient and family. Components of therapeutic relationships such as establishing trust, effective listening, and interviewing skills are required. A common mistake in the care of the pediatric patient and family is to blur the boundaries between the professional and social roles and to assist in decisions and care for the child and family in a role other than that of professional nurse (e.g., mother, friend).[28]

Behavioral Assessment Techniques

As compared to the adult patient who may consciously screen most behaviors and the spoken word, the young child does not. The young child, subconsciously, communicates behaviorally through verbal, nonverbal (body language, behaviors), and abstract cues (play, drawing, story telling) (Table 8-1). Although the child's behavior is more natural in

TABLE 8-1 Components of a Pediatric Behavioral Assessment

Verbal
    What is the child saying?
    Does the child understand what is being said?
    Do significant others understand the child?
    Does the verbal communication seem appropriate to the child's
        age?
Affective or nonverbal
    Posture
    Gestures
    Movements or lack of movement
    Reactions or coping style
    Facial expression (general, eyes, mouth)
Abstract
    Play or exploration or lack thereof
    Artistic expression through drawings or choice of color
    Storytelling
    Third-person techniques
Is there congruency among the types of behaviors?

Modified from Rosenthal CH: Pediatric behavioral assessment for the adult ICU nurse, Trends 1990 Conference, Philadelphia, 1990, SEPA Chapter, AACN.

TABLE 8-2 Contrasting Affective Nonverbal Behavioral Cues of the Healthy and the Critically Ill Child

Healthy	Critically ill
Posture	
Moves, flexes	May be loose, flaccid
	May prefer fetal position or position of comfort
Gestures	
Turns to familiar voices	Responds slowly to familiar voices
Movement	
Moves purposefully	Exhibits minimal movement, lethargy
Moves toward new, pleasurable items	Shows increased movement, irritability (possibly indicating cardiopulmonary or neurological compromise, pain, or sleep deprivation)
Moves away from threatening items, people	
Reactions/coping style	
Responds to parents coming, leaving	Responds minimally to parent presence, absence
Responds to environment, equipment	Responds minimally to presence, absence of transitional objects
Cries and fights invasive procedures	Displays minimal defensive responses
Facial expressions	
Looks at faces, makes eye contact	May not track faces, objects
Changes facial expressions in response to interactions	Avoids eye contact or has minimal response to interactions
Responds negatively to face wash	Minimally changes facial expression during face wash
Blinks in response to stimuli	Has increase, decrease in blinking
Widens eyes with fear	Avoids eye contact
Is fascinated with mouth	Avoids, dislikes mouth stimulation
Holds mouth "ready for action"	Drools, has loose mouth musculature
	Displays intermittent, weak sucks on pacifier

the home or a familiar environment, the cues available to the clinician can suggest how a child is feeling or perceiving an event or the presence of an individual.

In general, the child's behavior is more activity oriented and normally more emotional than adult behaviors. These qualities of a child's behavior should be viewed as normal in average, healthy children and may be used as parameters to contrast the critically ill child (Table 8-2).

Developmental Considerations

Children can be categorized into groups according to physical and cognitive age and common developmental capabilities, tasks, and fears. However, all children share common fears despite their cognitive or physical age. These fears include loss of control, threat of separation, painful procedures, and communicated anxiety.[42]

When the child's physical and cognitive age are the same, the nurse can generally predict the child's expected social, self-, language, thought, and physical development capabilities. If the child's physical and cognitive ages are discrepant, the assessment phase is critical to identify the level at which the child is functioning and to incorporate age-appropriate expectations and interventions into the plan of care.

Psychosocial and developmental assessment is beyond the scope of this reference. However, Table 8-3 summarizes specific age-group characteristics with common parental considerations and nursing interventions.

Family-Centered Care

The components of family-centered care are listed in the box on p. 597, but the most essential concept regarding family-centered care is to value, recognize, and support family members in the care of their child. The family is the "constant" in the child's life and is ultimately responsible for responding to the child's emotional, social, developmental, physical, and health care needs.[38] Table 8-4 includes some suggested methods of incorporating the family in the care of a critically ill child.

Appropriate support and incorporation of parents in the health care delivery system have the potential of buffering the threats of the ICU environment on the child. Parents may assist or influence the child's cognitive appraisal or evaluation of the environment, personnel, and events. The child often uses the reactions of the parent as a barometer in interpreting events from the range of threatening to beneficial.

Text continued on p. 598.

TABLE 8-3 Age-Specific Characteristics, Parental Concerns, and Associated Nursing Interventions

Age group characteristics	Identified parental considerations	Nursing interventions
Infants (birth to 12 mo)		
Develops sense of trust versus mistrust	Needs bonding	Recognize identifiable changes in status.
Is not able to provide self-care	Needs encouragement to do "passive physiotherapy" (range of motion, stroking)	Adhere to strict handwashing and limitation of visitors.
Requires expert respiratory management	Needs encouragement to do mothering tasks: feeding, touching, holding	Converse in a quiet, unabrupt manner.
Requires strict adherence to infection control		Encourage parents to do nonnursing aspects of care.
Needs stimulation through sight and sound		Act as surrogate in absence of parents.
Requires active play with toys		Provide mobiles to look at and toys to hold.

Toddler (1 to 3 yr)

Has prime concern of sense of autonomy and fear of separation	Needs encouragement to provide comfort measures and communication	Encourage parental participation through examples.
Is a dependent person but has own mind and will	Needs encouragement in holding child at bedside	Offer explanations of thoughts child must feel but cannot express (e.g., pain, Mommy not here).
Begins speech, albeit limited in use and vocabulary	Needs encouragement to participate in nonnursing aspects of care	Avoid participating in painful procedures; instead, offer comfort afterward by holding, stroking.
Is concerned about body integrity		Use sedation and restraints only as necessary for safety.
Protects self from environment through avoidance, escape, and denial		Demonstrate procedures and/or illness by dressing up toys and dolls, using puppets (child life worker).
Requires active play		Hold, stroke, spend time with child (especially at bedtime) if parents absent.
Regards parents as most significant persons		
Becomes especially lonely at bedtime		

From Soupios M, Gallagher J, and Orlowski JP: Nursing aspects of pediatric intensive care in a general hospital, Pediatr Clin North Am 27(3):628-629, 1980.

Continued.

TABLE 8-3 Age-Specific Characteristics, Parental Concerns, and Associated Nursing Interventions— cont'd

Age group characteristics	Identified parental considerations	Nursing interventions
Preschool (3 to 6 yr)		
Wants to maintain acquired skills of doing for self; immobility is frightening	Encourage participation in offering explanations of procedures and events, based on established trust with child	Demonstrate and discuss procedures using understandable adult vocabulary.
Has vivid imagination and sense of initiative	Encourage reading, game playing, activities based on limits of child's illness	Allow child to participate in acquired tasks.
Is acquiring language through limited use of words	Needs encouragement to participate in nonnursing aspects of care	Permit questions; understand denial through withdrawal.
Imitates adult behavior with potential accompanying sense of guilt	Encourage holding, stroking, communication	Dress up toys for child to demonstrate fears (child life worker).
Develops concept of self and nonself by exploring environment and body and by questioning		Use restraints only as necessary for safety, sedation for pain and to allay fear of immobility.
Regards family members as significant persons		Encourage emotional ties with home by encouraging parents to bring in child's favorite toys, games, pictures of pets and siblings, tape recordings.

School age (6 to 12 yr)

Needs recognition of accomplishment; has strong sense of duty	Encourage reading, game playing, activities based on limits of child's illness
Experiences inferiority through unattainable achievement, possibly depleting sense of identity	Needs encouragement to provide comfort measures; can act as go-between in communication for explanations and reinforcement
Is capable of verbalizing pain	
May demand overabundance of love and attention from mother and regress	Encourage holding, stroking
Requires that limits be set to foster a sense of security	Needs encouragement to participate in nonnursing aspects of care
Regards school and related events as main focus of significant persons	Assists in reality orientation with news of school and home

Ascertain child's level of understanding to identify and correct misconceptions and offer explanations at appropriate level.

Permit child participation in progressive self-care.

Understand and offer comfort for parental separation.

Be aware of verbal, nonverbal indications for pain and sedate accordingly.

Use child life worker for play therapy.

From Soupios M, Gallagher J, and Orlowski JP: Nursing aspects of pediatric intensive care in a general hospital, Pediatr Clin North Am 27(3):628-629, 1980.

Continued.

TABLE 8-3 Age-Specific Characteristics, Parental Concerns, and Associated Nursing Interventions—cont'd

Age group characteristics	Identified parental considerations	Nursing interventions
Puberty adolescence (12 to 19 yr)		
Seeks identity, independence, and clarification of role in society after separation from family	Needs to understand potential for regression	Treat as adult based on level of psychological adjustment.
Is especially vulnerable to depersonalization and regression	Needs encouragement to promote awareness of disease and prognosis	Recognize and foster independence through participation in care.
May experience loss of body control, destroying sense of pride in own sexuality	Encourage treating adolescent as an adult	Set limits but encourage decision making in planning of care.
Attempts to identify own sense of belonging, self-esteem	Can bring news of peer group and home events	Permit personal belongings at bedside.
Is concerned with body image change through surgery or illness	Encourage touching and communication	Include peers in visiting policies, since relationships are moving away from family.
Regards peer group as significant persons		Use music as comfort measure.

From Soupios M, Gallagher J, and Orlowski JP: Nursing aspects of pediatric intensive care in a general hospital, Pediatr Clin North Am 27(3):628-629, 1980.

Elements of Family-Centered Care

Recognize that the family is the constant in a child's life and that the service systems and personnel within those systems fluctuate.

Facilitate parent/professional collaboration at all levels of health care.

Honor the racial, ethnic, cultural, and socioeconomic diversity of families.

Recognize family strength and individuality and respect different methods of coping.

Share with parents, on a continuing basis and in a supportive manner, complete and unbiased information.

Encourage and facilitate family to family support and networking.

Understand and incorporate the developmental needs of infants, children, and adolescents and their families into health care systems.

Implement comprehensive policies and programs that provide emotional and financial support to meet the needs of families.

Design accessible health care systems that are flexible, culturally competent, and responsive to family-identified needs.

From National Center for Family-Centered Care: Key elements of family-centered care, Bethesda, Md, Association for the Care of Children's Health, brochure.

TABLE 8-4 Support Offered by Child's Parents, Suggested Activities, and Nursing Interventions

Support offered	Parent activity	Nurse intervention
Emotional	Parent presence	Support open visitation. Support parent and child while parent takes breaks. Assess parents' ability to care for themselves. Assess the status of siblings.
Tangible	Assist in physical care: bathing, turning, stroking, feeding Assist in diversional activities: play, reading, music	Assist parent to revise role of a parent of a well child to the role of a parent of a sick child.
Informational	Provide facts and knowledge that will assist the child in coping Provide feedback that the child is secure and will recover	Keep parents informed regarding rationale of events and child's progress. Support parents in providing appropriate feedback to child.

The presence and participation of parents in the care of their critically ill child offers three kinds of support: emotional, tangible and informational.[39]

Children can also offer support to the child hospitalized in the ICU. However, the child visitor may not know what to expect on entering nor what is expected while visiting the friend or relative. Therefore staff should be prepared to "educate" the young visitor about policies such as handwashing. In addition, unusual sights and sounds may need to be explained. The first visit can be individually structured based on the age and needs of the visitor. Direction should be provided during the visit (e.g., hang a picture that the child drew, count bandaids, hold the patient's hand, give kisses) to reduce fear or anxiety in both the patient and visitor. However, the pediatric patient's need or desire to have visitors such as a peer should be assessed and respected.

TABLE 8-5 Pediatric Vital Signs

Age	Heart rate	Respirations	Systolic BP
Newborn	100-160	30-60	50-70
1-6 wk	100-160	30-60	70-95
6 mo	90-120	25-40	80-100
1 yr	90-120	20-30	80-100
3 yr	80-120	20-30	80-110
6 yr	70-110	18-25	80-110
10 yr	60-90	15-20	90-120
14 yr	60-90	15-20	90-130

Modified from Seidel JS and Henderson DP: Prehospital care of pediatric emergencies, Los Angeles Pediatric Society, California Chapter 2, Los Angeles, 1987, American Academy of Pediatrics.

PHYSICAL ASSESSMENT SKILLS

In contrast to most adult patients, it is difficult to rationalize to a child the need for being in the ICU or the need for invasive or noninvasive interventions. Approaching the child in a therapeutic and age-appropriate manner will not only facilitate the assessment process but also lessen the threatening nature of the experience. The reader is encouraged to incorporate the essential psychosocial assessment skills previously discussed into the physical assessment process. Important physical assessment skills include the following:
1. Interpreting vital signs based on age-appropriate norms as well as the child's present clinical condition
2. Modifying assessment techniques based on the anatomical and physiological differences and similarities of the child and adult
3. Recognizing the decompensating child using a quick examination approach

Interpreting Vital Signs

Although assessment of the child requires a knowledge base of normal physiological parameters (Table 8-5), it is imperative to note the importance of observing the child before stimulation. Most physiological parameters such as respiration, heart rate, and blood pressure will vary with the presence of a foreign or threatening stranger. Baseline parameters are the most useful and are obtained at rest or sleep if possible. As in the adult, expect that pain, fear, fever, and activity will normally increase the child's vital signs.

It is important to compare the child's vital signs to no. only the age-appropriate "norms," but also to the present clinical condition.[16] In other words, normal vital signs may not be appropriate to the sick child. For example, the child who is ill should compensate by increasing heart rate, respiratory rate, and temperature in the presence of pneumonia. An inability to increase heart rate or a slowing in heart rate may not be congruent with compensation but may be a sign of noncompensation, especially in the face of a worsening clinical picture. However, trends in vital signs rather than single parameters are usually more reflective of the child's clinical course.

Anatomical and Physiological Differences in Children

An understanding of the anatomical and physiological differences in children is necessary to make appropriate modifications in assessment techniques and to interpret physical findings. The following are critical anatomical and physiological differences in the adult and child:

1. Neurological differences
   - Neurological functioning: At birth, the infant functions at a subcortical level composed primarily of brainstem functioning and spinal cord reflexes. Cortical development is 75% complete by 2 years of age.
   - Cranium: At birth, the child's cranial sutures are not completely fused. Complete fusion of the cranium is complete at 18 to 24 months of age, with posterior fontanel closing by 3 months and anterior fontanel closing at 9 to 18 months of age.
   - Rate of brain growth: Brain growth is rapid during the first few years of life. The newborn's brain is 25% of mature adult weight at birth, and at 2½ years, it has reached 75% of mature adult weight.
   - Reflexes: In addition to intact protective reflexes, several newborn reflexes are present. Moro reflex is present until 6 months of age. Rooting reflex is present until 4 months of age. Grasp reflex is present until 3 months of age. Babinski reflex is present until 9 to 12 months of age or at the time of walking.
   - Motor ability: Motor ability develops following the loss of newborn reflexes and the acquisition of voluntary motor skills.
   - Meningeal irritation: In addition to nuchal rigidity and Kernig's and Brudinski's signs, the young child may display paradoxical irritability, which is height-

ened irritability in response to normally soothing interventions, such as cradling.

- Response to injury: In response to trauma, the child has a lower incidence of mass lesions[4] and a higher incidence of intracranial hypertension[25] and is more likely to develop "malignant brain edema."[3]

2. Cardiovascular differences

- Heart rate: The infant and young child have a higher heart rate than the adult. The higher heart rate assists the child in meeting the need for a higher cardiac output despite a smaller stroke volume. As in the adult, coronary artery filling time occurs during diastole; in the young child, diastolic filling time is shorter.
- Skin (end-organ perfusion): The child's skin is thinner than that of the adult's; therefore it will display color changes rapidly and easily. Skin color, texture, and temperature is of great significance during assessment of the child.
- Peripheral perfusion: The presence and quality of peripheral pulses in the adult and young child are the same. Capillary refill is normally recorded in seconds rather than as brisk, normal, or slow. Normal capillary refill time in children is less than 2 seconds.
- Circulatory blood volume: The child has an estimated blood volume that varies with age. Despite a higher ml/kg of body weight volume, the overall total circulating volume is small. A small amount of blood loss can be significant in the child.
- Blood pressure: The child can compensate for up to a 25% blood loss before the systolic blood pressure falls.

3. Respiratory differences

- Basal metabolic rate: The newborn's metabolic rate is almost twice that of the adult's in relation to body size. This increased metabolic rate leads to a higher minute volume secondary to an increased respiratory rate and increased oxygen consumption.
- Airway patency: Due to the infant's large head (in proportion to body size); weak, underdeveloped neck muscles; and lack of cartilagenous support to the airway, the airway is easily compressible and obstructed by head and neck position alone. The narrowest part of the child's airway (until approximately 8 years of age) is at the level of the cricoid ring as opposed to the glottic opening in the adult.

- Airway size: The infant and young child's airways are smaller in diameter and in length and thus require smaller artificial airways. Airway compromise can be caused by the slightest amount of inflammation or edema and mucous plugs.
- Chest characteristics: The young child has a very thin, compliant chest wall that rises and falls easily with adequate ventilatory efforts. Due to the thin chest wall, breath sounds can be heard louder than breath sounds in the adult.
- Respiratory muscles: Both the accessory muscles of the neck and back and the intercostal muscles are poorly developed in the young child. As in the adult, the major muscle of respiration is the diaphragm. However, the child is more diaphragm dependent due to the weak accessory and intercostal muscles.
4. Gastrointestinal differences
   - Contour of abdomen: The abdomen of an infant and young child is normally soft and protuberant and becomes flat at approximately the time of adolescence.
   - Stomach capacity: Stomach capacities vary with the age of the child. A newborn's stomach capacity is 90 ml, a 1 month old's is 150 ml, a 12 month old's is 360 ml, and an adult's is 2000-3000 ml.
   - Stomach emptying time: The infant and young child have a gastric emptying time of approximately 2½ to 3 hours, which lengthens to 3-6 hours in the older child. The infant has an immature cardiac sphincter and may experience reverse peristalsis, leading to regurgitation.
   - Liver border: The position of the liver border beyond the costal margin varies with age. It is normally up to 3 cm below the costal margin in the newborn, 2 cm below the costal margin in a 1 year old, and 1 cm below the costal margin in a 4 to 5 year old.
   - Bowel function: Bowel function remains involuntary until 14 to 18 months of age, at which time myelination of the spinal cord is complete.
   - Nutritional needs: The child has larger obligate energy needs because the major metabolic organs make up a larger percentage of body weight. The child also has lower macronutrient stores (proteins, fats, and carbohydrates). The lack of stores and high metabolic rate

place the child at risk for protein calorie malnutrition. The child requires more calories per kilogram of body weight to meet these larger requirements.

5. Renal differences
   - Urine output: The infant has less ability to concentrate urine and therefore has a normal urine output of 2 ml/kg/hr. For the child and adolescent, normal urine output is 1 ml/kg/hr and 0.5 ml/kg/hr, respectively.
   - Body surface area (BSA): The infant and young child have a larger BSA in relation to body weight than the adult. Maintenance fluid requirements are precisely determined according to body weight or BSA.
   - Fluid volume status: The child's extracellular fluid compartment consists of a higher percentage of body fluids than adult's. In addition, the child has a higher insensible water loss because of the higher basal metabolic rate, higher respiratory rate, and larger BSA.

6. Endocrine differences
   - Glucose metabolism: Glucose production is increased in the neonate and the child up to 6 years of age (4-8 mg/kg/min), then slowly falls to adult levels (2 mg/kg/min).
     The infant and young child have smaller glycogen stores and an increased glucose demand because of the larger brain-to-body-size ratio.

7. Immunological differences
   - Inflammatory response: The newborn has fewer stored neutrophils and is less able to repeatedly replenish WBCs in the presence of overwhelming infection. Complement levels do not reach adult levels until 24 months of age, thus affecting chemotactic activity of phagocytes and opsonization of bacteria.
   - Humoral immunity: The newborn has a limited ability to differentiate B lymphocytes to mature plasma cells. Although the fetus and newborn synthesize small amounts of immunoglobulin, most is received via placental transfer from the maternal host.
     Physiological hypogammaglobulinemia occurs at approximately 4 to 5 months of age.
   - Cell-mediated immunity: Although the infant/child has all the components to perform cellular immunity, the opportunity to refine abilities to respond to bacteria, viruses, and fungi is nonexistent.

TABLE 8-6 Adult and Infant Glasgow Coma Scales*

| | Adult | | Infant |
Activity	Best response	Points	Best response
Eye opening	Spontaneous	4	Spontaneous
	To verbal stimuli	3	To speech
	To pain	2	To pain
	No response to pain	1	No response to pain
Motor	Follows commands	6	Normal spontaneous movements
	Localizes pain	5	Localizes pain
	Withdrawal in response to pain	4	Withdrawal in response to pain
	Flexion in response to pain	3	Flexion in response to pain
	Extension in response to pain	2	Extension in response to pain
	No response to pain	1	No response to pain
Verbal	Oriented	5	Coos, babbles
	Confused	4	Irritable crying
	Inappropriate words	3	Cries to pain
	Incomprehensible sounds	2	Moans to pain
	No verbal response	1	No verbal response

*Possible points of 3-15; score of <8 = coma.

Pediatric Head-to-Toe Assessment

Because of anatomical and physiological differences, assessment techniques must be modified. Although the following assessment is described in a systematic head-to-toe format, assessing the pediatric critically ill patient requires flexibility. As with the adult patient, the child's physical and psychological condition may dictate the priority and sequence in which the data are collected.

Neurological

LEVEL OF CONSCIOUSNESS

Level of consciousness is determined by assessing the state of arousal and orientation of the infant/child. (See Tables 8-1 and 8-2 to assess a child's behavior and interaction with the environment.)

Wakefulness or arousability is assessed in the same manner as in the adult and may vary from spontaneous arousability

TABLE 8-7 Average Head Circumference

Age	Mean (cm)	Standard deviation (cm)
Birth	35	1.2
1 mo	37.6	1.2
2 mo	39.7	1.2
3 mo	40.4	1.2
6 mo	43.4	1.1
9 mo	45	1.2
12 mo	46.5	1.2
18 mo	48.4	1.2
2 yr	49	1.2
3 yr	50	1.2
4 yr	50.5	1.2
5 yr	50.8	1.4
6 yr	51.2	1.4
7 yr	51.6	1.4
8 yr	52	1.5

Modified from Lowrey GH: Growth and development of children, Chicago, 1986, Year Book Medical Publishers.

to no response to noxious stimuli. In fact, fear alone may be a noxious stimulus that arouses the child. If it is necessary to assess the child's response to pain, the intensity of the sternal pressure must be modified to avoid injury to the skin or chest wall. Orbital and nipple pressure is not recommended in the pediatric patient. If examining a young child's eyes, care should be taken to avoid injury to the thin and fragile eyelids.

Orientation can be assessed by using the age-appropriate Glasgow Coma Scale. The adult and infant Glasgow Coma Scale are presented for comparison in Table 8-6.

HEAD CIRCUMFERENCE

Because brain growth is rapid during the first few years of life, measurement of head circumference is important in the child up to 2 years of age. The circumference of the child's head is related to intracranial volume and estimates the rate of brain growth. A measuring tape is held securely over the child's occipital protuberance and the forehead, but it should not cover the ears. The measurement is recorded in centimeters. Table 8-7 reviews the average head circumference of children, although abnormal trends found in sequential measurements are more significant than an isolated measurement.

FONTANELS

Fontanels provide a useful parameter to assess hydration or potential increased intracranial pressure. Bulging fontanels may be seen with increased intracranial pressure or with fluid overload. Sunken fontanels may be seen with fluid deficit.

NEWBORN REFLEXES

The newborn reflexes most commonly assessed are the Moro, rooting, grasp, and Babinski reflexes. The *Moro* reflex is tested by producing a loud noise such as hand clapping near the infant. The response should be abduction of the arm and shoulder; extension of the arm at the elbow; extension of the fingers, with a C formed at the thumb and the index finger; and later, adduction of the arm at the shoulder. In other words, in a normal response the infant moves the upper extremities out and then curls in as if to try and provide self-comfort.

The *rooting* reflex is tested by stroking one side of the infant's cheek. The normal response is for the infant to turn toward the stimulus and suck. The *grasp* reflex is tested by pressing a finger into the infant's palm. The normal response is for the infant to grasp the examiner's fingers. The *Babinski* reflex is tested by stroking the lateral aspect of the sole of the feet. The normal response in the infant is a fanning of the toes and dorsiflexion of the big toe.

MOTOR RESPONSE

Motor response can be assessed by evaluating muscle strength and tone as well as by using the Glasgow Coma Scale. If the infant/child moves the extremities spontaneously, movements should be of equal strength and tone. Although the expected findings are the same in the adult and child, the methods of assessment may be different. The infant/child may require a creative stimulus such as play as an encouragement to move.

Cardiovascular

HEART RATE

Heart rate (see Table 8-5 for normal ranges), although an important parameter, should not be assessed in isolation. *Tachycardia* is a nonspecific response to a variety of entities such as anxiety, fever, shock, and hypoxemia. Although the child is predisposed to bradycardia, tolerance is poor. Bradycardia often produces significant changes in perfusion, since cardiac output is heart rate dependent. *Bradycardia* is most often caused by hypoxemia but any vagal stimuli, such as suctioning, nasogastric (NG) tube insertion, and defecation, may precipitate an event.

PERIPHERAL PERFUSION

Decreased perfusion to the skin is an early and reliable sign of shock. Before assessing the skin, the examiner should note the room temperature, since some findings may be a normal response to the environment (such as mottling in a drafty operating room). Mottling in a bundled infant or in a warm environment is reason for further investigation. Assess skin temperature as well as the line of demarcation between extremity coolness and body warmth. Coolness or the progression of coolness toward the trunk may be a sign of diminishing perfusion.

Skin and mucous membrane color may vary from pink, dusky, pale, to ashen grey. Cyanosis can be peripheral or central. Peripheral cyanosis is normal in newborns but an abnormal finding in young children, as in the adult. Central cyanosis (circumoral) is always an abnormal finding. Cyanosis is a sign of poor perfusion, but it is a late and unreliable indicator.

PULSES

Carotid, brachial, radial, femoral, dorsalis pedis, and posterior tibial pulses are readily palpable in healthy infants and children. Note differences between peripheral and central (carotid, femoral) pulses. Peripheral pulses may be decreased because of hypothermia or may be an early sign of decreased perfusion. A loss of central pulses is a late sign of diminished perfusion. A capillary refill time longer than 2 seconds is also an early sign of decreased perfusion.

BLOOD PRESSURE

Normal ranges for blood pressure can be found in Table 8-5. Blood pressure should not be used as the sole indicator of systemic perfusion because a child's blood pressure may be within the normal range even though a state of diminished perfusion exists (e.g., weak pulses, cool skin, capillary refill >2 seconds). Pulse pressure, an index of stroke volume, may be used to assess the adequacy of systemic perfusion. A decrease in pulse pressure or an increase in diastolic pressure may be detected before a drop in systolic blood pressure. However, clinical manifestations of decreased perfusion should alert the clinician of cardiovascular compromise despite the presence of a "normal" blood pressure. Hypotension is a late sign and may signal impending cardiac arrest. Hypertension is rare in the critically ill child unless renal disease is present.

Pulmonary

RESPIRATORY RATE

The higher basal metabolic rate in the child accounts for a higher respiratory rate (see normal ranges in Table 8-5). The infant and child will increase their respiratory rates further to compensate for increased oxygen demand. Tachypnea is often the first sign of respiratory distress. A slow respiratory rate in a sick child often indicates impending respiratory arrest. Associated conditions such as fever and seizure activity, which further increase the metabolic rate, will also increase oxygen requirements. These conditions can cause rapid deterioration in an already compromised child.

AIRWAY

The infant is an obligate nose breather until 6 months of age, thus obstruction of nasal passages can produce significant airway compromise and respiratory distress. Secretions, edema, inflammation, and poorly taped NG tubes or occluded nasal cannulas can cause obstructed nasal passages in the infant.

The child's airway is small and can easily become obstructed. Whether the child is breathing spontaneously or has an artificial airway in place, it is critical to check airway patency. Avoid overextending or overflexing the neck because the airways are easily collapsible. Note the position in which the child is maintaining airway patency. The child who needs to sit up and forward to breathe is experiencing significant airway obstruction.

In positioning the decompensating child for optimal airway patency, place a small roll horizontally behind the child's shoulders. This will place the head and neck in a neutral position. An ideal-sized roll for the infant or young child is one or two adult pillow cases rolled up together.

The infant's airway is short—3.6 to 6 cm as compared to the adult's airway length of 11 cm.[50] If intubated, the child's head should remain in the neutral, midline position because repositioning the child's head can cause the endotracheal tube (ETT) to move. An ETT that is repositioned based on a chest radiograph taken while the child's head was not aligned properly can result in extubation or single lung ventilation.

THORAX

The thin, compliant chest wall normally allows for easy assessment of air entry. Air entry is assessed by observing the rise and fall of the child's chest. Unequal chest movement may indicate the development of a pneumothorax or atelectasis. Unequal chest movement may also indicate ETT obstruction or ETT displacement into the right mainstem bronchus.

Due to the child's flexible rib cage, which offers little stability to the chest wall, suprasternal, sternal, intercostal, and subcostal retractions may be seen in the child in respiratory distress. Assess for the presence and location of retractions.

The accessory muscles in the infant and young child are poorly developed and cannot be relied on for respiratory effort. The infant and the child use the abdomen to assist with breathing. This gives the appearance of "seesaw" breathing, a paradoxical movement of the chest and abdomen. Seesaw breathing becomes more exaggerated with respiratory distress or airway obstruction.

BREATH SOUNDS

Obstructed airways often produce sounds that are easily heard during assessment. Listen for expiratory grunting, inspiratory and expiratory stridor, and wheezing. Expiratory grunting is a sound produced in an attempt to increase physiological positive end-expiratory pressure (PEEP) to prevent small airways and alveoli from collapsing. As in the adult, stridor is usually heard with upper airway obstruction; wheezing is consistent with lower airway obstruction.

The infant and child's thin chest wall may allow the examiner to hear breath sounds over an area of pathology when sounds are actually being referred from another area of the lung. Listen for changes in the breath sounds as well as for their presence or absence.

Gastrointestinal

ABDOMEN

Although a protuberant abdomen is normal in the infant and young child, it is important to note if the abdomen is hard, firm, distended, or tender. Measure the abdominal girth at least every shift or more often if there is concern about abdominal distention. The measuring tape should be placed right above the umbilicus.

STOMACH

The stomach capacity of the infant and child is smaller than that of the adult (see p. 602), so caution must be taken when formulas or other fluids are instilled into the stomach. Bolus feedings should be of an appropriate amount, consistent with the child's stomach capacity. Fluids used with diagnostic tests, such as barium swallows, should also be of an appropriate amount.

Slower gastric emptying times must be taken into consideration with other nursing care activities. Allow an appropriate amount of time for absorption of formula before checking residuals. Residuals of greater than half of the child's hourly feeding may necessitate further evaluation. If at all possible, residuals should be re-fed to the child. When the child is receiving chest physiotherapy, allow enough time or check the gastric contents before starting the procedure so that problems with reflux and aspiration will be minimized.

LIVER BORDER

Determining the location of liver border should be part of the initial assessment and will establish a baseline for later comparison. The liver is normally not protected under the costal margin in the young child; thus when palpating the liver edge, it is wise to start at the iliac crest and move up until the liver border can be palpated.

If the liver extends 3 centimeters beyond the right costal margin, it may be an early sign of congestive heart failure, tumor, or hepatitis. Unlike adults, children sequester fluids in their liver during fluid overload, and liver enlargement may not be indicative of heart failure.

NUTRITION

The child has a high nutritional demand; therefore a thorough nutritional assessment is imperative. Table 8-8 lists the estimated nutrient needs per kilogram of body weight.

As in the adult, many parameters can be used to assess nutritional status in the child. Weight is a critical parameter. The child should be weighed daily at the same time and with the same scale. An unexplained weight loss of greater than 5% of the admission weight places the child nutritionally at risk. A weight loss of greater than 10% is associated with increased morbidity. A weight loss of greater than 30% is associated with increased mortality.[29]

TABLE 8-8 Recommended Dietary Allowances For Calories and Protein Based on Median Heights and Weights

Age	Wt (kg)	Ht (cm)	Kcal/kg	Kcal/day	Protein (g/kg)	Protein (g/day)
<6 mo	6	60	108	650	2.2	13
6-12 mo	9	71	98	850	1.6	14
1-3 yr	13	90	102	1300	1.2	16
4-6 yr	20	112	90	1800	1.1	24
7-10 yr	28	132	70	2000	1.0	28
11-14 yr (M)	45	157	55	2500	1.0	45
11-14 yr (F)	46	157	47	2200	0.8	44
15-18 yr (M)	66	176	45	3000	0.9	59
15-18 yr (F)	55	163	40	2200	0.8	44

M, Male; *F*, female.
Modified from Recommended dietary allowances, Washington, DC, 1989, National Academy Press.

Renal

URINE

Assessment of urine includes the amount, color, clarity, odor, specific gravity, pH and the presence of fluid, ketones, glucose, protein, and bilirubin. Because the infant has less ability to concentrate urine, a low specific gravity does not necessarily mean that the infant is adequately hydrated.

HYDRATION

The child's kidneys are not as mature as the adult's and may not process fluid as efficiently. This makes the child less able to handle sudden large amounts of fluid and more prone to fluid overload.

A higher percentage of total body water and higher insensible water loss predisposes the child to dehydration. Carefully measure fluid intake and output (I & O), including diapers and dressings. Sudden weight loss or gain indicates fluid imbalance (Table 8-9). Signs of dehydration include dry mucous membranes, decreased urine output, increased urine concentration, sunken fontanels and eyes, and poor skin turgor. Circulatory decompensation accompanies severe dehydration. Fluid overload is evidenced by bulging fontanels, taut skin, edema (usually periorbital and sacral), hepatomegaly, and other signs of congestive heart failure.

TABLE 8-9 Significant Weight Gain or Loss

Weight gain related to fluid overload	Weight loss related to dehydration
Infants	
>50 g/24 hr	Mild: 5% of body weight
	Moderate: 10% of body weight
	Severe: 15% of body weight
Children	
>200 g/24 hr	Mild: 3% of body weight
	Moderate: 6% of body weight
	Severe: 9% of body weight
Adolescents	
>500 g/24 hr	Mild: 3% of body weight
	Moderate: 6% of body weight
	Severe: 9% of body weight

Endocrine

GLUCOSE METABOLISM

The infant/young child's low glycogen stores and high glucose demand in average circumstances place the child at significant risk for hypoglycemia during states of psychological and physiological stress or prolonged fasting. Assessment of the length of the child's status without oral intake as well as quality and quantity of infusing intravenous (IV) fluids is paramount in assessing the child's risk for hypoglycemia. The presence of signs and symptoms of hypoglycemia should be noted, and serum glucose levels should be checked at regular intervals (box).

Immunological

INFECTION

Like the adult patient in the ICU, the pediatric patient is subjected to many situational aspects that carry the risk for infection. Admitting diagnosis, medical and nursing interventions, nutritional status, and stress may lead to an increased risk of infection. In addition, there are immunological, anatomical, and physiological differences that place the young child at risk. The infant experiencing an overwhelming infection may present without the normal systemic signs, specifically fever and leukocytosis. Therefore it is extremely important for the nurse to be astute to the subtle signs of infection in the infant, such as changes in feeding behaviors, altered glucose metabolism, and altered temperature regulation (hypothermia).

Signs and Symptoms of Hypoglycemia

Neonate	Infant/child
Pallor	Pallor, sweating
Tremors, jitteriness	Increased heart rate
Tachypnea	Nausea, vomiting
Feeding difficulties	Hunger, abdominal pain
Hypotonia	Irritability
Abnormal cry	Headache, visual disturbances
Apnea, cyanosis	
Convulsions	Mental confusion
Coma	Convulsions, coma

Until the child's humoral and cellular immunity matures, the child is susceptible to numerous infections. The child is particularly susceptible to infections caused by viruses, *Candida* species, and acute inflammatory bacteria during the period of physiological hypogammaglobulinemia.

Recognizing the Decompensating Child

A quick and systematic examination that is congruent with the American Heart Association's pediatric advanced life support standards can be used to rapidly recognize a child in distress. Using this approach to conduct ongoing assessments of the critically ill child may prevent subtle clues of deterioration from being overlooked. Table 8-10 outlines extremes in critical physiological functioning that can be used to determine the degree of decompensation and the child's response to therapy.

ENVIRONMENT

Psychosocial Environment

The components of psychosocial assessment skills are vital, but the atmosphere in which these skills are practiced is equally important. The psychosocial atmosphere of the unit should provide minimal opportunity for patients to experience communicated anxiety and reality distortion. There should also be an ongoing appreciation of the impact that the mixed population of patients has on the overall unit atmosphere.

Communicated anxiety

The tone and manner in which the clinician approaches the bedside of a pediatric patient and family is extremely important. Whether the nurse is an experienced pediatric clinician or an experienced adult clinician, approaching the bedside with the utmost confidence goes a long way in reinforcing the child's and family's confidence in the care that they will receive.

Communicated anxiety relates to the child's uneasy feelings in response to not only the parent's anxiety but also the anxiety of the health care team members in the child's immediate environment. Interventions to relieve the anxiety of parents and fellow health team members will have a direct impact on the child's well-being. Interventions may include but are not limited to assisting parents/staff in anticipating the child's responses to therapy and illness and guiding parents/staff in therapeutic communication techniques.

TABLE 8-10 Quick Examination of a Healthy Versus Decompensating Child

Assessment	Healthy child	Decompensating child
Airway		
Patency	Requires no interventions; child verbalizes and is able to swallow, cough, gag	Child self-positions; requires interventions such as head positioning, suctioning, adjunct airways
Breathing		
Respiratory rate	Is within age-appropriate limits	Is tachypneic or bradypneic compared to age-appropriate limits and condition
Chest movement (presence)	Chest rises and falls equally and simultaneously with abdomen with each breath	Has minimal or no chest movement with respiratory effort
Chest movement (quality)	Has silent and effortless respirations	Shows evidence of labored respirations with retractions
		Has asynchronous movement (seesaw) between chest and abdomen with respiratory efforts
Air movement (presence)	Air exchange is heard bilaterally in all lobes	Despite movement of the chest, minimal or no air exchange is noted on auscultation
Air movement (quality)	Breath sounds are normal intensity and duration per auscultation location	Has nasal flaring, grunting, stridor, or wheezing

Continued.

TABLE 8-10 Quick Examination of a Healthy Versus Decompensating Child—cont'd

Assessment	Healthy child	Decompensating child
Circulation		
Heart rate (presence)	Apical beat is present and within age-appropriate limit	Has absent heart rate, has bradycardia or tachycardia as compared to age-appropriate limits and clinical condition
Heart rate (quality)	Heart rate is regular with normal sinus rhythm	Has irregular, slow, or very rapid heart rate; common dysrhythmias include supraventricular tachycardia, bradyarrhythmias, and asystole
Skin	Has warm, pink extremities with capillary refill ≤2 seconds; peripheral pulses are present bilaterally with normal intensity	Has pallor, cyanotic or mottled skin color; has cool to cold extremities; capillary refill time is ≥2 seconds; peripheral pulses are weak, absent; central pulses are weak
Cerebral perfusion	Is alert to surroundings, recognizes parents or significant others, is responsive to fear and pain, has normal muscle tone	Is irritable, lethargic, obtunded, or comatose; has minimal or no reaction to pain; has loose muscle tone (floppy)
Blood pressure	Has blood pressure within age-appropriate limits	Shows fall in blood pressure from age-appropriate limits

Reality distortion

Most patients, including the young child, are observant to the sights and sounds of the unit, even during an acute illness. All ICU patients may distort reality, especially when experiencing fear, pain, medication administration, and cognitive immaturity. Minimize the instances that the patient may be exposed to procedures or to the procedures experienced by other patients. Despite minimal exposure, health team members should be prepared for the child to question the condition or status of other patients. This should be viewed as a window of opportunity to communicate effectively and honestly with the child.

Mixed population of patients

The presence of pediatric patients in the adult ICU influences adult patients and their families in addition to fellow health team members. It is a societal belief that children should not die and that parents should not outlive their offspring. Adult patients and staff are exposed to the sights and sounds of the critically ill child and may express concern and sadness for the child and family. At times the adult patient and significant other, including terminally ill patients, may experience a wide variety of emotions (such as guilt, anger, and nontherapeutic empathy) when exposed to the death or dying of a child.

Physical Environment

Planning a designated area

A specific area in the adult ICU should be designated and designed for the care of the child and family. The optimal solution is the design of glass-enclosed isolation rooms to physically separate the two populations of patients and to minimize the noise that is inherent in the care of children. Many adult ICUs allot a certain number of patient bedspaces in a specified location in the unit.

If a permanent, designated space in the unit is not possible, modification of an individual bedspace may include but is not limited to the addition of a pediatric supply cart, limitation of extraneous bedside equipment, and placement of the child in a bedspace of the unit that facilitates a balance between privacy and adequate observation by nursing staff.

Family support areas

Family support areas should be in close proximity to the unit. A waiting room, nutritional area, private consultation area, and sleeping accommodations are essential in meeting

Pediatric Supply Cart Contents

Drawer #1: intravenous therapy

20 ga 1″ Quick cath
22 ga 1″ Quick cath
24 ga ¾ ″ Quick cath
24 ga ¾ ″ Angiocath
21 ga Butterfly
23 ga Butterfly
25 ga Butterfly
Extension set with T connector
Syringes (1, 3, and 6 ml)
Suture kits
Infant/child soft restraints
Snoopy bandages
Infant/child arm boards
Tongue blades
5/16″ and ½ ″ penrose drains (infant/child tourniquets)
Safety pins

Drawer #2: respiratory

Oxisensors (pediatric, infant)
Oral airways (4-5-6-7 mm)
Nasopharyngeal airways
Tracheostomy tubes (pediatric 00, 0, 1, 2, 3)
Pediatric or small Yankaeur
Pediatric chest percussor (small, medium)
Junior or pediatric spirometer

Drawer #3: cardiovascular

Small electrodes
BP cuffs (newborn, child, young adult)
Pediatric stethoscope
Sets of pediatric blood tubes
Sterile mosquito clamps
Sterile needle drivers (small)

Drawer #4: GI/GU

Nasogastric tubes (5 feeding tube, 8, 10, 12 Fr)
Measuring tape
Bottle
Nipple
Pacifier
Urine bags
Foley catheters (8, 10, 12 Fr)

Pediatric Supply Cart Contents—cont'd

Drawer #5

Pediatric Thoraklex or Pleurevac
Trocar catheters (10, 12, 14, 16)
Pediatric trach tray
Pediatric LP tray
Buretrols
Radiation shield
Baby blanket, medium-sized diapers

---

basic physical needs of families as they support their child through the ICU experience. If the physical environment is not conducive to supporting parents or significant others, it is extremely important that these needs be recognized and addressed daily with a professional resource person.

Pediatric supply cart

In the adult-pediatric ICU, it is difficult to predict the number and acuity of the patient census; therefore a mechanism to facilitate bedside equipment access and supply is important. The development of a pediatric supply cart consolidates the required equipment and allows routine intensive care delivery to the infant, child, and adolescent within an adult-oriented unit. Just as the adult equipment is maintained at the bedside ready for use, it is helpful to organize the same supplies in the appropriate sizes for pediatric use in a cart that may be rolled to any bedside depending on the circumstances of a pediatric admission. Some suggested items to include on the pediatric supply cart are listed in the box.

EQUIPMENT

Physical Assessment Supplies

Supplies to perform a physical assessment on a pediatric patient are essentially the same as those for an adult patient. Equipment is selected considering the exact size of the patient, a factor that varies with age. Basic equipment for physical assessment includes a scale, stethoscope, blood pressure cuff, thermometer, measuring tape, and an otoscope with various size speculums.

Weighing devices

Because many therapies for the child, such as drug and fluids delivery, are weight specific, obtaining an accurate weight on

TABLE 8-11 Commonly Available Blood Pressures Cuffs

Cuff name*	Bladder width (cm)	Bladder length (cm)
Newborn	2.5-4.0	5.0-9.0
Infant	4.0-6.0	11.5-18.0
Child	7.5-9.0	17.0-19.0
Adult	11.5-13.0	22.0-26.0
Large arm	14.0-15.0	30.5-33.0
Thigh	18.0-19.0	36.0-38.0

From Horan MJ: Task force on blood pressure control in children: report of the second task force on blood pressure control in children, Ped 79(1): 3, 1987.
*Cuff name does not guarantee that the cuff will be appropriate size for a child within that age range.

or soon after admission is vital. Infant and adult scales should be available on the unit and should be able to measure in kilograms and grams, since the loss or gain of grams may be significant in a young child (see Table 8-9). Gram scales are also used to measure urine collected in a diaper or blood or body fluid loss on dressings and linen.

Stethoscope

Stethoscopes of any size can be used for auscultation; however, the small child has a more rounded chest wall, which may be auscultated more easily using a pediatric stethoscope with the smaller diaphragm and bell.

Blood pressure cuffs

The blood pressure cuff should be ⅔ to ¾ of the upper arm size, and the cuff bladder should completely encircle the child's arm only once. Various sizes should be readily available and used appropriately as determined by the size of the child. Table 8-11 reviews normal blood pressure cuff sizes in the pediatric patient.

Thermometer

If using the standard glass thermometer, avoid obtaining the young child's temperature orally. There is a high risk of the child biting and breaking the instrument. In obtaining rectal temperatures, use only rectal-tipped thermometers to minimize the risk of perirectal damage. Rectal temperatures are avoided until a newborn passes the first meconium stool and when a child has diarrhea, rectal irritation, neutropenia, or thrombocytopenia.

TABLE 8-12 Suggested Intravenous Catheter Sizes for Children

Age	Butterfly	Over-the-needle
Infant	25-27 ga	24 ga, usually 22-26
Child	23-25 ga	22 ga, usually 20-24
Adolescent	21-23 ga	20 ga, usually 18-22

Measuring tape

A nonstretch measuring tape that has units in both centimeters and inches should be available to record head circumferences and abdominal girths. Head circumferences are generally measured in children less than 2 years of age.

Otoscope

Due to the high frequency of ear infections in the pediatric population, an otoscope with appropriate-sized speculum covers should be available.

Peripheral Intravenous Access

Intravenous catheter selection

The optimal IV catheter size is one that is the smallest gauge to achieve the intended therapy but is small enough to avoid impairing blood flow around the catheter once placed in the intended vessel. Catheter types are the same as those found for the adult population: butterfly needles and over-the-needle catheters. Table 8-12 reviews suggested catheter sizes according to patient age.

Site selection

Each site for IV catheterization has its advantages and disadvantages. As in the adult patient, the clinician should consider the condition of the vessels, the purpose for the IV infusion, and the projected duration of the IV therapy.

Scalp veins are easily found in infants, but they require shaving a portion of the child's head and may be aesthetically unpleasant to the parents. These sites are rarely used and frequently do not last very long. Preferably, upper extremity sites are used and include the dorsum of the hand and the cephalic, median basilic, and median antecubital in the forearm. When selecting an upper extremity, the clinician should note the child's preference for right-sided or left-sided dominance and use the nondominant hand for the IV therapy.

Lower extremity sites are usually avoided in the adult

TABLE 8-13 Intravenous Catheter Insertion and Maintenance in Children

Difference	Result	Interventions
Cooperation	Difficulty is in accessing an uncooperative, moving target.	Explanation and preparation of infant is of minimal value, but prepare parent if present. Provide comfort and reassurance. Preparation of young child should be age-appropriate. Practice good positioning techniques of child (e.g., mummy wrap).
Security	Once IV is in place, difficulty is securing it due to small size of insertion site and frequent movement of child.	Prepare and use an arm board whenever possible. For infant, make arm boards out of padded tongue blades. Use soft restraints on affected extremity to minimize movement and risk of kinking or dislodging the catheter. Avoid circumferential taping. Obtain small latex drains or rubber bands for infants and small children.
Technique for venous distention	Because of young child's thin and sensitive skin, warm soaks may burn the patient and large tourniquets may be ineffective.	May use disposable diapers with warm water to wrap around extremity to dilate vessels, but keep the bed dry. Carefully check the temperature of any moist heat to avoid burning the child's thin skin.

population because of venous stasis and increased risk for thrombosis. Compliance with this standard is attempted in the pediatric population, especially if the child is near the age of walking. In the young infant, veins such as the saphenous, median marginal, and dorsal arch are used if necessary.

Patient management

The process of insertion and maintenance of IV catheters is essentially the same in the pediatric and adult patient. Table 8-13 reviews the essential differences in the pediatric patient and the associated, necessary interventions.

Difficulty in obtaining intravenous access

IV access in the infant and young child may be time consuming and difficult. A systematic approach should be in place to ensure efficient IV access in the event a pediatric patient requires resuscitation. Peripheral access is attempted for 1 to 2 minutes, and if access is unsuccessful, it is encouraged that medical personnel attempt a central access (femoral) in the child older than 3 years of age or intraosseous (IO) access in the child less than 3 years of age.

Intraosseous Access and Infusion

Description

Placing an access in the bone marrow cavity offers many advantages because an IO functions as a rigid vein that does not collapse in the presence of hypovolemia or circulatory shock. The marrow sinusoids drain into the venous systems, where fluid or medication can be immediately absorbed into the general circulation. Blood products, fluids, and medications may be administered through the IO route, although it is recommended that hypertonic and alkaline solutions be diluted before infusion.[11] Contraindications include osteogenesis imperfecta, osteoporosis, and a fractured extremity.

The optimal site for IO placement during a resuscitative effort is the proximal tibia (Figure 8-1), which precludes interference with ventilations and chest compressions. Reusable or disposable bone marrow needles, sizes 15 to 18 gauge, should be available.

Patient management

Once the IO access is in place, the needle should stand firmly upward without support, but it should be secured with tape and a sterile 2 × 2 to prevent dislodgement. As with any intravascular access, signs of extravasation and patency should be monitored. Heparin-saline flushes may discourage clotting of the access. The IO access is not meant to be a perma-

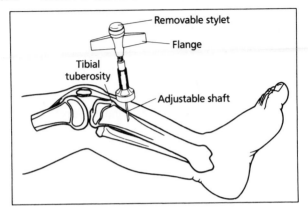

Figure 8-1 Intraosseous needle placement. Optimal needle insertion is in the medial, flat surface of the anterior tibia approximately 1 to 3 cm below the tibial tuberosity. The needle is directed at a 60- to 90-degree angle away from the growth plate to avoid the epiphyseal plate. (From Fiser D: Intraosseous infusion, N Eng J Med 322(22):1580, 1990.)

nent access; therefore attempts should be made to acquire other IV access and discontinue IO needle as soon as possible.

Complications
Complications related to the insertion and time-limited use of the IO access occur infrequently but may include subcutaneous infusion of fluid or leakage around the puncture site, cellulitis, and osteomyelitis.[5,11]

ECG Monitoring
Continuous display of the child's electrocardiogram (ECG) and a system to accurately and clearly record a paper tracing are essential. The optimal pediatric ECG machine must be able to monitor and record rapid heart rates of 250 to 300 beats per minute. Because of the infant's irregular respiratory rate and the infant's and young child's propensity toward respiratory rather than cardiac arrest, the machine should also have the capability of monitoring respiratory rate and breathing pattern.

Electrodes should be smaller than adult electrodes. The adhesive component of the electrode should allow for the sensitivity of the infant and young child's thinner skin. Skin preparation is essentially the same process and of equal importance in the pediatric patient. Electrode placement and chest landmarks are the same in the child and in the adult.

Noninvasive Blood Pressure

Blood pressure values obtained via the indirect method of mercury manometer and auscultation or palpation can be reliable. Repetitive measurements can be time consuming; thus, the use of automatic oscillometric monitors may be preferred. Although these machines appear efficient, there is some evidence that they are less reliable in the lower pressure range and may overestimate pressure in the infant experiencing hypotension.[8]

Pulse Oximeter

Pulse oximetry is essentially the same technique in the pediatric and adult patient, with a few exceptions. Because the skin is a reliable reflection of perfusion states, the child with poor peripheral perfusion is not an optimal candidate for pulse oximetry. In an impaired perfusion state the monitor will reflect inaccurate or unobtainable readings. In addition, the infant/young child tends to be more active, and movement of the extremity with the probe will lead to inaccurate readings.

End Tidal CO$_2$ Monitoring

The indications and methods for end tidal CO$_2$ monitoring are the same in the adult and pediatric patient.

Peripheral Artery Catheterization

Indications and site selection

The indications and sites for arterial cannulation and monitoring are the same as for the adult patient. The selection of an arterial site for arterial cannulation is determined by the stability of the artery and the availability of sufficient collateral circulation. Radial artery cannulation is the most commonly used site after verification of collateral ulnar artery circulation using the Allen test.

Patient management

The most important issues regarding arterial lines in the child are patency and security of the line, regulation of the amount and pressure of the flush solution, setting of appropriate alarm limits, and monitoring for complications. It is recommended that arterial lines be sutured at the insertion site in the young child to minimize the risk of accidental dislodgement. There should be a continuous administration of intraarterial solution to maintain patency. Consideration of not only the type of solution and need for heparinization but also the amount of fluid that the child receives hourly and daily are important.

For children who weigh less than 20 kg, it is recommended that the arterial line be placed on an infusion pump to regulate the flow and to avoid inadvertent administration of unnecessary fluid. Arterial lines should be flushed using a manual flush method rather than the pigtail flush method, regardless of the size of the child. Manual flushing facilitates accurate intake assessment, avoids unnecessary pressures on small, fragile vessels, and limits retrograde embolization into the central circulation. Alarms for all hemodynamic lines should be set for age-appropriate limits and should remain on at all times.

Complications

Complications are similar to those found in the adult; however, children have an increased risk of vasospasm and thrombosis.

Central Venous Catheterization

Insertion and maintenance of these lines are the same in the child as in the adult. Commonly used sites include the femoral and the external and internal jugular veins. The subclavian vein can be used; however, there is a high risk of complications associated with this location even by the expert clinician. This is due to the close proximity of the subclavian vein to the apex of the lung.

Pulmonary Artery Catheterization

Description

Pulmonary artery catheters are indicated in children who are receiving the most aggressive therapies, such as high ventilator pressures, massive hemodynamic support, and/or barbiturate therapy for increased intracranial pressure. Pulmonary artery catheters are available in four sizes. Table 8-14 lists

TABLE 8-14 Suggestions for Catheter Sizes

Age	Size
0-3 yr	5 Fr with 10 cm CVP
3-8 yr	5 Fr with 15 cm CVP
8-14 yr	7 Fr with 20 cm CVP
≥14 yr	7 Fr with 30 cm CVP

CVP, Central venous port.

suggestions for the selection of size of a pulmonary artery catheter.

Insertion

Pediatric pulmonary artery catheters are much smaller in diameter than adult catheters, yet they are not much shorter. The femoral vein is a commonly used vessel because it can accommodate the entire length of the catheter and allows for correct placement of catheter ports. Adult pulmonary artery catheters may also have an additional port for infusion of fluids and medications, which pediatric catheters do not. The CVP port of the 5 Fr catheter is extremely small and clots easily; therefore it is not an optimal port for blood component administration.

Normal values

The pressures of the cardiac chambers and great vessels are the same in the child as in the adult in the absence of congenital or acquired cardiac disease. Cardiac output varies greatly with size and body; therefore it is prudent to monitor cardiac index in children. The normal cardiac index ranges between 3.5 and 4.5 L/min/m^2.

Patient management

The same standards used for the management of arterial lines should be used for pulmonary artery lines (e.g., manual flushing, placing the catheters on infusion pumps for the child weighing less than 20 kg). In addition, the amount of solution used for cardiac output injectates is generally 5 ml rather than 10 ml and should be recorded as a part of the child's hourly intake.

Assistive Respiratory Devices

Manual resuscitation bags

Unlike the adult 1 liter manual resuscitation bag, pediatric manual resuscitation bags are available in infant (250 ml) and pediatric (500 ml) sizes. The resuscitation bag should be capable of delivering one and one-half times the child's tidal volume (V_T), or 10 to 15 ml/kg, as well as 100% oxygen. For the pediatric bags to consistently deliver 100% oxygen at rapid respiratory rates, the manual resuscitation bag should have an oxygen reservoir.

Most pediatric resuscitation bags are designed with a pop-off valve to prevent excessive pressure delivery with the average manual breath. Pop-off valves are normally activated with breaths requiring peak inspiratory pressures (PIPs) between 35 and 60 cm H_2O pressure, depending on the brand of resuscitation device. The pop-off valve is an operational device that reduces the incidence of barotrauma or gastric distention by releasing excessive pressure to the atmosphere rather than to the child. When manual ventilations are essential, this pop-off valve should be covered or deactivated to ensure maximal ventilation of the child, even if the lungs are stiff and require high PIPs. The pop-off valve is always open or activated unless covered with adhesive tape or the clinician's finger during manual breath delivery.

A pressure manometer is connected in-line to the manual resuscitation bag to minimize excessive PIPs and to provide breaths similar in pressure to the mechanical breaths received from the ventilator. This is especially helpful in a unit that provides care to a variety of patient populations and may minimize the incidence of excessively high-pressure breaths being delivered. Although a pressure manometer can assist in minimizing pressure and the reservoir can assist in providing 100% oxygen, the only indicator to ensuring adequate V_T delivery is a clinical one. The adequate amount of V_T delivered during a mechanical resuscitation breath is the amount that causes an observable rise and fall of the child's chest.

Resuscitation masks

Like bags, resuscitation masks come in a variety of sizes ranging from neonatal to young adult. The ideal mask is one that covers the child's nose and mouth yet avoids pressure on the eyes. Clear masks are preferred so that the presence of vomitus or a change in lip color can be observed immediately. Laerdal face masks are available in one size (adult) only. If absolutely necessary, the Laerdal face mask may be used upside down on the infant's face to completely cover the child's face while minimizing orbital pressure.

Artificial Airways

All pediatric airways are small compared to the overall body size of the patient. It is important to recognize that the smaller the airway, the more difficult it is to maintain position and patency.

Nasopharyngeal and oropharyngeal airways

The indications for the use of nasopharyngeal and oropharyngeal airways are identical in the pediatric and adult patient. The correct length for a nasopharyngeal airway in the infant or child is determined by measuring from the tip of the nose to the tragus of the ear. The diameter of the nasopharyngeal airway should be the largest size that easily inserts without causing blanching of the nares. The pediatric patient often has large adenoids and fragile nasal mucosa that can lacerate during the insertion process, causing significant nose bleeds. Nasopharyngeal airways should be maintained as patent as possible, since the infant is an obligate nose breather.

An oropharyngeal airway is particularly useful as an assistive device to bag-valve mask ventilations in the unconscious child. The proper size is estimated by placing the airway next to the child's face. The flange should be at the level of the central incisors, and the end should be approximately at the tip of the mandibular angle. Insertion is facilitated by using a tongue depressor to hold the tongue down onto the floor of the child's mouth. Because of the fragility of the child's oral mucosa, inserting the airway upside down and then rotating it 180 degrees is not recommended.

Endotracheal tubes

Unlike the adult patient, there are numerous sizes of ETTs available for the critically ill infant and child. To estimate the correct size of the ETT, choose a tube approximately the same size as the child's little finger, or use the following formula:

$$\text{Internal diameter} = \frac{16 + \text{age in yr}}{4}$$

It is important to recognize that both of these methods are estimations of the ETT size and that tubes one-half size (0.5 mm) larger and one-half size smaller should be available for immediate use. Generally, uncuffed ETTs are used in the child less than 8 years of age because the narrow cricoid cartilage provides an anatomical cuff in the presence of physiologically normal lungs. Pediatric endotracheal cuffs are available in cuffed tubes and may be indicated in the patient with stiff, noncompliant lungs.

Pediatric intubation

Although the nurse is not primarily responsible for intubating the pediatric patient, an understanding of the procedure will help prepare the nurse to assist with this life-saving measure. Every effort should be made to intubate the child under controlled conditions using appropriately sized equipment to prevent unsuccessful intubation or airway damage (see Table 8-16). Awake intubations should be considered only for resuscitation situations or when there is considerable question about whether the child can be ventilated by bag and mask when sedated and pharmacologically paralyzed. Rapid sequence sedation and paralysis with IV medications provide the clinician satisfactory visualization of the larynx in most cases. Cricoid pressure should be considered in all pediatric intubations to minimize aspiration.

Tracheostomy tubes

Tracheostomy tubes are available in neonatal and pediatric internal diameters. The difference between the neonate and pediatric sizes is in length of the airway. Pediatric-sized tracheostomy tubes are not available with cuffs unless the tube is custom ordered.

Patient management

HUMIDIFICATION

Humidity should always be provided with the use of any artificial airway. Respiratory distress can drastically increase the child's insensible water loss, increasing the vital significance of this intervention. Humidity will minimize excessive drying of respiratory secretions and the risk of occluding the artificial airway with mucous plugs. Humidity also prevents excessive drying and irritation of the airways.

SUCTIONING

Suctioning the child is the most common method used to determine patency of the artificial airway and to clear accumulated secretions.[50] Despite the frequency of this nursing intervention, care must be taken in the actual performance of the procedure to minimize complications.

Suction catheters are available in 6, 8, 10, and 14 French. The most common catheters used in the pediatric patient are the 8 and 10 French catheters. The selected catheter should be large enough to obtain secretions without completely occluding the child's artificial airway. Suction catheters should be no more than one-half the internal diameter of the ETT.

Each pass of the suction catheter should not exceed 10 seconds. During suctioning, the wall suction pressure gauge should not exceed 100 mm Hg so that airway damage is minimized. Another intervention to prevent mucosal damage that is practiced in some pediatric facilities includes measuring the suction catheter so that the catheter extends only beyond the end of the tracheostomy or ETT during the procedure. Once this measurement is determined, an example of the marked suction catheter should be posted at the child's bedside.

Mechanical Ventilation of the Child
The optimal ventilator

A ventilator must be able to deliver small but accurate V_{TS} (≤ 100 ml) against high airway resistance and low lung compliance because the young child has a higher basal metabolic rate, larger BSA, and a smaller airway diameter with higher airway resistance. Pediatric ventilators must be able to generate low and high inspiratory flow rates. A flow rate that is too high may result in the premature delivery of volume, the generation of unnecessary high pressures, and inadequate inspiratory/expiratory (I:E) ratios. A flow rate that is too low may not deliver the total V_T in the short inspiratory time available. Pediatric ventilators must have rapid response times or there will be poor coordination of the ventilator with the child's own breathing, thus increasing the child's work of breathing and the risk of not reversing the respiratory failure.

Modes of Mechanical Ventilation

Unlike the adult patient who is commonly ventilated using a volume-cycled ventilator, the pediatric patient may be ventilated using a variety of modes: volume cycled, pressure cycled, and time cycled.

Pressure-cycled ventilation is commonly used in the newborn or infant population because of the low V_{TS} needed and because a continuous-flow system requires no extra energy to initiate a breath.

However, *pressure-controlled ventilation* (using Siemens Servo C) is gaining popularity in the management of pediatric patients. This mode of ventilation permits airflow to reach a preset inspiratory pressure quickly in the inspiratory phase as opposed to near the end of the inspiratory phase (as occurs in pressure cycled). In pressure-controlled ventilation, the preset pressure is maintained during the inspiratory effort. This mode may be advantageous because it encourages partially collapsed alveoli to open with sustained inspiratory pressure. This mode of ventilation may decrease the mean airway pressure in some patients.

Volume-cycled ventilation may be used to ventilate even small children if proper consideration is given to the compression volume of the ventilator circuit. It is also important to assess whether the ventilator has a backup ventilator mode with parameters programmed that may be deleterious to the infant or child. For example, a machine with a backup ventilation mode that has a V_T of 500 ml could cause barotrauma in a child weighing 15 kg.

The choice of ventilator control may be critical to its success with a volume-cycled ventilator. Because small or weak children may have trouble opening the demand valve in the intermittent ventilation demand (IMV) circuit, hypoventilation is a real concern. Most current volume-cycled ventilators that are used in children have the options of assist control, IMV, synchronized IMV (SIMV), and pressure support. The use of SIMV with pressure support generally overcomes the problem of opening the demand valve and still allows the child the opportunity to breathe independently between ventilator breaths.

Time-cycled ventilation provides a continuous flow of gas in the respiratory circuit, which can decrease the work of breathing for the ill infant. In this situation the infant does not have to open a demand valve to access the next breath. The disadvantage to time-cycled ventilation is that the machine may have too low inspiratory flow capabilities and may not provide adequate flows for children who weigh more than 15 kg.

Indications for Mechanical Ventilation

In addition to the broad, generic reasons for mechanical ventilation such as respiratory failure, pediatric patients commonly require mechanical ventilation to decrease the work and the oxygen cost of breathing.

Initial ventilatory settings

RATE

The ventilator rate is determined by the child's age-appropriate respiratory rate, taking into consideration the underlying pathophysiology as well as the desired V_T. For example, if the child is to receive a V_T on the low range of normal (10 ml/kg), the rate may be set higher. If the child is to receive a V_T on the high range of normal (15 ml/kg), the rate may be set lower.

TIDAL VOLUME

The standard V_T used in the pediatric patient is between 10 and 15 ml/kg. Although the ventilator may be set to deliver a V_T, the actual volume that the child receives may vary because of air leaks around the ETT or compressible volume in the ventilator circuit. With the use of predominately uncuffed ETT, a portion of the set V_T will be lost around the tube. Even if a cuffed tube is used (where it is standard to maintain a minimal leak), some volume will be lost. Therefore it is necessary to monitor the exhaled V_T or returned volume to estimate the delivered V_T.[26]

It is important to use pediatric ventilator circuitry (e.g., small bore with minimal compliance factor [compliance factors vary from 0.5 to 2 ml/cm H_2O]) because the adult circuitry may significantly alter the V_T the child actually receives.

PEAK INSPIRATORY PRESSURE

As in the adult patient, PIP is predetermined in the pressure-cycled and pressure-controlled modes of ventilation. It is a measured end product of V_T and inspiratory time in other modes of ventilation. It is important to recognize that the respiratory compliance is similar in all age groups, so it takes about the same PIP to ventilate the lungs of a normal infant, child, and adult.

FRACTION OF INSPIRED OXYGEN (Fio_2)

As in adults, manipulations are made with various ventilation parameters to decrease the Fio_2 to below 40%.

POSITIVE END EXPIRATORY PRESSURE

Normally, physiological PEEP assists in stabilizing alveoli and maintaining the functional residual capacity (FRC). The young child has a greater tendency to collapse the alveoli than the older child or adult because of the underdeveloped collateral ventilatory channels. As soon as a child is intubated, physiological PEEP is lost, leading to the general recommendation that the young child routinely receive 2 to 3 cm H_2O PEEP.[26] With acute lung injury syndromes in which the FRC is low, higher levels of PEEP may be used similar to adults with acute respiratory distress syndrome (ARDS).

Complications

A common complication of ventilation devices in both pediatric and adult patients is barotrauma with air leaks. Although the treatments are identical (e.g., chest tubes), the etiologies and identification of the problem may be different. The infant not only sustains mechanical barotrauma but may experience spontaneous pneumothorax. Identification of the presence of air leaks in the pediatric patient may be challenging. Their thin chest walls may lead to referred breath sounds over collapsed lung fields, and the ability of pediatric patients to maintain their blood pressures for prolonged periods despite a tension pneumothorax may mask the classic

TABLE 8-15 Complications of Mechanical Ventilation

Complication	Developmental/situational risks	Interventions
Extubation (inadvertent)	Infant/child is cognitively too immature to understand rationale for tube placement and security. Infant/child is more activity oriented. Infant/child is usually intubated with uncuffed tube. Although cuffed tube does not ensure security, it does assist in stability.	Use soft restraints. Keep soft restraints for all extremities at the bedside. Provide adequate sedation and analgesia. Increase use of paralytic agents. Assess and document security of tube and markers at teeth/gums every hour.
Aspiration, gastric distention	Infant/child has delayed gastric emptying. Use of uncuffed ETTs is increased. Infant/child is prone to vomiting when extremely upset. Weak cardiac sphincter and large manual ventilation breaths increase the risk of introducing air into the stomach. Infant/child swallows air when upset and crying.	Place NG tube early. Facilitate gastric emptying with enteral medication delivery or feedings by placing patient on right side. Check residuals frequently. Assess stomach contents before upsetting procedures, Trendelenberg position, chest physiotherapy. Manually ventilate only with as much air that raises and lowers the child's chest.

signs of pneumothorax. Table 8-15 shows the two most common complications found in the child receiving mechanical ventilation, the developmental or situational aspects placing the child at risk, and the associated interventions.

Resuscitation Equipment and Supplies

Table 8-16 provides a list of essential resuscitation equipment based on the age and weight of the child. These supplies are recommended as contents in a resuscitation cart serving pediatric patients. The items are suggested as additions to other equipment listed in the chapter and are not inclusive. Additional recommended supplies include infant and pediatric internal and external defibrillator paddles and an external pacemaker machine with appropriately sized pacer electrodes.

Drainage Devices

Chest drainage systems

The indications and uses of chest drainage systems are identical in the adult and pediatric patient. Two primary differences include determining the size of the catheter and accurately measuring and interpreting the output. Various sizes are available to meet the needs of the different drainage purposes (air versus blood) and the size of the patient (see Table 8-16). Accurately measuring the hourly output from a chest drainage system is facilitated by numerical markings that are in small (1 to 2 ml) increments. It must be remembered that although the chest tube drainage may be small in absolute hourly output, it may be a significant proportion of the child's circulatory blood volume. A critical bleed following postoperative cardiac surgery is defined as 3 ml/kg of body weight for more than 2 hours and will require surgical intervention.[17]

Maintenance of chest tube patency is challenging in the presence of bloody drainage, since the lumen of these catheters are small. Chest tubes are not normally stripped because of the danger of creating excessively large negative intrathoracic pressures; however, in the presence of bloody chest drainage, gentle manipulation and stripping is imperative to maintain tube patency.

Gastrointestinal drainage devices

The indications and uses for gastrointestinal (GI) drainage devices are identical in the adult and pediatric patient but may have a greater significance in the pediatric patient because there is a greater incidence of aspiration and impe-

TABLE 8-16 Recommended Resuscitation Equipment for the Child

Age	0-6 mo	6-12 mo	1 yr	18 mo	3 yr	5 yr	6 yr	8 yr	10 yr	12 yr	14 yr
Weight (kg)	3-5	7	10	12	15	20	20	25	30	40	50
Resus mask	0-1	1	1-2	2	3	3	3	3	3	4	4-5
Laryngoscope (Miller/Mac)	0	1	1	1	2	2	2	2	2	2	3
ETT	3.0	3.5	3.5	4.0	4.5	5.0	5.5	6.0	6.0	6.5	7.0
Suction (ETT/trach)	6	6	8	8	10	10	10	10	10	14	14
Suction (OP/NP)	10	10	10	10	14	14	14	16	16	16	16
Chest tube	10-12	10-12	16-20	16-20	16-20	20-28	20-28	20-28	28-32	28-32	32-42
NG/OG	8	8	8	8	10	10	10	10	12	12	14
Foley	5	5	8	8	10	10	10	10	12	12	12
Trach (ped)	0	1	1	1-2	2-3	3	3	4	4	5	6

Modified from Widner-Kolberg MR: Baltimore, 1989, Maryland Institutes for Emergency Medical Services Systems.

dence to ventilatory efforts with abdominal distention. A variety of types and sizes of NG tubes are available (Table 8-16). The smaller sized tubes, such as the 5 French, are referred to as *feeding tubes* because they are primarily used for this purpose. Movement of the contents in these tubes is generally left to gravity, and they are manually irrigated as needed. Levine tubes are available in a variety of sizes and do not have a vent lumen. The ordinary Salem sump tubes with a blue vent lumen are available in sizes 10 and 12 French. These tubes may be connected to low intermittent wall suction, which should not exceed 100 mm Hg.

Due to the small lumen of the NG tubes, maintaining patency is challenging, especially if enteral medications are administered. Tube patency should be verified every 2 hours, and the tube should be irrigated if patency is questioned. Rather than irrigating with the standard 30 ml, it is wise to irrigate the pediatric NG tube with one and one-half times the deadspace volume of the tube to avoid excessive fluid administration to the child. All fluid entering and leaving the child's drainage system should be documented in the child's I & O record.

Urinary drainage devices

Urine output is an indicator of end-organ perfusion in the infant and young child and should be accurately measured every hour. Foley catheters are available in a variety of sizes (see Table 8-16) and do not differ from adult foley catheters other than the size of the lumen and the capacity of the balloon. The integrity and capacity of the balloon should be checked before insertion to avoid overdistending or breaking the balloon once in place. The double-lumen foley used for continuous irrigation is not available in pediatric sizes. In the newborn or small infant, a 5 French feeding tube may be used as a urinary catheter.

Urinary drainage bags or stoma bags may be used to collect urinary specimens or monitor urinary output. These devices are challenging to secure to the child, particularly the female patient. It is recommended that whatever urinary drainage device is chosen, a chux or diaper be placed under the child so that it can be weighed to determine any urine spillage or leakage. To test the specific gravity or pH of urine collected in a child's diaper, follow these steps:

1. Remove the top dry liner of the inside of the diaper to obtain urine-saturated fibers.

2. Place fibers into the barrel of a syringe.
3. Replace the plunger of the syringe and push the plunger, squeezing the urine from the syringe into a medicine cup.

Thermal Devices

Infants and young children have large BSAs in relation to body weight, which may place them at risk for hypothermia resulting in physiological instability. Infants cannot shiver to keep warm but rather undergo nonshivering thermogenesis to generate body heat. This is a limited capability because once the newborn burns brown fat, more cannot be generated. Furthermore, hypothermia shifts the oxyhemoglobin dissociation curve to the left, prevents the release of oxygen to the tissue, and increases oxygen consumption and glucose utilization in an effort to maintain the body's core temperature. The infant/young child who presents in respiratory distress may decompensate following exposure to the drafty ICU environment during invasive line placement. Thus, it is important to provide a temperature-controlled environment and monitor body temperature closely, particularly in the newborn and young child patient population.

Over-the-bed radiant warmers

The radiant warmer can provide an environment that allows access to the child while maintaining the child's normal body temperature. It is recommended that the child remain uncovered and that the warmer be used in the mode in which the child's temperature regulates the amount of heat rather than the machine delivering a certain percentage of power. Care should be taken to secure the skin temperature probe according to the manufacturer's directions and to frequently monitor both the skin probe temperature and the child's core temperature. Clinicians and parents should avoid using oil-based solutions on the child while under the warmer, since this may lead to thermal burns similar to sunburn.

Hypothermia/hyperthermia blankets and blood warmers

The indications, uses, and complications of thermal devices are the same in children and adults. Hyperthermia blankets are rarely used in the infant and young child because over-the-bed radiant warmers are so efficient. Cooling blankets are often helpful in controlling the body temperature of children who remain febrile despite antipyretic medications. If a thermal blanket is used, avoid placing the blanket on top of the child because the weight can impede ventilatory movement of the chest and abdomen.

DELIVERY OF FLUIDS, MEDICATIONS, AND BLOOD

Fluid Management

Fluid requirements by weight

Each child is individually assessed for the amount and type of prescribed IV fluid. The average child maintenance fluid requirements may be determined by body weight (Table 8-17).

Fluid requirements by body surface area

The child's maintenance fluid requirements may also be calculated according to BSA. (To determine BSA, see nomogram in Appendix E.) Maintenance fluid requirements are 1500 ml/m^2/day. For example, a child weighing 8 kg who is 35 cm long and has a BSA of 0.43 m^2 requires 645 ml/day (1500 ml $\times$ 0.43 m^2 = 645 ml) and an hourly rate of 27 ml (645 $\div$ 24 hr = 27 ml/hr).

Alteration in maintenance fluid requirements

Maintenance fluid requirements may be altered based on the child's disease state. Frequently, a child recovering from postoperative cardiac surgery, a neurological disorder, or a renal disorder is placed on variations of maintenance fluid requirements such as two-thirds maintenance fluid or replacement of insensible fluid loss only.

Accurate monitoring and delivery of fluid

It is imperative that fluid be administered accurately and safely to the critically ill child, since small fluid imbalances can be clinically significant. IV fluids are administered most commonly via an infusion device rather than by the gravity method. The gravity method is appropriate in very few instances due to the unreliability of the tubing clamps and patient and/or visitor exploration of the clamps.

Optimal pediatric infusion device

The optimal pediatric infusion device should have all the common safety alarms as well as the ability to accurately deliver small increments of fluid hourly (0.1 ml/hr). It is equally important, however, for the pediatric pump to deliver large, rapid fluid boluses (999 ml/hr). It is common for a nurse to use both macrorate and microrate devices at the bedside of a sick child.

Accompanying a pediatric infusion device should be the necessary IV tubing, small IV fluid containers, and buretrols

TABLE 8-17 Calculation of Daily Maintenance Fluid Requirements

Weight	Fluid requirement	Example
0-10 kg (>72 hr old)	100 ml/kg	Pt weight = 5 kg Pt wt (kg) × fluid requirement: 5 × 100 = 500 ml/day Hourly rate = 500 ÷ 24 = 21 ml/hr
11-20 kg	100 ml/kg for the first 10 kg or 1000 ml/day plus 50 ml/kg for each kg 11 through 20	Pt weight = 13 kg For the first 10 kg: 10 kg × 100 = 1000 ml For kg over 10 and ≤20 (total of 3): 3 kg × 50 = 150 ml 1000 ml +150 ml TOTAL 1150 ml/day Hourly rate = 1150 ÷ 24 = 48 ml/hr
21-30 kg	100 ml/kg for the first 10 kg or 1000 ml/day plus 50 ml/kg for each kg 11 through 20 plus 25 ml/kg for each kg 21 through 30	Pt weight = 26 kg For the first 10 kg: 10 kg × 100 = 1000 ml For kg over 10 and ≤20 (total of 10): 10 kg × 50 = 500 ml

For kg over 20 and ≤30 (total of 6):
6 kg × 25 = 150 ml

$$\begin{array}{r} 1000\ \text{ml} \\ 500\ \text{ml} \\ +150\ \text{ml} \\ \hline \text{TOTAL}\ \overline{1650\ \text{ml/day}} \end{array}$$

Hourly rate = 1650 ÷ 24
= 69 ml/hr

Pt weight = 32 kg
For the first 10 kg:
10 kg × 100 = 1000 ml
For kg over 10 and ≤20 (total of 10):
10 kg × 50 = 500 ml
For kg over 20 and ≤30 (total of 10):
10 kg × 25 = 250 ml
For kg over 30 and ≤40 (total of 2):
2 kg × 10 = 20 ml

$$\begin{array}{r} 1000\ \text{ml} \\ 500\ \text{ml} \\ 250\ \text{ml} \\ +\ 20\ \text{ml} \\ \hline \text{TOTAL}\ \overline{1770\ \text{ml/day}} \end{array}$$

Hourly rate = 1770 ÷ 24
= 74 ml/hr

31-40 kg

100 ml/kg for the first 10 kg or 1000 ml/day
plus 50 ml/kg for each kg 11 through 20
plus 25 ml/kg for each kg 21 through 30
plus 10 ml/kg for each kg 31 through 40

or solusets. IV tubing should ideally be microbore or contain the least amount of fluid as possible and have luer-locked connections. Attach an in-line buretrol so that the amount of fluid hanging at the child's bedside is not an inordinate amount. In case of pump malfunction or misprogram, the distal clamp of the buretrol will prevent delivery of the entire IV container to the child.

Administration of Fluid Boluses

Fluid boluses include the intermittent delivery of either colloid or crystalloid fluid in an attempt to restore intravascular volume. Pediatric advanced life support (PALS) standards recommend a fluid amount of 20 ml/kg of body weight. However, some children in the ICU may not tolerate a 20 ml/kg bolus because of existing or potential respiratory or cardiac failure. Generally, fluid boluses range between 10 and 20 ml/kg.

Important considerations regarding pediatric fluid boluses include (1) determination of the accurate amount and type of fluid, (2) rapid administration of fluid (given over 20 to 30 minutes), and (3) reevaluation of the patient for the need of another fluid bolus. Due to the small volumes of fluid and the small catheters with high resistances, gravity flow may not be sufficient to deliver a bolus efficiently. Fluid boluses are often drawn up in a 60 ml syringe and manually pushed.

Blood Component Administration

The fundamental principles in blood component administration are the same in the adult and pediatric patient. The primary difference is the prescribed dose, which is determined by the child's weight. Table 8-18 reviews blood component therapy, suggested dose, and rates of administration.

Medication Administration

Dose determination

Since a child may be significantly smaller or larger than the average child in the associated age group, medications are prescribed on a microgram, milligram, or milliequivalent per kilogram of body weight basis rather than on a standard dose according to age. Confirming the weight (in kg) that is being used to determine drug dosages is important. This same weight should be used during the child's entire hospitalization unless the child substantially loses or gains lean muscle mass.

Route determination

It is not the responsibility of the nurse to determine the route for medication administration. However, the nurse

TABLE 8-18 Blood Component Administration in Children

Blood component	Usual dose	Rate of infusion	Comments
Whole blood	20 ml/kg initially	As rapidly as necessary to restore volume and stabilize the child	Administration is usually reserved for massive hemorrhage.
Packed RBCs	10 ml/kg, not to exceed 15 ml/kg	5 ml/kg/hr or 2 ml/kg/hr if congestive heart failure develops	1 ml/kg will increase Hct approximately 1%. Infuse within 4 hr. If necessary, divide the unit into smaller volumes for infusion.
Platelets	1 unit for every 7-10 kg	Each unit over 5-10 min via syringe or pump	The usual dose will increase platelet count by 50,000/mm³.

Continued.

TABLE 8-18 Blood Component Administration in Children—cont'd

Blood component	Usual dose	Rate of infusion	Comments
Fresh frozen plasma	Hemorrhage: 15-30 ml/kg Clotting deficiency: 10-15 ml/kg	Hemorrhage: rapidly to stabilize the child Clotting deficiency: over 2-3 hr	Monitor for fluid overload.
Granulocytes	Dependent on WBC counts and clinical condition, 10 ml/kg/day initially	Slowly over 2-4 hr because of fever and chills, side effects commonly associated with infusion	Granulocytes have a short lifespan. Transfuse as soon after collection as possible. Type and cross match are not required.
Albumin 5%	1 g/kg or 20 ml/kg	1-2 ml/min or 60-120 ml/hr	Monitor for fluid overload. Type and cross match are not required.
Albumin 25%	1 g/kg or 4 ml/kg	0.2-0.4 ml/min or 12-24 ml/hr	Monitor for fluid overload. Type and cross match are not required.

TABLE 8-19 Intramuscular Injections According to Age Group

Age group	Needle length (in)	Needle gauge	Maximum volume (ml)
Infant	⅝	25-27	1
Toddler	1	22-23	1
Preschooler	1	22-23	1-1.5
School age	1-1.5	22-23	2
Adolescent	1-1.5	22-23	2

should recognize that drug absorption can be erratic if topical, rectal, oral, subcutaneous, or intramuscular (IM) routes are used. Delayed gastric emptying, less subcutaneous fat, and less-developed muscle mass are a few factors that can affect drug absorption in the critically ill child. Thus, medications should be administered via the IV route.

Oral medications

For administration of oral medications to the young child, it is important to account for the child's developmental capabilities. The developmental level will determine the method of administering the oral medication (spoon, cup, nipple, or single-dose system with needleless syringe). Generally, the child less than 8 years of age is unable to swallow a pill. Many dosage forms can not be crushed (e.g., sustained-released products); therefore it may be necessary to order the liquid dosage form.

Intramuscular medications

It is important to use the appropriate size syringe and needle to properly administer IM medications to the infant or young child. The amount of the medication, age of the child, and injection site are factors to consider (Tables 8-19 and 8-20). The gluteus maximus and deltoid muscles are avoided in the infant because these muscles are underdeveloped and nerves can be damaged.

Continuous infusions

For children weighing less than 40 kg, an easy method for preparing vasoactive continuous infusions is listed in Table 8-21. It is important to note that the mg or µg dose of the vasoactive medication is added to a buretrol first, and then the buretrol is filled with the selected admixture to the 100

Text continued on p. 651.

TABLE 8-20 Sites for Intramuscular Injections

Site	Landmarks	Interventions
Vastus lateralis: Preferred in children <3 yr (rectus femoris muscle also possibly used)	Greater trochanter and knee	Give injection in middle third of anterolateral aspect of thigh.

Greater trochanter

Femoral artery

Injection site (vastus lateralis)

Rectus femoris muscle

Give injection superior and lateral to imaginary line connecting landmarks.

Posterosuperior iliac crest and greater trochanter

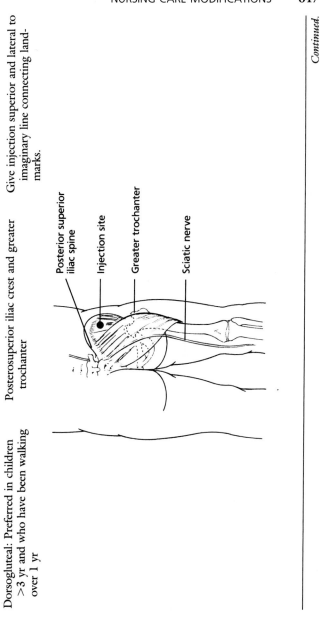

Posterior superior iliac spine

Injection site

Greater trochanter

Sciatic nerve

Dorsogluteal: Preferred in children >3 yr and who have been walking over 1 yr

Continued.

TABLE 8-20 Sites for Intramuscular Injections—cont'd

Site	Landmarks	Interventions
Ventrogluteal: Use in children >3 yr and who have been walking over 1 yr	Greater trochanter, anterior iliac spine, and posterior edge of iliac crest	Give injection at center of V that is formed when the index finger is placed on anterior iliac crest, middle finger on posterior iliac crest while palm of the hand is resting on greater trochanter. Use right hand to find landmarks when injecting into left ventrogluteal site; use left hand to find landmarks when injecting into right ventrogluteal site.

Iliac crest
Injection site
Anterior superior iliac spine

TABLE 8-21 Continuous Infusions

Drug	Dose*	Final preparation	Dosage range
Alprostadil PGE_1	$0.6 \times$ wt (kg)	1 ml/hr delivers 0.1 µg/kg/min	0.1-0.4 µg/kg/min
Dobutamine	$6.0 \times$ wt (kg)	1 ml/hr delivers 1 µg/kg/min	2-20 µg/kg/min
Dopamine	$6.0 \times$ wt (kg)	1 ml/hr delivers 1 µg/kg/min	2-20 µg/kg/min
Epinephrine	$0.6 \times$ wt (kg)	1 ml/hr delivers 0.1 µg/kg/min	0.1-1.0 µg/kg/min
Isoproterenol	$0.6 \times$ wt (kg)	1 ml/hr delivers 0.1 µg/kg/min	0.1-1.0 µg/kg/min
Lidocaine	$60 \times$ wt (kg)	1 ml/hr delivers 10 µg/kg/min	20-50 µg/kg/min
Nitroglycerin	$6.0 \times$ wt (kg)	1 ml/hr delivers 1 µg/kg/min	1-25 µg/kg/min
Nitroprusside	$6.0 \times$ wt (kg)	1 ml/hr delivers 1 µg/kg/min	1-8 µg/kg/min
Norepinephrine	$0.6 \times$ wt (kg)	1 ml/hr delivers 0.1 µg/kg/min	0.1-1.0 µg/kg/min

*Dose in mg added to the IV solution to make 100 ml.

TABLE 8-22 Pediatric Emergency Drug Dosages*

Drug	Usual IV dose	Comments
Atropine	0.02 mg/kg	Minimum dose is 0.15 mg.
Bretylium	Initial: 5 mg/kg	
	Repeat: 10 mg/kg	
Calcium chloride 10%	20 mg/kg (0.2 ml/kg)	Requires one to one dilution with 0.9% NaCl for final
Dextrose 50%	500 mg/kg	dose administration.
Diazepam	0.1 mg/kg	
Epinephrine	0.01 mg/kg of 1:10,000 solution	
Ketamine	1-2 mg/kg (normovolemia)	
	0.5 mg/kg (hypovolemia)	
Lidocaine	1 mg/kg	
Naloxone	0.01 mg/kg	
Phenobarbital	20 mg/kg	
Phenytoin	15 mg/kg	Use with 0.9% NaCl. Do not exceed 50 mg/min.
Procainamide	5 mg/kg	Do not exceed 50 mg/min.
Propranolol	0.1 mg/kg	Give slow IVP.
Sodium bicarbonate	1 mEq/kg	If child <1 yr, dilute one to one with D_5W.
Verapamil	0.1 mg/kg	Do not use if child <1 yr.

*Drug infusions can be found in Table 8-21.

ml mark. It is important that a clamp is placed between the admixture and the buretrol to avoid filling the buretrol with additional admixture and diluting the drug solution. A medication label should be placed on the buretrol rather than the admixture bag or bottle to accurately label the infusion.

Precalculated drug sheets

Pediatric dosages may be unfamiliar to the adult clinician; therefore a precalculated emergency drug sheet is very helpful. All emergency medication doses are based on the child's weight (in kg). The emergency drug sheet should include the recommended resuscitation medication dosages, medication concentration, and final medication dose and volume the individual child is to receive. The recommended dosages should reflect the American Heart Association's PALS standards.

Some hospitals have successfully incorporated the drug sheet into their existing computer system so that the calculations are made after entering the child's name and weight into the computer. The target user of the emergency drug sheet (pediatric code team or pediatric ICU team versus adult code team or adult ICU team) should be identified during the development and implementation of the drug sheet. If the emergency sheet is to be used primarily by adult clinicians, the drug sheet should reflect the adult perspective as closely as possible.

If the drug sheet is manually calculated, two registered nurses should verify the mathematical calculations and document the sheet's accuracy by signing and dating the sheet. A listing of pediatric emergency drugs and dosages can be found in Table 8-22.

Medication pitfalls

MULTIPLE CONCENTRATIONS

Several medications are available in multiple concentrations. For the child who weighs less than 20 kg, it is more efficient and accurate to use the lower concentration of the medication so that the dose in volume is not miniscule. Due to the mixed population of young children and adult patients, it may be necessary to have both concentrations available on the unit and code cart. Table 8-23 includes commonly used medications available in adult and pediatric concentrations.

DOSAGE CALCULATIONS

The risk for dosage calculation errors related to decimal point placement is greater when calculations are performed

TABLE 8-23 Recommendations for the Use of Medications with Multiple Drug Concentrations in Children

Drug name	Neonate/child (<20 kg)	Child (>20 kg)
Naloxone	Neonatal 0.02 mg/ml	Adult 0.4 mg/ml
Digitalis	Neonatal 0.1 mg/ml	Adult 0.25 mg/ml
Ketamine	Pediatric 10 mg/ml	Adult 100 mg/ml
Sodium bicarbonate	4.2% (0.5 mEq/ml)	8.4% (1 mEq/ml)

mentally. A calculator should be used to determine pediatric dosages.

Single-dose system

It is not uncommon for a nurse to administer a prescribed dose of a drug several times from the same syringe (e.g., 50 μg fentanyl from a syringe containing 200 mg) to an adult patient. A pediatric patient may require doses that are substantially smaller and thus more difficult to estimate from a multiple-dose syringe. Therefore a single-dose system is recommended for pediatric patients.

The *single-dose system* involves preparing one syringe to contain *only* the prescribed medication dose. The syringe should be properly labeled with the drug name and dose. The nurse administers the entire volume of the syringe to ensure that the prescribed dose has been given. The single-dose system prevents the nurse from overmedicating or undermedicating the patient, a hazard that can occur if a syringe containing a larger dose than prescribed is used.

After implementation of the single-dose system, it is important to realize that an unlabeled syringe can potentially contain any medication. *Nothing* should be administered to a child from an unlabeled syringe. All syringes must be labeled appropriately, including syringes of 0.9% sodium chloride used for flushing IV catheters.

Preparation of the first-course resuscitative medications

Administering medications during a resuscitative event using the single-dose system can be lengthy, especially for the inexperienced pediatric clinician. Thus, preparing and labeling syringes containing the child's first course of resuscitative drugs ahead of time can save time in the event of an emer-

---

First Course of Resuscitation Medications

Atropine   Sodium bicarbonate
Epinephrine   Dextrose*
Lidocaine

---

*Dextrose is drawn up as a first-course medication only if the patient is an infant or suffers from an acute metabolic problem.

gency (box). These syringes must be replaced every 24 hours because the medications contain no preservatives.

Sodium chloride flushes

Flushes (0.9% sodium chloride) are used to ensure delivery of medications. Manual flushing rather than gravity or pump-assisted flushing is preferred in the pediatric patient. The recommended volume for a flush should not exceed 3 ml for an infant and 5 ml for the child.[5] Flushes should be considered as intake and calculated in fluid intake totals.

SAFETY

Environmental Safety

In an environment that potentially contains critically ill patients of different ages and sizes, the importance of maintaining a safe and efficient environment cannot be overemphasized. It is recommended that a standard for an environmental safety check be developed and implemented. The box on p. 654 is an example of an environmental safety check standard adopted by the Critical Care Nursing Service, National Institutes of Health.

Soft Restraints

Soft restraints in the management of the adult ICU patient are most commonly used when the patient displays confusion, delirium, or combativeness. In an attempt to protect patient's civil rights, a medical order is required for the use of soft restraints, and this medical order cannot be written as a "prn" order. In the pediatric critical care setting the availability and use of soft restraints is generally considered a safety measure and used at the discretion of the bedside nurse. The critically ill child is unable to understand the rationale and maintenance of invasive and noninvasive equipment, so the use of soft restraints is common to ensure the security of artificial airways and intravascular lines.

Environmental Safety Check Standard

1. The safety check of the patient care environment will include verification of the following at the patient's bedside:
   a. Patient identification/allergy/typenex band present
   b. ECG, respiratory and hemodynamic monitor alarms activated with age-appropriate limits set
   c. Appropriate-sized manual resuscitation bag and oxygen-connecting tubing
   d. Appropriate-sized resuscitation mask
   e. Extra appropriate-sized artificial airways, if applicable
   f. Yankauer set-up with suction tubing and suction catheter
   g. Appropriate-sized blood pressure cuff
   h. Soft restraints at bedside
   i. Side rails positioned as appropriate to patient
   j. Patient call system in reach of patient/family
   k. Completed emergency drug sheet using child's dry weight in kilograms
   l. Bed in lowered position, as needed
2. If any component of the safety check standard is missing or incorrect, it is the responsibility of the on-coming nurse assigned to the patient to rectify the situation.

Parents often ask to loosen soft restraints stating that they will ensure restraint of the child's extremities. If parents were given this responsibility, they would feel an overwhelming sense of guilt if the child successfully pulled out a tube or catheter.

Phlebotomy Issues
Blood loss

Documenting the amount of blood loss via blood sampling should be included in the child's fluid balance. Each blood specimen contributes to blood loss, which can become significant during the child's hospitalization. Estimating the child's circulatory blood volume (Table 8-24) and comparing it with the total amount of blood withdrawn for analysis can assist the clinician to determine the severity of blood loss. When the volume of blood for analysis exceeds 5% to 7% of the circulatory blood volume or if there is a significant decrease in hematocrit levels, blood replacement should be anticipated.[14]

TABLE 8-24 Total Blood Volume

Age group	Approximate volume
Premature infants	100 ml/kg
Full-term infants	80-85 ml/kg
Children	80 ml/kg
Adults	70-75 ml/kg

Establishing minimum blood volumes for analysis

It is essential to establish minimum blood volumes required for laboratory tests and to ensure specimen quality, thereby minimizing the necessity for repeat testing. The established minimum blood volumes for analysis should reflect a joint effort between the ICU, existing general pediatric units, and the hospital laboratory. Microtubes and/or pediatric blood tubes should be available for pediatric blood samples. Reference sheets with the minimum accepted blood volumes necessary for laboratory analysis in both the adult and pediatric patient should be readily available at the bedside.

Pediatric sampling pitfalls

The majority of blood samples in the pediatric population are obtained through IV or intraarterial lines, increasing the chance of sampling error secondary to sample contamination by infusing fluids. An adequate amount of discard blood should be drawn to clear the infusing fluids from the sampling port of the catheter without contributing to excessive blood loss.

An optimal technique of blood drawing from intravascular catheters should minimize blood loss resulting from the actual amount of blood required for analysis and the need to remove discard blood from the intravascular access. In other words, the amount of the blood loss should equate the blood sample, not the blood sample plus the discard.[14]

In addition, the optimal technique should minimize fluid administration in "flushing" the intravascular access and should allow accurate measurements of the amount of flush solution administered with each sampling (Figure 8-2).[14]

Knowing the deadspace or priming volume of catheters is paramount to withdrawing the appropriate amount of discard blood and infusing the minimal amount of flush to

Text continued on p. 662.

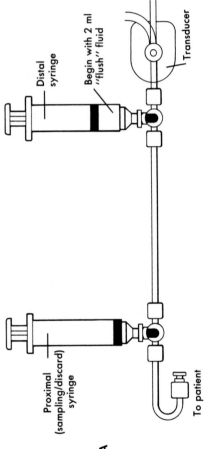

Distal syringe

Begin with 2 ml "flush" fluid

Transducer

Proximal (sampling/discard) syringe

To patient

A

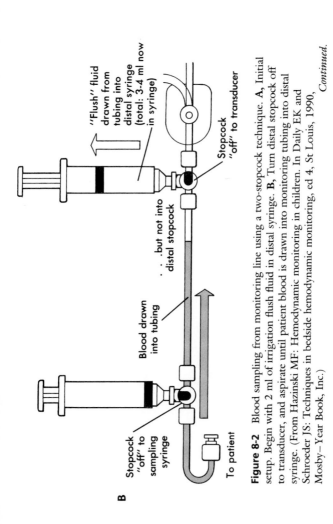

Figure 8-2   Blood sampling from monitoring line using a two-stopcock technique. **A,** Initial setup. Begin with 2 ml of irrigation flush fluid in distal syringe. **B,** Turn distal stopcock off to transducer, and aspirate until patient blood is drawn into monitoring tubing into distal syringe. (From Hazinski MF: Hemodynamic monitoring in children. In Daily EK and Schroeder JS: Techniques in bedside hemodynamic monitoring, ed 4, St Louis, 1990, Mosby–Year Book, Inc.)

Continued.

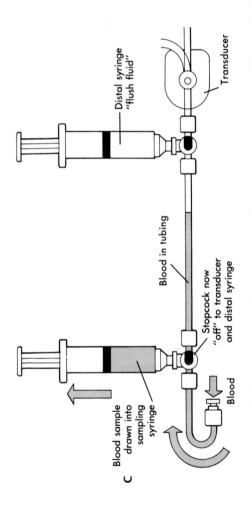

Distal syringe "flush fluid"

Transducer

Blood in tubing

Stopcock now "off" to transducer and distal syringe

Blood

Blood sample drawn into sampling syringe

C

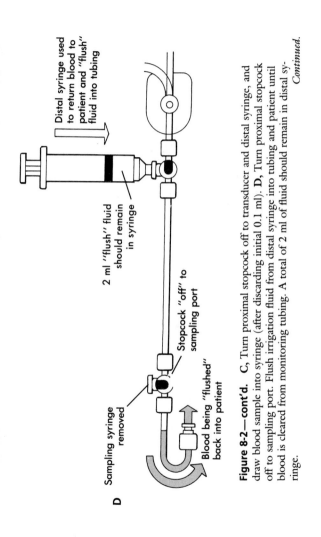

Distal syringe used to return blood to patient and "flush" fluid into tubing

2 ml "flush" fluid should remain in syringe

Sampling syringe removed

Stopcock "off" to sampling port

Blood being "flushed" back into patient

D

Figure 8-2—cont'd. **C,** Turn proximal stopcock off to transducer and distal syringe, and draw blood sample into syringe (after discarding initial 0.1 ml). **D,** Turn proximal stopcock off to sampling port. Flush irrigation fluid from distal syringe into tubing and patient until blood is cleared from monitoring tubing. A total of 2 ml of fluid should remain in distal syringe.

Continued.

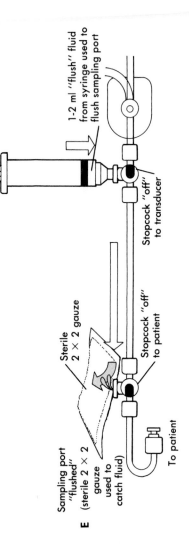

E

Sampling port "flushed" (sterile 2 × 2 gauze used to catch fluid)

Sterile 2 × 2 gauze

Stopcock "off" to patient

To patient

1-2 ml "flush" fluid from syringe used to flush sampling port

Stopcock "off" to transducer

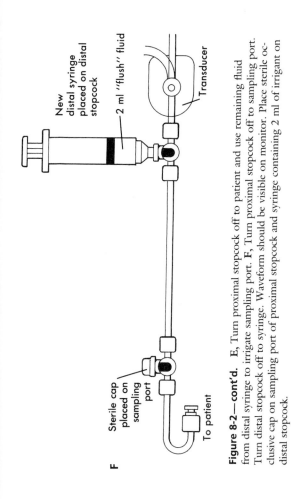

Figure 8-2—cont'd. **E,** Turn proximal stopcock off to patient and use remaining fluid from distal syringe to irrigate sampling port. **F,** Turn proximal stopcock off to sampling port. Turn distal stopcock off to syringe. Waveform should be visible on monitor. Place sterile occlusive cap on sampling port of proximal stopcock and syringe containing 2 ml of irrigant on distal stopcock.

Labels within figure:

New distal syringe placed on distal stopcock

2 ml "flush" fluid

Transducer

Sterile cap placed on sampling port

To patient

F

TABLE 8-25 Priming Volumes of Central Catheters—Pediatric

Catheter type	Size/length	Capacity/lumen (cc)
Triple-lumen	5.5 Fr/8 cm	0.2
	5.5 Fr/13 cm	0.2
	5 Fr/8 cm	0.2
	5 Fr/12 cm	0.3
	5 Fr/15 cm	0.3
Double-lumen	4 Fr/5 cm	0.1
	4 Fr/8 cm	0.2
	4 Fr/13 cm	0.3
	4 Fr/30 cm	0.6
	3 Fr/8 cm	0.1
Swan-Ganz	5 Fr/75 cm	0.6 blue
	5 Fr/80 cm	0.5 blue
Introducer	6 Fr/7 cm	1.2
Manifold		0.1 proximal
		0.2 distal
Broviac	2.7 Fr	0.15
	4.2 Fr	0.3
	6.6 Fr	0.7

Developed by Uhlman L, 10D Adult/Pediatric ICU, National Institutes of Health, Bethesda, Md.

clear the catheter. Table 8-25 shows an example of a reference that can be developed by clinicians to determine priming volumes of catheters commonly used in their institution.

VISITORS

Infection Control

The number of child visitors may increase when children are hospitalized in the adult ICU, necessitating a structured plan to address epidemiological issues and educational needs related to the child visitor. A child can be a carrier of organisms that pose a risk to pediatric and adult patients who are immunocompromised and/or critically ill. Rotavirus and respiratory syncytial virus (RSV) are seen in the adult population as secondary contacts from pediatric cases. Thus in a patient care setting with a mixed population, cross contamination must be prevented. To decrease this risk, a pediatric health screening tool (Figure 8-3) can be developed. The

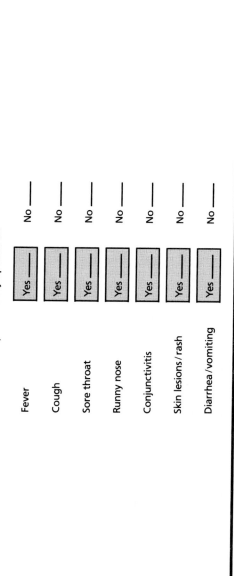

Health Screening Tool

Visitor's name: _____

Instructions: Interview the pediatric visitor or parent/caretaker of the prospective pediatric visitor. If any of the boxed answers are marked, the visitor is deemed ineligible to enter the patient care area.

Does the pediatric visitor have now or have had in the past week symptoms of:

	Yes	No
Fever	___	___
Cough	___	___
Sore throat	___	___
Runny nose	___	___
Conjunctivitis	___	___
Skin lesions/rash	___	___
Diarrhea/vomiting	___	___

Figure 8-3 An example of a health screening tool. (Critical Care Nursing Service, National Institutes of Health.)

Continued.

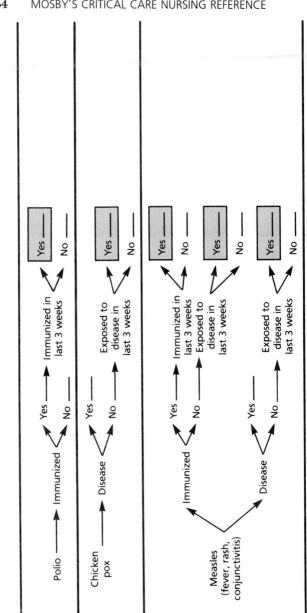

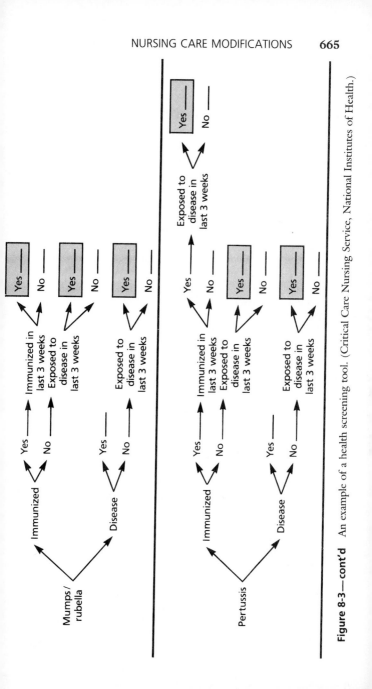

Figure 8-3—cont'd   An example of a health screening tool. (Critical Care Nursing Service, National Institutes of Health.)

tool can provide an objective measure to determine if the visitor is eligible to enter the ICU, and it can be easily implemented by ICU staff.

PREPARING THE CRITICALLY ILL CHILD FOR TRANSPORT

If a critically ill child must be transported to or from any critical care area within a hospital or to another health care facility, a safe transport must be planned. Optimal communication between hospital departments or the referring and receiving facilities is necessary for a successful transport. Guidelines and interventions that can be used for transporting the critically ill child include the following[47]:

1. Knowledge of the destination: To determine the length of time the patient will be at the alternate setting and what is needed, call ahead.
2. Evaluation of patient stability: Determine the risk/benefit of transport. Assess the level of intervention the patient has needed in the last 2 to 4 hours.
3. Maintenance of the airway: Anticipate potential emergencies and associated equipment needs. Secure ETT with tape that is well-anchored around the tube and face. Assign someone to manually hold the ETT while "bagging" and moving the patient.

   Disconnect the ETT from ambu bag when moving the patient to and from the stretcher.

   Suction the ETT just before leaving the unit. Take extra pediatric suction catheters and saline.

   Take a self-inflatable bag and correct size mask for all patients who have an ETT.

   Take an extra ETT for all intubated patients. Take pediatric intubation equipment if the patient is going to an area that is not familiar with pediatric patients. Take an extra trach tube and scissors for all patients who have a tracheostomy tube. Take full E-cylinder oxygen tanks. Check the gauge on the tank, and take oxygen masks for delivery of supplemental oxygen.
4. Continuous monitoring: Check battery on all portable ECG, respiratory, and pressure waveform monitors. Take vital signs every 15 minutes to ½ hour, including a check of neurological function. Monitor arterial pressure, intracranial pressure, or pulmonary artery catheters if applicable. Always take a blood pressure cuff. Monitor oximetry in selected cases.

5. Maintenance of IV access: Check for a blood return and check the skin around IV catheter site. Make sure IV is anchored to the skin and protected from dislodgement.

   Have extra vascular volume expanders (NS, lactated Ringers [LR], blood) for those patients who require frequent fluid boluses. IVs should be regulated by a pump if the patient is fluid restricted or has drip medications (attach more than one IV pump to one IV pole).

6. Immobilization: Immobilize combative or active patients to protect them from injury.

   For infants, use stockinette restraints for arms and legs. These can be safety pinned to the bedding, but detach them when transferring the infant out of the bed. For children, use arm and leg restraints (even on those patients who are recovering from anesthesia).

   Maintain C-spine precautions for all children with a suspected head or neck injury.

   For infants/toddlers, use two 10 lb sandbags, one on either side of the head, taping across the forehead to each sandbag. For older children, maintain neck collar placement. Notify physician to help move the patient. Secure drainage bags to the bed or stretcher. Avoid securing items to the side rail.

7. Temperature regulation: Cover the child sufficiently with blankets. For infants, swaddle them in blankets and use head covering (stockinette caps). Have warming lights/blankets/radiant warmers ready on return from the transport.

8. Medications: Emergency IV push medications include atropine, epinephrine 1:10,000, sodium bicarbonate, and 50% dextrose. Have a pediatric emergency drug card with drug doses calculated for the patient's weight, and have narcotics, sedatives, or anticonvulsants available for combative or seizing patients.

REFERENCES

1. Behrman RE, Vaughan VC, and Nelson WE: Nelson textbook of pediatrics, ed 13, Philadelphia, 1987, WB Saunders Co, p 1814.
2. Brown PA et al: Quick reference to pediatric intensive care nursing, Rockville, Md, 1989, Aspen Publishers, Inc.
3. Bruce D et al: Diffuse cerebral swelling following head injuries in children: the syndrome of "malignant brain edema," J Neurosurg 54:170, 1981.

4. Bruce D et al: Pathophysiology, treatment and outcome following severe head injury in children, Child's Brain 5:174, 1979.

5. Chameides L: Textbook of pediatric advanced life support, Dallas, 1988, American Academy of Pediatrics and American Heart Association.

6. Crowley C and Morrow A: A comprehensive approach to the child in respiratory failure, Crit Care Q 3:27, 1980.

7. Davis R et al: Head and spinal cord injury. In Rogers MC (ed): Textbook of pediatric intensive care, Baltimore, 1987, Williams & Wilkins, Inc.

8. Diprose GK et al: Dinamapp fails to detect hypotension in the very low birthweight infants, Arch Dis Child 61:771, 1986.

9. Disabato J and Wulf J: Nursing strategies: altered neurologic function. In Foster R, Hunsberger M, and Anderson J (eds): Family centered nursing care of children, Philadelphia, 1989, WB Saunders Co.

10. Fields AI: Respiratory support and mechanical ventilation, Pediatric Critical Care Clinical Review Series: Part I, Society of Critical Care Medicine, pp 75-81, 1989.

11. Fiser DH: Intraosseous infusion, N Engl J Med 322(22): 1579-1581, 1990.

12. Golden GS: Textbook of pediatric neurology, New York, 1987, Plenum Medical Book Co.

13. Guyton A: Textbook of medical physiology, ed 7, Philadelphia, 1986, WB Saunders Co.

14. Hazinski MF: Hemodynamic monitoring in children. In Daily EK and Schroeder JS (eds): Techniques in bedside hemodynamic monitoring, ed 4, St Louis, 1989, The CV Mosby Co, pp 247-315.

15. Hazinski MF: Understanding fluid balance in the seriously ill child, Ped Nurs 14(3):231-236, 1988.

16. Hazinski MF: Nursing care of the critically ill child, ed 2, St Louis, 1991, The CV Mosby Co, pp 1-11.

17. Hazinski MF: Critical care of the pediatric cardiovascular patient, Nurs Clin North Am 16(4):671-697, 1981.

18. Hunsberger M and Isseman R: Nursing strategies: altered digestive function. In Foster R, Hunsberger M, and Anderson J (eds): Family centered nursing care of children, Philadelphia, 1989, WB Saunders Co.

19. Kennedy J: Renal disorders. In Hazinski MF (ed): Nursing care of the critically ill child, St Louis, 1984, The CV Mosby Co, pp 455-546.

20. Kidder C: Reestablishing health factors influencing the child's recovery in pediatric intensive care, J Ped Nurs 4(2):96-103, 1989.

21. Kirsch CSB: Pharmacotherapeutics for the neonate and the pediatric patient. In Kuhn MM (ed): Pharmacotherapeutics: a nursing process approach, ed 2, Philadelphia, 1991, FA Davis Co, p 319.

22. Landier WC, Barrell ML, and Styffe EJ: How to administer blood components to children, MCN 12(3):178-184, 1987.

23. Lowrey GH: Growth and development of children, ed 7, Chicago, 1978, Year Book Medical Publishers, Inc.

24. Mayer T: Emergency management of pediatric trauma, St Louis, 1985, The CV Mosby Co.

25. Mayer T and Walker M: Emergency intracranial pressure monitoring in pediatrics: management of the acute coma of brain insult, Clin Pediatr 21:391, 1982.

26. McWilliams BC: Mechanical ventilation in pediatric patients, Clin Chest Med 8(4):597-609, 1987.

27. Moloney-Harmon PA: The pediatric trauma patient. In Welton RH and Shane K (eds): Case studies in trauma nursing, Baltimore, 1989, Williams & Wilkins, Inc, pp 279-287.

28. Petrillo M and Sanger S: Emotional care of hospitalized children: an environmental approach, ed 2, Philadelphia, 1980, JB Lippincott.

29. Pollack M: Nutritional failure and support in pediatric intensive care. In Shoemaker W et al (eds): Textbook of critical care, ed 2, Philadelphia, 1989, WB Saunders Co.

30. Pollack M et al: Malnutrition in critically ill infants and children, JPEN 6:20, 1982.

31. Raphaely RC et al: Experience with pulmonary artery catheterizations in critically ill children, Crit Care Med 8:265, 1980.

32. Reily MD: The renal system. In Smith JB (ed): Pediatric critical care, New York, 1983, John Wiley & Sons, Inc, pp 305-414.

33. Rennick J: Re-establishing the parental role in the pediatric intensive care unit, J Pediatr Nurs 1:40-44, 1986.

34. Rosenthal CH: Pediatric critical care nursing in the adult ICU: essentials of practice, National Conference on Pediatric Critical Care Nursing, New York, 1990, Contemporary Forums.

35. Rosenthal CH: Immunosuppression in pediatric critical care patients, Crit Care Nurs Clin North Am 1(4):775-785, 1989.

36. Rossetti V et al: Difficulty and delay in intravascular access in pediatric arrests, Ann Emerg Med 13:406, 1984 (abstract).

37. Rubenstein J and Hageman J: Monitoring of critically ill infants and children, Crit Care Clin North Am 4:621, 1988.

38. Rushton CH: Family-centered care in the critical care setting: myth or reality? Child Health Care 19(2):68-78, 1990.

39. Schaefer C, Coyne JC, and Lazarus RS: The health-related functions of social support, J Behav Med 4:381-399, 1982.

40. Shelton T, Jeppson E, and Johnson B: Family centered care for children with special health care needs, Washington, DC, 1987, Association of the Care of Children's Health.
41. Slota M: Pediatric neurological assessment, Crit Care Nurse 3:106, 1983.
42. Smith JB (ed): Pediatric critical care, New York, 1983, John Wiley & Sons, Inc, pp 1-20.
43. Soupios M, Gallagher J, and Orlowski JP: Nursing aspects of pediatric intensive care in a general hospital, Ped Clin North Am 27(3):621-633, 1980.
44. Sperhac AM and Harper J: Physical assessment. In Mott SR, James SR, and Sperhac AM (eds): Nursing care of children and families, ed 2, Redwood City, Calif, 1990, Addison-Wesley, pp 343-400.
45. Susla GM and Dionne RE: Pharmacokinetics-pharmacodynamics: drug delivery and therapeutic drug monitoring. In Holbrook P (ed): Textbook of pediatric critical care, Philadelphia, WB Saunders Co (in press).
46. Tietjen SD: Starting an infant's IV, Am J Nurs May, pp 44-47, 1990.
47. Tomkins J: Guidelines for intrahospital transport, Ped Nurs 16(1):50-53, 1990.
48. Trad PV: Psychosocial scenarios for pediatrics, New York, 1988, Springer-Verlag.
49. Tribett D and Brenner M: Peripheral and femoral vein cannulation, Prob Crit Care 2(2):266-285, 1988.
50. Turner BS: Maintaining the artificial airway: current concepts, Pediatr Nurs 16(5):487-489, 1990.
51. Van Lente F and Pippenger CE: The pediatric acute care laboratory, Pediatr Clin North Am 34(1):231-246, 1987.
52. Wofford LG: The pediatric patient. In Price MS and Fox JD (eds): Hemodynamic monitoring in critical care, Rockville, Md, 1987, Aspen Publishers, Inc.

Glossary

afterload The force the ventricles must overcome to eject blood

angioedema Giant wheal, reaction of the subcutaneous or submucosal tissue resulting in localized edema

antrectomy The surgical excision of the pyloric part of the stomach

anuria Absence of urine formation, usually < 75 ml/day

areflexia Absence of reflexes

asterixis Flapping tremor, usually a sign of neurological irritation

atelectasis Collapse of alveoli that results in a loss of surface area available for gas exchange

autoregulation The body's ability to control blood flow despite changes in arterial blood pressure

azotemia Presence of nitrogen compounds in the blood (elevated BUN level)

Brudzinski's sign Flexion of the knee and hip in response to bending the patient's head toward the chest, a sign of meningeal irritation

cardiovert Application of electrical current synchronized to the QRS complex to terminate a tachydysrhythmia

carpopedal The wrist (carpal) and foot (pedal)

Chvostek's sign Spasm of facial muscles elicited on tapping the area over the facial nerve, sign of tetany

circumoral Around the mouth; circumoral pallor or cyanosis refers to paleness or bluish color around the mouth

colloid Solutions that cannot pass through semipermeable membranes (e.g., dextran, albumin), usually retained in the intravascular space and used to restore volume

contractility Ability of the cell to shorten and lengthen its muscle fiber

contralateral Pertaining to the opposite side

crystalloid Solutions that can pass through semipermeable membranes (e.g., D_5W, NS)

decerebrate Bilateral extension, internal rotation, and wrist flexion; bilateral extension, internal rotation, and plantar flexion of lower extremities

decorticate Bilateral adduction of shoulders; extension, internal rotation, and plantar flexion of lower extremities; pronation and flexion of elbows and wrists

defibrillate Application of nonsynchronized electrical current to the myocardium to terminate a life-threatening dysrhythmia

dehiscence Separation or splitting open of a surgical wound

dermatome Area of skin supplied by nerve fibers

distal Farthest from the point of origin

dysesthesia Impaired sensation (out of proportion to the stimulus)

dysphasia Impairment of speech (e.g., inability to arrange words in the proper order)

dysrhythmia Any disorder of rate, rhythm, electrical impulse origin, or conduction within the heart

ecchymosis Nonraised, purplish hemorrhagic spot larger than a petechia

ectopy Arising from an abnormal site (e.g., ectopic beats are impulses arising outside the normal electrical conduction system of the heart)

empyema Pus accumulation in a body cavity

encephalopathy Degeneration of the brain caused by several conditions or diseases

endocardial Layer of cells that line the cavity of the heart

escharotomy Surgical incision of the burned body part to reduce pressure on tissues and restore blood flow

eupnea Normal respiration

flaccid Weak muscles

gastroduodenostomy Surgical connection of the duodenum and stomach (Billroth I procedure)

gastroenterostomy Surgical connection of the stomach and intestine

gastrojejunostomy Surgical connection of the stomach and jejunum (Billroth II procedure)

gastroparesis Paralysis of the stomach

gavage Feeding through a tube

hemianopsia Blindness in half of the visual field

hemoptysis Blood in sputum, coughing up of blood

hypercapnea Elevated carbon dioxide in the blood

hypercarbia Elevated carbon dioxide in the blood

hyperpyrexia Elevated temperature, fever, hyperthermia

hypertonic An osmolality greater than fluids it is being compared to (i.e., hypertonic IV fluids such as D_5NS and $D_{10}W$ refer to an osmolality > 300 and, if infused, can cause cells to shrink and circulatory overload)

hypokinesia Decreased movement or motion (e.g., a hypokinetic ventricle refers to decreased contraction [motion] of the ventricle)

hypotonic An osmolality less than fluids it is being compared to (i.e., hypotonic IV fluids such as 0.45NS refer to an osmolality < 300 and, if infused, can cause cells to swell, hypotension, and fluid depletion)

hypoxemia Deficient oxygenation in the blood

hypoxia Reduced oxygen availability to the tissues

inotropic   Pertaining to the force or strength of muscular contraction

ipsilateral   Pertaining to the same side

isotonic   The same osmolality of fluid it is being compared to (i.e., isotonic IV fluids such as 0.9NS and lactated Ringers refer to solutions that do not affect flow of water across the cell membranes)

Kernig's sign   Inability to completely extend the leg when the thigh is flexed on the abdomen

lateralizing   Pertaining to one side

lavage   Irrigation of a cavity or organ such as the stomach

leukocytosis   Increase in number of leukocytes (basophils, eosinophils, neutrophils, monocytes, lymphocytes)

leukopenia   Decrease in number of leukocytes (usually < 5000/μl)

myoglobinuria   Presence of myoglobin (globulin from muscle) in the urine

nuchal rigidity   Stiff neck

oliguria   Urine volume < 400 ml/day

otorrhea   Discharge from the ear

papilledema   Edema of the optic disk

paraplegia   Paralysis of the lower extremities

parenchyma   The essential elements of an organ

petechia   Nonraised, round, purplish spots caused by intradermal or submucous hemorrhages

pheochromocytoma   A tumor of the adrenal medulla that secretes epinephrine and norepinephrine, resulting in severe hypertension, increased metabolism, and hyperglycemia

photophobia   Intolerance to light

polydipsia   Excessive thirst

polyuria   Excessive urination

postictal   Following a seizure

preload   Volume of blood in the ventricles at the end of diastole

proprioception   Pertaining to the position of the body; involves balance, coordination, and posture

proximal   Closest or nearest to the point of origin

pyloroplasty   Surgery involving the pylorus, usually to enlarge the communication between the stomach and duodenum

quadriplegia   Paralysis of all four extremities

rhabdomyolysis   Skeletal muscle injury that results in release of substances such as myoglobin that are potentially toxic to the kidney

rhinorrhea   Discharge from the nose

stomatitis   Inflammation of the oral mucosa

thrombocytopenia   Reduction in the number of platelets

tonic-clonic   Involuntary muscular contraction and relaxation in rapid succession

Trendelenberg Position in which the patient is supine and the head is down

Trousseau's sign Carpal spasm on compression of the upper arm, sign of tetany

urticaria Hives, vascular reaction that results in wheals and itching (pruritus)

vagotomy The surgical interruption of the vagus nerve, usually performed to reduce gastric secretions in the treatment of ulcers

ventilation Movement of air between the lungs and environment

*ACLS Algorithms**

Asystole

If rhythm is unclear and VF is possible,
defibrillate as for VF—If asystole is present*

↓

Continue CPR

↓

Establish IV access

↓

Epinephrine, 1:10,000, 0.5-1.0 mg IV push†

↓

Intubate when possible‡

↓

Atropine, 1.0 mg IV push (repeated in 5 min)

↓

(Consider bicarbonate)§

↓

Consider pacing

Figure A-1 Asystole (cardiac standstill). This sequence was developed to assist in teaching how to treat a broad range of patients with asystole. Some patients may require care not specified herein. This algorithm should not be construed to prohibit such flexibility. Flow of algorithm presumes asystole is continuing.
VF, Ventricular fibrillation; *IV,* intravenous.
*Asystole should be confirmed in two leads.
†Epinephrine should be repeated every 5 minutes.
‡Intubation is preferable; if it can be accomplished simultaneously with other techniques, the earlier the better. However, cardiopulmonary resuscitation *(CPR)* and use of epinephrine are more important initially if patient can be ventilated without intubation. (Endotracheal epinephrine may be used.)
§Value of sodium bicarbonate is questionable during cardiac arrest, and it is not recommended for the routine cardiac arrest sequence. Consideration of its use in a dose of 1 mEq/kg is appropriate . Half of original dose may be repeated every 10 minutes if it is used.

From American Heart Association: Textbook of advanced cardiac life support, Dallas, 1987, American Heart Association.

Ventricular Fibrillation

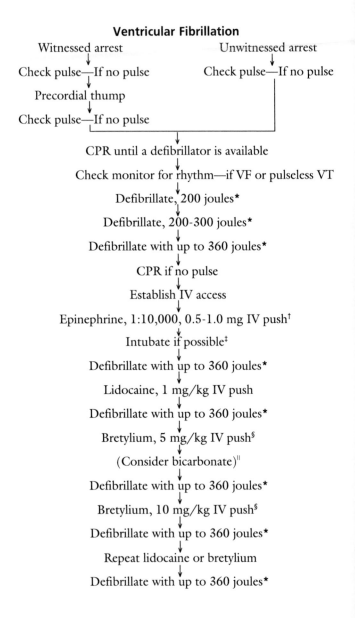

Witnessed arrest   Unwitnessed arrest

Check pulse—If no pulse   Check pulse—If no pulse

Precordial thump

Check pulse—If no pulse

CPR until a defibrillator is available

Check monitor for rhythm—if VF or pulseless VT

Defibrillate, 200 joules*

Defibrillate, 200-300 joules*

Defibrillate with up to 360 joules*

CPR if no pulse

Establish IV access

Epinephrine, 1:10,000, 0.5-1.0 mg IV push†

Intubate if possible‡

Defibrillate with up to 360 joules*

Lidocaine, 1 mg/kg IV push

Defibrillate with up to 360 joules*

Bretylium, 5 mg/kg IV push§

(Consider bicarbonate)‖

Defibrillate with up to 360 joules*

Bretylium, 10 mg/kg IV push§

Defibrillate with up to 360 joules*

Repeat lidocaine or bretylium

Defibrillate with up to 360 joules*

Figure A-2   Ventricular fibrillation (and pulseless ventricular tachycardia). This sequence was developed to assist in teaching how to treat a broad range of patients with ventricular fibrillation *(VF)* or pulseless ventricular tachycardia *(VT)*. Some patients may require care not specified herein. This algorithm should not be construed as prohibiting such flexibility. Flow of algorithm presumes that VF is continuing. Pulseless VT should be treated identically to VF.
CPR, cardiopulmonary resuscitation.
*Check pulse and rhythm after each shock. If VF recurs after transiently converting (rather than persists without ever converting), use whatever energy level has previously been successful for defibrillation.
†Epinephrine should be repeated every 5 minutes.
‡Intubation is preferable. If it can be accompanied simultaneously with other techniques, the earlier the better. However, defibrillation and epinephrine are more important initially if the patient can be ventilated without intubation.
§Some may prefer repeated doses of lidocaine, which may be given in 0.5 mg/kg boluses every 8 minutes to a total dose of 3 mg/kg.
‖Value of sodium bicarbonate is questionable during cardiac arrest, and it is not recommended for routine cardiac arrest sequence. Consideration of its use in a dose of 1 mEq/kg is appropriate at this point. Half of original dose may be repeated every 10 minutes if it is used.

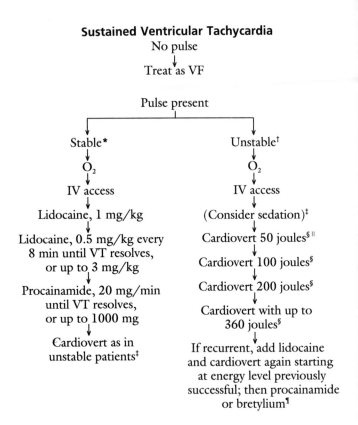

Sustained Ventricular Tachycardia

No pulse
↓
Treat as VF

Pulse present

Stable*
↓
O₂
↓
IV access
↓
Lidocaine, 1 mg/kg
↓
Lidocaine, 0.5 mg/kg every
8 min until VT resolves,
or up to 3 mg/kg
↓
Procainamide, 20 mg/min
until VT resolves,
or up to 1000 mg
↓
Cardiovert as in
unstable patients‡

Unstable†
↓
O₂
↓
IV access
↓
(Consider sedation)‡
↓
Cardiovert 50 joules§ ‖
↓
Cardiovert 100 joules§
↓
Cardiovert 200 joules§
↓
Cardiovert with up to
360 joules§
↓
If recurrent, add lidocaine
and cardiovert again starting
at energy level previously
successful; then procainamide
or bretylium¶

Figure A-3 Sustained ventricular tachycardia *(VT)*. This sequence
was developed to assist in teaching how to treat a broad range of patients with sustained VT. Some patients may require care not specified
herein. This algorithm should not be construed as prohibiting such
flexibility. Flow of algorithm presumes that VT is continuing.
VF, Ventricular fibrillation.
*If patient becomes unstable† at any time, move to "Unstable" arm of
algorithm.
†Unstable indicates symptoms (e.g., chest pain or dyspnea), hypotension (systolic blood pressure <90 mm Hg), congestive heart failure,
ischemia, or infarction.
‡Sedation should be considered for all patients, including those defined as unstable, except those who are hemodynamically unstable
(e.g., hypotensive, in pulmonary edema, or unconscious).
§If hypotension, pulmonary edema, or unconsciousness is present, unsynchronized cardioversion should be done to avoid delay associated
with synchronization. *Continued.*

Electromechanical Dissociation

Continue CPR

↓

Establish IV access

↓

Epinephrine, 1:10,000, 0.5-1.0 mg IV push*

↓

Intubate when possible†

↓

(Consider bicarbonate)‡

↓

Consider hypovolemia,
cardiac tamponade,
tension pneumothorax,
hypoxemia, acidosis,
pulmonary embolism

Figure A-4 Electromechanical dissociation. This sequence was developed to assist in teaching how to treat a broad range of patients with electromechanical dissociation. Some patients may require care not specified herein. This algorithm should not be construed to prohibit such flexibility. Flow of algorithm presumes that electromechanical dissociation is continuing.

CPR, Cardiopulmonary resuscitation; *IV,* intravenous.

*Epinephrine should be repeated every 5 minutes.

†Intubation is preferable. If it can be accomplished simultaneously with other techniques, the earlier the better. However, epinephrine is more important initially if the patient can be ventilated without intubation.

‡Value of sodium bicarbonate is questionable during cardiac arrest, and it is not recommended for routine cardiac arrest sequence. Consideration of its use in a dose of 1 mEq/kg is appropriate at this point. Half of original dose may be repeated every 10 minutes if it is used.

Figure A-3—cont'd.

‖In the absence of hypotension, pulmonary edema, or unconsciousness, a precordial thump may be employed before cardioversion.

¶Once VT has resolved, begin intravenous *(IV)* infusion of antidysrhythmic agent that has aided resolution of VT. If hypotension, pulmonary edema, or unconsciousness is present, use lidocaine if cardioversion alone is unsuccessful, followed by bretylium. In all other patients, the recommended order of therapy is lidocaine, procainamide, and then bretylium.

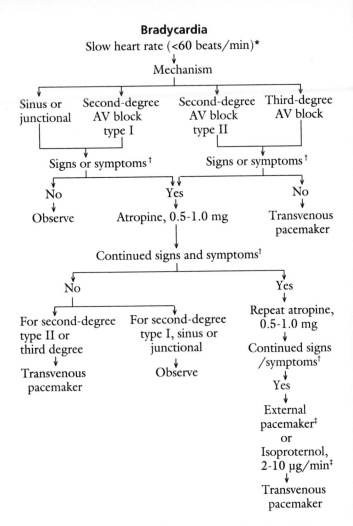

Bradycardia

Slow heart rate (<60 beats/min)*

↓

Mechanism

Sinus or junctional | Second-degree AV block type I | Second-degree AV block type II | Third-degree AV block

Signs or symptoms†   Signs or symptoms†

No → Observe

Yes → Atropine, 0.5-1.0 mg

No → Transvenous pacemaker

Continued signs and symptoms†

No

Yes

For second-degree type II or third degree → Transvenous pacemaker

For second-degree type I, sinus or junctional → Observe

Repeat atropine, 0.5-1.0 mg

↓

Continued signs /symptoms†

↓

Yes

↓

External pacemaker‡ or Isoproternol, 2-10 µg/min‡

↓

Transvenous pacemaker

Figure A-5 Bradycardia. This sequence was developed to assist in teaching how to treat a broad range of patients with bradycardia. Some patients may require care not specified herein. This algorithm should not be construed to prohibit such flexibility.

AV, Atrioventricular.

*A solitary chest thump or cough may stimulate cardiac electrical activity and result in improved CO and may be used at this point.

†Hypotension (blood pressure <90 mm Hg), premature ventricular contractions, altered mental status or symptoms (e.g., chest pain or dyspnea), ischemia, or infarction.

‡Temporizing therapy.

Ventricular Ectopy

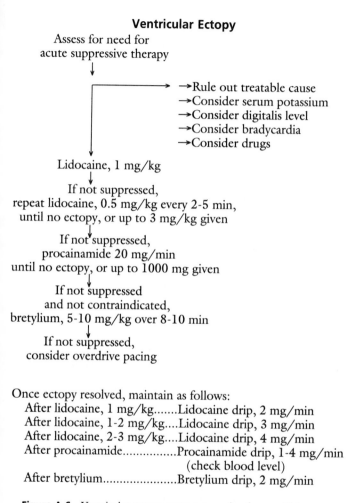

Assess for need for
acute suppressive therapy

→Rule out treatable cause
→Consider serum potassium
→Consider digitalis level
→Consider bradycardia
→Consider drugs

Lidocaine, 1 mg/kg

If not suppressed,
repeat lidocaine, 0.5 mg/kg every 2-5 min,
until no ectopy, or up to 3 mg/kg given

If not suppressed,
procainamide 20 mg/min
until no ectopy, or up to 1000 mg given

If not suppressed
and not contraindicated,
bretylium, 5-10 mg/kg over 8-10 min

If not suppressed,
consider overdrive pacing

Once ectopy resolved, maintain as follows:
After lidocaine, 1 mg/kg.......Lidocaine drip, 2 mg/min
After lidocaine, 1-2 mg/kg....Lidocaine drip, 3 mg/min
After lidocaine, 2-3 mg/kg....Lidocaine drip, 4 mg/min
After procainamide................Procainamide drip, 1-4 mg/min
(check blood level)
After bretylium.......................Bretylium drip, 2 mg/min

Figure A-6 Ventricular ectopy: acute suppressive therapy. This sequence was developed to assist in teaching how to treat a broad range of patients with ventricular ectopy. Some patients may require therapy not specified herein. This algorithm should not be construed as prohibiting such flexibility.

Paroxysmal Supraventricular Tachycardia

Unstable	Stable
↓	↓
Synchronous cardioversion 75-100 joules	Vagal maneuvers
↓	↓
Synchronous cardioversion 200 joules	Verapamil, 5 mg IV
↓	↓
Synchronous cardioversion 360 joules	Verapamil, 10 mg IV (in 15-20 min)
↓	↓
Correct underlying abnormalities	Cardioversion, digoxin, ß blockers, pacing as indicated
↓	
Pharmacological therapy+ Cardioversion	

Figure A-7   Paroxysmal supraventricular tachycardia (PSVT). This sequence was developed to assist in teaching how to treat a broad range of patients with sustained PSVT. Some patients may require care not specified herein. This algorithm should not be construed as prohibiting such flexibility. Flow of algorithm presumes PSVT is continuing. If conversion occurs but PSVT recurs, repeated electrical cardioversion is *not* indicated. Sedation should be used as time permits.

Laboratory Values

COMPLETE BLOOD COUNT

RBC	$4.25\text{-}5.5 \times 10^6/\mu l$ (males)
	$3.6\text{-}5.0 \times 10^6/\mu l$ (females)
WBC	$5\text{-}10 \times 10^3/\mu l$
Hgb	13.5-17.5 g/dl (males)
	12-16 g/dl (females)
Hct	40%-54% (males)
	37%-47% (females)

COAGULATION

Plts	$150\text{-}350 \times 10^3/\mu l$
PT	10-14 sec
PTT	30-45 sec
APTT	16-25 sec
ACT	92-128 sec
FSP	<10 μg/dl

CHEMISTRY

Albumin	3.5-5 g/dl
Alkaline phosphatase	25-97 U/L
Alanine aminotransferase (ALT/SGPT)	4-35 U/L
Ammonia	18-54 μmol/L (males)
	12-50 μmol/L (females)
Amylase	4-25 U/ml
Anion gap	8-16 mEq/L
Aspartate aminotransferase (AST/SGOT)	8-33 U/L
Bilirubin	
Direct	0-0.2 mg/dl
Total	0.2-1.0 mg/dl
Indirect	Total − direct
BUN	10-20 mg/dl
BUN:Cr ratio	10:1-15:1
Calcium	8.5-10.5 mg/dl

Cholesterol . . . . . . 120-200 mg/dl
  HDL . . . . 26-63 mg/dl (males)
  . . . . 39-92 mg/dl (females)
  LDL . . . . 70-180 mg/dl
  . . . . <130 is desirable
  LDL/HDL ratio . . . <3.0
  Cholesterol/HDL ratio. <4.5
Chloride. . . . . 98-106 mEq/L
CO_2 . . . . 24-32 mEq/L
Creatinine . . . . 0.7-1.3 mg/dl (males)
  . . . . 0.6-1.2 mg/dl (females)
Glucose . . . . 70-110 mg/dl
Iron . . . . 50-150 μg/dl
Lactate . . . . 0.5-2.2 mEq/L
Lactic dehydrogenase
(LDH) . . . . 70-250 U/L
Lipase. . . . . 4-24 U/L
Magnesium . . . . . . 1.3-2.1 mEq/L
Osmolality. . . . . . . 275-295 mOsm/kg
Potassium . . . . 3.5-5.0 mEq/L
Phosphorus . . . . . . 2.5-4.5 mg/dl
Protein . . . . 6-8 g/dl
Sedimentation rate . . . 0-10 mm/hr (males)
  . . 0-15 mm/hr (females)
Sodium . . . . 135-145 mEq/L
T_3 . . . . 0.8-1.1 μg/dl
T_4 . . . . 4.5-11.5 μg/dl
Triglyceride . . . . . . 46-316 mg/dl (males, 30-40 yr)
  . . . . . . 75-313 mg/dl (males, >50 yr)
  . . . . . . 37-174 mg/dl (females, 30-40 yr)
  . . . . . . 52-280 mg/dl (females >50 yr)
Uric acid . . . . 3.5-8 mg/dl

CARDIAC PROFILE
SGOT (AST) . . . . . 6-18 U/L (females)
  . . . . . 7-21 U/L (males)
  With MI
    Onset . . . . . . 12-18 hr
    Peak . . . . . . 24-48 hr
    Duration . . . . . 3-4 days
CK . . . . 96-140 U/L (females)
  . . . . 38-174 U/L (males)

With MI
   Onset . . . . 4-6 hr
   Peak . . . . 12-24 hr
   Duration . . . . . 3-4 days
CK-MB 0%
  With MI
   Onset . . . . 4-6 hr
   Peak . . . . 12-24 hr
   Duration . . . . . 2-3 days
LDH . . . . 70-180 mg/dl
  With MI
   Onset . . . . 24-48 hr
   Peak . . . . 3-6 days
   Duration . . . . . 7-10 days
LDH_1 . . . . 17.5%-28.3% of total LDH
LDH_2 . . . . 30.4%-36.4% of total LDH
  With MI
  $LDH_1 > LDH_2$
   Onset . . . . 12-24 hr
   Peak . . . . 48 hr
   Duration . . . . . Variable

URINE ELECTROLYTES

Na . . . . 40-220 mEq/day
K . . . . 25-125 mEq/day
Cl . . . . 110-250 mEq/day

CSF

Pressure (initial) . . . 70-180 mm H_2O
Albumin . . . . 11-48 mg/dl
Cell count . . . . . . 0-5 mononuclear cells
Chloride . . . . 120-130 mEq/L
Glucose . . . . 50-75 mg/dl
IgG . . . . 0-8.6 mg/dl
Protein . . . . 15-45 mg/dl

DRUG LEVELS

Digoxin . . . . 1-2 ng/ml
Phenytoin . . . . . . 10-20 µg/ml
Theophylline . . . . . 10-20 µg/ml
Barbiturate coma . . . . 10 mg/dl
Gentamicin
  Trough . . . . 1-2 µg/ml
  Peak . . . . 6-8 µg/ml

Lidocaine . . . . .1.5-5 µg/ml
Tobramycin
  Trough . . . . .1-2 µg/ml
  Peak . . . . .6-8 µg/ml
Vancomycin
  Trough . . . . .5-10 µg/ml
  Peak . . . . .30-40 µg/ml

BLOOD GASES
Arterial
O_2 sat 95%
P_{O_2} . . . . .80-100 mm Hg
P_{CO_2} . . . . .35-45 mm Hg
pH 7.35-7.45
HCO_3 . . . . .22-26 mEq/L

Venous
O_2 sat 60%-80%
P_{O_2} . . . . .35-45 mm Hg
P_{CO_2} . . . . .41-51 mm Hg
pH 7.31-7.41
HCO_3 . . . . .22-26 mEq/L

Organ/Tissue Donation

Organs including the kidneys, heart, pancreas, and liver can be donated for transplantation. A heart-beating, brain-dead cadaver is mandatory, and blood type is required.

Tissues including skin, bone, eye, ear, heart valves, and soft tissues can also be transplanted. Tissue donation does not require a heart-beating cadaver because the tissues are avascular when transplanted. Organs and tissues may also be donated for medical research.

Potential Donor Identification

a. Brain-dead patients (see p. 11 for brain-death criteria)
b. No active infection
c. No history of transmissible disease
d. No previous disease of the organ/tissue (e.g., renal disease, insulin-dependent diabetes mellitus, rheumatoid arthritis, malignancy [except brain tumor], bone disease)
e. Any age (physiological age is considered)
f. Anyone, regardless of medical history or age, is eligible for eye donation, and donation of organs and tissues for biomedical research.

Resources Available

a. Contact your local organ-procurement organization
b. Call the national 24-hour donation hotline: 1-800-24DONOR
c. International Institute for Advancement of Medicine (donation for research): 215-363-3600
d. National Disease Research Interchange (donation for research): 215-557-7361

General Guidelines: Care of the Donor*

Respiratory function

OUTCOMES

- pH 7.35-7.45
- Pao_2 70-100 mm Hg
- O_2 sat $\geq$ 95%
- Absence of peripheral cyanosis
- Absence of adventitious lung sounds

INTERVENTIONS
- Regulate ventilator settings as needed.
- Monitor peak inspiratory pressure and suction prn.
- Assess nail beds.
- Auscultate lung fields.
- Turn patient frequently, if appropriate.
- Assess chest wall excursion.
- Prevent or aggressively treat pneumothorax.

Cardiovascular function

OUTCOMES
- SBP $\geq$ 100 mm Hg

INTERVENTIONS
- Administer crystalloids/colloids to keep SBP $\geq$ 100 mm Hg.
- Administer PRBCs if Hct < 30%.
- Administer dopamine to keep SBP $\geq$ 100 mm Hg, if necessary.
- Monitor fluid losses.
- Monitor for fluid overload (CVP).

Renal function

OUTCOMES
- u/o ~ 100 ml/hr
- CVP: 8-10 cm H_2O
- BUN: 10-20 mg/dl
- Creatinine: 0.6-1.2 mg/dl

INTERVENTIONS
- Assist with CVP insertion.
- Administer fluids such as Ringers lactate, hespan, plasmanate to maintain CVP.
- Administer dopamine if necessary to increase renal perfusion.

- Administer diuretics (mannitol, furosemide) to increase u/o if patient is hydrated and BP stable.
- Monitor BP, CVP, u/o q1h.
- Monitor kidney function (BUN, Cr) and electrolytes.

If diabetes insipidus occurs:

- Administer aqueous pitressin as an infusion and titrate to keep u/o between 200-400 ml/hr.
- Replace u/o ml for ml.
- Administer additional fluids as necessary.

*Organ-specific protocols are used—contact your local organ-procurement agency.

Guidelines for Avascular Tissues

Cornea

- Apply ophthalmic saline solution to eyes; tape eyes closed.
- Apply cold compresses to eyes.
- Elevate HOB.

Skin

- Turn patient frequently.
- Assess for skin breakdown/infection.

REFERENCES

Hagan T: Personal communication, Arizona Organ Bank, Phoenix, May, 1990.

Kozlowski L: Case study in identification and maintenance of an organ donor, Heart Lung 17(4):366-371, 1988.

Norris MK: How to manage tissue donation, Am J Nurs 89(10):1300-1302, 1989.

Organ and tissue donor manual: Arizona Organ Bank, Dec 1988, Phoenix.

Snyder L and Peter N: How to manage organ donation, Am J Nurs 89(10):1294-1298, 1989.

Scoring Tools

TRAUMA SCORE

Assessment parameter		Trauma score
Glasgow coma scale	14-15	5
score	11-13	4
	8-10	3
	5-7	2
	3-4	1
Respiratory rate	10-24	4
	25-35	3
	>35	2
	1-9	1
	0	0
Respiratory expansion	Normal	1
	Shallow	0
	Retractive	0
Systolic blood pressure	>90	4
	70-90	3
	50-69	2
	1-49	1
No carotid pulse	0	0
Capillary refill	Normal	2
	Delayed	1
	None	0

From Champion HR, Gainer PS, and Yackee E: A progress report on the trauma score in predicting a fatal outcome, J Trauma 26:927-931, 1988; and Champion HR et al: Trauma score, Crit Care Med 9(9):672-676, 1981.

TRAUMA SCORE

Projected estimate of survival	
Trauma score	**Percentage survival**
16	99
15	98
14	96
13	93
12	87
11	76
10	60
9	42
8	26
7	15
6	8
5	4
4	2
3	1
2	0
1	0

THERAPEUTIC INTERVENTION SCORING SYSTEM (TISS)

4 Points

a. Cardiac arrest and/or countershock within past 48 hr*
b. Controlled ventilation with or without PEEP*
c. Controlled ventilation with intermittent or continuous muscle relaxants*
d. Balloon tamponade of varices*
e. Continuous arterial infusion*
f. Pulmonary artery catheter
g. Atrial and/or ventricular pacing*
h. Hemodialysis in unstable patient*
i. Peritoneal dialysis
j. Induced hypothermia*
k. Pressure-activated blood infusion*
l. G-suit
m. Intracranial pressure monitoring
n. Platelet transfusion
o. IABA (intraaortic balloon assist)
p. Emergency operative procedures (within past 24 hr)*
q. Lavage of acute GI bleeding
r. Emergency endoscopy or bronchoscopy
s. Vasoactive drug infusion (>1 drug)

2 Points

a. CVP (central venous pressure)
b. 2 peripheral IV catheters
c. Hemodialysis—stable patient
d. Fresh tracheostomy (less than 48 hr)
e. Spontaneous respiration via endotracheal tube or tracheostomy (T-piece or trach mask)
f. GI feedings
g. Replacement of excess fluid loss*
h. Parenteral chemotherapy
i. Hourly neuro vital signs
j. Multiple dressing changes
k. Pitressin infusion IV

3 Points

a. Central IV hyperalimentation (includes renal, cardiac, hepatic failure fluid)
b. Pacemaker on standby
c. Chest tubes
d. Intermittent mandatory ventilation (IMV) or assisted ventilation*
e. Continuous positive airway pressure (CPAP)
f. Concentrated K^+ infusion via central catheter
g. Nasotracheal or orotracheal intubation*
h. Blind intratracheal suctioning

1 Point

a. ECG monitoring
b. Hourly vital signs
c. 1 peripheral IV catheter
d. Chronic anticoagulation
e. Standard intake and output (q24h)
f. STAT blood tests
g. Intermittent scheduled IV medications
h. Routine dressing changes
i. Standard orthopedic traction
j. Tracheostomy care

From Keene AR and Cullen DJ: Therapeutic intervention scoring system: update 1983, Crit Care Med 11(1):2, 1983.

*Therapeutic Intervention Scoring System explanation code:

4-Point Interventions: (a) Point score for 2 days after most recent cardiac arrest. (b) Does not mean intermittent mandatory ventilation (3-point intervention). Means that regardless of the internal plumbing of ventilator, the full ventilatory needs are being supplied by the machine. Whether the patient is ineffectively breathing around the ventilator is irrelevant as long as it is providing the needed minute ventilation. (c) For example, D-tubocurarine chloride, pancuronium (Pavulon), metocurine (Metubine). (d) Use Sengstaken-Blakemore or Linton tube for esophageal or gastric bleeding. (e) Pitressin infusion via IMA, SMA, gastric artery catheters for control of gastrointestinal bleeding, or other intraarterial infusion. Does not include standard 3 ml/hr heparin flush to maintain catheter patency. (g) Active pacing even if a chronic pacemaker. (h) Include first 2 runs of acute dialysis. Include chronic dialysis when medical situation renders dialysis unstable. (j) Continuous or intermittent cooling to achieve temperature <33° C. (k) Use of a blood pump or manual pumping in those requiring rapid blood replacement. (p) May be the initial emergency procedure—precludes diagnostic tests.

3-Point Interventions: (d) The patient is supplying some ventilatory needs. (g) Not a daily point score. Patient must have been intubated in the ICU (elective or emergency) within previous 24 hr. (i) Measurement of intake/output above normal 24-hr routine. Frequent adjustment of intake according to total output. (x) Includes Rheomacrodex. (bb) For example, Stryker frame. CircOlectric.

2-Point Interventions: (g) Replacement of clear fluids over and above the ordered maintenance level.

1-Point Intervention: (k) Must have a decubitus ulcer. Does not include preventive therapy.

Continued.

THERAPEUTIC INTERVENTION SCORING SYSTEM (TISS)

3 Points—cont'd

i. Complex metabolic balance (frequent I & O)*
j. Multiple ABG, bleeding, STAT studies (>4/shift)
k. Frequent infusions of blood products (>5 units/24 hr)
l. Bolus IV medication (nonscheduled)
m. Vasoactive drug infusion (1 drug)
n. Continuous antiarrhythmia infusions
o. Cardioversion for arrhythmia (not defibrillation)
p. Hypothermia blanket
q. Arterial line
r. Acute digitalization—within 48 hr
s. Measurement of cardiac output by any method
t. Active diuresis for fluid overload or cerebral edema
u. Active Rx for metabolic alkalosis
v. Active Rx for metabolic acidosis
w. Emergency thoracentesis, paracentesis, pericardiocentesis
x. Active anticoagulation (initial 48 hr)*
y. Phlebotomy for volume overload
z. Coverage with more than 2 IV antibiotics
aa. Rx of seizures, metabolic encephalopathy (48 hr of onset)
bb. Complicated orthopedic traction*

1 Point—cont'd

k. Decubitus ulcer*
l. Urinary catheter
m. Supplemental oxygen (nasal or mask)
n. Antibiotics IV (2 or less)
o. Chest physiotherapy
p. Extensive irrigations, packings, or debridement of wound, fistula, or colostomy
q. GI decompression
r. Peripheral hyperalimentation/intralipid therapy

For table footnote, see p. 693.

APACHE III SCORING COMPONENTS

Age Points

≤44	0
45-59	5
60-64	11
65-69	13
70-74	16
75-84	17
≥85	24

Chronic Health Points

Cirrhosis	4
Immunosuppression	10
Leukemia/multiple myeloma	10
Metastatic cancer	11
Lymphoma	13
Hepatic failure	16
AIDS	23

APACHE III Physiological Scoring for Vital Signs and Laboratory Tests

Pulse

8	5	0	1	5	7	13	17
≤39	40-49	50-99 beats/min	100-109	110-119	120-139	140-154	≥155

Mean BP

23	15	7	6	0	4	7	9	10
≤39	40-59	60-69	70-79	80-99 mm Hg	100-119	120-129	130-139	≥140

Temp

20	16	13	8	2	0	4
≤32.9	33-33.4	33.5-33.9	34-34.9	35-35.9	36°C-39.9°C	≥40

Respiratory rate*

17	8	7	0	6	9	11	18
≤5	6-11*	12-13	14-24 breaths/min	25-34	35-39	40-49	≥50

PaO_2†

15	5	2	0
≤49	50-69	70-79	≥80 mm Hg

A-aDO_2†

0	7	9	11	14
<100	100-249	250-349	350-499	≥500

Hct

3	0	3
≤40.9	41%-49%	≥50

WBCs

19	5	0	1	5
<1	1-2.9	3-19.9/mm³	20-24.9	≥25

Cr‡

3	0	4	7
≤0.4	44-132 µmol/dl 0.5-1.4 mg/dl	133-171 µmol/dl 1.5-1.94	≥172 ≥1.95

Creatinine§ (with ARF)

Points	0 Cr§	10
	0-132 μmol/dl	≥133
	0-1.4 mg/dl	≥1.5

Urine output (u/o, ml/day)

15	8	7	5	4	u/o 0	1
≤399	400-599	600-899	900-1499	1500-1999	2000-3999 ml/day	≥4000

BUN

BUN 0	2	7	11	12
≤6.1 mmol/L	6.2-7.1	7.2-14.3	14.4-28.5	≥28.6
≤16.9 mg/dl	17-19	20-39	40-79	≥80

Na

3	2	0 Na	4
≤119	120-134	135-154 mmol/L	≥155
≤119	120-134	135-154 mEq/L	≥155

Albumin

11	6	0 Albumin	4
≤19	20-24	25-44 g/L	≥45
≤1.9	2.0-2.4	2.5-4.4 g/dl	≥4.5

Bilirubin

0 Bilirubin	5	6	8	16
≤34 μmol/L	35-51	52-85	86-135	≥136
≤1.9 mg/dl	2.9	3-4.9	5-7.9	≥8.0

Glucose

8‖	9‖	Glucose 0	3	5
≤2.1	2.2-3.3	3.4-11.1 mmol/L	11.2-19.3	≥19.4
≤39	40-59	60-199 mg/dl	200-349	≥350

Modified from Knaus WA et al: The APACHE III prognostic system, Chest (in press).
BP, Blood pressure; *Temp*, temperature; *PaO₂*, arterial oxygen tension or partial pressure; *A-aDO₂*, alveolar-arterial oxygen gradient; *Hct*, hematocrit; *WBC*, white blood cells (count); *Cr*, creatinine; *u/o*, urine output; *BUN*, blood urea nitrogen; *Na*, sodium.
*For patients on mechanical ventilation, no points are given for respiratory rates 6-12.
†Only use A-aDO₂ for intubated patients with FiO₂ ≥0.5. Do not use PaO₂ weights for these patients.
‡Creatinine without acute renal failure (ARF). ARF is defined as creatinine ≥1.5 dl/day and urine output <410 ml/day and no chronic dialysis.
§Creatinine with ARF.
‖Glucose ≤39 mg/dl is lower weight than 40-59.

Acid-Base Points

pH	Paco$_2$	Points
<7.2	<50	12
<7.2	≥50	4
7.2-<7.35	<30	9
7.2-<7.3	30-<40	6
7.2-<7.3	40-<50	3
7.2-<7.3	≥50	2
7.35-<7.5	<30	5
7.3-<7.45	30-<45	0
7.3-<7.45	≥45	1
7.45-<7.5	30-<35	0
7.45-<7.5	35-<45	2
7.45-<7.5	>45	12
7.5-≥7.65	≥40	12
7.5-<7.6	<40	3
≥7.6	<25	0
≥7.6	25-<40	3

Neurological Scoring*

	Oriented, converses	Confused speech	Inappropriate words and incoherent sounds	No response
Obeys verbal command	0	3	10	15 16†
Localizes pain	3	8	13	15 16†
Flexion withdrawal/ decorticate rigidity	3	13	24 24†	24 33†
Decerebrate rigidity/no response	3	13	29 29†	29 48†

*Points assigned if eyes open spontaneously or to painful/verbal stimulation.
†Points assigned if eyes do not open spontaneously or to painful/verbal stimulation.

BSA Nomogram

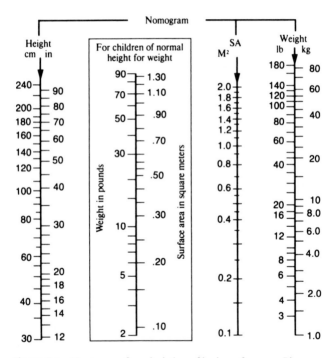

Figure E-1 Nomogram for calculation of body surface area. Place a straight edge from the patient's height in the left column to the weight in the right column. The point of intersection on the body surface area column indicates the body surface area. (From Behrman RE and Vaughn VC, eds: Nelson's textbook of pediatrics, ed 12, Philadelphia, 1983, WB Saunders Co.)

Index